HEALTH CARE FINANCIAL MANAGEMENT FOR NURSE MANAGERS:
MERGING THE HEART WITH THE DOLLAR

JANNE DUNHAM-TAYLOR, PhD, RN

JOSEPH Z. PINCZUK, MHA

JONES AND BARTLETT PUBLISHERS
Sudbury, Massachusetts
BOSTON   TORONTO   LONDON   SINGAPORE

World Headquarters
Jones and Bartlett Publishers
40 Tall Pine Drive
Sudbury, MA 01776
978-443-5000
info@jbpub.com
www.jbpub.com

Jones and Bartlett Publishers Canada
2406 Nikanna Road
Mississauga, ON L5C 2W6
CANADA

Jones and Bartlett Publishers International
Barb House, Barb Mews
London W6 7PA
UK

Jones and Bartlett's books and products are available through most bookstores and online booksellers. To contact Jones and Bartlett Publishers directly, call 800-832-0034, fax 978-443-8000, or visit our website www.jbpub.com.

Substantial discounts on bulk quantities of Jones and Bartlett's publications are available to corporations, professional associations, and other qualified organizations. For details and specific discount information, contact the special sales department at Jones and Bartlett via the above contact information or send an email to specialsales@jbpub.com.

Library of Congress Cataloging-in-Publication Data
Dunham-Taylor, Janne.
 Health care financial management for nurse managers : merging the heart with the dollar / Janne Dunham-Taylor, Joseph Z. Pinczuk.-- 1st ed.
  p. cm.
 Includes bibliographical references and index.
 ISBN 0-7637-3149-8 (pbk.)
 1. Nursing services--Business management. 2. Medical economics. I. Pinczuk, Joseph Z. II. Title.
 RT86.7.D855 2004
 362.1'068'1--dc22

                    2004019592

Production Credits
Acquisitions Editor: Kevin Sullivan
Production Director: Amy Rose
Associate Production Editor: Tracey Chapman
Associate Editor: Amy Sibley
Marketing Manager: Emily Ekle
Manufacturing and Inventory Coordinator: Amy Bacus
Composition: AnnMarie Lemoine
Cover Design: Kristin E. Ohlin
Printing and Binding: Malloy, Inc.
Cover Printing: Malloy, Inc.

Printed in the United States of America
09 08 07 06 05   10 9 8 7 6 5 4 3 2 1

Dedications

This book is dedicated to the many nursing administration students and nurse administrators who have touched out lives. We learned a lot from you and we salute you.

—JDT & JZP

Thanks to Mom, Dad, and the family for all your support and encouragement in completing this venture.

—JDT

I want to thank Rosemary, my wife and best friend, for encouraging me in this labor of love. It is through her patience and understanding that I was able to complete this project.

—JZP

Contributors

Paul Bayes, D.B.A. Accounting, M.S. Economics, B.S. Accounting. Dr. Paul Bayes is Chair and Professor of Accountancy at East Tennessee State University. Dr. Bayes earned his Bachelor and Doctorate degrees in Accounting from the University of Kentucky. He also holds a Master's in Economics from Indiana State University. He is active in accounting practitioner organizations holding several offices including president of the Mountain Empire Institute of Management Accountants Chapter. He is also active in academic organizations and has served on several national committees. Dr. Bayes has published and presented over 50 articles for both practitioner and academic organizations and has published an Accounting Information Systems Case textbook with co-author Dr. John Nash.

Sandy K. Calhoun, MSN, RN, CPHQ earned a Master of Science in Nursing degree with a concentration in nursing administration from East Tennessee State University (ETSU), Johnson City, Tennessee. She is currently pursuing a Doctorate of Science in Nursing with a focus in education at ETSU. Ms. Calhoun has 30 years of nursing experience, focusing on nursing administration, quality management, and education. She is employed as a full-time instructor at ETSU and serves as Extern/Intern Coordinator for Mountain States Health Alliance, located in Northeast Tennessee.

Janne Dunham-Taylor, PhD, RN is currently the Chair of Adult Nursing at East Tennessee State University, teaching nursing administration graduate courses at both master's and doctoral levels. Previously she has been a head nurse, nursing supervisor, and director of nursing in a state hospital, a university hospital, and a teaching hospital. She has been an assistant dean and has held two acting dean positions, as well as being a chair, in university settings. She has taught nursing administration courses for 19 years. Her research has been concerned with transformational leadership at the CNO level nationally. She has numerous publications on various nursing administration topics.

Sharron Rutledge Grindstaff, MSN, BSN, RN is a registered nurse with 20 years of professional nursing experience. As a staff nurse, her practice included medical-surgical, orthopedic, and urology nursing. She has worked as a coordinator for a patient classification and scheduling system implementation project and as the nurse liaison and system analyst/builder for a hospital information system implementation team. She has worked as a relief House Supervisor, Patient Care Services Quality Improvement Coordinator, and an Interim Director of Support Services for a large medical center in Tennessee. She is currently the Chief Nursing Officer for Unicoi County Memorial Hospital, Inc. and Administrator for Unicoi County Home Health in Erwin, Tennessee. She holds a Bachelor of Science in Nursing, a Master of Science in Nursing and a Healthcare Graduate Management Certificate from East Tennessee State University in Johnson City, Tennessee. She is the 2004–2005 President of the Tennessee Organization of Nurse Executives

(TONE). She is also a member of AONE, Tennessee Center for Nursing (TCN) board member, Tennessee Nurses Association (TNA), Sigma Theta Tau – Epsilon Sigma Chapter, and the American College of Healthcare Executives (ACHE).

Patricia A. Hayes, PhD, RN is an Associate Professor of Nursing at East Tennessee State University. Her current research centers on the development and implementation of a case management model for the frail elderly in public housing, which won the Virginia Stone Scholar Award of the American Nurses Foundation. She teaches case management and philosophy of nursing science, as well as theory and research.

J.D. Kleinke is a medical economist with an MSB in finance (Johns Hopkins) and a BS in economics (University of Maryland), J.D. Kleinke is a frequent contributor to the *Wall Street Journal*, *JAMA*, *Barron's*, *Modern Healthcare*, *Business and Health*, *Managed Healthcare*, *Health Affairs*, and *Compensation and Benefits Management*. He also serves on the editorial board of *Health Affairs*. During the 1990s, Kleinke was a driving force growing HCIA from a small firm engaged in data analysis for the health care industry into a publicly traded corporation providing analysis and software products to a broad spectrum of health care providers. Kleinke's background also includes experience with Sheppard Pratt Health Systems, where he was instrumental in developing and managing a provider-based, managed health care system. Sheppard Pratt, the largest psychiatric hospital in the United States, was the first to develop such a system.

Janelle Krueger, BS, RN. Senior Consultant, Kathy Malloch Associates, Louisville, KY is senior consultant for Kathy Malloch & Associates. Ms. Krueger has extensive experience in critical care and operational system management. As a registered nurse for 18 years, she has held corporate and regional level clinical and quality positions. Her experiences include program management for ENEPCS, training and education of clinical information systems, and hospital administrative roles. She has her CCRN certification and is currently pursuing an MBA degree.

Catherine B. Leary, MSN, RN, CNAA serves as Chief Operating Officer of Hillcrest Hospital. She is responsible for ensuring the delivery of high-quality care of Hillcrest Hospital patients and its community-based services.

Ms. Leary holds a Master of Science in Nursing degree, a nursing diploma, and a Bachelor of Arts degree in Psychology. In addition, she has completed numerous graduate semester hours in the areas of education and business. She holds a nursing license in the State of Ohio and is a member of Sigma Theta Tau International honorary nursing society. She holds certification in Nursing Administration, Advanced. In 1998 she was recognized as a Woman of Professional Excellence by the Greater Cleveland YWCA.

Ms. Leary is a member of the Cleveland Clinic Home Health Professional Advisory Board, Cuyahoga Community College Nursing Education Advisory Committee, the American Organization of Nurse Executives, and the Ohio League for Nursing. She is on the Executive Committee of the Board of Directors of the Greater Cleveland Chapter of the American Red Cross. She is an adjunct clinical faculty member of the Kent State University School of Nursing and Ursuline College Breen School of Nursing. She is the Chairman of the Hillcrest Hospital Community Leadership Council. She is a member of the Executive Board, Mayfield Area Business Education Community Alliance Foundation, and a member of the Board of Directors, Mayfield Area Chamber of Commerce.

Hillcrest Hospital has earned the distinction of the 100 Top Hospitals Award, HCIA in 2000, 1999, 1998, 1996, 1995. In 2001 the hospital earned an Ohio Award for Excellence.

Catherine B. Leary is a nurse who continues to be proud of her profession. She is a role model for many others as she touches their lives.

Linda Nash Legg, MSN, RN is a registered nurse with a total of 27 years in the nursing profession. During her career she has been employed in the positions of Perinatal Staff Nurse, Maternal-Child Clinical Educator, Nurse Manager of Obstetric and Pediatric Nursing Units, Nurse Educator, and Director of Planetree and Volunteer Services. She has experienced first-hand the multitude of challenges that nurse executives, and the health care industry as a whole, have faced over these past years as they strive to maintain quality, patient-centered care in a health care environment consisting of increasing nursing shortages and budgetary cutbacks. She states, "The good news is, as with all challenges, knowledge grows. This chapter contains budgetary strategies that have been formulated as we, nursing administrators, have continued to become more efficient, work smarter, focus, and strive to meet the needs of our patients in a manner that preserves the overall meaning of 'providing patient care in a nurturing, healing environment.'"

Dru Malcolm, MSN, RN, CPHRM is currently Director of Clinical Integration at Indian Path Medical Center, a facility of Mountain States Health Alliance. She celebrates 25 years of nursing experience with a focus in emergency nursing, emergency preparedness, quality, and risk management. She holds a Master of Science in Nursing Administration, certification as a health care professional in risk management, has been selected as an examiner for TNCPE, and serves as adjunct faculty at East Tennessee State University.

Kathy Malloch, PhD, MBA, RN, President, Kathy Malloch Associates, Glendale, AZ is president of Kathy Malloch & Associates, a national health care consulting firm that provides services to assist leaders in challenging status quo systems and creating new models. Successful innovations include healing model management, matrix performance measurement, and expert nurse patient classification systems. Prior to her focus on consulting and education, she held positions of staff nurse, nurse manager, director of nursing, and Vice-President for Patient Care Services. Most recently, Dr. Malloch co-authored *Quantum Leadership: A Textbook of New Leadership* with Dr. Tim Porter-O'Grady.

R. Penny Marquette, DBA, presently retired, was a KPMG Peat Marwick Faculty Fellow in Accounting and a Professor in Accounting at the University of Akron, Akron, Ohio. She has also taught at Cleveland State University in Cleveland, Ohio, and at Kent State University in Kent, Ohio. She has a DBA in Accounting with a Finance Minor at Kent

State University; an MBA at the University of Akron in Accounting; and a BS in Journalism and English from the University of Florida in Gainesville. She has authored numerous publications.

Jo-Ann Summitt Marrs Ed.D., APRN, BC is presently Associate Dean of Academic Programs and Student Services and is Chair of the Professional Roles and Mental Health Nursing Department at East Tennessee State University College of Nursing.

Jo-Ann holds a Doctor of Education in Public Health and a Master of Science in Nursing from the University of Tennessee. She acquired her Family Nurse Practitioner certificate from Pittsburg State University and is presently practicing in one of the College of Nursing's nurse managed clinics for Hispanic women and children. She has served in an administrative capacity since 1987.

Her main interest is in the area of moral turpitude and licensure for nurses. She has led a national campaign for background checks and fingerprinting to be a requirement for admission to nursing schools.

Joseph Z. Pinczuk, MHA presently retired, held executive positions overseeing finance, administration and operations for twenty-nine years. He has a Masters of Professional Management in Hospital Administration from Indiana Northern University and a Bachelors of Business Administration in Accounting from Cleveland State University. He has been a CFO in hospitals ranging in size from 55 beds to serving as the CFO of the Tri-County Hospital Group in Ohio consisting of three hospitals with a total of 254 beds. He also served as CFO of a Continuing Care Retirement Community (CCRC) consisting of 285 resident units, 75 skilled nursing and 24 assisted living beds. He is a member and had served as a Director on the Board of the Healthcare Financial Management Association (HFMA), NE Ohio Chapter and received the Follmer Bronze, Reeves Silver and Muncie Gold Awards for his contributions to the organization. A former Adjunct Professor of Nursing, College of Nursing, University of Akron and a co-author of an article "Surviving Capitation", American Journal of Nursing (March 1996).

Tammy Samples, MSN, RN, received her masters with a concentration in Nursing Administration. Her past 19 years experience is mainly in neonatal intensive care nursing. Her management experience includes shift leader for a neonatal intensive care unit, unit leader for Pediatrics and Pediatric Intensive Care Unit and House Supervision. She also has experience as the Clinical Educator for a children's hospital. Currently she provides outreach neonatal education to hospitals in referral areas.

Norma Tomlinson, MSN, RN, CNA is a registered nurse with over 30 years of professional nursing experience. As a staff nurse, her practice included medical-surgical and orthopedic nursing, children's psychiatric nursing, and geriatric skilled nursing. She has been a staff development instructor in a general hospital and developed and administered a Medicare-certified, hospital-based home health agency. She has experience as the Director of Medical-Surgical Nursing in both a large urban hospital as well as in a hospital system. She has served as the Vice-President of Clinical Services in hospitals in Ohio and Michigan. She is currently the Vice-President of Clinical Services and Operations for Wellmont Holston Valley Medical Center in Kingsport, Tennessee. She holds an Associate degree in Nursing from Purdue University, a BSN from Youngstown State University, and an MSN from the University of Akron. She is a member of Phi Kappa Phi, Sigma Theta Tau, AONE, and TONE. She served for several years as the president of the Akron-Canton Regional Organization of Nurse Executives and on the Board of OONE.

Patricia M. Vanhook, MSN, APRN, BC, Magnet Coordinator, Mountain States Health Alliance, Johnson City, TN. Acknowledgement and gratitude to Mountain States Health Alliance, Kathryn Wilhoit, RN, MSN, CNAA, FAHCE; Debbie McInturff, RN, Financial Analyst; Karen Cober, RN, MSN, Director, Medical Center HomeCare Services; Paula Claytor, MBA, Senior Director of Managed Care; and Alicia Vanhook, Systems Analysis; at Mountain States Health Alliance for their assistance and guidance.

Rick Wallace, MA, MDiv, MAOM, MSLS, AHIP is the Outreach and Public Services Librarian for the Quillen College of Medicine Library. He provides library services to hospitals and clinics in 17 east Tennessee counties. Also, he serves as project director for the library's consumer health information service, is clinical librarian for ETSU medical residents, and oversees the library's document delivery service.

Martha Whaley, MSLS has worked in the Quillen College of Medicine Library since 1976. As Technical Services Coordinator she manages the selection, acquisition, cataloging, and processing of print and electronic library materials. She is director of The Museum at Mountain Home, which is housed in an early 20th century clock tower building at the James H. Quillen VA Medical Center. The Museum chronicles the development of health care in South Central Appalachia. She also manages the Library's historical book and journal collection which is housed in an early 20th century Carnegie Library.

Contents

Part VII **Determining and Evaluating Staffing** **711**

Chapter 19 *Patient Classification Systems* *713*
KATHY MALLOCH AND JANELLE KRUEGER

Preface

Janne and Joe have been working together for years. It all started when the CNO at Joe's hospital invited Janne (an experienced nurse administrator teaching at the local university) to come and work with the nurse managers to enhance their knowledge about budgeting. When Janne met Joe (the CFO) she realized that he was an unusual CFO as he both understood and supported the "care" side of health care. Come to find out, he was a former respiratory therapist and married to a registered nurse. Joe thought that Janne's information for the nurse managers was important, and it was evident that the CNO and CFO worked well together.

Then Joe began to regularly come to talk to graduate nursing administration students in Janne's fiscal course. He could clearly explain financial terms, the way the finance department worked, and the future implications of reimbursement and how it would affect the health care organization, nurses, patients, and community.

Gradually the ideas for this book began to take root and blossom. We knew that we did not want to create the typical financial book that kept finances in a silo. Instead, we wanted to present finances in the larger dimension—as a part of a greater whole. We also both felt strongly that regular dialogue and respect between finance and nursing was critical to the success of a health care organization. Our goal was to provide nurse administrators with information so they can be more effective in their roles.

This book has been a labor of love but has been fraught with delays. Janne moved to another state. The original contract was with Aspen Publishers and when halfway finished, there was an 18-month delay until Jones and Bartlett purchased Aspen's book division. Then when finished, the book was too long, so what started as one book became two— both titles starting with *Health Care Financial Management for Nurse Managers*. This became the first book, *Health Care Financial Management for Nurse Managers: Merging the Heart with the Dollar*, with a broader focus of all that affects finances in an organization. The second book is *Health Care Financial Management for Nurse Managers: Applications in Hospitals, Long-Term Care, Home Care, and Ambulatory Care*, providing specific financial applications in those settings.

This book is made richer by the many contributors who have shared their expertise on certain subjects. We thank them for all their time, knowledge, and dedication to this book.

We hope that this book is both practical and helpful for you. We have tried to provide other wonderful references—but, of course, cannot possibly do justice to the many additional resources available.

Acknowledgments

We would like to thank the other people who made this book possible. First, a big thanks to Mrs. Gina Rose, always there to help—creating tables, searching out the appropriate sources for permissions, finding sources on the Internet, and generally supporting the authors in this endeavor. Thanks to both Dr. Joellen Edwards and Dr. Pat Smith, the College of Nursing Administration Team, the Adult Nursing Department faculty, and other nursing faculty for their support and encouragement. Thanks to Mrs. Dru Malcolm and Ms. Billie Sills for their valuable feedback on chapters as the book was being written. Thanks also to Mrs. Karen Deyo, who has helped convert files, copy, etc; and to Ms. Lana J. Seal and Ms. Megan Alexander who helped with library work, checking references, and copying.

Every Management Decision Has Financial Implications—Every Financial Decision Has Management Implications!

This book addresses health care financial management issues for nurse managers. Although, in many cases, this information is also helpful for the chief nursing officer or other nurse administrator roles. Nurse managers, or nurse administrators, can be found in a variety of settings—hospitals, ambulatory/outpatient clinics and centers, long term care, and home care. This is written to provide helpful information that pertains to each of these settings.

To be successful in financial management, nurse administrators must understand, regardless of setting, what impacts the health care environment, and the financial implications that will result from these forces. The nurse administrator needs to express what must happen not only for good nursing practice, but also for the financial aspects involved. To be most effective in this new century the nurse administrator needs to operate from a new knowledge base using different skills. This is further complicated by the financial implications.

Leaving Our Silos Behind!

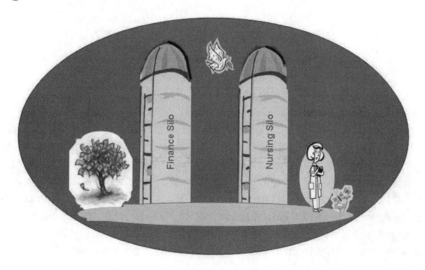

One change we are facing is that we all need to break down our silos. The problem with the financial aspect of health care is that it is often viewed as a separate silo—a silo where nurses do not enter, and one where financial personnel reside. Meanwhile, nurses are in their own silo, and financial personnel are not found there. As co-authors of this book we, a nurse administrator and a chief financial officer, believe that it is time to break down, and to end, this silo mentality. Our effectiveness in health care demands that we interface regularly with each other, and truly have dialogue about the issues that we both face. We are most effective if we can face these issues together using the strengths of both our professions.

> *Nurse administrators are more effective when they express themselves using financial principles and data.*

Nurses need to express themselves more effectively using financial principles and data; financial personnel need to more effectively understand the "care" side of health care. Because this book is written for the nurse administrator, we will give our emphasis to the first. We hope that a book written for financial personnel will be forthcoming and will emphasize the importance of financial personnel understanding how the care side impacts finances.

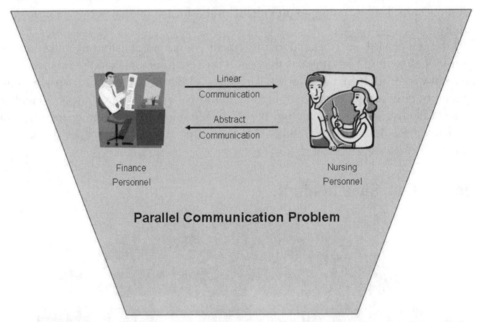

Parallel Communication Problem

One of the problems that occurs when nurses and financial people try to have dialogue together is that financial officers often think in a linear way. When they talk to each other, they talk about numbers, ratios, and stats. On the other hand, nurses think in an abstract, interpersonal way. When nurses talk to each other they talk about how someone feels, how someone will be affected by a certain treatment, or whether tasks have been accomplished.

The breakdown in communication occurs when nurses talk to financial people and use abstract language, and financial people, when they talk to nurses, use linear language. The conversations run parallel to each other, with both sides not understanding what the other side is talking about. Nurses complain that financial people never think about anything but the bottom line; financial people complain that all nurses do is whine about quality. True dialogue and communication do not occur.

This book will give examples that nurses can use to better communicate with financial personnel, as well as with other linear-thinking administrators. In addition, we recommend that if a nurse administrator really wants to talk effectively with financial administrators, he/she should think of ways to communicate the abstract information using linear language (i.e., numbers that will be affected by something that has occurred or that is being planned, specific amounts of money needed to implement a project, and so forth).

> *When discussing issues with financial personnel, nurse administrators are more effective expressing abstract information using linear language.*

Abstract thinking is an effective way for communication with nurses and physicians. However, it is often ineffective when communicating with the finance department. And concepts like "care" will not have meaning to a finance officer. Caring is an abstract term. Exceptions occur when a financial person experiences a serious illness, or when, in the past, the financial officer has been a health care professional.

At times this communication problem can be compounded by simple differences in male and female communication (remember *Men Are From Mars, Women Are From Venus?*), especially if the chief financial officer (CFO) is male and the chief nursing officer (CNO) is female. This is changing with less gender-specific roles in the workplace. In the past, a male CNO often had an edge because he could be "one of the boys." This is also slowly changing.

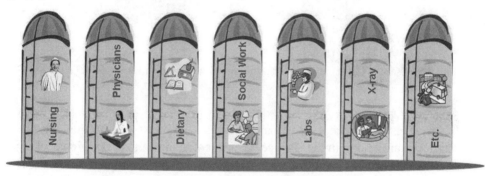

Organizational Silos

Other silos can impact a health care team's effectiveness. Chances are, other departments have structures that need to be broken down as well. This book will discuss various organizational processes that can actually cause errors to happen, putting a patient's life at stake—not to mention resulting law suits occuring from the errors. Although one person may have made the mistake, when the team analyzes what occurred, most often personnel from several departments and/or physicians, contributed to the error. We advocate that if each member can bring his/her expertise to the table and work as members of a team, everyone benefits—patients, staff, physicians—as well as the bottom line. Additionally, all the team members get a larger, more accurate assessment of the organization as a whole.

> *Solutions are more effective when all the staff and administrators involved in a situation work together to come up with the best way to accomplish the work.*

Solutions are always better when the people directly involved are part of the team that is coming up with the solutions. Therefore we advocate that staff, as well as administrators, come to the table on issues, and decide upon the best way to accomplish the work. This gets rid of another silo—that administrators are to handle all this, not delegate to others. And under the old system, staff are to implement whatever the administrator decides is best and blindly follow the administrative edicts. This old patriarchal (or matriarchal in nursing) authoritarian model is not effective. This is another silo that is disintegrating and needs to disappear. It is a leftover from the previous century.

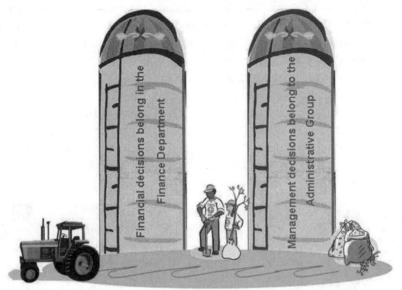

Another silo is the concept that finances are a separate issue. By this, we mean that financial decisions belong in the finance department, management decisions belong to the administrative group, and so forth. The reality is that *every financial decision has management implications, and every management decision has financial implications*. If we properly prepare the nurse manager, or nurse administrator, this person must be able to make the interface between finances and nursing management, and make decisions based upon both perspectives. This person needs to understand both the financial situation and the nursing situation. In addition, both groups need to have a better overall organizational perspective as there are other stakeholders in the mix.

To break down this silo we turn to clinical decision making. In the Budget Strategies section we discuss the importance of staff having a heightened awareness of the financial implications involved in clinical practice. This is another area that the nurse manager will need to work on with staff.

Financial Know How

Knowledge of the current health care financial overview will allow nurse managers to effectively manage *and anticipate* appropriate actions in response to a changing financial environment. But understanding is not sufficient. In order to respond effectively, and to work successfully with the financial arm of the health care entity, nurse managers must understand financial concepts such as staffing, budgeting, identifying and analyzing variances, measuring productivity, costing, accounting, and forecasting.

A critical element for success is the ability to effectively interface with finance department personnel. An unusual feature of this book is that it will contain both typical nursing administration terminology and financial accounting terminology. Suggestions will be given to the nurse manager to more effectively communicate, and to maximize understanding of concepts and issues, with financial personnel who may come from different backgrounds and attach different meanings to the same terms. This book will provide nurse managers with a view from both the nursing and the financial sides—and give suggestions for successfully integrating these viewpoints. This realistic integration of nursing and finance will enhance nurse manager effectiveness.

This book will cover a wide range of financial information. All chapters cover information that is important regardless of health care setting. Concepts will be presented followed by examples. Although many of the examples will have an inpatient focus, there will also be examples from other health care settings such as ambulatory care, home care, and long-term care. For example, individual chapters on health care finance, economics, budgeting, staffing, patient classification systems, and productivity will present good basic information applicable to all settings.

As information is presented in each chapter, it is important to note that much of this information is interrelated. For example, when discussing budgeting, one must be concerned with staffing, patient acuity, and productivity of staff, as well as with quality standards. Although finance and accounting terminology will be interspersed throughout all the chapters, specific chapters on accounting and assessing financial performance will be included.

In the complementary text, *Health Care Financial Management for Nurse Managers: Financial Applications in Hospitals, Long-Term Care, Home Care, and Ambulatory Care*, specific examples are given that illustrate the nurse manager role in specific settings. This information expands and tailors the principles in this book to the unique rules and regulations, or the way of measuring services, for hospitals, long-term care, home care, and ambulatory care.

An enormous challenge in the current health care climate is achieving quality service while keeping expenses down. There are an infinite number of strategies that can be employed toward achieving this end. The health care industry has a long way to go, and every nurse manager and every health care administrator will need creative solutions to better meet the goal of quality service at an acceptable cost. This book will discuss strategies used within the health care industry as a whole, as well as specific strategies for the nurse manager.

A Systems Approach

This book will take a *systems approach* to analyzing the financial impact of health care decisions. Although there will be specific chapters on certain financial aspects, a nurse manager cannot make the mistake of ignoring the whole while dealing with the individual parts. After all, *every management decision has financial and budgetary implications; every financial decision has management implications.* Too often decisions are made in isolation, ignoring the secondary, or *feedback* effects of those decisions. Often, such isolated decisions yield short-term improvement followed by a long-term worsening of the underlying situation.

> *Every management decision has financial and budgetary implications. Every financial decision has management implications.*

For example, prospective payment has mobilized administrators in health care organizations to identify effective and efficient processes that cost less yet deliver quality care. Nursing comes under scrutiny because a large part of the operating budget is devoted to nursing staff costs. When health care administrators do not really understand the patient care side of business, it is easy for them to come to the conclusion that considerable cost savings can be realized by cutting the nursing service budget. And if nursing is not paying attention to efficiency, and cannot articulate effectively how massive cuts will impact the organization, chances are that big cuts will occur—and not necessarily in ways that will best serve the patient.

It has become essential that the nurse administrator understand, and can articulate, how the dollars and cents of the health care business impact the entire business. And, in the process, it may be necessary to more directly show other administrators what patient care is really about and how cost cutting needs to account for patient outcomes.

By viewing the health care organization as an integrated system, and involving staff who directly work with patients, we can help nurse managers avoid these pitfalls. In *an integrated system*, no one department, profession, or organization can stand alone. To be most effective, there needs to be constant dialogue between all segments of the organization, along with an open dialogue with the community being served.

There is a ripple effect. If one department is not functioning adequately, the whole organization is affected. Worse yet, patients receiving services are affected. The impact may extend beyond the health care entity to affect suppliers such as physicians. Ultimately, the long-term effects could include decreased patient safety, more patient complications, less patient satisfaction with services, fewer patients coming to the health care organization, physicians choosing to refer patients elsewhere, more lawsuits, increased staff turnover, and other problems. Obviously, this cycle can dramatically affect revenues. If competing sources are available and the problems are significant enough, the health care organization could even go out of business.

It is easy for nurse managers to get so caught up in the day-to-day details of running their department or division(s) that they become isolated from the larger picture. This is dangerous and can have deleterious effects on the organization. Let's take an example.

A Staffing Problem From a Systems' Perspective

Imagine a new nurse manager, down two full-time positions, and faced with the decision of how to effectively staff for a large patient load. There are several possible options: ask existing staff to work overtime, call in part-time or prn personnel to work additional hours, call in agency personnel, "go short," or float staff from somewhere else in the organization. Perhaps the nurse manager is not overly concerned about the shortage because the nursing supervisor will send staff from another unit. At first, the serious ramifications of this situation are unclear, but left unchecked, this situation can quickly become a larger problem.

The first system-wide problem will be felt by other nurse managers, who have staffed adequately, but are now constantly having their staff pulled to the unit with the shortage. Resentments will begin to build. There will be quality care issues as well. The staff members being floated may not be adequately oriented to the new unit, may not have taken care of that kind of patient before, or many not understand physician expectations. Soon the floating staff members will also resent having to constantly staff the unit experiencing the shortage. Patients may not receive the quality of care that one would desire, physicians will be unhappy, nursing turnover will increase, and so it goes.

This downward spiral will continue until the first nurse manager fixes the problem, or the person supervising that nurse manager dialogues, counsels, or eventually replaces the nurse manager.

A More Complex View of the Problem

Let's expand the above example by looking at some of the financial and economic decisions that also complicate the problem of how to cover for two missing staff members. First, assume the nurse manager is aware that the health care organization is in a state of financial crisis because Medicare and Medicaid reimbursements have been less than what was anticipated at the beginning of the budget year. Perhaps the nurse manager has taken over a chaotic situation where unit staff are not working well together, and the two staff members who recently left did so because they wanted to work in a more stable environment.

In this situation (*which hardly strains credibility*), there are many management and financial implications that the nurse manager will need to consider. *For the short term*, how much staff, and what staff mix, will be necessary to safely care for the patients? We have already looked at the problems associated with floating staff from other units, but perhaps there is another unit that could help care for some of these patients. And, if these potential problems are considered *before* the staff are floated, many pitfalls can be avoided.

Since the health care organization is probably cutting costs due to lower-than-anticipated reimbursements, any action that will increase cost may be frowned upon by upper level administration. Nevertheless, while overtime will be viewed as an increased cost, it can still save money when compared with incurring the salary and benefit costs for the two missing full-time staff members. Not to mention the costs of hiring agency personnel! If the nurse manager plans to "sell" the overtime solution to the administration, it would be wise to have the costs associated with these alternatives at hand when the meeting occurs.

It is equally important to do something immediately to lessen the chaotic conditions on the unit and get staff working together more effectively. When staff are not working together effectively, the quality of patient care will suffer. More mistakes and increased legal problems occur when chaos becomes the norm. From a financial point of view, these potential costs overwhelm concerns about overtime or agency personnel. And, more importantly, how does one ever measure an unnecessary illness or death? In deciding how to approach the problem of staff cohesion, another critical factor involves the amount of support the nurse manager will receive from both the immediate supervisor and from the higher level administration.

For the long term, there will continue to be less reimbursement for Medicare and Medicaid patients. What is the ratio of these patients to private-pay patients? If over 50% of the patients are on Medicare or Medicaid, payments to the health care organization will be delayed and will not cover actual costs. How can costs be cut further, while achieving an adequate standard of care? In the long run it is also important to take an accurate inventory of your resources, the most valuable being the people who work in the organization. Involving every person in the organization is critical to maximize effectiveness. Staff who actually do the work are often the best source of information on how to become more cost effective and improve service delivery.

> *The way staff are valued and treated will reflect the way the patients are valued and treated.*

Taking care of one's staff is always important, but given the existing nursing shortage crises, combined with an environment of diminished reimbursement, having staff leave in frustration is certain to further exacerbate all problems and diminish organizational effectiveness. Failure to retain staff *always* results in additional costs—both financial and service quality—to the facility. A good rule of thumb is that *the way staff are valued and treated will reflect the way that patients are valued and treated.*

Walking the Tight Rope

From these issues, one can see that it is impossible to cleanly separate financial from management decisions. In many situations, the nurse manager must take some action that has both management and financial implications. If the nurse manager does nothing, *that is still an action*—this could have patient implications. Nurse managers need to be actively involved in all aspects of the nursing care, and that includes financial issues.

Nurse managers frequently feel that they are "between a rock and a hard place." On the one hand, they are involved in patient care, constantly working with staff members who provide direct service to patients. On the other hand, they must effectively interface with other disciplines and with administrators at higher levels in the organization, individuals who are somewhat distanced from patient care. Often the nurse manager is caught between two groups wanting diametrically opposed solutions to existing problems. The best way to resolve such dilemmas is to get back to basic values—*what is best for the patient?* The purpose of this book is to help the nurse manager increase her/his knowledge base, learn techniques and develop additional skills to be more effective in acting as the link between direct patient care, and the financial administration of the entity.

For effective financial management, it is necessary for the nurse manager to:

- *Be an effective leader;*
- *Have an organizational/systems perspective;*
- *Achieve quality standards;*
- *Be conversant in financial practices and techniques; and*
- *Understand how all this fits within the community and society.*

It is a tall order for a person who may have had no management training.

> *When the nurse administrator is caught between two diametrically opposed solutions to existing problems, the dilemma is best solved by asking, "What is best for the patient?"*

PART ONE

Necessary Essentials for Financial Viability—or If Not Fixed It Will Cost More Money

Some may wonder why we have included the chapters in Part I in a financial management book. After all, why aren't we getting right into finances and budgeting? Actually, we have started with these chapters for a very specific financial reason. As will become clear in later chapters, any time that we make the financial part come first, we will create more financial problems—*things will become more expensive.* So for the most effective bottom line, the bottom line *cannot* be first priority! It has to become second behind some VERY important issues discussed in Part I.

Part I was given first placement in this book because these are the issues that are the most important. If we do not pay attention to every aspect in Part I, we will lose money! While if these aspects are in place, we will do much better financially.

Part I starts with a letter to nurses about doing what is right for the patients, written by a hospital Chief Operating Officer who is also a nurse. The message behind the letter: If we do what is right for the patient, the money will follow. We found this letter to be energizing and personally moving. We hope that you do too.

> *For the most effective bottom line, the bottom line cannot be the first priority! It has to become second priority behind some VERY important issues discussed in Part One.*

The second chapter is concerned with quality issues. The most important quality issue is to know what the patient wants and values. Often we do not even ask this question! We, as nurses, are often stuck in our 'task' box. In addition, we have a TREMENDOUS problem with patient safety—at least 4% of the patients we treat will die from our mistakes! We would never choose an airline with that kind of record! So why should patients choose *our* services? In fact, a lot of the patient safety issues are caused by a series of events or organizational processes that are broken. IT IS TIME TO FIX THIS PROBLEM, to leave blame behind (after all, we are all human and, chances are, one person did not cause the

11

problem alone). Every single one of us needs to do everything in our power to be sure that our patients are safe. Another quality problem is that we treat dis-ease, and do not do much to encourage health.

Leadership is the topic of the third chapter. If administrative leadership is broken at the top, everything else is broken within an organization, and the organization will lose A LOT of money. *Fish rots from the head.* But money is only a minor problem compared with patient outcomes. Patients will be more in jeopardy if the leadership is inadequate. This chapter is next deliberately because we need to fix our administrative leadership before we can expect others in our employ to improve! If the administrative leadership is broken at any level in the organization, other financial problems will occur that could have been prevented if we had fixed the leadership problem(s). For example, it is hard to achieve effective teamwork when there is a problem with the administrative leader.

Leadership starts from within, so the first part of the third chapter is concerned with personal mastery. The second part of leadership involves the effectiveness of our relationships with others. Our leadership role has changed and will continue to change. Can we keep up with it? Authoritarian leadership, along with "control" and language like "subordinates" and "superiors," are a thing of the past. Can we let all that go, and truly empower and trust others to give their best?

The fourth chapter is concerned with organizational strategies. First, it is important that all live by the core values. Second, an administrator needs to accurately assess the organization and can only accomplish this if one does regular, frequent rounds. Next it is important to examine organizational processes or relationships that can be impeding progress. Shared governance, interdisciplinary teamwork, and promoting healthy collaborative cultures are all part of our administrative work as we design the organization. As we deal with needed changes, we must avoid "quick fixes" that will worsen problems rather than fix them, and we may need to effectively turn dysfunctional groups around.

The fifth chapter is about ethics. Whenever there is money to be made, ethics quickly can be skirted. However, this is a trap. If our administrative actions are unethical, the rest of the organization is broken, and money will be lost. Can we feel good looking at ourselves in the mirror every morning? Health care is fraught with ethical dilemmas—between patients and families, between patients and health care providers, between members of the interdisciplinary team, between staff and administrators or board, between staff and physicians, between caregivers and finance, and between executive team members. This chapter is concerned with the nurse administrator role with ethics.

Unfortunately within our current health care system, there are many examples of fraud and abuse in health care that go way beyond the nurse administrator role. Sometimes nurses will become involved with these, so it is important to be aware of them, and to avoid getting involved with them at all costs.

The Centers for Medicare and Medicaid Services (CMS) describes *fraud* as "the intentional deception or misrepresentation that an individual knows to be false or does not believe to be true and makes, knowing that the deception could result in some unauthorized benefit to himself/herself or some other person" or agency.

Fraud typically involves:

- *Overutilization*—providing unnecessary services . . . ;
- *Upcoding*—assigning a Current Procedure Terminology (CPT) code that reflects a higher level of service than actually was provided . . . ;
- *Billing for services not provided*— . . . the only issue to be resolved is whether the bill was submitted intentionally or through oversight . . . ;
- *Failing to provide necessary services*—[capitation] penalizes the health care professional for overutilization; thus, providers may be monetarily encouraged to [underserve patients]. . .;
- *Filing false cost reports*—typically filed by providers who are paid under Medicare Part A, including hospitals, skilled nursing facilities and home health agencies . . ., e.g., disguising an unallowable cost as an allowable cost;
- *Enrolling fictitious participants in HMOs* (Lovitky, 1997, pp. 42–44);
- *Misrepresenting the patient's diagnosis* to justify the services or equipment furnished;
- *Unbundling* or *exploding*—Altering claim forms or billing for separate parts of a single procedure to obtain a higher payment or using split-billing schemes;
- *Looping*—Using insurance benefits of one member for billing for services provided for another. This is known to be more frequent when services are provided for more than one family member at the same time;
- *Double Billing*—Deliberately applying for duplicate payment, that is, billing Medicare and a private insurer for the same services;
- *Phantom Billing*—Billing for services rendered by an agency that is not certified as a Medicare participant through one that is certified; or
- *Kickbacks*—Soliciting, offering, or receiving rebates/remunerations and bribes from other healthcare agencies or durable medical equipment companies (Tahan, 1999, p. 19).

A Medicare statute, "otherwise known as the Anti-Kickback Act" (Lovitky, 1997, p. 44) now deals with this last issue. Examples of this are when a physician refers a patient for laboratory tests to a lab owned by the physician or a family member; or "several physicians have been prosecuted for accepting payment from hospitals in exchange for referring Medicare patients to those hospitals. Similar types of prosecutions have occurred with respect to illegal payments made by durable medical equipment suppliers to nursing homes and home health agencies" (Lovitky, 1997, pp. 44–45). Furthermore:

> Distinguishing between fraud and mere negligence is imperative. Fraud generally occurs when individuals knowingly disregard the truth by submitting intentionally false claims. A mere oversight or an inadvertent error will not rise to the level of fraud; however, a pattern of oversights or errors may increase the likelihood of fraud liability. One cannot escape liability merely by intentionally not learning the truth about health claims being submitted. The government will prosecute "ostrich" behavior. Similarly, liability may not be avoided merely by outsourcing billing functions to a billing company. Typically, the government will assert its claims against both the principal and the agent in this type of circumstance (Lovitky, 1997, pp. 42–44).

Abuse, which is not easy to prove, is billing for excessive charges, services not provided or not medically necessary, or undocumented care. CMS defines abuse as "incidents or practices . . . that are inconsistent with accepted sound medical practices, directly or indirectly resulting in unnecessary costs… or improper payment… for services that fail to meet professionally recognized standards." A familiar example is the unnecessary surgery issue with hysterectomies, tonsillectomies, ceasarean sections, and coronary bypass surgeries; unnecessary hospitalizations, unnecessary tests, unnecessary medications, or unnecessary physician visits are also abuse examples. Abuse can also occur when patients are denied their rights, experience verbal or physical abuse, or are restrained unnecessarily.

Fraudulent claims are probably costing billions of dollars—both for insurance companies and from our tax dollars. Medicare fraud was found to be 14 percent when the federal government did the first comprehensive audit of Medicare. This prompted the federal government to start The National Health Care Anti-Fraud Association in 1985, both to discover fraud and abuse and to teach about it. Several additional Acts have aimed at increasing the federal government's effectiveness in this issue. Meanwhile, both the Attorney General's office and the Department of Health and Human Services have begun investigating and heavily fining persons or organizations involved in fraudulent claims.

In 1998 "as part of its Medicare fraud-busting campaign, [CMS] launched a program… that enlists the country's 39 million Medicare beneficiaries. As the program's 'eyes and ears in the field,'… seniors can report a suspected case of fraud to the agency and collect a bounty of up to $1,000. The money comes from funds recovered from providers.… [Seniors are doing just that, and] not all of them want money.… They see it as their personal responsibility" (Haugh, 1999, p. 16). This is called the "qui tan whistleblower statute." This law allows private individuals to sue on behalf of the United States government when they become aware of fraudulent activities. The private citizen bringing the suit obtains a reward—usually 15 percent to 30 percent of any amounts collected by the government. Qui tam suits have resulted in several large dollar awards in which millions have been paid to the whistleblower" (Lovitky, 1997, pp. 42–44).

> Where does the nurse come into all this?
>
> The ethos of the corporation and the urgency for profit maximization place pressures on health care corporations to act in a way that may be incompatible with ethical practice. Profit-driven incentives often result in corporate deviance and criminal behavior. Nurses may be pressured to go along with schemes that may be unethical or illegal and because of shaky job markets may be unable to adhere to professional ethical guidelines.… Dirty hands cases are those instances in which one agent is morally forced by someone else's immorality to do what is, or otherwise would be, wrong.… Problems of this kind have been labeled by some as "dirty hands" situations, because the circumstances are such that the agent is left with a "moral stain" after taking an action (Mohr and Mahon, 1996, pp. 28–29).

This is important background information to keep in mind before reading Chapter 5 on Ethics.

These first five chapters set the stage for the basics for effective financial management. Financial viability follows all this. It never should be top priority, or all the rest of this will not be in place and finances will suffer.

CHAPTER 1

An Open Letter to Nurse Leaders
If We Do What Is Right for the Patients,
Financial Well-Being Will Follow

Catherine B. Leary, MSN, RN, CNAA

DRG, RBRVS, BBA, APC, ABN, HMO, MCO, OSHA, LMRP, HIPAA . . . in the final years of the twentieth century our daily bread was served up with a bitter alphabet soup. The same trend continues at the start of this new millennium. Program after program is launched to control the run-away costs of health care and to increase fiscal accountability for the use of the health care dollar.

These years have been hard for nurses. Our health care organizations reacted to diminishing fiscal resources by down-sizing and re-engineering. Doing more with less became a route to survival. In this time of crisis, we nurses have come close to the edge—the edge of losing control of our values and of our ability to make a difference.

Nurses are good people—compliant to the rules. We want to do the right thing and be team players. In these years of declining reimbursement, however, we have sometimes been led to believe that we should make our decisions on behalf of dollars instead of patients. We have become followers instead of leaders.

This letter is a call to leadership and a call to believe in yourself and the nurses you lead. As the gospel hymn says, "We are the people we've been waiting for."

Our calling in life is to do what is right for our patients. And it has been my experience (and that of many others) that doing what is right for the patient leads to a positive bottom line. *Make decisions on behalf of the patients and the dollars will follow*; "a good outcome leads to a good income" as one of my friends declares.

All nurses know that this is true—we have seen it with our own eyes. The relative value of nursing care is huge. There is no substitute and there are no short cuts. It is up to you and other nursing leaders in your organization to carry this message to all corners of your realm of influence—to the community in which you work, to the board which directs your organization, to the physicians, to the patients, and to the nurses whom you lead.

Now is the time. We are fortunate to be experiencing a return to a values-based workplace in this country. Scan the shelves of the business section in your local bookstore. People are seeking a reconnection between their personal and work lives. We are awakening to a need for principles and values to breathe spirit and meaning into what we do with our lives. This belief is a natural fit for nurses since it is what we have always believed.

It is easy to catch the wave, but difficult to stay on top of it. It takes courage, persistence, and a lot of hard work. It requires that you align your daily work with the dictates of your heart. Having blind faith without looking back helps a lot when you champion a cause. Always remember that you and your nurses embody the standard of care. Couple that thought with the message that a high standard of care will lead the organization to a profitable position. *Reflect upon what is right for the patient in everything you say and do.* It is a winning formula. I guarantee it. Say it out loud a lot. People want to hear it. And best of all, it is catching. Soon you will hear people around you saying it and acting it out.

Another current trend that supports the cause is patient safety—the prevention of errors. The research literature, as well as the popular media, conclude that patients must be put first. Errors not only harm patients, but also cost more. Doing what is right for the patient saves money. Staffing with an adequate number and mix of registered nurses prevents errors. Arm yourself with all the objective data and information you can get your hands on to prove your point. We nurses have always known this information in our guts; now there are studies to prove it. There are a few other ways to prepare yourself for this crusade on behalf of the patients. Know your business. Be credible. Be smart. And most of all develop relationships. Health care (as with most things in life) is about relationships. Let me explain what I mean.

Mission

To be successful, know (and feel) the relationship between the organization's mission and your own mission. **Exhibit 1–1** illustrates this idea.

Spend some time thinking about this, reflecting on it, and discussing it with others in your work place. It is important to personally embrace the alignment and to understand how what you do supports the mission. To feel a resonance between your spirit and the cause of the organization is very powerful. If you believe in what you are doing, work becomes a joyful thing. Your role as a nurse leader is to develop a unit-based mission that supports the organization's mission and strategy. The most effective approach is to engage your team in this effort. Personal involvement for each nurse will lead inevitably to buy-in and success. It takes a lot of time up front but there is a huge return on this investment, as each heart connects personally to the mission. **Exhibit 1–2** is an example of a hospital's mission and scorecard.

You can see how this can be carried to the unit level. Regular and timely reporting on progress toward goals helps to keep nurses engaged in the process. Pride in their unit grows with the realization that everyone has value to the organization as a whole.

Exhibit 1–1 Translating a Mission into Desired Outcomes

Mission	Why we exist
Core Values	What we believe in
Vision	What we want to be
Strategy	Our game plan
Balanced Scorecard	Implementation and focus
Strategic Initiatives	What we need to do
Personal Objectives	What I need to do

Strategic Outcomes

Satisfied Shareholders	Delighted Customers	Effective Processes	Motivated and Prepared Workforce

Reprinted by permission of *Harvard Business School Press*.
From: Kaplan, R. & Norton, D. (2001), *The Strategy-Focused Organization: How Balance Scorecard Companies Thrive in the New Business Environment*, p. 73.
Copyright © 2004 by the Harvard Business School Publishing Corporation; all rights reserved.

Staffing Model

Another key to success is to thoroughly know and understand how your area delivers patient care. What exactly are the needs of each patient population that your unit serves? What are the needs of the unit as a whole? Ask all the questions you need to develop a comprehensive construct of staffing requirements. Next, sort this out in terms of skill mix. What delivery-of-care method should you use? Try several ideas. How many registered nurses do you need? Be reasonable. There really is a shortage of labor and revenue. Be able to justify your request for high-priced personnel to senior management. Know the hours per patient day (HPPD) or relative value units (RVUs) that are required to deliver excellent patient care. Know this by day, by shift, and by hour. Know exactly what skill mix you need. Be able to visualize who will do what on each shift. What exactly is the role of the Registered Nurse (RN) and what exactly is the role of everyone else? And finally, how do these roles mesh to deliver safe, seamless care that satisfies the customer? This exercise, of course, is the first part of the budgeting process. To do it as a group project with your staff is the most effective method. Everyone can then understand where the budget (the staffing) comes from and how important it is to work as a team to care for patients. When they are involved in the process, nurses start to feel more like participants and owners of the process and less like victims of it.

Exhibit 1–2 Duke Children's Hospital—Balanced Scorecard

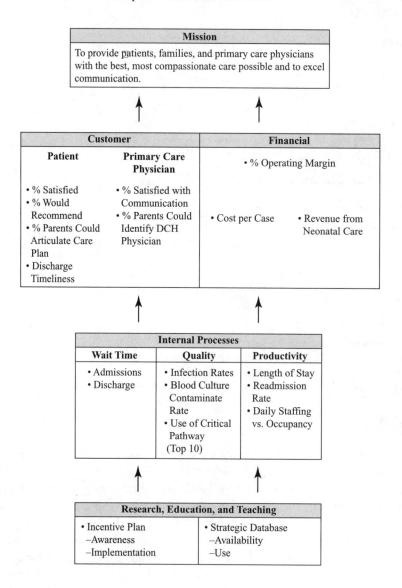

The Budgeting Process

Often, the annual budget is developed without input from managers. Historical performance is used in the forecast, and some adjustments are made based on economic predictions. If this is the case for you, you still have two opportunities for influence.

To be effective you need to have inside knowledge of the budgeting process. Find out who develops the wage and salary budget. It may be a management engineer or someone in the human resource department. The best way to find out is to ask the Chief Financial Officer. CFOs are usually delighted that someone is interested in learning more about the budgeting process. It is likely that he or she will candidly and eagerly answer all of your questions.

Developing a partnering relationship with the CFO is key. You need each other to be successful. The CFO is often the pivotal contact between the board and the organization. Even if most board members have little health care experience, they usually have a lot of expertise with financial reports. Therefore, they scrutinize expenditures and want explanations. The budget for nursing is often one of the biggest, and the CFO must be prepared to defend it. With input from the Chief Nursing Officer (CNO) as a primary "business partner," the CFO is well-equipped to defend the nursing budget—pointing out the direct link between nursing care and excellent patient outcomes.

Get involved in forecasting the budget at the very beginning. If your organization's fiscal year coincides with the calendar year, this may be as early as the middle of the third quarter. Make recommendations to the appropriate person for the staffing your unit needs. Be detailed—include full time equivalents (FTEs), skill mix per shift, allocation to each shift, etc. Be sure to include a line item for education and development. It is a good idea, too, to compare your staffing tables to benchmarks that are recognized as respectable in the industry. This helps you verify your work to yourself, your nurses, the CFO, and the board. You may not find exact comparisons, but you will be able to find scenarios close enough to your own to be helpful. If you can get both staffing numbers and information about patient outcomes from the benchmark, you are well on the way to building the case for putting patients first.

Most organizations expect managers to review the first draft of the budget before it is finalized. This is another opportunity for you to give valuable input. However, you may need to negotiate with your peers at this late point in the allocation process. In other words, the size of the pie has been determined. All that remains to decide is the size of the slice for each department.

The Nursing Team

There is significant power in having a strong nursing leadership team. Rally around each other. Know your strengths. Know your plan. Stand as one. In unity there is strength. Be the world's best champion for front-line nurses and for patients. Be quite clear on who your customers are and how to delight them. Meet frequently as a team and share your progress toward goals. Celebrate. Have fun. Incredible synergy and creativity will emerge. Get worked up. Be excited. Your work is very meaningful. It is a cause worthy of your best effort. Nursing is the most noble calling—serving human kind. What could be more important? Be positive and optimistic! Fall in love with nursing again. A strong visionary team can master any challenge.

Group Think

A potentially powerful attribute of having a strong leadership team is the ability to make good decisions. When resources are scarce, every decision about their use must be a careful one. A team that recognizes the strengths of each member, and is open and trusting, is a vehicle to success. Problems can be explored from different perspectives. Divergent opinions and disagreements can stimulate spirited dialogue and new ideas will emerge. Concurrence and convergence on a plan of action will result in an even stronger team. Every decision should be tested for its possible short-term and long-term consequences. For example, a short-term plan of conservative staffing to save money may result in a long-term result of poor staff retention and cost more money in the long run. The more good minds you bring to bear on a problem, the better your decisions will be, as long as you are nimble and quick in getting to the plan of action.

Other Relationships

Depending on how you look at it, or what your perspective is, just about everyone is your partner and/or your customer. The personal relationships you develop with each and all are an important part of your base of power. Nursing leaders usually have excellent interpersonal skills; building relationships is probably second nature. Capitalize on this skill. Use every opportunity to communicate and educate. You are the nursing expert. You, better than anyone, can explain why nursing is the back-bone of the organization—the key to impeccable patient care and financial health.

Following are some suggestions on leaders in your organization who can be pivotal to your (nursing's) success. Cultivate these relationships:

- **Chief Administrator (CEO, COO, CAO).** This person wants to be credible in the eyes of the board and the physicians. His or her goal is to assure that high-quality health care is provided in a fiscally responsible manner. If you succeed in this goal it is a done deal.
- **Chief Nursing Officer (CNO).** The same thoughts apply here. If you report to the CNO always know what goals the CNO is working toward and mesh into those.
- **Human Resources Director.** There are several key roles here—recruiting the best people, establishing competitive wages, offering benefits that retain and satisfy employees, developing feedback methods that reinforce goal-oriented performance, gathering information about employee satisfaction, and helping in the process of severing from the organization employees who do not share the values and the goals of the organization.
- **Staff Educators.** These people need to be your best friends. The nurses of the organization are their most important asset. Invest in their education heavily. Start with a stellar orientation—a little extra time and effort up-front will pay off handsomely. Offer education abundantly. Nurses like to keep learning. They also like to teach. Pay

them a stipend when they mentor new employees. Excellent experienced nurses are the standard of care. Reward them for passing on their knowledge.

- **Chief Information Officer.** An important key to the future lies here. We need to push the "e-envelope" for nurses. Time-saving and error-preventing information systems, monitoring systems, and documentation systems are an absolute necessity. Ideally, you will find a nurse on your staff, or on your leadership team, who is a nursing informatics fanatic. Get this person involved in decisions about the organization's investment in information systems that ease the paper burden on our nurses.
- **Physicians.** As our colleagues at the bedside, if you consistently provide excellent patient care, they can be your greatest ally. It is more effective if they are beholden to you and not the opposite. Nursing alone cannot be successful. Everyone needs to embrace the thought that patients come first. Your job is to get all departments to support the work of the nurses. This is not easy to do if you appear superior or demanding. Express your appreciation. Celebrate successes. Share progress toward goals as a mutual endeavor and accomplishment.
- **The Governing Board.** The governing board is our ultimate partner and customer. Remember that the Joint Commission on Accreditation of Healthcare Organizations (JCAHO) requires that the voice of nurses be heard at the board level. Ideally the CNO attends all board meetings. At the least, the CNO should report regularly to the board. Use this forum wisely. Report progress on established goals. Emphasize improved performance. Using objective data, make your needs known—better staffing, better wages. No whining allowed. Never undercut the CEO. Rehearse your presentations. Remember that you are equal. Do not be intimidated. Study after study has shown us that nurses are the most respected of all professionals. Let your presence reinforce that well-deserved stature.

Keep Your Promises

Strive tirelessly to meet and exceed the goals you establish. This is sometimes the hardest part—especially if you have set "stretch" goals (and you should). In linking mission to strategy to goals, you develop a dashboard of indicators that help you steer your course. These should include patient outcomes that reflect excellent nursing care, such as skin integrity, patient education, etc. Keep track of indications of the well-being of your nurses—things like retention rate, employee satisfaction, hours of nurse education, etc. And, of course, keep track of data that tells you about adherence to your staffing plan—hours per patient day, skill mix, agency hours, over-time hours, etc. Review your progress frequently. It is essential that you share timely information with your staff. Celebrate successes. Develop action plans with staff input when you get off track. A good rule of thumb is that three data points are a trend. If you have three data points off track, it is time to act. Remember also that flexibility is important. That is not to say that you should ever lower the standard of care. Impeccable patient care is sacred. However, health care is changing so fast these days that a goal established six months ago may no longer be applicable. Change your plan if the plan no longer fits.

Though objective measurable goals are essential in securing the resources you need and in measuring your success, subjective feedback is also very valuable. Listen carefully to what your customers are saying—the patients, their families, your nurses, the physicians. You will hear compliments and complaints. Pass the compliments on to those who have earned them. Consider the complaints as gifts. This is often free advice on how to make things better. There is a grain of truth in every complaint. Do not let complaints get you down. Remember this: when people bring their concerns to you, they believe in you. They know that you have the power to make a difference. I believe that, too. Godspeed.

There is one question, one answer, one passion: **What is right for the patient?**

CHAPTER 2

Providing Value-Based Services while Achieving Quality And Financial Accountability

Janne Dunham-Taylor, PhD, RN

Dru Malcolm, MSN, RN

Sandy K. Calhoun, MSN, RN, CPHQ

The top priority in any health care setting is to find out what the patient values; to provide that care in a loving, safe, excellent way when possible, and to strive to constantly improve our care delivery. This is true for both staff and physicians at the point of care, and for us as administrators in all our decisions and actions.

Introduction

What a tall order!! Thankfully, at times this is achieved. At this point both patient and care-givers feel like it has all been worthwhile. If you need an uplifting experience, read Bargmann's, *The Top Hospital in America: The Heart and Soul of a Great Medical Center* (2002). Additionally, a few health care organizations have been awarded the Malcolm Baldridge Award, and a compelling book, *Radical Loving Care: Building the Healing Hospital in America,* provides some answers on ways to achieve this goal. Although the above-mentioned are about hospitals, they could just as easily describe long-term care, home care, ambulatory care, and primary care settings. We will return to achieving all this after discussing the present situation and some of the problems that have surfaced.

Thus there are three enormous challenges confronting us in health care today. These are:

- ***We must regularly determine what our patient/client/resident wants and values.***
  We often have totally missed the mark on this challenge. Many of us do not know how to find this information. We have not been good listeners—and that starts with those

of us in administrative roles. The way we treat employees is the way the employees will treat patients. Quality constantly boils down to what the patient values and wants. Because this is such a misunderstood concept, we will devote a section of this chapter to it.

- *We provide the very best care quality, once we know what the patient values, and once we have assured patient safety.*
The quality of the care still must take what the patient values into account. Otherwise, it is possible that what we think is quality actually goes against what the patient wants. Quality, as measured by the patient perception, is what we are stressing here in this chapter. However, we realize that the patient may not always realize what is the best quality and we must ensure that we are using mechanisms such as providing evidenced-based care.

- *We must keep our patient/client/resident safe.*
To accomplish this, every one of us in health care needs to constantly strive to think of ways that will improve safety. This means the small things from wiping up a water spill someone has left on the floor, to purchasing technology, and implementing systems that all of us need to follow to the letter. Collins and Porras (1994) describe three characteristics of premier companies[1] that support this second mandate:

1. Because the visionary companies have such clarity about who they are, what they're all about, and what they're trying to achieve, they tend to not have much room for people unwilling or unsuited to their demanding standards, both in terms of performance and congruence (p. 121). Visionary companies impose tight ideological control and simultaneously provide wide operating autonomy that encourages individual initiative.... We found that the visionary companies were significantly more decentralized and granted greater operational autonomy than the comparison companies (p. 137).

2. A visionary company creates a total environment that envelops employees, bombarding them with a set of signals so consistent and mutually reinforcing that it's virtually impossible to misunderstand the company's ideology and ambitions (p. 121).

3. In examining the history of the visionary companies, we were struck by how often they made some of their best moves not by detailed strategic planning, but rather by experimentation, trial and error, opportunism, and—quite literally—accident (p. 141).

---

[1] These premier companies have lasted 50 to 100 years, and are at the top when compared with like companies.

We Have a L-O-N-G Way to Go to Fix our Health Care System

Many times there are BIG problems in health care. More often than not care is fragmented and depersonalized. We may do harm at the patient's expense. At times patients become worse rather than better when they come in contact with us. And we even do things that are against the patient's wishes. We have SO much more work to do. Is there ever a need for change! Statistics show that the United States ranks 37th in overall quality of health care, according to the World Health Organization, but spends more per person on health care than any other country.

Patient Safety Issues

It is estimated that there are 98,000 hospital deaths per year from avoidable hospital errors, not to mention errors occurring in other health care settings. In fact, more people die from avoidable hospital errors than the number that die from breast cancer or motor vehicle accidents.

The patient safety scandal is inexcusable. Patients coming to us for treatment could experience a life-threatening event due to our error. The present error rate is way too high. The Harvard Medical Practice Study reported that nearly 4 percent of hospitalized patients experienced an adverse event–injury caused by treatment (Buerhaus, 1999). The study further identified that two thirds of these adverse events could have been prevented.

> The ideal system is one in which there are very few errors and every one of them is reported and discussed and something is done about them. We have not accomplished the first part of this, and, frankly, if we had a system in which every error was reported, we would be deluged. Every hospital would have many more errors than it could handle. It's a sad commentary but our high error rate is one of the ways the health care industry differs from other hazardous industries, such as aviation (p. 284).

This study was followed by the Institute of Medicine (IOM) report, *To Err Is Human* (2000)—followed by *Crossing the Quality Chasm: A New Health System for the 21st Century* (2001)—saying that medical errors in U.S. hospitals kill at least 44,000 people. In fact, this figure may be as high as 98,000. They also likened the medical error situation to the airline industry. If an airline said that 4 percent of the planes crashed—while the others arrived safely—we certainly would not want to fly on that airline.

Safety-Centered Solutions reports that after tracking 250,000 medical errors, 25 percent were from adverse drug events, 20 percent were surgical incidents, 20 percent were patient falls, and 15 percent were nosocomial infections. *These figures are a disgrace.* This report also examined the costs of these events: 25 percent of the costs resulted from surgical incidents, 25 percent from nosocomial infections, 15 percent from adverse drug events, and 15 percent from patient falls (Haugh, 2000).

These complications are expensive in actual dollars, not to mention the unmeasurable costs of patients' lives, or the amount of time and treatment necessary to improve, and the additional worry on the part of patients and families. The Advisory Board (2000) reported that nine complications from greatest to least expense (decubitus ulcer, septicemia, post-operative pulmonary complications, postoperative infections except pneumonia and wound, aspiration pneumonia, postoperative gastrointestinal hemorrhage, reopening of surgical site, postoperative pneumonia, and shock or cardiorespiratory arrest in-hospital) were in the highest cost level when examining the hospital experience. These alone cost an additional $16,889 to $28,681 per patient discharge, and increased length of stay from 6.4 days to 20.5. This does not take into account the additional expense that could occur post-hospital discharge, i.e., long-term care, home care, medications, the need for a caregiver in the home, additional physician visits, and so forth.

Many of these complications could either be prevented, or detected early, if the patient received excellent nursing care. This would mean that the nurses were regularly assessing the patients, were using critical thinking to identify and treat patients, and were communicating effectively across all shifts, including weekends and holidays.

"The Institute for Safe Medication Practices says medication errors can be reduced by 85 percent using simple technology like handheld scanners and bar codes" (p. 45). The Food and Drug Administration (FDA) followed up on this recommendation by mandating that barcoding be on all single-unit packages of prescription drugs, over-the-counter drugs commonly used in hospitals, vaccines, and biologics such as blood by the end of 2003. (Barcoding is further explained in the next section, and in Chapter 12, Budget Strategies.) However, so far, many hospitals and long-term care facilities have not implemented such procedures, nor have many of them purchased the equipment necessary to use the barcoding mechanism.

Another issue is a shortage of emergency rooms and hospital beds. "More than 1,000 hospitals and 1,100 Emergency Departments (EDs) have closed in the past ten years, leaving a capacity shortage…. Perpetually backlogged EDs and a marked increase in diversion status usage demonstrate the lack of available and staffed beds for patient placement. In fact, a survey of 1,501 hospitals with EDs that describe themselves as either at or over capacity identifies several reasons for instituting diversion status, including the lack of critical care and general acute beds" (Nooner, 2004, p. 39).

In fact, this shortage is such a serious problem that various pieces of legislation, as well as Medicaid regulations, require that patients have a right to obtain medical information, explanations, and instructions in their own language. The general public is aware of this problem, as shown by reading such things as **Exhibit 2–1**, or CHIPS Network News Headlines (news@chipsnetwork.com) that reflects Americans' dissatisfaction with healthcare.

Sub-Standard Care

Bad as it may be, patient safety is not the only problem. Even when patients have a safe episode of care, they often feel depersonalized, experience long waits, and think that the health care provider does not listen nor care about either what is wrong, nor about what the patient actually wants or needs. Worse yet, a number of patients receive substandard care—especially if they are in a lower socioeconomic group or if they are a racial or ethnic minority.

Exhibit 2–1 Gun Owners vs. Doctors

- Number of physicians in the United States 700,000
- Accidental deaths caused by physicians per year 120,000
- Accidental deaths per physician 0.171
- Number of gun owners in the United States 80,000,000
- Number of accidental gun deaths per year (all age groups) 1,500
- Accidental deaths per gun owner 0.0000188

PLEASE ALERT YOUR FRIENDS TO THIS ALARMING THREAT. WE MUST BAN DOCTORS BEFORE THIS GETS OUT OF HAND. AS A PUBLIC HEALTH MEASURE I HAVE WITHHELD THE STATISTICS ON LAWYERS FOR FEAR THAT THE SHOCK COULD CAUSE PEOPLE TO SEEK MEDICAL ATTENTION.

From: Alternative Medicine Magazine (www.alternativemedicine.com)

According to a report released this spring by the Institute of Medicine, 'racial and ethnic minorities tend to receive lower-quality health care than whites do, even when insurance status, age and severity of conditions are comparable.' The report asserts that low-quality treatment contributes to higher death rates for minorities (Kelly, 2002, p. 24).

Let's review the numbers:

- United States residents speak at least 329 languages.

- 44 million Americans do not have health insurance.

- Latinos are twice as likely as other Americans to lack health care coverage.

- By 2030, the Hispanic population will increase 113% and the Asian American population by 132%.

- African Americans' infant mortality rate is 2.5 times greater than that of Caucasians.

- African Americans' death rate from HIV/AIDS is seven times greater than that of Caucasians. Their homicide rate is six times greater.

- Native Americans are 2.4 times more likely than Caucasians to die from diabetes, and three times more likely to die of cirrhosis.

- Vietnamese women have a five times greater incidence of cervical cancer than Caucasian women.

- Less than 2% of health care CEOs and COOs are non-Caucasian.

New technologies and worldwide epidemics bring us into a global spotlight. Our colleagues and patients come from all over the planet. Whether immigrants, refugees, or natural-born citizens, they require careful consideration and respectful treatment (Alexander, 2002, pp. 30–31).

Bottom-Line Orientation Loses—Both Quality and Money

Many health care administrators have made the bottom line their first priority, with doing what is right for the patient a poor second. Research (see Chapter 14, Budget Strategies) tells us that when the bottom line is first, this results in financial disaster for the organization because everything spirals downward. If we do not pay attention to quality, safety, and value, patients suffer, staff and physicians are unhappy, and costs increase significantly. Obvious costs include longer patient lengths of stay, improper use of supplies and equipment, more patient complications, or, worse yet, deaths. Then there are the hidden, or less obvious, costs such as poor leadership, legal issues caused by poor practice combined with unhappy patients and families, potential clients who do not want to come to the facility, physicians who choose to practice elsewhere, greater staff turnover—not to mention hiring and orienting costs, and staff not working effectively as a team. These issues can result in loss of services offered by the facility or culminate and pose a threat to the viability of the facility, adding to the continuum of inaccessible health care, increased costs, increased length of stay, and overall dissatisfaction with services rendered. This is how the spiral works. If allowed to continue, the organization will eventually go out of business.

Poor Administrative Leadership

Even when the bottom line is not first priority, some really important problems can be causing serious monetary losses. For example, in Chapter 3 we discuss the importance of effective administrative leadership from the top down because poor leadership creates financial disasters. Actually, if leadership is really effective, the patient is at the top of the organizational chart with the CEO and Board being at the bottom, serving everyone else. In Chapter 4 we discuss the importance of having a systems perspective, being careful not to make "quick fix" solutions that end up costing more in the long run. Often an inventory of processes reveals that considerable dollars could be saved simply by making the processes more efficient.

Historically, authoritarian leadership style prevailed—withholding information, top-down communication, and not expecting first-line managers to have anything to do with the budget. Today these methods are obsolete and will lead to financial ruin. We are now experiencing changes that can affect both quality and the bottom line. It is important that we share information, and have honest dialogue with, and between, staff members.

It is precisely this authoritarian leadership and bottom-line orientation that produces unhealthy work environments. This problem is exaggerated by an aging workforce with the average nurse being mid-forties, the average nursing faculty being 56 years old. Additionally, there is presently a workforce shortage which drives costs up. Then there are the generational differences. What baby boomers were willing to sacrifice in terms of work environment and work hours, the later generations are not willing to do. And nurses are complaining.

In an American Journal of Nursing (AJN) survey of over 7,000 nurses, "nearly two out of five nurses said they wouldn't want a family member to receive care at their organization.... Over half of the nurses reported less continuity of care and an increase in unexpected readmissions" (Shindul-Rothschild, et al., 1996, p. 25). The nurses went on to report the following quality issues: "The incidence of complications secondary to admitting diagnosis (53%), medication errors (54%), nosocomial/wound infections (58%), pressure ulcers/skin breakdown (59%), injuries to patients (66%), and unexpected patient deaths (74%)" (p. 33). Not to mention losing dentures, glasses, and other belongings while patients are receiving inpatient care in any setting.

Perhaps these issues occurred because most RNs reported "less time to teach patients and their families (73%), comfort and talk to patients (74%), provide basic nursing care (69%), document care (66%), and consult with other members of the health care team (57%)" (p. 31). All this has caused nurses to say that they are less satisfied with their work. Isn't this a sad commentary? What are we administrators doing about it? You see, the way we health care administrators treat health care staff is the way the staff will treat patients. It keeps coming back to us!

Regulatory Issues

One regional and national trend, discussed more in Chapter 6, is all the regulation that has occurred because people's needs have not been met adequately or safely. The regulations present problems of their own. They are designed to serve populations of people and do not take into account individual preferences. They define specific policies that need to be enforced yet do not take into account the exceptions that are needed when following these policies. The regulations have become so cumbersome that a health care organization cannot possibly follow all of them, even when we have hired specific people who just deal with meeting regulations. This system of regulations, although it gives a lot of business to lawyers, is not benefiting us as citizens. Granted, some regulations have resulted in better practice, so we do not want to throw out the baby with the bathwater! But there needs to be a better balance between what is best practice and what is overkill. Our profession must get more involved with social policy.

Besides regulation, the government has taken over much of the health insurance system through Medicare and Medicaid. (This is further explained in Chapter 6.) As health care expenses rise, and the elderly group eligible for Medicare grows, governments are faced with finding the money to cover the expenses these large systems have incurred. Thus it has been necessary to curtail health care expenses. Heaven knows what will happen by 2010 because, chances are, we will be unable to pay for it all.

Technology Costs

As health care monies are curtailed or cut, another problem has surfaced. We are in the information age, yet *when* we have computer systems, they cannot talk to one another (they are not *integrated*), purchased information systems *quickly become obsolete*, and information system companies fold and leave us holding the bag. Yet, if we want prompt payment we must use a computerized system to report care given, and the current movement for patient safety involves many necessary technological purchases. Then, to add insult to injury, the government insisted that we meet Health Insurance Portability and Accountability Act of 1996 (HIPAA is explained in Chapter 6) requirements while keeping down health care costs with the Balanced Budget Act. The dilemma is that all these technology purchases need to be made at a time when reimbursements are curtailed.

Is It Possible to Achieve Quality when We Are Having to Cut Costs?

Some people will tell you that it is very difficult, if not impossible, to achieve quality while cutting costs in health care. However, just because money is cut does not automatically mean that quality will suffer. Quality and money, although linked, are really two separate issues. For instance, say administrative leadership has been a serious problem. Chances are, if the administrative leadership is improved, or replaced by more effective administrators, a lot of money will be saved—this change will turn a downward spiral upwards. All sorts of other issues will begin to improve, and costs will decrease as care gets better. Fewer dollars does not have to mean that quality gets worse.

Reframing the Cost-Quality Dilemma to Value-Based Care

Porter-O'Grady and Malloch (2002) suggest that we should reframe the cost-quality dilemma by asking a *value question*. "The problem… is how to provide value-based, high-quality care that is affordable and at the same time make money" (p. 316).

> Given the constraints caused by balanced budget initiatives, leaders are often caught in a cost-quality balancing act and are not always sure how to achieve *value-based care.…* Perhaps it would be helpful to reframe the quality question as a value question. Value is determined by the three elements of cost, quality, and service. Cost is driven by the available resources.… Quality is partly determined by the outcomes of care. Service is a matter of the time and type of care provided. Thus the question becomes, *Are health care leaders obligated to provide value-based services to patients and family members?* The issue of spending money on quality is now linked to both cost and service.

> Achieving value-based health care faces an additional challenge: drawing conclusions about quality initiatives and return on investment when there are multiple factors involved. A further complication is the extensive use of a type of cost-benefit analysis that is not sensitive to health care objectives. If the benefits of a program can be priced in dollars, then a cost-benefit analysis will be able to identify the alternative with the largest benefit-to-cost ratio.

Definition

Value
- Cost
- Quality
- Service

However, many decisions involve benefits that are not easily quantifiable in monetary terms or otherwise, such as psychological benefits and environmental benefits (clean air and water).

Health care leaders and providers are now required to examine services using the value equation and make decisions accordingly. If resources are limited, leaders must ask whether every patient sign and symptom require intervention, particularly if minimal or no improvement in the patient's clinical condition is the likely outcome. Paying close attention to the health improvement value of health care services is an incredibly difficult challenge for providers and leaders schooled in the doctrine that increasing access to health care and growth in the health care system were absolute goods. Unfortunately, accountability and control were absent from the cost-based payment system, and the results are well known—exhaustion of resources. Health professionals are currently challenged to move from "rich" care to "wise" care (pp. 316–317).

What has value makes a difference. For example, a young woman discovers that she has slight scoliosis after seeing a health care provider for a painful back. Perhaps "wise" care begins with health. Dr. Fritz Smith, an osteopath, invented a treatment process called *zero balance* that works with the skeletal system to get it moving properly. A practitioner doing the zero balance procedure with this young woman on a regular basis can actually begin to straighten this young woman's back. The traditional alternative is to do extensive surgery. Which might the young woman value most? In this case the cost of the zero balance is not as great as the surgery, and the zero balance procedure is not as invasive.

This points out other problems with our current health care system. The first problem is that our tertiary reimbursement system might not cover the zero balance treatment yet will reimburse for surgery. In many cases today, the patient will decide to pay for the zero balance as an out-of-pocket expense. Second, the surgeon may be unaware of the zero balance option, or may just think that this information is not accurate. After all, the surgeon was not taught this in medical school. The surgeon might also see doing this surgery as a source of revenue that would be lost if all scoliosis patients could be helped by a less invasive procedure. So this value question can lead to ethical implications if the surgeon continues to recommend and perform surgery, even when aware that there is another less invasive option.

The nurse manager has a tremendous impact with this "wise" patient care issue. Being closer to the patient, the nurse manager has a good handle on what patients want and need. If the nurse knows about zero balance, the nurse may choose to tell the patient about it. This could incur the wrath of the surgeon. Or, if left up to the patient, the patient might choose the surgery anyway, believing in it more than the new concept of zero balance. But if the nurse does not tell the patient about zero balance, the nurse has violated his/her ethical principles. It's a dilemma.

Porter-O'Grady and Malloch (2002) observe:

> What one does and what difference it makes are the key issues for all providers. If an organization provides 1,000 services and only 25 make a difference, then the other 975 services must be considered for elimination—even if the 975 services have billing codes that render them reimbursable.
>
> Provider accountability for contributions to patient care outcomes is a missing piece of health care. All professional care providers must focus their actions on achieving desired outcomes and only implement interventions that have a basis in science or a realistic chance of benefiting patients.
>
> The measurement of health care outcomes is gradually becoming more meaningful and reflective of patient needs. Unfortunately, indicators are often looked at in an order that fails to take into account the basic goal of health care—health improvement. For example, productivity measures are typically examined prior to clinical outcomes. If productivity targets are exceeded, increases in productivity are mandated without consideration of their potential impact on care provision (p. 316).

It is important that the nurse manager constantly be thinking, *"What does the patient value?"*— along with *"safety, safety, safety"*—*"quality, quality, quality,"* while thinking, *"cost effectiveness, cost effectiveness, cost effectiveness."* Make sure that the services provided are only the ones that are *valuable* to the patients. And the expectation is that staff at the point of care are thinking the same thing. Tall order. This is a change for most of us who are used to providing care *as we know it*.

So far we have not found out what the patient wants and values, and there are no outcome measurements that can tell us how successfully we have accomplished this goal. Instead our measurements are complications that may have occurred, or financial ratios, or staffing or turnover numbers—none of which tells us what the *patient wanted* and did the *patient get it*?

The problem is that we need to figure out, and be creative enough, to find the ways to achieve and measure what the patient values. It is *not* by *doing it the way we have always done it*. Perhaps the best way comes back to the cost, quality, and service elements that O'Grady and Malloch discuss. This means we need to find out what the patient wants and values, then examine whether and how we can provide it. What is the cost? What quality components are needed? Are we providing the services needed?

We administrators are not alone in needing to make this change in perspective. All staff, the board, the executive team, and physicians will need to learn to think this way. Everyone has to get into the act of providing valuable services that provide quality in a cost-effective way. After all, everyone contributes to achieving this goal, and we can always do better. Paying attention to *value* as first priority, with safety and quality a part of this, helps us to make better decisions.

Value has another implication. We all must understand the importance of including our patients in the decision-making process. The patient has to be involved in deciding what services will be provided, taking into account the costs. Quality relates to an awareness of alternatives such as providing evidence-based practice. We need to change to determine what will be best for the patient. If we are deciding whether to go ahead with a new service, we may decide to do this based on what patients have told us about their needs. The bottom line will follow. It is not the top priority but is secondary to what is valued. As we effectively deliver what is valued, we can figure out how to do this in a cost-effective way.

Such a challenge! Or, let's change the way we think about this. Such an opportunity! It is exciting to be part of the cutting edge of true *health* care, based on what has value for the patient. This is a pivotal point that will change health care as we know it. The choice is to pay attention to it or to become obsolete. So the first issue is to find out what the patient values, or really wants; couple this with quality—that elusive thing that no matter how wonderful we are, there is always more that we can do—and loving service. Quality also means safety. Cost effectiveness comes third—it follows the value and quality/safety issues. When we provide valuable services, the outcome *always* has to be what is best for the patient. And as Leary points out in Chapter 1, *that* is what makes money. The bottom line always follows, and is never first.

So we need to get out of the box. An important part of our administrative role is to pay attention to ways that we can reframe our work to better achieve our patient's goals. This is complicated because often staff do not want to get out of the box, and part of our job as administrators is to encourage them to leave this comfortable, unchanging zone to try uncharted territory. This can be a tall order for administrators, and can even jeopardize our job if there is a general staff revolt. But if we choose *not* to pay attention to getting out of the box, our job and workplace will be jeopardized as the work becomes obsolete. Another dilemma! Some of these changes will result in our providing services at less cost while, at the same time, better quality or higher levels of safety are achieved.

Another trap we can get into is to say that because we have inadequate resources there is no way that we can make improvements. In this case, we do not even *try* to do anything, bemoaning the fact that reimbursements are not as high as they should be. We need to throw away this crutch (the excuse of inadequate resources) and instead ask, *how we can make a difference?*

We should also remember that if we cannot figure out a way to do things better, someone else will. After all, we do not want to be like the manufacturer of buggies, in the horse and buggy era, who did not want to have anything to do with the car! Someone will always figure out a way to do things better—and they might even save money doing it. Take the freestanding surgery centers, for example. They can do some of the same surgery procedures at less cost than the hospital OR. Yes, it is partly because the overhead is cheaper in a surgery center. ***So why does overhead in a hospital have to be so much higher??***

Another issue in health care relates directly to the value question. Patients are often expected to fit the health care provider's schedule. Say our patient has a full-time job days Monday through Friday but needs to make an appointment with a provider who offers no weekend or evening appointments. So our patient has to take sick time, or take unpaid time off, missing work to go to the appointment. Then a doc-in-a-box center opens where our patient can get the same services in the evening or during the weekend. Now there is a choice. Does our patient choose to miss work and lose pay/use sick time, or go after hours for an appointment? What the patient values most must be considered.

In Chapter 1, Leary, a chief operating officer, discusses how *when we do what is right for the patient, we will make money*. The finances will follow as second priority. Although she does not actually call doing what is right for the patient *value*, this is implied. If we do what the patient values and then consider finances, patients will receive good care and have faith in the organization, staff will be proud to work there and work more effectively as a team, physicians will want to bring their patients to the facility, and everyone wins as well as meeting the budget. Research supports this.

So Where Do We Start?

> No problem can be solved from the same consciousness that created it.
> We must learn to see the world anew.
>
> —*Albert Einstein*

What are we doing about the present mess in our health care system? Not nearly enough. We have an ENORMOUS amount of work to do. First, there is the value issue; second, we have the patient safety scandal. Third, we have health care providers still treating patients the same way they learned to in school—even though it is twenty years later. Finally, the system has become so depersonalized that patients dread having to come to us, and nurses want to leave. Where do we start?

One thing that has always been true of Americans is that during times of turmoil, we pull together to fix the problem. We need to start doing things differently. It needs to start within our ranks as administrators. How effective is our leadership? Chapter 3 is extensive because this is *so* important—including the financial impact. The process needs to start internally with us. Chapter 4 follows with organizational problems because a lot of what needs to be fixed we use when we provide services with our patients.

So, in this chapter, we want to take a different look at what quality is really all about. Perhaps it starts with the radical loving care described by Chapman (2004). He advocates what we already know in our nursing role. This means that we listen to each patient, that we read between the lines. The physical diagnosis may not be the most important issue for the patient. Instead, we should find out what the patient values and provide this when possible. Not only is care safe, but excellent, following evidence-based practice guidelines coupled with what the patient wants. While this happens we are constantly improving what we do.

As we redefine quality, there is one ray of hope. In a recent Gallup poll, nurses (83%) fare better than physicians (68%) as the public rates them on being the most honest and ethical. In fact, nurses were above most professions—veterinarians, dentists, pharmacists, policemen, clergy, and college teachers. HMO managers only got 9 percent! So as we fix this mess, there is a lot that we, as nurses, can do because the public is more likely to trust us in this process. Let's not lose this trust, but, instead, guard it carefully and live up to this expectation.

As we resolve our present problems, we must be attentive to the next group of issues to be fixed or repaired, always keeping in mind that:

> Our top priority in any health care setting is to find out what the patient values; provide that care in a loving, safe, excellent way when possible; and strive to constantly improve our care delivery—true for both staff and physicians at the point of care, and for us as administrators in all our decisions and actions.

The Patient Value Perspective—Our First Priority

This chapter immediately follows Chapter 1 because quality from a patient value perspective is the most important issue in health care. Everything else follows, and supports, this quality initiative. When we are effective in the quality arena, our every decision, and every action, strive to provide the care that is needed in the safest, most effective way. But what exactly is quality?

> In 1990, the Institute of Medicine (IOM) proposed that 'quality of care is the degree to which health services for individuals and populations increase the likelihood of desired health outcomes and are consistent with current professional knowledge.'... It does correspond with the definition of quality used by the Joint Commission. The more prevalent belief is that an explicitly common definition of quality is lacking. Even the Joint Commission raises pertinent concerns regarding the IOM definition of quality, noting quality requires a judgment. Quality is then in the eyes of the beholder, meaning different things to different people because assessing quality entails a subjective evaluation.
>
> Yet, the absence of a definition of quality need not be an absolute roadblock to future efforts. All individuals involved with examining quality—purchasers, payers, providers, patients, and health care executives—need to accept that the components of quality will vary depending on the stakeholder. An obligation exists to acknowledge explicitly and consistently from whose perspective quality is being examined. Performance measures then must be constructed to tap into the particular view of that constituency (Jennings and Staggers, 1999, p. 19).

Thus the definition of quality has been inadequate. In fact, most of it has not considered the patient's perspective, but relies heavily upon the health care professional's perspective, or that of the payer or regulator. We have forgotten the most important person in the equation—our patient, our client, our resident. Frequently, the health care professional never consulted the patient to find out what the patient wanted, needed, or valued. Perhaps this is captured in the definition in the book, *Through the Patients' Eyes* (1993):

> Quality . . . has two dimensions. One has to do with technical excellence: the skill and competence of professionals and the ability of diagnostic or therapeutic equipment, procedures, and systems to accomplish what they are meant to accomplish, reliably and effectively. Borrowing the language and conceptual models of industrial engineering, we speak in this sense of 'quality control,' 'quality assurance,' and 'quality improvement.'
>
> The other dimension related to subjective experience—its texture and substance, its sentient quality. In this sense, we speak of the quality of a sensation or experience or the quality of human relationships. In health care, it is quality in this subjective dimension that patients experience most directly—in their perception of illness or well-being and in their encounters with health care professionals and institutions (p. xi).

The Institute of Medicine has recommended that for this new century, we commit to six goals for improvement that will change this perspective to what the patient wants and values:

> Advances must begin with all health care constituencies—health professionals, federal and state policy makers, public and private purchasers of care, regulators, organization managers and governing boards, and consumers—committing to a national statement of purpose for the health care system as a whole. In making this commitment, the parties would accept as their explicit purpose 'to continually reduce the burden of illness, injury, and disability, and to improve the health and functioning of the people of the United States.' The parties also would adopt a shared vision of six specific aims for improvement. These aims are built around the core need for health care to be:
>
> • *Safe:* avoiding injuries to patients from the care that is intended to help them.
>
> • *Effective:* providing services based on scientific knowledge to all who could benefit, and reframing from providing services to those not likely to benefit.
>
> • *Patient-centered:* providing care that is respectful of and responsive to individual patient preferences, needs, and values, and ensuring that patient values guide all clinical decisions.
>
> • *Timely:* reducing waits and sometimes harmful delays for both those who receive and those who give care.
>
> • *Efficient:* avoiding waste, including waste of equipment, supplies, ideas, and energy. (Efficiency is discussed in Chapter 21, Productivity, with additional information in Chapter 14, Budget Strategies.)

- *Equitable:* providing care that does not vary in quality because of personal characteristics such as gender, ethnicity, geographic location, and socioeconomic status.

A health care system that achieves major gains in these six areas would be far better at meeting patient needs. Patients would experience care that is safer, more reliable, more responsible to their needs, more integrated, and more available, and they could count on receiving the full array of preventive, acute, and chronic services that are likely to prove beneficial. Clinicians and other health workers also would benefit through their increased satisfaction at being better able to do their jobs and thereby bring improved health, greater longevity, less pain and suffering, and increased personal productivity to those who receive their care (*Crossing the Quality Chasm: A New Health System for the 21st Century*, 2001, pp. 2–3).

In this chapter, we are choosing the "patient-centered" aim as the core of quality with every other aim following it. In fact, all the other aims are really subsumed by being patient centered. The patient wants safe care; this responsibility lies with us, the health care providers, to make sure this is the case. We equate effectiveness with the quality initiative. If we are patient centered, the timely and equitable parts will automatically follow. However, both the timely and equitable aspects will suffer if we are centered on other things such as the bottom line or ourselves.

What Do We Mean by What the Patient Values?

If we are patient centered, we are *listening* to what each patient wants, and the answer may surprise us. The patient might not agree with our definition of what has value. In fact, the patient might value something entirely different than the care we are providing! What do patients value? It is best to ask them. Often patients value different things at different times. For instance, when a patient is in critical condition, the patient wants a highly skilled, prompt, technologically–advanced, yet kind care giver; while a non-acute patient wants a rapid turnaround with a kind, personable care giver.

But it is more than that.

The answer to the value question will depend upon how the patient defines *quality of life*. Take some examples:

- The 400-pound patient with a heart attack appreciates care for the heart attack but may not value or want to be put on an 800-calorie diet and be weighed on the laundry scales.
- The patient may value the provider who takes the time to listen and bring a warm blanket when needed, more than whether there was IV access on the first attempt. And if both are achieved, so much the better!
- The African-American patient wants loving care that does not discriminate.
- The poor patient hurts as much as the wealthy one.

- Some patients want a peaceful death, i.e., a patient with a gangrenous leg in renal failure that chooses not to have surgery, or patients who know that they are not going to get better and want to choose the way to live for the rest of their lives. Or the patient may not want any heroic measures as she or he lies dying.
- A heart patient may not want to start using healthy practices and chooses to smoke, eat too much fatty food or junk food, not exercise, and not lose weight. This person has chosen not to change, and then will face the reality that this lifestyle will cause. The patient has valued the present life style over health. The choice is the patient's, not ours.

Values pivot on the circumstances at hand and whose point of view is considered. *Patient perceptions, and what the patient wants, are more important than what we think the patient **should** want* when determining quality indicators. We are not the patient's parents! Our old patriarchal (or matriarchal) systems need to die with the previous century. For example, once we have determined what evidence-based care might be for a specific patient, there is still more to do. We need to then offer the patient choices in specific remedies and therapies that fall under that evidence-based care rubric. And as we have previously stated, the patient has a right to turn down all of it and proceed with life, or face death, without our having given the patient anything—if that is what the patient has chosen. We presently fail in health care delivery because we often consider what we would want instead of consulting the patient and finding out the patient's wishes.

In health care, it is easy to get caught up in our routines and *forget* to ask patients what they want, and to forget the family or other significant people around the patient. Regardless of whether the patient and family are loving and functional or dysfunctional, they are a unit. The family may experience a number of conflicts that we will need to deal with as we are working to provide care for the patient. In fact, at times a family member will determine what is best for the patient (i.e., with a pediatric patient or in certain cultural situations). Determining the family's relationships, and understanding the patient's perspective, is all part of the value component. Our reward for valued, safe care is satisfied patients—and best of all we can look ourselves in the mirror every day and know that we have given our best.

Paying attention to value and quality puts us in an interesting dilemma. *Value and quality are those elusive things that we never totally achieve. So why should we spend so much time and effort striving to achieve them??* Working to achieve better value and quality sounds like a frustrating experience, yet, at the same time, when we feel that we have done our best, we achieve our most satisfying work experiences. When excellent, safe care is delivered, and the patient has valued the service, everyone on the health care team feels good about his/her work, and, most importantly, the patient benefits by experiencing the best we can offer.

Reframing from the Health Perspective

As we ask patients what they value, we find that some patients leave the health care decisions up to us, or will choose our present illness model, simply because that is all they know, or they may believe that we can cure them. However, there has been a groundswell of interest in the general public about moving toward a health perspective.

How Does One Achieve Health?

Even though we call it "health" care, our present system is actually an "illness" system. (See Chapter 6 for an historical overview that shows how we got into our present system.) We in the nursing and medical professions deliver illness-care. We focus on diagnosis and treatment of disease and chronic illness. We identify nutritional screening and identification of risk factors, such as smoking or consumption of alcohol, in clinical assessments but often do not do anything, or offer any services to the patient, to help the patient overcome these problems. Payment is made to treat disease. Think about that word. Wouldn't we rather experience *ease* than *dis-ease*? Doesn't *ease* really mean health? Our present system is not based on what makes health. Don't we need to reframe this illness orientation?

Many people don't think too much of our illness box. It is invasive—we hurt people with some of our procedures; it may be unsafe; it may be unfriendly or unhelpful; it may not cure us; the treatment may create more medical problems; we give medications that can have some very dangerous, irreversible side effects. We may not explain what we will do; one's life savings can be used up entirely for one episode of illness; and the patient might feel worse when he/she is discharged! When a patient has to go to inpatient facilities, the food is generally neither very healthy nor nutritious; there is no opportunity for exercise; the environment is often loud and unpleasant, especially if a television is blaring; we wake up patients out of a healing sleep to do activities on our schedules, not theirs; we do not listen to what the family or patient requests. The list goes on. Our treatment is based on treating disease. The issue of how to achieve health is not even asked. We take all this for granted in our illness box, as this is our present reality.

This leaves much room for improvement. Think about that. Is this really the reality we want to create? Where is the caring part of nursing in all this? After all, think about all these undesirable realities our patients—and we ourselves face— if we experience illness this way. Isn't it comforting to think about having a less invasive procedure done to treat a problem? Don't we hate it when we really cannot help a patient get better? Perhaps we need to revise our present care system and make "health" the basis of the system. This totally upends our illness-care box! To change venues and concentrate on wellness, maintenance of health, and prevention of disease would be a complete change of paradigm for most health care providers.

Yet, if we pay attention to *value*, we must determine what achieves health. Many people *are* choosing health. In fact, the public is ahead of many of us in the "health" (it is really "illness") care professions on this issue. People are choosing to spend billions of their own dollars on care that helps them to achieve health. This includes such things as alternative therapies, vitamins, healthy foods, exercise, meditation/prayer, acupuncture, and massage, to name a few. In fact, there are even studies illustrating the positive effects of 15 seconds of laughter a day. Many people have figured out the importance of health and are looking for ways to maintain it throughout their lifetime. The means to achieve and maintain health are available. If we really want to achieve the value part of health care, we, as health care providers, need to regroup and provide this education because our customers are finding it elsewhere. Even the regulators are getting into the act. For instance, JCAHO has adopted new standards that address various screening processes to identify risks and promote a healthier lifestyle.

Our nursing profession teaches about health, as well as illness, so we are partially ahead of other health professions on this issue. However, many of us continue to have a dis-ease approach to care.

Instead we need to ask first, what does the patient want? Then we can determine if the patient would rather come from a *health* perspective. Think about the elderly person coming into our system that has been exercising regularly, eating nutritious foods, living independently, and suddenly this person has a stroke that limits mobility and the ability to communicate. This person's quality of life has suddenly imploded. This person is going to want to know if it is possible to ever get back to where she or he was before. Can she or he be healthy again? What will be her or his quality of life? Can she or he continue to live an independent lifestyle?

The health approach is more holistic in nature. Alternative therapies, holistic medicine, and herbal remedies are more accessible. When a person experiences an illness, there are alternative therapies to consider. Better yet, if a person has a history that seems to predisposition a possible illness, there might be more the person could do to prevent this illness from ever occurring.

This health approach not only needs to be directed toward patients/clients/residents, but must also be applied to employees. What a wonderful message for the establishment/administration/employer to send to employees—*Your health and quality of life is important and we want to assist you in reaching your optimal level of health.* This premise could be reflected in the mission, vision, and value statements of the organization, and it is helpful when there are incentives provided within the organization to reach optimal health. By promoting wellness, including smoking cessation, weight control, exercise programs, and routine screenings, the organization is investing in its employees, and, hopefully, increasing quality of life. It benefits the employees as well as the facility. Some organizations have offered reduced, or free, memberships to wellness facilities, or employees can receive therapeutic massage on site. Others have financial incentives, or reduced health premiums, for eliminating risk factors. Happy, healthy employees are more productive, use less sick time, and reflect the image the organization promotes. In Sweden, everyone takes a coffee break together to not only reduce stress but promote teamwork.

What is health? There has been a lot of research on this. Health has several components. First, let's look at food. Eating nutritious food that has not been tampered with is really a more healthy practice. We are seeing teenagers on junk food diets experience the acute and chronic illnesses that adults were not experiencing until mid-life a generation or two ago, including the early onset of diabetes due to the vast amounts of sugar and refined flour consumed (cupcakes and a carbonated sweet drink for breakfast, and so forth), or the early onset of cardiac problems from consuming high fat, high salt fast foods. We are now getting food that has been tampered with genetically as well as chemically. This is not healthy for any of us.

Whole-grain, natural, organic, unprocessed foods are healthiest. There is a reason for the food pyramid, currently being reviewed, and, whether or not we agree with it, many Americans would be a lot healthier if they followed it rather than the poor diet they presently eat. Many Americans believe that adding vitamin and mineral supplements is necessary for better health because our foods are not always grown under ideal conditions that achieve the highest nutritional value.

Another factor in health includes the benefits of exercise. More people are doing it— have you noticed all the people walking in the mall in the morning? There are various theories about what type of exercise is best. A lot of it is personal preference. The main idea is, *use it or lose it.* Our body needs regular exercise to keep maximum function.

Health also involves dealing effectively with stress. For instance, playing certain music during surgery and recovery enhances healing; having loved ones present when one is sick enhances healing; having soft light and beautiful surroundings enhances healing; and having pets present can enhance healing. Many nurses have learned therapeutic touch, give back rubs, or use other healing methods such Reiki that can bring comfort to patients. Exercise can help as can relaxation techniques, prayer, and meditation. Being around water can be soothing, which is probably why waterfalls are so popular both indoors and in the landscape. In China, the government has recommended that everyone participate in Qigong because it helps to prevent many chronic diseases. Qigong or ChiGong, originating in Chinese medicine, is a series of specific physical exercises that affects and improves physical, emotional, mental, and spiritual levels, as well as being a wonderful stress reliever. We can deal with our thoughts more effectively to lessen stress. For instance, worry can cause stress while positive thoughts can decrease it; we can perceive that many of the minor irritations are only that and will be forgotten by next year; or we may find that presently we can be calm with events that would have stressed us earlier in life.

Another aspect related to health is our spiritual beliefs. Have you ever noticed the special energy present in certain locations of the world such as on mountains, or when walking beside an ocean, or in churches, temples, synagogues, and mosques? Our spiritual beliefs can give us hope and comfort that we are not alone. It can provide a reason to live in a different manner. *Love one another* is a recurring theme spiritually. (See Barnum's (2003) *Spirituality in Nursing: From Traditional to New Age*, 2nd ed. for additional information on spirituality.)

The Healing Relationship

We have been discussing "loving" care in this chapter. Love is necessary for healing. By love, we are not meaning a sexual dalliance, but a *meaningful caring relationship*. Jean Watson has examined the relationship between caring and curing in her book, *Postmodern Nursing and Beyond* (2004). Here she examines both the technical side of nursing and the holistic side more traditionally associated with *caring*. Over the years there has been a lot of emphasis on the caring component of nursing practice.

Another excellent resource is *Radical Loving Care: Building the Healing Hospital in America* by Eric Chapman (2004). He makes the connection between loving and healing, stressing the importance of listening to the patient:

> A veteran housekeeper swings her mop rhythmically along the linoleum-coated 7th-floor hallway of a large urban hospital. From a nearby room the cry of an old man who is confused by age and illness carves a ragged hole in the hallway air. He is begging for his absent daughter.
>
> Calls of anguish and confusion come frequently from hospital rooms across America, but they are often ignored. The staff members are busy with other things.
>
> After a little while, as the man continues to cry out, the housekeeper does something that is very unusual in the contemporary American hospital. Instead of ignoring the call or waiting for a nurse to respond, she puts down her mop, walks into the old man's room, and gently takes his hand in hers. The old man calms down immediately and soon goes off to sleep. The housekeeper returns to mopping the floor.
>
> The housekeeper has quietly created what we call in a Healing Hospital a Sacred Encounter. Need has been heard and has been answered with love. For a few moments, she and the confused, sick old man have entered love's endless and immortal stream. In these moments the housekeeper has broken through the traditional bonds of her work, freed herself from the fear of being punished by a supervisor for stepping outside her job description, and responded to a human cry for help. The old man's call for love was answered—not by a drug or a patient restraint, but by the soothing touch of a loving hand (pp. 3–4).

Chapman emphasizes not seeing a patient as a stranger but as a brother or sister. He encourages us to see that what the patient needs goes beyond the physical needs to the emotions behind it. Significant life changes may be thrust upon a patient. Pain may be occurring, and pain is a lonely experience. "Radical loving care" is about making a significant connection with each patient:

> As I used to say regularly to new employee partners in orientation, 'Today is the last day on earth for two people within these walls, and they are spending that last day with us. And today is also the first day on earth for seventeen people. They are spending it with us as well. What could be more sacred than to be with people on their first or last day on earth? And what could be more meaningful than to be present with them when they may be in their greatest pain or highest joy?' (p. 45).

Chapman describes a trinity that one wants to have present in a health care organization: The Golden Thread (the loving thread that connects us); The Sacred Encounter (this is what the housekeeper did); and The Servant's Heart (we are serving others):

> Loving care has a long and beautiful tradition in human history. In these pages the heritage of loving care is symbolized by the image of a Golden

Thread, which is also a symbol of faith in God. It represents the positive tradition of healing versus the negative tradition of transaction-based behavior (p. 10).

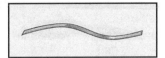

A second symbol, a pair of intersecting circles, signifies the merging of love and need in the Sacred Encounter, which is the fundamental relationship between caregiver and patient. This symbol also signifies hope—the hope that comes into our hearts when we experience loving encounters (p. 10).

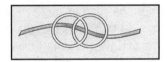

The third symbol, a red heart, signifies the nature of the Servant's Heart. It also symbolizes love and is love's greatest expression. This expression, although it specifically references the heart, assumes the full involvement of our best thought processes. Loving care is not loving if it fails to engage the best skills and competency of caregivers (p. 10).

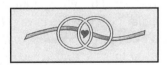

There is so much we could do that would promote a healing environment. For instance, Murphy (2000) suggests the following:

- Patients with a window view have shorter postoperative stays, experience fewer complications, and need less pain medication.
- Full-spectrum lighting increases efficiency and reduces fatigue for clinical staff and provides benefits for patients and families.
- Nature plays a key role in healing. A nine-year study of American hospitals conducted by Texas A&M University showed that when patients looked at scenes of trees, water, or gardens for as little as five minutes, their blood pressure dropped and tense muscles relaxed. Patients who looked out windows with views of tree-filled lawns instead of brick walls had fewer postoperative hospital stays and a reduced need for strong analgesics.

- Blue hues create a calming atmosphere and benefit those acute care patients who are sedated.
- Patients recuperating from surgery or illness need an energizing environment. Colors that evoke the outdoors such as sky blue, pale peach, and muted green provide stimulation.
- A 1995 study showed that open-heart surgery patients healed faster and required fewer painkillers when they had pictures—particularly soothing scenes of lakes and forests—in their rooms (Murphy, 2000, p. 38).

Carpenter (2002) describes giving patients their choice in DVDs or music during imaging exams.

As we define health, many have said that there is a *mind-body connection* with health. This has been shown in several ways, such as Valerie Hunt's research at UCLA about auras. She uses Kirlian photography to take pictures of various people or things and show an aura color that surrounds our bodies. The aura color changes based on what we are currently feeling and thinking. When feeling love, it is yellow or gold that both surrounds our loved one and ourselves; while other emotions such as anger is a red color that surrounds our body. Love heals while anger brings disease. This makes sense. Think about how we feel when we get angry. Our body becomes rigid, our emotions are highly involved, and, if continued long enough, our body's physical weak point will begin to exacerbate disease. This disease can be healed by love, by hope, by balance. She also found that nutritious foods have an aura while junk foods do not. Isn't that interesting?

The mind-body connection has been demonstrated through other research studies. An excellent reference that both explores the mind-body connection and reports research findings in this area is Targ and Katra's (1998) *Miracles of Mind: Exploring Nonlocal Consciousness and Spiritual Healing*. Healing can occur because of so many factors going on within a person, and can also be affected by others at great distance. Perhaps this is why prayer chains have become so popular now that we have internet capability. Bill Moyers (1993) narrates a set of five video cassettes on *Healing and the Mind* that explores healing practices around the world. Given that the imbalance of our minds and emotions can cause disease, the reverse seemingly must also be true. We can improve our health with positive thoughts and emotions. In the future, health care most likely will be based on balancing the mind-body connection instead of treating only the physical symptoms. There is an interesting book by Louise Hay (1988), *Heal Your Body*, that lists many different diseases in different parts of the body, then lists the thought that may have caused this disease, and gives a new thought that might better replace the old one to achieve better health. For example, if one has pneumonia, one might be thinking, "Depression. Grief. Fear of taking in life. Not feeling worthy of living life fully" (p. 48). We could replace this thought with, "I have the capacity to take in the fullness of life. I lovingly live life to the fullest" (p. 48). The message is that, *if we change our thoughts, we can improve our health*.

Cultural Diversity

Another value factor is cultural diversity. We are increasingly seeing a worldwide crossover of people and cultures. Here in the United States, by the year 2050, the non-white population is expected to more than triple as a result of increased immigration and rising birth rates (Powell, 2000). It is not uncommon to see Spanish-speaking television stations, or to buy something and have the instructions be given in several languages.

This diversity constitutes a new perspective toward not only culturally diverse patients, but also toward culturally diverse staff. We are often unaware of specific cultural beliefs, values, and lifeways, and may, inadvertently, tread on those beliefs and practices. Like patient safety, there is a lot of room for improvement.

Everywhere we turn there are differences between us. There are male/female differences, there are differences in religions or spiritual beliefs or rejection of such beliefs, there are differences in the way we perceive illness and health. These differences can lead not only to wars, but can lead to inadequate or improper care in our health care systems. We have discovered that different cultural groups receive a different quality of care.

As health care professionals it is important to recognize the wonderful differences that exist between different cultures, and we support these cultural beliefs. For instance, a couple from Afghanistan just had a baby and put a red string on the baby's wrist. The nursery nurses kept cutting off the string, the couple kept getting upset and putting it back on. In Afghanistan they believe that the red string on the baby's wrist keeps the soul in the body. Why wasn't the nurse listening?

> The cause of ill-health in many folk medical traditions is often supernatural, metaphysical, or interpersonal. In traditional Hispanic cultures, the source of sickness could be a 'hot' and 'cold' imbalance, or the dislocation of internal organs, or it may have a magical or emotional origin. … Hispanic patients may speak of *susto*, an illness arising from fright, or *empacho*, stomach cramps believed to be caused by a ball of food sticking to the wall of the stomach.… Chinese patients may believe that illness is caused by an imbalance of *yin* and *yang*. Many Native Americans feel that the source of sickness lies in a lack of harmony or an imbalance with natural or supernatural forces.… Black Americans from the rural South may believe that sickness is a divine punishment for sin or a sign of disharmony with the forces of nature.… Yet even patients from social and educational backgrounds broadly similar to those of their caregivers often have different explanatory models that affect their understanding of illness and their behavior (Gerteis, et al., 1993, p. 22).

To offer quality of care for all patients, health care service and support systems should inherently recognize that:

- Each culture defines the family as the primary support system and preferred intervener.

- Most racial and ethnic minority populations speak more than one language and this may create a unique set of mental health issues to which the system must be equipped to respond.

- Patients and their families make different choices based on cultural focus.

- Culturally preferred choices, not culturally blind or culturally free interventions, drive practice in the service delivery system.

- All cross-cultural interactions offer dynamics that require acknowledgment, adjustment, and acceptance.

- Health care systems must sanction or mandate the inclusion of cultural knowledge in practice and policy making.

An individual's social status almost always hinges on his or her socioeconomic status. In fact, 90% of a person's health status is determined by household income, not actual access to care (Alexander, 2002, pp. 31–32).

It is important to educate all staff about cultural differences, and have systems in place that will encourage everyone to respect and give radical loving care to each person based on that person's cultural beliefs. Alexander (2002) recommends that this needs to "include the following core components: cultural/racial/ethnic identity, language/communication ability and style, religious beliefs and practices, illness and wellness behaviors, and healing beliefs and practices" (p. 32).

Virtually all of the conventions of everyday life, as well as those relating to illness in particular, are defined by culture, and the success of any social encounter depends on a common, or compatible, understanding of these conventions. They include all the unspoken norms that govern forms of address, attitudes toward authority, directness of speech, and displays of emotion; the norms that delineate 'personal space' and define hygienic and dietary practices, as well as taboos about nudity and sexuality; and the norms that define gender, social, and family roles and the rituals pertaining to sickness and death....

Misunderstanding about culturally sanctioned customs and behavior are also prevalent. Some Native Americans burn sage during purification rituals, for example, but they may be accused of smoking marijuana when they do this in a hospital setting. In Western society, eye contact indicates sincere interest or understanding, but in other cultures, it may show disrespect. Compared to those from Eastern cultures, Westerners tend to interpret gender roles liberally; health care practitioners should not be surprised to find an African or Asian man refusing to be examined by a female doctor, or an African or Asian woman expecting her husband to be present throughout a consultation.... In many Far Eastern cultures, it is inappropriate for a female patient to discuss 'female problems' in the presence of a male stranger—and this may pose particular problems of communication when a male interpreter is used. Russian immigrants may feel that handshaking and smiling signify frivolity and immaturity, and they may therefore have no confidence in a clinician who displays such behavior.... In Eastern cultures, rectal examinations and therapeutic agents (enemas, suppositories) are all taboo, and a psychiatric referral may make a person ineligible for an arranged marriage (Gerteis, et al., 1993, pp. 24–25).

We have a lot of work to do to achieve better cultural understanding. There are some wonderful references available. The following describe different cultures, and give a description of how nursing care will need to differ depending upon a person's ethnic/cultural/regional background:

- Giger and Davidhizar's book, *Transcultural Nursing: Assessment and Intervention.*
- St. Hill, Lipson, and Meleis's book, *Caring for Women Cross-Culturally.*
- Purnell and Paulanka's book, *Transcultural Health Care: A Culturally Competent Approach.*
- Culhane-Pera, Vawter, Xiong, Babbitt, and Solberg's book, *Healing by Heart: Clinical and Ethical Case Stories of Hmong Families and Western Providers.*

These books are a must read. They provide information that is unknown to many health care providers.

> When individuals of dissimilar cultural orientations meet in a work or therapeutic environment, the likelihood for developing a mutually satisfying relationship is improved if both parties in the relationship attempt to learn about each other's culture. The literature reports many definitions for the terms *cultural awareness*, *cultural sensitivity*, and *cultural competence....* Cultural awareness has more to do with an appreciation of the external signs of diversity, such as arts, music, dress, and physical characteristics. Cultural sensitivity has more to do with personal attitudes and not saying things that might be offensive to someone from a cultural or ethnic background different from the health-care provider's. Increasing one's consciousness of cultural diversity improves the possibilities for health-care practitioners to provide culturally competent care. Cultural competence... means:
>
> 1. Developing an awareness of one's own existence, sensations, thoughts, and environment without letting it have an undue influence on those from other backgrounds.
>
> 2. Demonstrating knowledge and understanding of the client's culture, health-related needs, and meanings of health and illness.
>
> 3. Accepting and respecting cultural differences.
>
> 4. Not assuming that the health-care provider's beliefs and values are the same as the client's.

5. Resisting judgmental attitudes such as 'different is not as good.'

6. Being open to cultural encounters.

7. Adapting care to be congruent with the client's culture. Cultural competence is a conscious process and not necessarily linear.

... One progresses from unconscious incompetence (not being aware that one is lacking knowledge about another culture), to conscious incompetence (being aware that one is lacking knowledge about another culture), to conscious competence (learning about the client's culture, verifying generalizations about the client's culture, and providing culturally specific interventions), and finally, to unconscious competence (automatically providing culturally congruent care to clients of diverse cultures)....

An understanding of one's own culture and personal values, and the ability to detach oneself from 'excess baggage' associated with personal views, are essential to cultural competence. Even then, traces of ethnocentrism may unconsciously pervade one's attitudes and behavior. *Ethnocentrism*, the universal tendency of human beings to think that their ways of thinking, acting, and believing are the only right, proper, and natural ways, can be a major barrier to providing culturally competent care. Ethnocentrism perpetuates an attitude in which beliefs that differ greatly from one's own are strange, bizarre, or unenlightened and, therefore, wrong (Purnell and Paulanka, 2003, p. 4).

Can you see how many of us are ethnocentric in giving care to clients when we do not find out what clients value? And when we do not take the time to learn about their cultural or ethnic differences?

Giger and Davidhizar (2004) provide a cultural assessment model and intervention strategies using six cultural phenomena: communication, space, social organization, time, environmental context, and biological variations. Many health care providers do not conduct a cultural assessment of their clients, and thus can inadvertently not support a client's cultural norms and values. This book also examines different spiritual or religious beliefs that can have a significant impact on both how a person responds to disease, and how our cultural perspective affects our response to the disease. We must base our care on the client's cultural and spiritual perspectives.

As we give care based on cultural differences, it will affect nutrition (for instance, what about the vegetarian client, or someone who is used to highly spiced Indian foods?); family functioning (who in the family makes the decisions about the client's care—it may not be the client); lifestyle differences (having a large extended family live together or visit the ill family member); spiritual or religious differences (such as Islam); biological variations (African American propensity for sickle cell anemia); the way one relates to both health and disease (being stoic versus very emotive); communication issues (including language differences); differences in locus of control (destiny or karma versus religious faith); differences in views about independence versus collectivism (Eastern cultures make decisions based on what is best for the population as a whole); and socioeconomic differences (not being able to afford certain medications or something like chiropractic treatment).

Differences also occur within the same culture. For instance, male and female differences in communication can create communication problems when one does not understand the other. The book, *Men Are From Mars, Women Are From Venus*, became popular because it described these differences. Another book which reports male-female communication research that has been done, is *You Just Don't Understand* by Tannen. She says:

> Having done the research that led to this book, I now see that my husband was simply engaging the world in a way that many men do: as an individual in a hierarchical social order in which he was either one-up or one-down. In this world, conversations are negotiations in which people try to achieve and maintain the upper hand if they can, and protect themselves from others' attempts to put them down and push them around. Life, then, is a contest, a struggle to preserve independence and avoid failure.
>
> I, on the other hand, was approaching the world as many women do: as an individual in a network of connections. In this world, conversations are negotiations for closeness in which people try to seek and give confirmation and support, and to reach consensus. They try to protect themselves from others' attempts to push them away. Life, then, is a community, a struggle to preserve intimacy and avoid isolation. Though there are hierarchies in this world too, they are hierarchies more of friendship than of power and accomplishment.
>
> Women are also concerned with achieving status and avoiding failure, but these are not the goals they are focused on all the time, and they tend to pursue them in the guise of connection. And men are also concerned with achieving involvement and avoiding isolation, but they are not focused on these goals, and they tend to pursue them in the guise of opposition (pp. 24–25).

In addition to these two references, there are some excellent videotapes available such as *Gender Differences in the Workplace Series* by Dr. Pat Heim. To be effective in communication with the opposite sex, it is actually a cross-cultural experience because there are distinct gender differences. Heim applies this content to the workplace showing how these differences can affect teamwork.

Another cultural difference is between physicians, nurses, and non-clinical administrators. Physicians learn right from medical school that they are autonomous, independent (although this is changing with group practices), and it is easy for some to be autocratic and domineering because they never learned about team work and collaboration. Nurses can often feel that they are in a one-down position in a hierarchy of importance, because administrators tend to give more importance to the physicians and tend to give physicians more of what they want. When all come from the same core values and work together to provide care for patients (see Chapter 4), these differences can be overcome. When the administration does not support core values and gives too much autonomy to physicians, disruptive physician behaviors may be allowed to continue, creating a less effective work environment. Care can be compromised when this occurs.

This cultural diversity section, obviously, could be a whole book, as there are so many cultural differences surrounding us every day. It is of the utmost importance that cultural differences are recognized and respected within our health care system and that each person receives loving care specific to his/her expectations.

Replace Patient Compliance with What the Patient Values

As we have been defining what has value to the patient, the phrase *patient compliance* must be eliminated from our health care dictionary! The term is a throwback to the patriarchal medical system. It assumes that we know better than the patient what is good for the patient. In fact, the patient has a choice and may be making the "noncompliant" decisions for good reasons. Let's take some figures that the American Heart Association released:

- 50% of all patients, across a wide range of diseases, are not compliant with prescription treatment regimens.
- 43% of Americans over age 50 have chosen not to fully comply[2] with their medication regimens. Almost one-third stopped taking their medicine before it ran out, and 22% took less than prescribed on the label. 12% decided not to take it after they filled it.
- 14% to 21% of patients never fill their original prescriptions.

Why are patients "*noncompliant?*" Think of all the side effects that can occur with medications. For instance, so many people say that their doctors have ordered a drug—for instance a steroid—and they know that they have such bad side effects that they don't want to take the medication. Maybe being "noncompliant" is smart, and is safer! The American Heart Association noted the following:

- As many as half of all medications are taken incorrectly leading each year to an estimated 9 million adverse drug reactions and a quarter of all nursing home admissions. [This means that] of the 2 billion prescriptions filled each year, approximately half are taken improperly.
- The failure of patients to follow doctor-recommended medical treatment costs the U.S. economy $8.5 billion annually in additional hospitalizations and physician visits, and roughly $100 billion a year in other health care and productivity costs (*Patient Compliance*, 2000).

Another "*noncompliance*" issue is the cost of our services. Still using medications as an example, I can't help but think of a scenario recently observed in the local pharmacy. An elderly woman was talking to the pharmacist. He had just told her that her medications were $568. She said, "I am on a fixed income. I don't have that much money." He said, "Well, your doctor insists on not using generic medications so there is nothing I can do to bring the cost down." What they finally agreed to do was for her to pay for a week's worth

---

[2] Note the word, *comply*. The meaning is that we know better than the patient what medication regimen is best.

of medications and wait for her next Social Security check. I wondered, if she used the Social Security check for the medications, how was she going to pay for the other necessities, such as eating for the month. I'm sure the physician thought that the generic medications were not as effective. However, was the physician really taking into account the value question, i.e., this woman's situation? Should the pharmacist have called the physician to discuss the possibility of using generic drugs to save costs for the client? And even if generic drugs were used, can this woman afford to buy the medications and still have food and a roof over her head? Were all these drugs necessary? Do the drugs have to cost so much?

This example also exemplifies another problem. Prescription drug costs have been rising above the level of inflation. There are some ethical issues here with drug companies because most of our elderly, often on fixed income, are on more medications. There is still a lot of wining and dining that goes on with physicians from the pharmaceutical companies; many physicians expect this! However, on the other side of the coin, some physicians distribute pharmaceutical samples to the elderly. The health care professions should join this discussion as well. This is an example of a societal problem that needs to be fixed. If patients really need medication, surely there is a less expensive way to provide it.

Continuing with the noncompliance issue, there are larger societal issues adding to this problem. First, think of how difficult it is for many patients to get back in to see their doctors when they experience problems. Additionally, they are charged for another office visit. And in an HMO system if they need to be transferred to a specialist, they may or may not be able to get beyond the gatekeeper to get the care they need. Once in the health care system, many of us do not understand the importance of patient teaching. This is compounded by not really listening to the patient; and by our only treating disease without much emphasis on teaching, or on prevention. So the public deals with this issue by being "noncompliant," by reading the internet and other literature on health and on their illnesses—sometimes being better informed than we are—and by turning to alternative medicine.

Perhaps the most important "compliance" issue is that we forget that patients have the right to make choices. Note the following:

- In dietary studies for blood pressure reduction of people in the 30s to early 50s, only 50 percent to 60 percent are typically able to stay on track for six months. By the end of three years, the number is down to about 20 percent.
- Two-thirds of all heart failure patients do not comply with treatment recommendations in regard to smoking cessation, reduced alcohol consumption, and prescription medications (*Patient Compliance*, 2000).
- Obesity has become a national problem, but so many nurses and physicians are overweight that there is a reluctance to address this issue. Another facet of this problem are school lunches and obesity in children.

We, in the medical professions, are just as "guilty" of lack of "compliance" as the general public! It is hard to give up smoking, for instance, because it is a major addiction. So is alcohol. Remember: You can lead a horse to water, but you cannot make the horse drink!

It is so important to discuss treatments, including medications, with patients. We need to do a better job of patient (and family) teaching. We must encourage the patient (and family) to ask questions and to understand how to best deal with health problems. The nurses need to have time to do this activity, and to be expected to teach patients.

Once we have thrown out the "patient compliance" patriarchal system, we need to replace it with what the patient values. We need to redesign our health care delivery systems. The Institute of Medicine recommends ten rules to achieve this redesign:

1. *Care is based on continuous healing relationships.* Patients should receive care whenever they need it and in many forms, not just face-to-face visits. This implies that the health care system must be responsive at all times, and access to care should be provided over the Internet, by telephone, and by other means in addition to in-person visits.

2. *Care is customized according to patient needs and values.* The system should be designed to meet the most common types of needs, but should have the capability to respond to individual patient choices and preferences.

3. *The patient is the source of control.* Patients should be given the necessary information and opportunity to exercise the degree of control they choose over health care decisions that affect them. The system should be able to accommodate differences in patient preferences and encourage shared decision making.

4. *Knowledge is shared and information flows freely.* Patients should have unfettered access to their own medical information and to clinical knowledge. Clinicians and patients should communicate effectively and share information.

5. *Decision making is evidence-based.* Patients should receive care based on the best available scientific knowledge. Care should not vary illogically from clinician to clinician or from place to place.

6. *Safety is a system property.* Patients should be safe from injury caused by the care system. Reducing risk and ensuring safety require greater attention to systems that help prevent and mitigate errors.

7. *Transparency is necessary.* The system should make available to patients and their families information that enables them to make informed decisions when selecting a health plan, hospital, or clinical practice, or when choosing among alternative treatments. This should include information describing the system's performance on safety, evidence-based practice, and patient satisfaction.

8. *Needs are anticipated.* The system should anticipate patient needs, rather than simply react to events.

9. *Waste is continuously decreased.* The system should not waste resources or patient time.

10. *Cooperation among clinicians is a priority.* Clinicians and institutions should actively collaborate and communicate to ensure an appropriate exchange of information and coordination of care (*Crossing the Quality Chasm: A New Health System for the 21st Century*, 2001, pp. 3–4).

PATIENT AND FAMILY ADVISORY COUNCILS

One way to find out what patients want and need is to have focus groups with patients and families. For example, Ponte, et al., (2003) established two Patient and Family Advisory Councils, one for pediatrics and one for adults. It probably would be helpful to establish one for the elderly as well.

> At Dana-Farber Cancer Institute in Boston, we have been engaged for more than 5 years in a process of rethinking and redesigning many of our most critical operations in order to integrate the voices of patients and families into virtually everything we do. Although this work is far from complete, we believe we have made significant progress in crafting a new paradigm of care: one that places the patient and family in an entirely new position within the organization's operational and care structures....
>
> By working through the councils, the voices of patients and families are blended with those of clinicians, administrators, and other staff as the processes and systems of care are designed and delivered. Patients provide input on organizational policies, are placed on continuous improvement teams, and are invited to join search committees and develop educational programming for staff. Members of the councils also sit on the Joint Committee on Quality Improvement and Risk Management, a board-level committee that approves the institute's quality improvement plan, evaluates outcomes of quality improvement activities, and reviews reports regarding sentinel events.
>
> Creating this level of integration requires important preliminary work within the organization. There must be a shared understanding of the critical components of patient-centered care. There must be strong advocacy for the concept at the highest levels of the administrative leadership team. And there must be in place a strong, interdisciplinary work team, for it is premature to think about integrating patients and families into a team if the underpinnings of effective teamwork are not yet in place (pp. 82–83).

There is a wonderful book, *Through the Patient's Eyes: Understanding and Promoting Patient-Centered Care* (Gerteis, Edgman-Levitan, Daley, and Delbanco, 1993), that reports on results from focus group data collected in 1989 with 6,455 patients, and with approximately 2,000 of their identified care partners. This was a random sampling of patients from across the country that, within six months, had experienced a hospitalization. This book provides a framework of questions that could be used with focus groups, and suggests that the questions differ when used with patients versus with other family members. It states that:

> For the most part, those who work in the health care field do not need to be convinced that what patients think, feel, and experience is important. Health professionals are, by nature, a kind and sensitive lot, motivated

by an honest desire to help people and ease their suffering. But if they
recognize the intrinsic importance of patients' subjective experience to
the quality of care, why has that experience not figured more promi-
nently in shaping health care services and institutions? Why has there
not been a more systematic effort to incorporate patients' experiences
and judgments into planning and quality assessment? In part, the answer
lies with the fundamental tension between the objectively analytical tendencies of medicine as science and the subjective and personal nature of
medicine as practice. The ideology of science, which has shaped medical training for most of this century, values that which is quantifiable,
generalizable, and amenable to technical intervention. The qualitative,
individual, and human aspects of the patient's experience are hard to
describe or evaluate in a way that is accepted as scientifically valid, even
when they are acknowledged to be important.... The practical difficulties that clinical decision analysis have encountered in their attempts to
quantify individual utilities reflect this dilemma (Gerteis, Edgman-
Levitan, Daley, and Delbanco, 1993, p. 4).

As one plans advisory groups, some useful questions are found in *Through the Patients'
Eyes*: "We defined seven dimensions of patient-centered care, including (1) respect for
patients' values, preferences, and expressed needs; (2) coordination and integration of
care; (3) information, communication, and education; (4) physical comfort; (5) emotional
support and alleviation of fear and anxiety; (6) involvement of family and friends; and (7)
transition and continuity" (p. xii). They found that there was real discord between the
patient's perceptions of *illness* and our clinical objective approach to *disease*:

To a patient, illness entails not only the physical discomfort of ill health,
but all of the social and psychological ramifications of being unwell.
And the broader meaning of illness in this emotional and social context—its effect on their lives and on the lives of those around them—
may be far more important to patients than the physical impairment
itself.... Modern medicine has been described, with only a hint of jest,
as so disease oriented that the ideal situation would be to have patients
leave their damaged physical vessels at the hospital for repair, while taking their social and emotional selves home (p. 21).

What Do We Mean by Quality Care?

After we have determined what the patient values, we need to make sure the care we provide is of the highest quality, as we provide the care the patient needs. How do we achieve
this?

The first choice that the patient makes is where to go for health care. What doctor does
the patient choose? Which health care organization will the patient choose? At times, this
is determined by the insurance plan, but often the patient can make choices.

> Satisfied patients will reenroll with a particular provider or health plan; dissatisfied patients will disenroll or vote with their feet. This decision making is influenced largely by advice from people the patients trust, predominantly family and friends. Word-of-mouth information has an enormously persuasive and largely ignored impact on patient choice (Jennings and Staggers, 1999, p. 24).

The author is reminded of her father telling her not to take him to one hospital in another state "because people die there."

Patients are also finding that they can get on the Internet and find report cards on facilities, or find information about the particular health problem they are experiencing. This information can also influence their choice, and be a factor why they leave certain practitioners if what is offered does not agree with what the patient wanted.

Once the patient chooses a facility, each person who has contact with her or him influences the patient's impression of what the facility is like. The employees can make or break an organization, although the ultimate responsibility comes back to us—the administrative team. Are we educating our team about their influence, do we treat them as valuable employees, are the expectations of caring and listening emphasized? It starts with us—and our words and our actions must be in alignment.

Educating front-line staff at the point of care is why more health care organizations, including the Malcolm Baldridge winners, are turning to scripted ways of handling situations. The most important two characteristics with all employees—including us—are *caring* and *listening*. We have been stressing the listening characteristic in the previous section. The caring aspect is what helps to heal.

Reframing/Our View of the World

As we examine quality, we may need to reframe our quality perspective. Do you notice how often the word *reframe* is appearing? As we experience changes, our view of the world changes. Our perspective becomes reframed to a different picture of reality.

> Leaders too may be victims of their own perspectives. Too much dependence on past successes creates a definition for success that may no longer by sustainable. The greatest impediment to future success is past success.... Whatever defines the contextual framework of success in the past can be temptingly easy to use as the measure of current success, resulting in the wrong measure for the right issue (staffing ratios, more staff, keeping patients longer, more money, etc.). Clinical leaders must see the approaching challenges within the context of their becoming, not through the eyes of past experience, old solutions, and historical triumphs....
>
> Imagine for just a moment how painful this message of deconstruction and reformatting is to the serious and talented men and women who devoted their lives to building the current health system infrastructure. Think also about the many nursing heroes who have fought to build the

current foundations for nursing practice. The challenge confronting the
requirement to tear practice apart and examine care practices anew is all
but overwhelming. This, however, is what the vision of creating a new
and pertinent future infrastructure calls nurses to do and is now the
major work of the time (Porter-O'Grady, 2003, pp. 62–63).

As administrative leaders, one of our roles is to communicate a vision that stretches us
but remains possible to achieve. Many of our present practices are like the horse and
buggy; they are quickly becoming obsolete. So where do we need to go? This entire book
provides answers to more effectively do our administrative work. For example, first, we
need to examine our leadership (Chapter 3), second, we need to make sure we can do an
organizational assessment and learn how to identify and make systems changes effectively
(Chapter 4), and third, we need to know how to find information (Chapter 8). Porter-
O'Grady and Malloch (2002) define what they see as our major administrative tasks in the
21st century:

- Deconstructing the barriers and structures of the 20th Century,
- Alerting staff about the implications of changing what they do,
- Establishing safety around taking risks and experimenting,
- Embracing new technologies as a way of doing work,
- Reading the signposts along the road to the future and translating the emerging real-
  ity into language the staff can use,
- Demonstrating personal engagement with the change effort,
- Helping others adapt to the demands of a changing health system,
- Creating a safe milieu for the struggles and pain of change,
- Enumerating small successes as a basis for supporting staff, and
- Celebrating the journey and all progress made (p. 19).

Along with our administrative role, an educational role is needed for nurses and other
health-care providers to help them change their perception of reality. Otherwise, some will
leave, and have left, our profession in frustration. As we educate nurses, they need to learn
about all these new realities, because it is probable that our big buildings, and present
health care system procedures, won't even exist in the future, and neither will our educational systems! Instead, much of the care and education may take place in chatrooms or
virtual realities. Or take genomics—it is possible that we can treat patients by just tweak-
ing the DNA. Or maybe, when a patient needs treatment, we can use the, "Beam me up,
Scotty" routine, from *Star Trek*, to either send the caregiver to the patient, or the patient to
the caregiver. Our education needs to help nurses be more open to things happening outside their nursing boxes because a good proportion of what we teach today will be obsolete tomorrow.

Recognition of Value and Quality

There are a number of programs in health care, some that have gained national awareness,
that pay attention to both the value and quality issues from the patient perspective. We have

already described Eric Chapman's *Radical Loving Care*, and the patient issues identified in *Through The Patient's Eyes*. We describe a few more programs here.

THE PLANETREE MODEL

Planetree acknowledges the importance of environment, providing a more humanistic, personalized, patient-centered experience. The delivery is holistic, encompassing mental, social, and emotional dimensions as well as physical symptoms. The goal is to maximize health care by combining medical therapy with complementary alternatives utilizing architectural and environmental designs in the process. Planetree embraces a novel concept in that the provision of compassionate, nurturing, personalized care is designed not only for patients and patient families, but also for staff. Thus, using the Planetree approach, the organization must embrace a culture that nurtures staff as well as patients (www.planetree.org/brochure).

The Planetree philosophy consists of nine components. Planetree facilities are challenged to incorporate these components to provide appropriate humanistic health care delivered in a caring environment.

The nine components are:

- Human interaction,
- Empowerment,
- Social networks,
- Human touch,
- Spirituality,
- Architecture,
- Healing arts,
- Nutrition, and
- Complementary therapy (www.shands.org/hospitals/AGH/Planetree.htm).

Planetree also provides measurement tools for continuous evaluation of quality of care including patient satisfaction surveys and community image assessment.

THE EDEN ALTERNATIVE

A philosophy similar to the Planetree model, instituted in long-term care, is the Eden Alternative. Developed by Dr. William Thomas, geriatrician, it is based on his belief that the focus of long-term care should be *care* and not treatment. Thomas further elaborates that the major problems in nursing homes are loneliness, boredom, and helplessness; the residents are overmedicated, deprived the enjoyment of a pleasant meal by unnecessary dietary restrictions, and subject to endless activity programs developed to meet regulatory compliance rather than provide entertainment for the residents. His solution was the creation of an environment that allowed people to flourish by inundating them with life in the form of plants, animals, and children. The Eden Alternative offers a more humanistic, home-like environment; it offers residents opportunities to maintain and control the environment, and encourages interaction and compassion (Thomas, 1996).

Although outcome measures have not been established, the program was piloted in the Chase Memorial Nursing Home and resulted in a decline in patient mortality, decline in medication use, and a decline in nurse aide turnover (Bruck, 1997).

Magnet Hospital Status

Earning the esteemed designation as a Magnet Hospital has become a renowned indicator of quality. This is an expensive process in terms of both money and resources for the facility. A Magnet Hospital voluntarily endures a strenuous evaluation of nursing services, and successfully meets all criteria determined by nursing services and patient care in a hospital setting.

Program objectives are to:

- Recognize nursing services that use the scope and standards for nurse administrators to build programs of nursing excellence in the delivery of nursing care to patients.
- Promote quality in a milieu that supports professional nursing practice.
- Provide a vehicle for the dissemination of successful nursing practices and strategies among institutions utilizing the services of registered professional nurses.

Designation as a Magnet Hospital is the most rigorous quality award relevant to nursing and can enhance a hospital's ability to recruit professional staff. The designation is valid for a four-year period and reflects the scope and standards championed in the quality arena and supported by credentialing agencies. Presently, approximately 450 hospitals have Magnet Hospital status, with the number growing.

The Malcolm Baldridge Award

The Malcolm Baldridge Award is another prestigious quality indicator available for outstanding performance in manufacturing, service, small business, education, and health care. It requires detailed preparation, applications, and on-site visits, and is considered America's highest honor for performance excellence. SSM Health Care, based in St. Louis, was the first health care organization to win this coveted award followed by St. Luke's Hospital in Kansas City, MO, and Baptist Hospital in Pensacola, FL.

Evidence-Based Practice

Now that we have discussed listening to the patient and providing a caring environment, we turn to quality dimensions—*to provide the most up-to-date care and treatment*. Research shows that practitioners—physicians and nurses—still provide care that is similar to what they learned in school, even though there may be a much more effective treatment that is presently used. Now that we are in the information age, it has become impossible for us (the practitioners) to stay current because there is too much information. So how do we achieve this goal? Enter the Internet, and the explanation in Chapter 8 of what is available, and how to sift through the information to select what is valid and reliable. As administrators we must both provide access and encourage practitioners to use this information highway regularly. This is what evidence-based practice is all about.

Evidence-based practice (EBP) is a synthesis of research and clinical expertise demonstrated to be successful that result in a plan of care specific to particular conditions. We may not always know what is best for a certain individual with a particular need. Research has shown that both physicians and nurses plan care and treatment based on what was done when they graduated from school. This is where the information highway is important. We need to have access to the latest research on that problem, and/or treatment of the problem, and use that information to determine the most appropriate care for our patient. It is important to note here:

> Many clinicians confuse the terms "evidence-based practice" and "research-based practice" and use the terms interchangeably. Research-based practice refers to the use of knowledge based on systematic studies and does not take into account the clinician's expertise or the individual patient preferences (Barnsteiner and Prevost, 2002, p. 18).

For instance, there is a lot of research currently available on patient outcomes. As a physician or nurse practitioner writes a medication order, they may not know which of several drugs might be most effective. This person can immediately access research data bases that answer this question, even though a person is at a rural location. Then the physician or nurse practitioner can provide evidence-based care to the patient. In the same way the nurse at the bedside can look up patient diagnoses, preferred treatments, preferred medications, contraindications, side effects, etc., to more safely care for our patients.

Chapter 8 is devoted to describing how to access the latest information quickly and at the moment it is needed. The chapter is written by librarians that have worked to make this information available using a just-in-time method.

Why is evidence-based practice so important? "The literature indicates that at least *one-third* of the time, health-care providers do not follow even uncontroversial, evidence-based recommendations" (Barnsteiner and Prevost, 2002, p. 18). One big problem is that providers do not realize how easily information can be accessed, or do not take the time to look up the current research results (which is where the just-in-time information discussed in Chapter 8 can be so helpful). All the provider needs is a computer with internet access to get this information quickly and easily.

Administratively, we must encourage evidence-based practice: teaching nurses what it is and how to find it on the Internet, providing computer access, and giving nurses time to look up information on their patients (Barnsteiner and Prevost, 2002; Lopez-Bushnell, 2002). Also, as one is measuring quality effectiveness, comparing actual treatment to evidence-based practice could provide a useful indicator, provided that patient preferences and idiosyncrasies along with the economic factors that may have influenced the care given are considered as part of evidence-based practice.

CLINICAL PATHWAYS/PROTOCOLS

Evidence-based practice can also be achieved by using *clinical pathways* or *clinical protocols* when delivering care, as long as the pathways or protocols are kept up to date.[3] An effective clinical pathway is the result of interdisciplinary teamwork; the team includes the physician, nurse, social worker, dietitian, and patient, and may include other members such as chaplain, or nurse aide or significant family members. Protocols that physicians have agreed upon can automatically be implemented without an order.

---

[3] An example of a pathway or protocol can be found in Chapter 1 in Dunham-Taylor and Pinczuk, *Health Care Financial Management for Nurse Managers: Applications in Hospitals, Long-Term Care, Home Care, and Ambulatory Care*. (2006). Sudbury, MA: Jones and Bartlett.

Care is more streamlined and timely when the pathway, or protocol, is followed. When implemented correctly, a standard of excellence is in place, and enhanced quality is achieved. Everyone knows what to do and does it at the specified time. The patient benefits with better care—care that is more timely; less is forgotten or postponed, resulting in greater patient satisfaction; costs are saved as length of stay is decreased; physician and nurse charting time is decreased; and nurses do not have to find physicians, or other interdisciplinary team members, to implement the care or write orders. Everybody wins.

The main problem is that implementation time is needed to get everyone together, to get physician buy-in, and to deal effectively with conflicts that occur. Conflict resolution is necessary before a successful pathway can be reached. Presently, there are some pathways where physicians and/or patients have not been involved in the process. This is not advantageous because physician buy-in is critical for successful implementation of the pathway. Additionally the pathways have not taken into account what is valuable to the patient. Existing pathways will need to be reexamined to make sure that these factors are included. As we establish new pathways, it is helpful to include both patients and physicians on the interdisciplinary committee forming the pathways. Periodically, all pathways should be reviewed in light of new research and ongoing clinical evidence to maintain pathway effectiveness.

The only caution to clinical pathways is that all the caregivers continue to take into account patient idiosyncrasies or differences that might change the pathway. For instance, a patient allergy to certain antibiotics might preclude using the standard antibiotic recommended in the pathway. Or, the patient might prefer a different setting upon discharge than is the usual placement. The patient's values must remain the *first* priority with a clinical pathway or protocol.

Getting Out of the Box

The times are changing; we need to change with it. We can do it kicking and screaming, or we can look around us for clues as to what we might expect. In this section, we discuss some of the clues that are present. Since we are all in the health care box, some of these changes are hard to perceive because they are outside our view of reality.

Nursing Is Changing Whether We Want It To Or Not!

We are moving into a new information age that requires different approaches and perspectives.

> Moving into a new age does not mean leaving everything behind. It does mean thinking about what needs to be left behind and reflecting on what does go with us as we move into an age with a different set of parameters (Porter-O'Grady and Malloch, 2002, p. 10).

We are facing many significant changes that affect the care we give, the systems that are in place to deliver care, and even the present perspectives we have on the world in general. It is easy to be complacent and not pay attention to the changes. However, they are all around us:

This is the beginning of the end of nursing care as we have all become accustomed to providing and using.... The hospital-based, sickness-oriented, late-stage model of nursing service delivery is no longer either appropriate or prevailing. Nurses now must determine what traditional practices and functions are no longer relevant or sustainable and let them go. At the same time, nurses must discern what is emerging on the practice horizon that must now become increasingly a part of nursing practice. Influences like genomics, nano-therapy, fiberoptics, pharmacotherapeutics, virtual care models, early-stage interventions, patient managed delivery, [alternative therapies], etc. are now pressing on the periphery of the profession and will dominate nursing adaptation for the next 2 decades. The technology of the time is quickly moving the health professions into a context where the kind of therapies that will be used require less mechanical and manual intervention and a greater use of other innovative approaches. This transition makes it possible to treat illness at an earlier stage and either eliminate or alter the need for more mechanical (surgical) interventions that are more intensive and costly. It is quickly becoming a time of ending for the health care system as we know it. Furthermore, it is the end of the Newtonian, 20th century medical and nursing practice, and other health-related practices, as those disciplines have historically understood them.

The work of the time for the clinical leader is helping colleagues and patients end their attachment to the kind of health care system they have grown comfortable with. So many nurses are mourning the loss of something they think should not have passed or should be retained. Many nurses are mourning the loss of those very practices, sentiments, or roles that brought them to nursing in the first place. Some even wish those traditions would return. The truth is that most of what is being mourned should neither be retained nor protected. Neither the times nor yesterday's circumstances will return, nor should they.... Those ideals that brought many of us to nursing (enough time for good care, long stays, detailed care processes, residential models of care, heavy emphasis on manual procedures, compliant and passive patient roles, etc.) no longer exist. The question is not will these processes return but instead: what is nursing now becoming and how must I adapt?

A major role of the clinical leader in this day and time is engaging others around the reality of their own change. Complacency at this time of radical shifting is a strategy that guarantees failure. The leader must take whatever action is necessary to impress upon those he or she leads that this is a time of great mobility and shifting foundations (Porter-O'Grady, 2003, p. 62).

This is an exciting, challenging time when we, as nurse professionals and as nurse (or health care) administrators, can be forging new roles that better fit the new realities. The only constant in our present reality is that it will change. We are at a crossroads. We can lament what we are losing, or have lost, or we can begin to design where we need to go next. (There is nothing wrong with doing a little mourning, but life goes on.) In addition to the traditional nursing role changing, our leadership roles are changing as well. The question is, do we remain stuck in our past, or can we move into an exciting, unknown future?

As we face all this change, there is hope. After all, think of what our ancestors faced. My grandmother, born in 1886, faced electricity, short skirts, phones, and automobiles all hitting her present reality before she turned forty. In fact, my great aunt talked about driving a Model-T Ford for the first time and realizing when she reached her destination that no one had told her how to stop the car! So she let it coast to a stop. We are facing changes like that. We won't necessarily know what to do, so at times we will have to make it up as we go along.

However, there are some present clues about the new reality we face. For instance, as previously mentioned, health care is not as invasive now as it was ten years ago. Think of *Star Trek* where the doctor rarely does anything invasive—no IVs, little surgery—and mainly uses technology to determine what is wrong with the patient. The treatment is generally not invasive either. From the patient's perspective, that sounds wonderful! That is a reality that we can glimpse from the media. Or going on with this analogy in *Star Trek: The New Generation*, there is a room where people can experience a virtual reality that they can create. Gene Roddenbury, who initially wrote *Star Trek*, incorporated present capabilities and new scientific developments that many of us did not know about, and designed the systems used in this story based on the new emerging reality.

Utilization Management

> *Utilization management* is 'the review of services delivered by a health care provider to determine whether, according to preestablished standards, the services were medically necessary.' … The major functions of this department are conducting inpatient and outpatient reviews; examining length-of-stay issues, payer contacts for precertification, and continued stays; responding to peer review organizations, preparing peer review organization denial appeals, and eliminating avoidable days (Meisenheimer, 1997, p. 150).

Historically, over the last quarter-century, hospitals established a person(s), or department, assigned to do utilization review (UR)—relaying clinical information to payers so the payers could determine whether they would pay for additional care for patients. In the managed care climate (managed care is further explained in Chapter 6), one cannot give the care and then submit the bill, but instead must get pre-approval for the care. The payers determine whether the care is allowable. Once the payers determine that the care meets their criteria, the patient is certified for payment.

Often the utilization reviewers are RNs. In this time of nursing shortages, this use of available registered nurses for UR is starting to be questioned. As case management has evolved (this is further explained in Chapter 16, Case Management), case managers have become involved with utilization review.

Murray (2001) reported research on reviews in one hospital with a 1 percent denial rate, a very low rate not often achieved. This study found that the usual reason for denial was that the care needed was not included in the insurance contract purchased by the patient's employer. Unfortunately, Murray also found that psychiatry, neurology, and rehabilitation had the most frequent denials.

STANDARDS AND SCOPE OF PRACTICE ISSUES

Standards and scope of practice for licensed professionals are defined by their licensing agency with standards exemplified by best practices and supported by professional/facility/community expectations. See the large number of nursing scope and standards for various nursing specialties in the references at the end of this chapter. Policies and procedures need to reflect standards and scope, and be in compliance with regulatory agencies such as JCAHO, OSHA, and CMS, further defined in Chapter 6. The idea behind both standards and definitions of scope of practice help us to determine what is considered to be quality practice. Most health care organizations have policies that define specific standards. In addition, most health care organizations not only must determine that staff work within the scope of practice, but that staff remain updated in their skills.

EVIDENCE-BASED PRACTICE IN ADMINISTRATION

Chapter 8 also discusses ways that we can more effectively use research and administrative practice knowledge to improve the way we lead and use organizational strategies. Many of us are not current in our administrative practice, just like the practitioners who are still treating patients based on what they learned 20 years ago.

Providing Patient Safety

Another VERY IMPORTANT mandate with quality is always to provide a safe environment. In the past, the traditional approach to patient safety was to identify what an individual practitioner had done wrong. When very serious, this resulted in occurrences being "reported to the board for disciplinary investigation because of an error or breach in the standards of safe practice" (Woods and Johnson, 2002, p. 45). It is easy to get into blame and punishment with errors. This only encourages a person to hide errors and not report them.

A more effective solution is to report the error and undertake a root cause analysis to determine what each person could have done differently to prevent this from happening again. After all, *usually medical errors involve more than one person and require a systems approach in finding solutions*.

It makes far more sense to be more *proactive* about patient safety by involving everyone in critically evaluating current practice patterns, current processes being used, potential environmental hazards, and anything else that might result in an unsafe situation *before* any incident occurs. The information can be included in the Performance Improvement goals, strategies can be implemented for prevention, and our patients will be safer.

Remove Blame—Replace with "What Could We Have Done to Prevent the Error from Occurring??"

Blame and punishment are best left behind, finding a more effective way to handle errors. The Institute of Medicine study pointed out that often we blame and punish people for errors, but we do not look at the most important issue about those errors—*what could we have done to prevent the error from occurring?* Blame will not accomplish anything except to encourage people to hide errors.

Johnson (2000) advocates starting with the cultural issues surrounding the safety problem; we have to stop being punitive about error reporting. We have to turn this around. Blame-free reporting is stressed to identify trends that are responsible for errors. This can be a difficult issue for an administrator who has some authoritarian tendencies as actions speak louder than words. If we call someone out on a medication error, or our tone of voice is punitive, the damage is done. Errors will continue to be hidden and not discussed. This is very dangerous. The first part of the problem is finding out what is happening so we can fix it.

Instead, we need to set an example by owning up to our own errors and encouraging others to do the same. Each error indicates something that is wrong with our system and is an alert that we need to make a change for a safer environment. Unfortunately, there is nothing worse than realizing that you have just made an error that could cause harm to someone else!

Encourage Error Reporting

Both the Institute of Medicine report and the Harvard study advocate eliminating the authoritarian way of doing business encouraging *everyone* to speak up about errors. Even anonymous reports should be dealt with. We need to investigate each incident, do what we can immediately for the patient, and then think of ways we could prevent this incident from ever happening again. Often people across the entire organization need to make changes. After all, we are all people who can make mistakes.

When we make a patient safety error, we must admit that we have made a mistake. It is our practice responsibility. Practice responsibility refers to the socially embedded knowledge, notions of good, and skill lodged in a health care team of local practitioners. Practitioners have a practice responsibility to learn from experience and make that learning available to other practitioners; that way, experiential learning is cumulative and collective and shapes the research agenda.

RISK MANAGEMENT/INCIDENT REPORTS/SENTINEL EVENTS

Incident reports and risk management have been around for years, but often have not been used as effectively as they could be. It is most often the incident report that alerts risk management personnel about significant problems:

> Risk management 'serves to prevent the loss of financial assets resulting
> from injury to patients, visitors, employees, independent medical staff,
> or from damage, theft, or loss of property. Risk management also

includes transfer of liability and insurance financing to cover unavoidable injuries or claims for damages.'... Although the health care manager's current functions and responsibilities may vary from organization to organization, generally the risk manager is responsible for risk financing and risk transfer—through the purchase of insurance or the management of self-insurance, loss control. This responsibility involves the management of claims and lawsuits arising from allegations of negligence as well as proactive risk management, which involves the identification and management of situations within the organization that may give rise to patient injury or harm. It is this function that requires the highest level of integration with quality management and utilization management (Meisenheimer, 1997, p. 148).

However, incident reports provide a source of errors, and usually provide clues about unresolved systems problems—*if we pay attention to them*. Let's look at some examples:

- You're helping a post-op patient walk from his bed to the bathroom, and he stubs the big toe on his right foot on the IV pole he's pushing.

- When you check on an elderly patient recovering from a mild CVA, you find her on the floor, her left arm apparently fractured. She tells you she was looking for her dog.

- In the process of reconstituting a vial of cefazolin (Ancef, Kefzol) to administer to a patient with pneumonia, you sneeze as you're about to pierce the vial's stopper to add sterile water, nicking your thumb with the needle.

If you were the nurse involved in any of these scenarios, would you file an incident report? In all three cases, your answer should be "Yes."

An incident report should be filed whenever an unexpected event occurs. The rule of thumb is that any time a patient makes a complaint, a medication error occurs, a medical device malfunctions, or anyone—patient, staff member or visitor—is injured or involved in a situation with the potential for injury, an incident report is required (Brooke, 2002, p. 4).

Incident reports, even for minor incidents, provide clues about what needs to be fixed.

If we pay attention, nothing more serious will happen. When the incidents are more important, including sentinel events, everyone needs to participate in a root-cause analysis of the incident. More serious incidents usually involve several people, even though one person may look like s/he caused the problem. Usually there is an organizational systems process that went wrong, or a new process needs to be implemented. (Systems problems are discussed in more detail in Chapter 4.)

"A *Sentinel Event* is an unexpected occurrence involving death or serious physical or psychological injury, or the risk thereof. Serious injury specifically includes loss of limb or function. The phrase 'or the risk thereof' includes any process variation for which a recurrence would carry a significant chance of a serious adverse outcome" (JCAHO, 2000,

p. 51). When these events occur, they need to be immediately addressed. The cause must be determined along with what could have been done to prevent it happening again. Generally, such an event involves a group of people within the organization that all need to participate in this procedure. JCAHO calls this process a *root cause analysis*. As with patient safety issues, the idea is not to blame anyone, but it is to examine the processes that might have contributed to the event, as well as to identify processes for prevention. Then this is shared with all staff, implemented, and, hopefully, will keep another similar event from occurring. Generally, mandates exist so that this data must be reported to accrediting agencies as well as to many state health departments.

Since this has been mandated, JCAHO has identified that patient falls were a serious problem for inpatient facilities; that half of the patients were over 80 years old; that often previous falls had occurred; that often either chronic mental illness or sedation were factors; and that death was more likely when anticoagulation medication was being used. Falls were more likely to occur at night, on weekends and holidays, and were often accompanied by a "recent environmental change and urinary urgency." A frequent problem that occurred was that staff communication was incomplete between shifts and between facilities, and that many times patient assessment had been inadequate.

The following are additional risk reduction strategies that were identified to prevent falls:

- Installing bed alarms or redesigning bed alarm checks and tests.
- Installing self-latching locks on utility rooms.
- Restricting window openings.
- Installing alarms on exits.
- Adding fall prevention to education of patients, residents or individuals served and their families.
- Improving and standardizing nurse call systems.
- Using "low beds" for those at risk for falls.
- Revising staffing procedures.
- Counseling individual caregivers.
- Revising the competency evaluation process (JCAHO Sentinel Event Alert, 2000).

The Institute of Medicine advocates developing both mandatory and voluntary error-reporting systems for serious adverse events, defined broadly as death or injuries resulting from medical interventions. Most states have laws about this issue. The voluntary systems would be protected from legal discoverability.

Identify Trends Causing Errors

Although we will list some common errors in the next section, generally, there is no one person at fault in an error situation—nor is it one factor that caused the error. It is really a combination of factors, or lack of proper systems, that have caused the error.

As people identify errors, gather the data and examine it carefully for patterns or trends that provide clues for immediate action. As with sentinel events, conducting an investigation to determine the *root cause analysis* of the error is important. Chances are there are safer systems that can help to prevent other practitioners from making the same mistake.

For example, perhaps drug packaging looks the same for different drugs, or drug names that are very similar but have very different uses. We may need to change the packaging, or set up check points so we do not give a different drug than intended. Barcoding can make a tremendous difference with this example.

Another possible cause of errors is abbreviations, symbols, and dose designations. The way these are written can cause errors (i.e., 1.0 mg can be mistaken as 10 mg. It is better to write 1 mg.) JCAHO published a list of abbreviations, symbols, and dose designations, and has mandated that they *not* be used as of 2004. The list can be found at www.jcaho.org.

Another cause of errors is lack of critical thinking. Sometimes it can be simple things like a dehydrated patient who is admitted for another diagnosis and no one thinks to start an IV. Or using the dehydrated example, a physician orders insertion of a PEG tube while the patient is in long-term care. So the patient goes to the local hospital for another physician to insert it. This second physician finds that the patient's stomach is drastically enlarged so that a PEG tube cannot be inserted, and the staff send the patient back to the long-term care facility. No one has called the first physician about this, no one has started an IV, and no one has made other recommendations as to treatment, or the urgency of the need for treatment. Everyone was so segmented and task oriented in their roles that the care was not adequate.

> Nursing tasks, important to achieving physiologic homeostasis and ultimate well-being, have also become a comfortable, safe routine or substitute for critical thinking. This has left nurses in a confusing position. Helping RNs understand their impact on outcomes and their accountability for achieving the planned results through expert team leadership renews excitement and enhances their professional role (Hansten and Washburn, 1999, p. 25).

We need to revisit our professional role (the professional role of the nurse is discussed further in Chapter 20, Staffing), encourage or teach critical thinking, and give nurses the time to be able to do this adequately.

Sometimes communication is a problem. For instance, often LPNs give medications while nurse aides are responsible for other aspects of the patient's care, with an RN being accountable for the overall care. With several people potentially involved, something can either be easily missed, or may not be communicated, and could cause a serious patient error.

Another potentially dangerous time is when staffing is inadequate, when the RN never does rounds or talks with patients, when care groups do not function using good teamwork, or when the RN does not assume leadership of the team. Any of these situations are fraught with potential safety and quality issues for the patients.

In one research study, Woods and Doan-Johnson (2002) analyzed 21 disciplinary case files from nine state boards of nursing to develop a taxonomy of nursing practice errors, their causes, patient outcomes, and disciplinary actions. We can use this data as a starting point in Performance Improvement efforts to proactively prevent these from occurring as much as possible.

They found eight categories of nursing errors, each of which has system, individual, and practice contributions to error:

- Lack of attentiveness,
- Lack of agency/fiduciary concern,
- Inappropriate judgment,
- Medication errors,
- Lack of intervention on the patient's behalf,
- Lack of prevention,
- Missed or mistaken physician or health care provider orders, or
- Documentation errors (p. 46).

Let's consider each individually as they are beginning clues as to what we need to do for prevention.

LACK OF ATTENTIVENESS

It is important that each nurse at the point of care is finding out, and remembering, assessment data on each patient; is putting this into a physiological, psychological, sociological, cultural, and spiritual context; and is then "paying attention to the patient's clinical condition and response to therapy, as well as potential hazards or errors in treatment" (p. 46).

> Lack of attentiveness can be caused by system level problems such as understaffing, high staff turnover, or sudden shifts in the acuity levels of patients without an increase in nursing staff.
>
> A distinction between monitoring unpredictable and predictable conditions was made because each has different implications for error reduction strategies. For example, *missing predictable complications*, such as postoperative hemorrhage, indicates a lack of monitoring and accurate assessment of the postoperative patient; it may also indicate possible breakdowns in communication of patient assessments. Intermittent in-service education on detecting postoperative complications, along with case studies of missed post-operative hemorrhage or other complications, is needed to sustain appropriate levels of vigilance and clinical judgment. *Early detection of unpredictable conditions*, such as an acute myocardial infarction or a cerebrovascular accident (CVA) for long-term patients, requires different educational strategies and regular particularized assessments of all patients (p. 46).

LACK OF AGENCY/FIDUCIARY CONCERN

This gets back to the piece about what the patient values. In the nurse's relationship with the patient, the nurse must be a patient advocate for whatever the patient values. Often, the relationship extends to family or significant others as well.

> When the nurse fails to question an inappropriate physician or prescriber order, or fails to call a physician for a patient whose vital signs or labo-

ratory reports are critical, or fails to heed patient or family requests for assistance, the nurse's lack of fiduciary concern and moral agency on behalf of the patient causes harm and may be considered a source of substandard or erroneous nursing practice.

Breach of confidentiality is also a breach of fiduciary concern for the patient's privacy and dignity. *Unintentional breach of confidentiality* occurs when the nurse discusses a patient's condition at the nurse's station and the family, patient, or visitor overhears the communication. *Intentional breach of confidentiality is…* when nurses deliberately share patient information with news media or deliberately check patient records for personal information about the patient (pp. 46–47). (This has ethical implications as well, see Chapter 5.)

INAPPROPRIATE JUDGMENT

This is a very broad category that probably will need to be further refined. So much of a nurse's actions are inherent on clinical judgment. This is where critical thinking comes in. This means the nurse is not doing tasks or rote procedures but instead is taking into account various factors that will determine what care is appropriate for that moment in time. Unfortunately, many associate degree RNs do not have coursework on pathophysiology or pharmacology. They have learned tasks and rote actions. So unless they have gotten the information some other way, they may not be able to do the critical thinking that is required for patient safety. A lot of nurse education is necessary to rectify this problem.

> Various types of inappropriate judgment were identified, including inadequate assessment; faulty logic due to the use of rote habitual action or convention; an unwarranted or faulty intervention, such as giving too much pain medication or giving a medication despite a patient's allergy; and unreasonable expectations for lesser-trained staff, such as when the nurse delegates an action beyond the practice scope, training, and experience of another staff member. In addition, a subclass of inadequate assessment was identified as the nurse not knowing or recognizing the implications of signs and symptoms identified in the assessment (p. 47).

MEDICATION ERRORS

More has been reported on medication errors than any other error, yet we know that many medication errors are never reported. Woods and Doan-Johnson recommend that the definition provided by the National Coordinating Council for Medication Error Reporting and Prevention be used:

> *A medication error is any preventable event that may cause or lead to inappropriate medication use or patient harm while the medication is in the control of the health care professional, patient, or consumer. Such events may be related to professional practice, health care products, procedures, and systems, including prescribing; order communication;*

> *product labeling, packaging, and nomenclature; compounding; dispensing; distribution; administration; education; monitoring; and use* (p. 47).

Woods and Doan-Johnson, and the Joint Commission on Accreditation of Healthcare Organizations identified different types of medication errors:

- Missed doses of medication.
- Wrong time of administration of medication, either more frequently or less frequently than ordered.
- I.V. rate too fast, delivering too much medication.
- Wrong concentration or dosage of medication delivered I.V.
- Wrong route of administration... or wrong medication administered.
- Wrong medications delivered due to misidentifying the patient.
- Medications with similar names [being confused].
- Medications with similar packaging [being confused].
- Medications that are not commonly used or prescribed [so staff do not know how it is to be used, contraindications, or possible side effects].
- Commonly used medications (such as antibiotics, opiates, and nonsteroidal anti-inflammatory drugs) to which many patients are allergic.
- Medications that require testing (such as lithium, warfarin, digoxin, and theophylline) to ensure that proper (nontoxic) therapeutic levels are maintained (Woods and Doan-Johnson, p. 47).

LACK OF INTERVENTION ON THE PATIENT'S BEHALF

Again, this is where the nurse's judgment and clinical expertise is important. Often symptoms that the nurse does not recognize, or does not recognize in time, occur so a complication or death results when, with earlier intervention, it could possibly have been avoided. Once again, critical thinking, along with additional education for nurses who do not think in this way, needs to be encouraged.

LACK OF PREVENTION

Woods and Doan-Johnson point out that in this area it is hard to identify preventive actions that worked because if the patient outcome is good, it is not always clear that some specific action caused this outcome. It becomes very noticeable when something goes wrong. The main point here is to teach all employees to identify any potential problems and rectify them as soon as the problems are noticed. Woods and Doan-Johnson have identified three areas of concern:

> *Breach of infection precautions* is one of the major threats to patient safety in hospitals and long-term-care facilities. *Lack of prevention of hazards of immobility/decreased mobility* covers a broad range of patient complications, such as pressure ulcers, stasis pneumonia, and patient falls. *Lack of provision of a safe environment* includes the large variety of potentially dangerous environmental hazards to patients (for example, electric shock, patient burns, lack of bed side rails, spills on the floor, and inadequate assistance/supervision with patient ambulation) (p. 48).

MISSED OR MISTAKEN PHYSICIAN/HEALTH CARE PROVIDER'S ORDERS.

This is another cause of errors that a computerized documentation system could more effectively prevent.

DOCUMENTATION ERRORS.

There are two identified problems in this area:

- *Charting procedures or medications before they were completed.* Such a documentation error can cause a patient to miss a dose of medication or a treatment and can confuse, misrepresent, or mask a patient's true condition.
- *Lack of charting of observations of the patient* causes serious harm when a nurse fails to chart signs of patient deterioration, pain, or agitation or particular signs of complications related to the illness or therapies (p. 48).

Again, educating nurses about these issues is very important.

Set up Systems to Prevent Mistakes

The question is: how can we set up systems to prevent mistakes from occurring? Mechanisms to bring about patient safety are being published daily. For instance, the Leapfrog Group, a coalition of large public and private payers, was formed after the Institute of Medicine published the patient safety study. They published three standards that all hospital providers must meet to get business from the Leapfrog Group coalition:

- Implement a computerized physician order entry (CPOE) system.
- Meet volume thresholds for certain complex procedures, such as coronary artery bypass grafts and esophageal surgery.
- Hire intensive specialists (intensive specialists are discussed in more detail in Chapter 14 on Budget Strategies) (Sarudi, May 2001, p. 32).

We need to continually identify additional issues. So far we have only identified the tip of the iceberg. We follow with a few safety devices that will help improve patient safety. As an administrator we need to make sure that we are including these safety devices in budget requests. We need to be assertive and argue the importance of these expenditures! Let's start with computers and the information age.

What Does It Mean to Be in the Information Age?

Now that we are in the *information* age, there is too much information in our reality, and the way we perceive information has changed. The question is not necessarily how much information we can learn, retain, and use. Instead it is how well we can *access* the needed information. Baby boomers are having difficulty with this reality, but the newer generations are already experiencing, and living it. There is a disconnect between generations at present. In health care this reality has great implications for the future, causing health care systems to move to integrated computer systems, a costly venture. We are limping presently because so many of our computer programs cannot talk to one another. This will change very quickly. If we ignore this, our health care organization will become obsolete. This is a major financial question as these computer systems are expensive. Where will smaller facilities get the money to purchase this new reality?

This question gives us another clue. We can approach this problem by saying, "We don't have the money for this." Which leads us to obsolescence. Or we can reframe the question, "How can we get this new system?" If we *believe* there is a way, there *will* be a way.

ONLINE CLINICAL DOCUMENTATION SYSTEMS

The Leapfrog Group identified the importance of a computerized physician order entry (CPOE) system. Actually, there are entire online clinical documentation systems that are even better with physician order entry as a part of the larger system. Online documentation provides *integration of documentation* from all disciplines. Because all disciplines chart together, there is immediate access to relevant information, as well as better continuity of care. In addition, preformatted charting presents an easier, timesaving format for the clinician to follow, and helps to achieve patient safety by indicating all possibilities associated with symptoms. Built-in clinical alerts identify abnormal results, allergies, stop dates on medicines, incompatible medicines, alerts that it is time to give medications, and a variety of other safeguards that promote patient safety and optimize quality.

Online systems also provide immediate and virtual access to laboratory and radiology results in both the health care facility and the physician's office. In addition, physicians can initiate computerized physician order entry (CPOE) from their office location. Prescriptions and discharge instructions can be generated. From a safety standpoint, the liability from legibility problems is decreased.

Using these systems, documentation is thorough and better reflects patient status, resulting in increased reimbursement from accurate coding. The systems can even link cost and quality data. Note here that in long-term care, this already occurs with the RUGS/MDS system. (As you will read in Chapter 19 on Patient Classification Systems, these systems can also provide patient classification data without the nurses having to fill out separate forms.)

An alert to clinicians using computers when in the patient's presence: a study found that patients often thought that clinicians were doing some computer activity not related to that patient, because clinicians gave no explanation of what they were doing. So it is important to explain to the patient that we are documenting care.

BARCODING

We discussed barcoding for medication administration (more in Chapter 14, Budget Strategies). A closed-loop system comprised of a scanner to barcode the medication, the clinician administering the medication, and the patient's armband has been piloted in many trial studies, and has proven very successful in reducing medication errors related to the five rights of medication administration: right patient, right route, right dose, right time, and right medication. Pyxis medication dispensers are available in many facilities to assist with medication administration. The medicine is categorized in drawers and the appropriate drawer opens when the patient name and medication name are entered. Some facilities have implemented robotics to assist with medication identification in the pharmacy as well as with delivery from the pharmacy. This has greatly decreased the possibility of error. Although cost is significant, the savings realized from diverted errors, increased patient satisfaction, and promotion of quality more than substantiates the expense. In this era of health care shortages at crisis proportions, robotic help is needed.

LAPTOP COMPUTERS WITH INTERNET ACCESS/ PERSONAL PALM DEVICES.

Laptop computers and personal palm devices are being used more frequently to promote efficiency and decrease transcription errors. Access is available from remote locations and to decrease redundancy of information regarding demographics and insurance status asked during registration processes. In addition, clinicians can look up information about medications, diagnoses, and other health information immediately as needed. (This is discussed in more detail in Chapter 8 on capabilities of present information technologies, and is also discussed further in Chapter 14, Budget Strategies.)

Get Everyone in on the Act!

Everyone in health care organizations needs to be cognizant of both patient safety and quality issues with the aim that all are constantly thinking, *how can we be safer in our patient care?* This really needs to be a Performance Improvement goal. Administratively, we need to stress the importance of patient safety through our actions and words. Then we need to listen to everyone's ideas, and implement the suggestions that make sense. The old authoritarian system is dead. Information needs to be shared with all staff. Dialogue about solutions is the best way to directly confront the safety issue.

Patient safety and quality are an issue for every staff member to work on—both thinking of better solutions, and then implementing or trialing the solutions. Encourage everyone to comb literature and the internet. Safety and quality can always be improved. Safety is like quality—we never totally get there but we sure can get a whole lot better in safeguarding our patients. Hopefully, we will make wonderful progress.

Change Organizational Processes

All staff have common issues with quality, including patient safety. Everyone, and all processes, in the organization need to be involved with promoting quality and safety. These issues often will cross department lines, and must be dealt with organizationally. All health care personnel can make helpful contributions for improvement. As we go through a day at work, we need to constantly identify what could be improved. For example, as shift report occurs nurses may need to discuss outcomes instead of tasks (Hansten and Washburn, 1999).

In the administrative and unit team meetings, share information and results with everyone. Set up rewards, or even give awards, to people as they discover, create, and improve on both safety and quality issues. Make sure to note success in employee evaluations. Post current information in the department or unit. Update staff on new medications, sentinel event alerts, and other quality or patient safety issues. Get their help in determining how such incidents can be prevented in the future. Encourage discussion about patient safety in all staff meetings. Get other interdisciplinary team members, including physicians, involved in the safety issue. We are all in this effort together. Quality and safety are the most important issues we have as an administrator.

Quality and safety does not stop with employees of the organization. Patients and their families need to be involved. They have some wonderful ideas. For instance, with all the safety issues about *getting the right medication, right dose, right route, to the right patient at the right time,* the patients are often the best source on what medications they take and how they take them. Patients know what their current medications look like and can identify that something is not right. And, equally important, patients need to know about new medications—and how these medications might interact with other medications, herbs, or other over-the-counter drugs.

Communicate, Communicate, Communicate!

No matter how much we communicate, there is always more we need to communicate. Communication is at least a two-way exchange of both people listening to each other and having dialogue together. As quality and safety issues are considered often there are many people involved—both across shifts and across departments, not to mention the physicians and the patients plus significant others. We are part of a service industry, and we have not communicated enough unless dialogue has occurred with every person who might be involved in the safety issue. Tall order!

Take one example: Miscommunication occurs between professional groups. Markey and Brown (2002) noted that a team of RNs, physical therapists, occupational therapists, patient care assistants, and physicians, when working together on teams, discovered that each discipline had a different vocabulary for the same items:

> Each department had its own activity and mobility vocabulary and because staff members' duties for mobilizing patients were not defined, creating a common language and clarifying responsibilities were essential to ensuring effective patient mobility plans. The group developed seven standard descriptions of mobility and activity levels ranging from 'Total 100%/Be prepared to do everything' to 'Independent/No assistance needed.' With dressing, for instance, a patient who needs 'total assistance' would meet the description, 'Patient needs to be dressed,' while a patient who needs 'moderate' assistance would be noted as 'Get dressing articles ready. Can put limbs in clothing but can't pull on completely' (p. 1).

They found that specific guidelines were most helpful in carrying out the activities specified by nurses, physicians, physical therapists, or occupational therapists. These guidelines were also shared with patients and families, accomplishing better consistency when working with patients, as, for example, the nurse aide understood specifically what to have the patient do, and what the aide should do for the patient.

These guidelines provided a set of *scripted behaviors* that achieved a more consistent approach. This scripted format is becoming more popular in every health care setting, including the hospitals receiving the Malcolm Baldridge Award. In fact, part of their success is because the scripted format provides more consistent care regardless of the provider.

As we receive more information from focus groups of patients and families, and share the information with all the staff at the point of care, this melds what the patients want and need with staff behaviors. It also makes the work more meaningful to staff.

Employee Issues

When discussing value and quality, we cannot ignore employees. When employees are not valued, they will not treat others as having value. Put in a positive way, when administrators value employees, employees will value patients. Thus, this section includes issues in the value and quality arena that pertain to employees.

OSHA Standards for Employee Safety

The first employee issue is employee safety. There are so many possible hazards in the health care industry. The Occupational Safety and Health Administration (OSHA) (www.osha-sic.gov), provides nationally-mandated ongoing standards for the workplace. Thus health care staff must regularly orient to current OSHA standards. In addition, OSHA has record-keeping forms that someone in the organization must keep updated to document that OSHA standards have been followed. In larger health care systems, both quality and infection control personnel are often concerned with workplace compliance with OSHA standards. In smaller systems, this becomes another responsibility of staff who assume many roles. Either way, the nurse manager needs to be aware of the current standards, must make sure that staff have been oriented to these standards, and must be sure that the unit is in compliance with the standards.

Promoting a Healthy Workplace

Achieving a healthy workplace includes *examining how the environment affects all present*. It can be quite complicated. For instance, a nurse experiencing a needle stick when the patient has AIDS or hepatitis is a major hazard. We also have members from the general public visiting or being admitted into health care facilities. These people may have a number of issues that could endanger others, i.e., have a gun, bring infections, threaten staff, and so forth. We have a responsibility to protect staff as well as patients in this environment.

Bioterrorism

A new issue that must be addressed in relation to patient and staff safety is bioterrorism. The intentional introduction of anthrax, smallpox, or other disease entities as a biological weapon would certainly play havoc on already short-staffed, financially burdened health care facilities. Procedures to address the identified emergency would be dictated by the

Federal Emergency Management Administration (FEMA), but facility-related issues such as lack of available nurses, and methods to contain or quarantine would be facility specific, and should be addressed in policy prior to the need. Thus disaster planning, and preparedness, has assumed new significance. Sadly enough, this needs to also be considered at budget time to designate appropriate funds for protective apparel, vaccinations, preparation and training for staff, and public education.

Performance Improvement

The question is always, *are we doing our best as a total organization in achieving quality?* Of course, the answer is always that we could do better. All organizations need *performance improvement* to examine current quality and safety issues as well as to identify opportunities to enhance quality. It is a *proactive* process, meaning that everyone not only identifies problems but has suggestions for improvements. Performance improvement may have been implemented with varying success by many health care organizations and businesses.

The reason for variance in the success of these programs is that many times there are administrative leadership problems that are not being fixed, that many organizational processes need to be fixed and may negatively impact the success of the performance improvement plan, and that performance improvement is not perceived as being important. Interestingly, when performance improvement is effective, it often decreases expenses as well. Additionally, it produces a more efficient practice that results in increased patient satisfaction and quality.

The performance improvement concept began in the business literature with Dr. William Demming, the guru of continuous improvement (Walton, 1986). He viewed production as having three elements: 1) why we make what we make, 2) how we make what we make, and 3) how we improve what we make. For business success, it is important to continually be thinking about all three as an integrated whole.

Performance Improvement can be called by various names—Continuous Improvement, Continuous Quality Improvement (CQI), and Total Quality Measurement (TQM), to name a few. Different methodologies may be employed to initiate Performance Improvement, but many health care organizations use focus PDCA, or some similar designation, to address quality improvement.

P . . . Plan, determine what the improvement will be and the method for data collection.

D . . . Do, implement the plan.

C . . . Check, review and analyze the results.

A . . . Act, hold the gain and continue with the improvement (Al-Assaf and Schmele, 1993; Meisenheimer, 1997).

In other words, to *plan*, one would identify the issue or problem, identify customers (stakeholders), flow chart the current processes, determine the cause and effect of why you do what you do (identifying barriers), and then flowchart a streamlined process removing wasted efforts or steps. This process has everyone involved in the dialogue thus producing even more ideas. Everyone is a problem solver, decision maker, and implementer. Only the core value, explained in Chapter 4, remains stationary. Everything else can be improved and changed.

Next, one implements the plan (*do*), making sure that all staff involved in the implementation phase are aware of the plan, and that the administrative team is supporting the plan, keeping records of what actually happens as the plan is implemented. Then one would need to *check*, or review and analyze the results by finding out from the people involved what happened, identifying the positives and negatives that happened, including any measurements that could be taken to determine whether the outcome was a success or whether additional changes were needed. The final step (*act*) then continues with the successful components of the plan, and/or corrects the plan, and continues the improvement.

For the most effective performance improvement, everyone in the facility needs to be involved. Thus an interdisciplinary team should facilitate performance improvement. Opportunities for improvement come from any source—staff, patients or patient satisfaction surveys, accrediting criteria, complaints, physicians, family members, even the housekeeping staff. The team determines the method of data collection and analysis, as well as the thresholds and control limits for review. Many Performance Improvement tools are available to evaluate trends and patterns and assist in determining the need for further action. The results are forwarded to the facility-wide Performance Improvement committee, and are often benchmarked against like organizations for best practice standards.

A new form of performance improvement is called Six Sigma, previously used in other non-health care businesses. Six Sigma provides a systematic approach used to improve patient outcomes. It is now being implemented in many hospitals to reduce errors. This performance improvement tool incorporates massive data analysis to identify and reduce variation. Created by Motorola in 1985, there are six steps to define the process and streamline variability. The Six Steps to Six Sigma are:

- Identify the product you created or the service you provide. In other words,...What do you do?
- Identify the customer(s) for your product or service, and determine what they consider important [this would identify what the patient values]. In other words,...Who uses your products or services? [We would suggest asking, *What do the customers value?*]
- Identify your needs (to provide product/ service so that it satisfies the customer). In other words,...What do you need to do your work?
- Define the process for doing your work. In other words,...How do you do your work?
- Mistake proof the process and eliminate wasted effort. In other words,...How can you do your work better?
- Ensure continuous improvement by measuring, analyzing, and controlling the improved process. In other words,...How perfectly are you doing your customer focused work? (Six Sigma and SPC, http://www.sixsigmaspc.com/six-sigma/six-sigma.html).

Six Sigma utilizes a scientific process to identify variation in the workplace, magnifying the potential for error. By reducing variability and promoting standardization, the potential for errors is greatly decreased, resulting in increased patient safety and a better product. *Standardization* is an important concept here. For instance, because we have different people interacting with patients in our service industry, we want all staff to be cognizant of, and use, certain customer service behaviors and scripting responses. This means that customer service is standardized so that no matter who the patient comes in contact with, the customer service behaviors are present.

The idea behind performance improvement is that it results in changes in practice that provide better quality or value to the patient. An excellent example of a performance improvement project that determined a change in practice is the implementation of a service guarantee in various emergency departments across the country. CentraState, Oakwood Healthcare System, and St. Joseph Health Center examined practices in their emergency departments to determine what was effective and what resulted in patient dissatisfaction. A major complaint was wait time in the department before being seen by a physician or a provider. These facilities instituted processes enabling them to offer a service guarantee stating that a provider would see the patient, and/or treatment would be started, within thirty minutes. This has not only been an excellent success for the department, but has improved patient satisfaction, staff morale, and resulted in increased volume/revenue for each facility in the organization. (And we need to find additional ways to decrease wait time!)

Input and participation by staff are essential to the success of the project. Front-line staff are more familiar with the problems and opportunities in the department than anyone else, and can be instrumental in identifying and implementing change, or in orchestrating sabotage when not consulted. Involvement in performance improvement programs is often mandated in annual evaluations, and reflected in bonuses for incentive plans.

Former patients are particularly valuable members on performance improvement committees. After all, the improvement effort is meant to improve the way we treat patients, and these committee members know what was important to them during their illness. It is also helpful if committee members have had a loved one experience all the difficulties inherent in a health care crisis within the health care system. Input from both patients and committee members who have had this experience is invaluable. They have the best ideas as to what needs to be done, or changed, to achieve value.

Performance Measurement

> Performance measurement is simply a means of compiling data.
> Converting the data into information and using them to make decisions
> is at the heart of the value of performance measurement (Jennings and
> Staggers, 1999, p. 27).

One helpful resource on available tools is the *Handbook for Improvement: A Reference Guide for Tools and Guides*, 2nd ed. (1997).[4]

In an effort to contain costs, performance measurement became popular in the early 1990s when companies purchasing health plans could examine cost and quality data to determine which plan was best for the dollars spent. At first these plans were called report

---

[4] This is available from Executive Learning, 7107 Executive Center Dr., Suite 160, Brentwood, TN 37027.
  Phone: 615-373-8483.

cards, and published only summaries of various performance data. Report cards then started to be used internally by health care organizations to improve services. (For an example, see http://www.healthgrades.com). The idea behind performance measurement was that the patient outcomes could determine the effectiveness of organizational performance. Although this measurement was an improvement from past practices, there were several problems with this measurement: 1) future performance cannot be determined from the historical data; 2) no one asked the patient what the patient wanted or valued; 3) at times organizations were swimming in data that was collected, but no one figured out how to analyze it or use it effectively; and 4) sometimes this data was used punitively when outcomes were not met, which only impeded future improvement occuring.

Examples of using report card data include:

- Van Servellen and Schultz (1999) reviewed the literature to see if there was a relationship between hospital characteristics and inpatient mortality. They found three significant results:
  1) physician board certification was significantly and inversely associated with mortality;
  2) as RNs increased, patient mortality decreased; and
  3) as operating expenditures rise, the mortality rate drops.
- McCue, Mark, and Harless (2003) found a statistically significant increase in operating costs when registered nurse levels increased, but no statistically significant decrease in profit, when examining 422 hospitals from 1990 to 1995.

Performance improvement often involves interdisciplinary teams committed to solving problems. For instance, Hypnar and Anderson (2001) describe a team—home health care, physical therapy (acute care), finance, public relations, operating room, nursing, and a physician—that met when the hospital was losing money on patients having major limb reattachment procedures of the lower extremity (DRG 209) to find a way to better deal with these patients. Their plan not only saved money, it gave better, more consistent care to the patients and resulted in lower lengths of stay and fewer complications, as well as produced greater employee and physician satisfaction. (Chapter 4 gives more details on conducting such meetings.)

Sentara Healthcare (2002) established performance improvement goals, and then went one step further. They tied it with the incentive plan. (We would take it one step further, and tie it in with an incentive plan for *all* staff.)

> Our chief medical officer, who has worked in four institutions, said that this is the only place he's worked where he actually gets calls from the non-medical managers asking if we are making progress in the clinical quality indicators because their compensation is tied to these improvements. So it's a system to foster innovation with built-in accountability aimed at increasing the quality of care.... A good example is our remotely monitored electronic ICU. Intensive care specialists monitor ICU patients 19 hours a day for timely intervention. [From 7 a.m. to noon, physicians make rounds in the actual units.] The physician has

computer access to the patient's records, including lab or radiographic tests, and can view the patient and talk with staff via in-room, high-resolution video cameras. The system enhances traditional rounds and on-site monitoring. Patient mortality rates have dropped 25 to 35 percent and it's achieved a 155 percent payback (Grayson, 2002, p. 36).

Payers also got involved in the cost-quality initiatives. For example, a payer might specify a *carepath* in order to obtain reimbursement. If the carepath is not followed as specified, the health care organization does not receive reimbursement for the care. In other words, if antibiotics are not given within two hours of a pneumonia diagnosis (the carepath specification), the payer will not reimburse the hospital. In this case, the clinician needs to be timely in treating the patient or everyone loses, including the patient.

PATIENT SATISFACTION

Patient satisfaction has been one early performance measurement that pays attention to what the patient values. Patient satisfaction instruments are a beginning measurement of value, although they take place after the health care experience. Hospitals, particularly, have used patient satisfaction measurement for some time because measuring patient satisfaction has been an important core outcome measure for JCAHO accreditation. A survey regarding patient satisfaction, initiated by *Hospitals and Health Networks*, was sent to a random sample of hospital administrators. A response rate of 15.7 percent was noted representing 783 completed questionnaires. "Almost 95% say they measure patient satisfaction in their organization. Over 99% say there are many opportunities to improve patient satisfaction." When asked if they are doing a better job than ten years ago, less than 40 percent stated this was the case (Hoppszaliern, 2001).

In this survey, 71 percent of the hospitals used an outside vendor to conduct the patient satisfaction survey with hospitals under 100 beds spending on average $23,611, and hospitals having 600+ beds spending $184,433. "The amount of money spent is directly proportional to competition in the service area and the size of the hospital. The frustration comes with not having the resources and staff time to reach goals" (Hoppszaliern, 2001). Companies that provide patient satisfaction instruments, or services, to health care organizations include both Gallop and Press Ganey. Generally, hospitals pay these companies to actually collect and tabulate the data as patients are more likely to be honest with an outside group asking the questions.

Even the patient satisfaction instrument misses many patient value issues. For instance, in an inner-city emergency room, patient satisfaction scores can go down if street people addicted to drugs are not given additional narcotics. Or, a patient in a rehab hospital may have had an aide that did all the activities of daily living for the patient, when the patient wanted to be more independent and re-learn how to care for him/herself. And from the patient perspective:

> Few patients would agree that they are in fact the focus of services or in control of anything.... They could cite facts such as these:
>
> • Providers continue to prescribe treatments without discussion with the patients.

- Visiting hours are still in effect.

- Appointment times for services are based on Monday through Friday schedules.

- Patient procedures and their scheduled times are determined by providers without input from patients or families.

Leaders have plenty left to do to transform the health care system into one that is truly based on the will of the patient. A good place to begin is the Internet, [although many elderly are not computer literate] which should be pushed as a proactive means of assisting consumers in interpreting health care information. Other strategies leaders should use to increase the patient focus of health care include these:

- Find the courage to continue the journey to creating a better system. Avoid the tendency to believe that the system is as consumer focused as it can be.

- Recognize that personal experiences as a patient can be invaluable for learning the truth about health care service delivery.

- Remain committed and focused when complaints override positive feedback. Resist the temptation to retire from health care.

- Never stop asking patients to share their experience of the health care system. Learn from them and share the information gained with other health professionals to improve the system.

- Believe that every health professional possesses courage, passion, energy, and self-discipline but may need reassurance and encouragement to exhibit them fully (Porter-O'Grady and Malloch, 2002, p. 322).

To adequately assess patient satisfaction, both the patient's and the provider's expectations must be clearly identified. Typically in the past patients were seen as customers in need of health care; now they are informed consumers looking for quality of care and noticing the method of delivery. Health care has become a competitive business. Many facilities are using contract agencies to market their services and measure their success; they have implemented service excellence initiatives to improve patient satisfaction. Some even have scripted behaviors and protocols to handle dialogue in difficult situations. (This is an example of the standardization issue discussed previously.)

The problem is that we are dealing with people. What has value to one person may not have value with another. For example, one person may welcome talking about their emotions with a health care giver, while another person may find this invasive. One person may respond to pain by grinning and bearing it, while another who experiences even mild pain, loudly expresses this to all.

Staff, or department, evaluations may be directly linked to satisfaction results. When this occurs, staff should be aware of this so they can take ownership for improvement. Too often a paradox exists: "Non-management staff—those who are most likely to have patient contact—are least likely to see the patient satisfaction data. Less than 25 percent of non-management staff see the data, compared with almost 80 percent of managers" (Hoppszaliern, 2001).

Results from patient satisfaction surveys can be very useful, and can be used to:

- Improve and measure the quality of care;
- Manage complaints;
- Implement strategic planning and marketing decisions;
- Evaluate and/or provide bonuses to departments or individual (physician and non-physician) staff;
- Enhance public relations;
- Meet accreditation standards;
- Monitor for risk management;
- Link survey results to clinical data;
- Use survey results for contract payer negotiations;
- Compare the results for benchmarking; and
- Link the results to financial data.

JCAHO Expands Performance Measurement

As report card data became available, JCAHO expanded performance measurement to include a set of standardized screening indicators. At this point a health care organization has to select a minimum of four screening indicators—two from a clinical/service list and two human resource indicators. The organization then needs to look at the relationship between them. **Exhibit 2–2** lists JCAHO's screening indicators.

JCAHO also set up a data system called ORYX™ to track performance data that participating health care organizations report to JCAHO. This is being used for site visits, and can show trends, either positive or negative, that a health care organization will need to respond to on an ongoing basis. Eventually JCAHO is planning to expand the measure sets to include: clinical performance; patient perception of care, treatment and services; health status; and administrative or financial measures. (For more information on this, see http://oryx@jcaho.org.)

CMS Gets Involved

Then CMS got into the act. They are requiring hospitals to submit performance data for ten quality measures on all patients, not just on Medicare patients, in order to receive full funding. Hospitals who do not choose to do this will receive 0.4 percent less funding on Medicare patients. To see a sample of this, go to www.cms.hhs.gov/quality/hospital.

Performance Measurement and Patient Value

Jennings and Staggers (1999) point out that performance measurement might totally miss the boat because we may not have captured what the patient values.

> The cost of care in a pain clinic affords a good example of one aspect of
> data quality and how the focus of data collection that is based on the unit
> of analysis can affect decision making. If the goal of the clinic is pain

Exhibit 2–2 JCAHO's Screening Indicators

Clinical/Service Indicators	Human Resource Indicators
• Family complaints	• Overtime
• Patient complaints	• Staff vacancy rate
• Patient falls	• Staff satisfaction
• Adverse drug events	• Staff turnover rate
• Injuries to patients	• Understaffing as compared to hospital's
• Skin breakdown	staffing plan
• Pneumonia	• Nursing care hours per patient day
• Postoperative infections	• Staff injuries on the job
• Urinary tract infections	• On-call or per diem use
• Upper gastrointestinal bleeding	• Sick time
• Shock/cardiac arrest	
• Length of stay	

> relief, then dollars per patient day would not be the preferred way to
> approach the cost analysis. Instead, the actual cost per discharged patient
> whose pain is relieved would reflect the concept better (p. 27).

We need to keep coming back to what the patient values. If we lose sight of this, all our statistics are useless. We may be making a profit and have wonderful patient outcome statistics, such as preventing complications, but if the patients are not getting what they want or need, it is their choice whether or not to come back next time. This comes back to the patient and family advisory focus groups that we discussed earlier in this chapter. The data received from this group provides rich resources of data for both performance improvement and performance measurement.

As one collects data from focus groups, or even as one organizes the groups, it is important to think about the data in terms of populations served, or the amount of data may easily get out of hand. This means that our focus moves from thinking about individuals to considering similar needs of larger groups of patients. If we examine populations of patients, it probably needs to go beyond groups with a certain disease or problem to some kind of subgroup population with similar concerns. For instance, parents of young children would have different concerns than older adults experiencing chronic diseases on a fixed income, or from certain populations who are more concerned with maintaining health. The focus group participants may need to be organized in a different way to better identify these populations.

Jennings and Staggers (1999) describe the results from one focus group:

> In a group of senior citizens, for example, alternate therapies such as
> acupuncture and over-the-counter remedies, including supplemental
> vitamins and minerals, were of substantial interest to health care users.
> Furthermore, only 1 of their 10 top health concerns related to chronic
> disease despite the prevalence of chronic problems in older persons. The

patients were more concerned about joint pain, stress, being overweight, back pain, and lack of energy… An important message to all individuals involved with users of the health care system is *the necessity of listening to patients regarding what matters to them* (pp. 23–24).

BENCHMARKING

Many health care organizations are benchmarking quality measures with other similar organizations. Often, when benchmarking, the organization sets a goal, such as to be in the top 25th quartile. However, be aware that benchmarking can be fraught with problems. Rudy, et al. (2001) report that:

> Benchmarking is a common approach to establishing quality. However, the conclusions drawn from benchmarking depend heavily on whether the benchmark is obtained from the literature, from hospital-specific sources, or from an integrated hospital system. Benchmarking using the literature may appear the simplest, but often a literature-based benchmark is not available, is not sufficiently relevant, or differs in definitions, populations, or clinical practice…. An important but rarely addressed issue in literature-based benchmarking is assessing uncertainty, such as the standard error, in the benchmark itself.
>
> Internal benchmarking is available to hospitals with the relevant databases and statistical expertise, but it can provide an invalid assessment of performance when compared to other institutions….
>
> System benchmarking appears to avoid the pitfalls of these other two methods, but it requires coordinated database resources and sophisticated statistical analyses. System-based benchmarks without adequate adjustments for acuity put hospitals with higher acuity at a disadvantage. Hospitals with smaller censuses may have larger differences between hospital-specific and system-based estimates than do those with larger censuses (p. 189).

There is an additional problem with benchmarking. *It compares current **practices**, not what has value from the patient perspective.* For instance, we benchmark the wait time for emergency rooms. An hour wait time is considered normal. Think about this statement from the patient perspective. Does the patient enjoy experiencing an hour or more waiting to be seen in the emergency room? From a value perspective, wouldn't it be better to measure by eliminating the wait time and seeing the patient immediately? After all, some are already using 30 minutes as the benchmark, and even 30 minutes is not as valuable to the patient as no wait time! Remember if we don't achieve it, someone else will!

Using a Balanced Scorecard System

As we work on Performance Improvement, a new system, called the balanced scorecard, can help to draw all the organizational or performance improvement components together.

The Balanced Scorecard is more than a measurement system. Innovation companies use the framework for their management processes. Organizations use the system to define objectives, focus on their strategy, and communicate that strategy throughout the organization. The power of the Balanced Scorecard occurs when it is transformed from a measurement system to a management system. Critics note that nearly 70 percent of scorecard implementations fail due to lack of dedication to the theory driving the scorecard. Implementation is a 25–26 month process and requires a significant commitment from everyone involved. The scorecard enables the organization to become aligned and focused. Used in this manner, the Balanced Scorecard is the foundation for managing organizations in the information age.

Kaplan and Norton developed scorecards (also known as dashboards, instrument panels, and data display devices) in 1991. The use of the Balanced Scorecard remains unchanged—it is the provision of a strategic management and performance management tool. Measurement of key financial, quality, market and operational indicators provide management with an understanding of performance in relation to established strategic goals and graphically displays a snapshot of the institution's overall health (Health Care Advisory Board, "Balanced Scorecards," 1999). In "Poor Performance Measurement Can Drive Financial Crisis," the Health Care Advisory Board (2002) noted in their study of hospital downturns that "inadequate performance measurement" ranked fifth as the root cause of financial flashpoints.

Successful implementations have been documented using the following process:

- The implementation (this process is further explained in Chapter 15, Forecasting) for a health care facility is a 25–26 months process. Commitment from senior leadership, and education for this group regarding the process and outcomes prior to initiation, prevents ambiguity.
- In months one and two, a strategic planning retreat is conducted involving the entire organization (those who are unable to attend provide input and are given feedback). This retreat is critical, as consensus is sought regarding the organization's vision, strategic goals and objectives.
- During months three and four, a strategic planning committee is selected to identify objectives for each perspective in the balanced scorecard.
- In the next two months, the strategic planning committee communicates and seeks commitment from the staff for the selected scorecard.
- In the following month, the scorecard is revised based on staff input.
- In months eight and nine, the revised scorecard is deployed to employees. Each unit/department and employee is required to develop a scorecard that supports the strategies identified on the facility scorecard.
- For the next two months, the strategic planning committee reviews individual and department balanced scorecards and suggests revisions.
- At the one-year point, senior leadership formulates a five-year plan based on the finalized scorecard.
- During months 13–24, departmental and organizational progress is reviewed quarterly to identify opportunities to improve.

- At months 25–26, the hospital evaluation committee assesses staff performance based on the individual balanced scorecards.

Based on the results, retention, promotion, salary increases and other rewards are realized. The strategic planning committee revises the balanced scorecard and five-year plan based on the results of the metrics, and after scanning the environment for needed adjustments (Health Care Advisory Board, "Balanced Scorecards," 1999). The cycle continues in the following years.

Theurer (as cited in Health Care Advisory Board, "Balanced Scorecards," 1999) recognized that the following pitfalls should be avoided when creating indicators for a balanced scorecard:

1. Lack of context—measures should tie to strategic goals and drive organizational strategy and resource allocation.
2. Benchmarks are vital to understanding metrics as they rank the organizations against peers.
3. Leadership must empower employees and provide sufficient resources to develop unit level performance measures.
4. Without sufficient resources, the staff will simply recycle existing measures.
5. Bureaucratic uniformity will squelch the individualized nature of each unit and should be avoided so that each unit can be measured based on its unique attributes.
6. Indicators must be used as tools for continuous improvement, not as tools to punish poor performance.
7. Key stakeholders should provide positive reinforcement for improvements realized.

Critics note that nearly 70 percent of scorecard implementations fail. Most often, the failure is due to lack of true dedication to the theory driving the scorecard; with the resulting matrix perceived as little more than the latest business fad. The Health Care Advisory Board noted in "#2 'Metric Austerity' Ensures Big Picture Awareness" that dashboards should be limited to 15 to 30 metrics. Drill-down data should be reserved for situations when a more comprehensive assessment is warranted.

Chow (as cited in Health Care Advisory Board, "Balanced Scorecards," 1999) noted that one of the most difficult tasks in developing a balanced scorecard is organization. Most scorecards are housed in a one-page format. Plotting an organization's strategy, mission, vision, and key metrics in an "at-a-glance" format provides a challenge. Because dashboards are designed to focus attention on potential problems, replacement of raw numbers with graphics facilitates the recognition of patterns and trends. Experienced health care facilities have found two types of graphics particularly effective—spider charts (which compare performance across all metrics and all categories), and bar or line graphs (display trends in individual indicators) (Health Care Advisory Board, "#3 Graphic Display Facilitates Prompt Recognition of Trends," 2002).

In "#1 Metric Balance Avoids the Vulnerability of Narrow Focus," the Health Care Advisory Board (2002), identified that best practice dashboards (scorecards) track indicators in four areas: finances, operations, quality, and satisfaction. Indicators in these four parameters provide a balanced view of the organization. Performance must be viewed at an organizational level (from different perspectives), as performance problems are not always apparent from a single viewpoint.

Generally, *financial indicators* appear first on the scorecard. Financial indicators include profitability, cash flow, and actual/budget comparison. Redundant financial indicators guard against misperceptions based on individual indicators. Key measures of operations demonstrate cost containment efforts and business growth. Vigilant performance monitoring can detect minor deviations which translate into substantial deficits in financial projections. One Midwestern system experienced a 3.6 percent decline in inpatient volume in a one-year span, which translated to a $9 million loss in operating profit (Health Care Advisory Board, "Current Conditions Require Vigilant Performance Monitoring," 2002).

Patient care, the key product of health care organizations, often comes next. Clinical quality metrics directly affect revenue growth (Health Care Advisory Board, "#1 Metric Balance Avoids the Vulnerability of Narrow Focus," 2002). Examples of clinical quality metrics include mortality, morbidity, medication error rates, and fall rates.

Service quality must also be measured. Satisfaction measures assess staff loyalty and gauge the organization's ability to maintain competent staff. *Goal congruence* brings the employee's and the organization's wants and desires together. It is essential that employees buy into the organization's plans. Employees must feel that when the organization is successful, they too are successful. *Goal divergence* places employees and the organization at odds. Motivated employees and management are key to the success of the organization. Unmotivated employees are unlikely to meet the organization's plans, thus the company is unlikely to meet established goals (Finkler, 2001). To attract customers, grow the business, and increase revenue, patient and physician satisfaction are critical. Employee and physician satisfaction are predictors of volume and financial health (Health Care Advisory Board, "#1 Metric Balance Avoids the Vulnerability of Narrow Focus," 2002).

In August of 1999, the Health Care Advisory Board noted in "Balanced Scorecards," four basic perspectives for balanced score cards: *customer, finance, innovation and learning,* and *internal business.* Indicators are designed to measure key aspects from each category. Indicators must be quantifiable, objective, and actionable. These indicators are benchmarked against organizational goals, competitors, and best practice. Benchmarking provides management with the "big picture" prospective of the organization at a given time, as well as an understanding of how an organization compares to peers. When benchmarking, ensure that only like quantities are compared. An example includes: if turnover is measured, does it include temporary or part-time workers, or only full-time employees.

While indicators act as an early health care performance measurement, to benefit from a balanced scorecard, one must develop organizational-specific metrics. Individualized metrics can represent a significant learning curve for organizational leadership, and because performance measurement is not an exact science, administrators must experiment to create the right balance for their organization. The process usually involves both department heads and senior leadership. Significant commitment is required from everyone involved (Health Care Advisory Board, "Balanced Scorecards," 1999).

Rivers' "Developing Performance Metrics" flowchart (as cited in Health Care Advisory Board, "Balanced Scorecards," 1999) describes the process of developing both strategic and tactical performance metrics. The beginning step is a clearly stated and understood mission statement. Next, strategic objectives are completed and key business units or departments are identified. Performance measures are selected for each unit/department with comparative "best practice" benchmark organizations selected. Staff education and system deployment follows. Measures that do not support the goals of the organization should be rejected. A comparison is then completed to assure that business units do not have competing goals. Adjustments are made to the system as required. Data is then collected, analyzed, and published. If improvements are on track, the cycle continues. If not, an assessment is made to assure the metrics support goals and/or the mission statement. The process supports continuous improvement for the health care organization.

Chandrasekhar (as cited in Health Care Advisory Board, "Balanced Scorecards," 1999) proclaims that the answers to four fundamental questions aid leadership to develop appropriate performance measures for incorporation into the scorecard. These are:

- **Customer perspective:** "How do customers see us?"
- **Financial perspective:** "How do board members see us?"
- **Innovation and learning perspective:** "Can we continue to improve and create value?"
- **Internal business perspective:** "What are our goals?" (p. 5).

These questions should be answered in light of the organization's mission, vision and values. Each question will be analyzed for incorporation into the balanced scorecard.

CUSTOMER PERSPECTIVE

In their 1990 publication, "Medicare: A Strategy for Quality Assurance, Volume I," the National Academy of Sciences, Institute of Medicine (IOM) charged future quality assurance programs to require balance between regulation and professionalism, provider and patient orientation, and processes of care and desired health outcomes. In this publication, the IOM defined quality of care as "the degree to which health services for individuals and populations increase the likelihood of desired health outcomes and are consistent with current professional knowledge" (National Academy of Sciences, IOM, "Medicare: A Strategy for Quality Assurance, Volume I", 1990, p. 4). The IOM (1990) noted that net benefits reflect consideration of patient satisfaction and well-being, health status, quality-of-life outcomes, and the processes of patient care and decision making—all intangible assets necessary for successful organizations in the information era.

The IOM definition of quality of care is widely accepted and provides a foundation for a customer perspective in health care organizations. Too often the important *value* dimension is excluded. As yet *we have neither adequate measurements of what the patient wants and values, nor what the patient can afford.* This is because we often do not even ask what the patient wants or values; this leaves us with no data to analyze. Therefore, our measurements are an elusive process and can always be improved. (Add that to the Performance Improvement list!)

One of the best ways to see if we have made a difference is to first identify and record what the patient values, and second, to measure the effects before and after the treatment the patient valued was given. Organizationally, one could measure the before and after effects when an improvement suggested by the Patient and Advisory Council is implemented. Although some benefits, including patient satisfaction, can be measured quantitively, this measurement cannot because we must get the patient's perspective. But one benefit might be that the patient has a better quality of life. If the quantitative questions are not appropriate, one might miss this benefit entirely. Remember that the patient satisfaction level does not necessarily get at whether what the patient valued has been achieved.

Additional customers that must be considered include purchasers of health care coverage: employers, labor unions, and private group purchasers. An escalating petition from this group is demanding high-quality health care for the dollars they spend—this mandates attention from health care organizations. Providers are not alone in their zeal for balanced scorecards. Private purchasers of health care are developing quality improvement programs and report cards to assure the health care coverage they purchase is based on quality, not just cost and benefits. Companies such as GTE, General Motors, and Digital Equipment Corporation, invest resources to drive these efforts to improve care, to increase satisfaction, and to reduce costs for the employees and their respective organizations (Challenge, 1998). An official of GTE noted, "We think that improved quality inherently costs less. Improve the quality of health care and, in turn, improve the quality of life" (*The Business Roundtable*, 1997).

Health care organizations exist to improve the quality of life, thus the effects on individual and societal well-being are important measures of success (in addition to the financial results of operations). Managers must have outcomes, output quality and quantity data, and units of input other than dollars and costs of outputs (Herzlinger and Nitterhouse, 1994).

FINANCIAL PERSPECTIVE

Although their importance is widely recognized, performance measures are not reported in the audited general-purpose financial statements. Neither is it expected to be in the foreseeable future. Many organizations include unaudited data about their accomplishments in internal statements and annual reports. Managerial accounting and measuring and analyzing actual results or outcomes are used. Revenues received, the financial value of the services provided, are important for health care organizations (Herzlinger and Nitterhouse, 1994).

Financial performance measures indicate whether or not an organization's strategy, implementation, and execution are contributing to bottom-line improvement. Measures typically relate to *profitability*—total margin, return on investment, PLA, and operating margin, *liquidity and cash flow*—days cash on hand, all sources; current ratio of assets for one year; and days in accounts receivable; and *capital structure*—debt service coverage, average age of plant, and bad debt expense (Ohio Hospital Association, 2003). See **Exhibit 2–3** for an example using actual statewide data. From this information one can see how the Balanced Budget Act lowered profitability for health care systems.

INNOVATION AND LEARNING PERSPECTIVE

Performance improvement studies demonstrate that poor quality is expensive. Quality health care does not have to increase expenses. Quality improvements can increase revenues and decrease costs, both of which have a positive impact on the bottom line. Word-of-mouth approval from the community improves market share, which can provide a positive revenue stream. When processes of care are streamlined and errors are

Exhibit 2–3 Statewide Financial Performance Measures Using Ohio Data

	1998	2002
Profitability		
Total Margin	4.29	2.44
Return on Investment, PLA	8.60	7.51
Operating Margin	1.90	2.21
	(for 2000 as 1998 data is not available)	
Liquidity and Cash Flow		
Days Cash on Hand, All Sources	128	109
Current Ratio of Assets for One Year	1.90	1.90
Days in Accounts Receivable	70.60	55.16
Capital Structure		
Debt Service Coverage	3.74	3.25
Average Age of Plant	9.73	9.99
Bad Debt Expense	4.77	4.54

From: Ohio Hospital Statewide Financial Performance. (2003). *Vital $igns: Indicators of Ohio Hospital Financial Viability*. Columbus, OH: Ohio Hospital Association.

decreased, the cost of failures declines, and the added labor costs and resources needed for rework are saved. The cost of quality can be defined as the point when optimal quality is obtained at minimum costs. Increased quality is observed when prevention and appraisal costs increase. Likewise, as preventive costs rise, the number of failures declines. Lower quality equates to a higher number of failures, which increases costs. The total quality management journey provides a system for meeting and exceeding customer needs and expectations (Windemuth, 1994).

The scorecard link to learning reveals significant investments in reskilling employees to generate innovation and improvement for business processes, customers, and stakeholders. Employee-based measures include employee satisfaction, retention, training and skills as well as specific drivers for these measures. Alignment of employee incentives with overall organizational success factors effect customer and internal processes, thus they are key to the organization's strategy (Kaplan and Norton, 1996).

INTERNAL BUSINESS PERSPECTIVE

Assessments of internal business perspectives guard the organization's viability. The strategic planning process outlines goals for the organization—how will the organization know when these goals are met? Health care organizations can no longer simply measure the number of patients treated. Better measures of the organization's health, growth, and improvement are required. Key metrics include comparison of actual outcomes to expected outcomes, i.e., are benefits for the organization what were expected? Careful analysis of these variances determines the reasons for performance outcomes and allows for remedial actions. Health care organizations have an additional obligation to society. Measurement of public good is difficult and proxies are frequently used (Finkler, 2001).

Health care organizations must be both effective (accomplish outcomes) and efficient (use minimum resources to accomplish these outcomes). (This is discussed in Chapter on Productivity.) The organization must choose metrics that are a balance of the two to assure internal business goals are met; otherwise the organization may be effective and not efficient, or efficient and not effective. Quality as well as quantity must be measured in order to provide a balance of the two metrics (Finkler, 2001).

Herzlinger and Nitterhourse (1994) describe four categories of outcomes, each measuring different aspects of the business. The four categories are presented in descending order of measurement validity (Category 1 is easier to delineate than Category 4). Category 1 *measures outcomes.* Generally inputs are used, but one could also use the costs of resources consumed. An example would be if the nursing department expenditures grew 20 percent to $500,000 in 2003, compared to 2002. It would seem that the nursing department output grew by 20 percent. This is not necessarily true, as costs and outcomes do not grow in parallel. In health care organizations, input measures do not measure societal benefits, quality, or efficiency or effectiveness—these are usually financial measures.

Category 2, *processes of delivering care*, is often specified with implicit measurement of certain steps in the process. The assumption is that following a particular process leads to a certain level of outcome. This is not always true in health care, thus some process measures capture efficiency of service and the quantity produced. This could include factors like decreasing length of stay, productivity measurements, turnover rates, or usage of agency staff. They do not measure quality, benefits, effectiveness, or financial terms. The National Quality Forum provides a framework that can be used to measure nursing care performance. See **Exhibit 2–4**.

Category 3, *program output*, measures actual numbers of outputs in a given program. This could include number of patients served within a DRG designation. Though these measures do not explicitly measure societal benefits and effectiveness, it does focus on achievements of the organization.

Category 4, *program effects*, measures the impact of services and ideally relates these effects to their costs. Some of the clinical quality data relating to complications (medication errors, patient falls, nosocomial infections, decubitis ulcers, pneumonias) are negative effects of the program. What positive effects did patients experience? This relates directly to finding out what the patient valued. If there are problems with the care, there may even be physician dissatisfaction or flight if other facilities are available. This category is difficult to obtain and interpret correctly, but when captured and interpreted correctly, it is the most valuable of the four categories for measuring outcome.

The utility of the balanced scorecard is more than an operational measurement system. Innovative companies use the balanced scorecard as a strategic management system for long-term viability of the organization. The measurement focus of the balanced scorecard system accomplishes the following critical management processes:

- Clarifying and translating the organization's vision and strategy,
- Communicating and linking strategic objectives and measures,
- Planning,
- Target setting,

- Aligning of strategic initiatives,
- Enhancing strategic feedback, and
- Learning (Kaplan and Norton, 1996).

Clarifying and Translating the Vision and Strategy

The balanced scorecard process begins with senior leadership working together to establish the organization's strategy and translating these strategies to the unit/department level strategies. Indicators are selected based on those processes that are most critical for achieving breakthrough performance for customers and stakeholders. The process of building a balanced scorecard clarifies strategic objectives and defines the metrics used to assess performance (Kaplan and Norton, 1996).

Communicating and Linking

Exhibit 2–4 National Quality Forum's Framework of Nursing-Sensitive Performance Measures

Evidence-Based Performance Measures—Acute Care
1. Death among surgical inpatients with treatable serious complications (failure to rescue).
2. Pressure ulcer prevalence.
3. Falls prevalence.
4. Falls with injury.
5. Restraint prevalence.
6. Urinary catheter-associated urinary tract infection for intensive care unit (ICU) patients.
7. Central line catheter-associated blood stream infection rate for ICU and high-risk nursery patients.
8. Ventilator-associated pneumonia for ICU and HRN patients.
9. Smoking cessation counseling for acute myocardial infarction.
10. Smoking cessation counseling for heart failure.
11. Smoking cessation counseling for pneumonia.
12. Skill mix.
13. Nursing care hours per patient day.
14. Practice Environment Scale—Nursing Work Index (composite + five subscales).
15. Voluntary turnover.

Evidence-Based Performance Measures—Chronic Care
1. Residents whose need for more help with daily activities has increased.
2. Residents who experience moderate to severe pain.
3. Residents who were physically restrained during the seven-day assessment period.
4. Residents who spent most of their time in bed or in a chair in their room during the seven-day assessment period.
5. Residents with a decline in their ability to move about in their room or the adjacent corridor.
6. Residents with a urinary tract infection.
7. Residents with worsening of a depressed or anxious mood.

Modified from: www.qualityforum.org. (2004).

The balanced scorecard is communicated throughout the organization using multimedia systems such as bulletin boards, newsletters, videos, and intranet sites. All employees reach an understanding of the critical objectives that must be met for the organization's strategy to succeed. The scorecard provides a vehicle for enhancing communication and gaining commitment from units/departments to senior leaders. Dialogue is encouraged for breakthrough performance, not just short-term financial objectives. This enhanced communication and alignment of efforts and initiatives clarifies the unit/department and the organization's long-term goals and strategies for achieving the goals (Kaplan and Norton, 1996).

PLANNING, TARGET SETTING, AND ALIGNING

The greatest impact of the balanced scorecard is when it is deployed to drive organizational change. Stretch targets (meaning that although we have not yet achieved this, the goal is that we will reach the goal) are identified from customer expectations (both existing and potential customers should be queried), or from benchmarking with best practice peers. Once targets are set, managers align strategies to achieve breakthrough objectives. In addition, the balanced scorecard allows the organization to integrate strategic planning with the budgeting process. Both short-term and long-term targets are established, as well as the mechanisms and resources needed to accomplish these outcomes (Kaplan and Norton, 1996).

ENHANCING STRATEGIC FEEDBACK AND LEARNING

The final process of the balanced scorecard is the strategic learning framework. It is, perhaps, the most important and innovative aspect of the scorecard system. Monitoring allows for adjustments in strategy and, if necessary, fundamental changes to the strategy. Monthly and quarterly management reviews examine results—financial, customer, internal processes and innovation—for employees, systems, and procedures. Strategic learning continually occurs. Strategies for the information age must consider the turbulent environments, when senior leaders need feedback about complicated strategies. Planned strategies, though initiated with the best of intentions and with the best information available, may not be appropriate or valid for contemporary conditions (Kaplan and Norton, 1996).

Duke Children's Hospital (DCH) in Durham, North Carolina, touted their financial turnaround to be the result of implementation of a balanced scorecard system. Between 1993 and 1996 DCH's cost per case increased $4,389, while reimbursement declined, leading to a negative net margin in 1996 of $11 million dollars. During this same period, nurse productivity declined from the 80th percentile to the 70th percentile, while patient and staff satisfaction declined to record lows. Prompted by these events, the facility implemented a balanced scorecard system with the philosophy that clinical concerns did not take precedence over business concerns, nor did business concerns take precedence over clinical concerns. According to the project leader, the scorecard allowed senior leaders to realize new strategies to improve the business. The net margin rebounded from a $11 million dollar loss in 1996 to $4 million dollar gain in 2000. Cost per case decreased from $14,889 in 1996 to $10,500 in 2000. Likewise, nursing productivity improved from 71 percent in 1996 to 100 percent in 2000 (Health Care Advisory Board, "Balanced Scorecard Guides Duke

Children's Hospital to Financial Turnaround," 2001). DCH overcame resistance from both the medical (cookbook medicine) and hospital staff (power shift). Additional quantitative results include an 18 percent increase in customer satisfaction and a 1.8-day length of stay decrease from 1996 to 2000 (Health Care Advisory Board, "Harvard Business Review: Corporate Scorecard Model Helped Duke Children's Hospital Reverse Fortunes," 2000).

BALANCED SCORECARD EFFECTIVENESS

While much information and research is available regarding quality assurance/quality improvement tools and techniques, presently the major sources of literature on balanced scorecards are from the Health Care Advisory Board and the system's founders Kaplan and Norton. Intuitively (and by applying total quality management principles) the system is sound; however, the literature regarding quantifiable data or research on the topic is scant. The authors were unable to locate data regarding a cost-benefit analysis of the system.

The outlined implementation processes seem protracted in this day of rapid response time. On the other hand, the outline provides an excellent roadmap to assure the organization remains "on track." The system provides a framework for a health care organization's management processes—tying objectives with strategy, and providing a forum for communication throughout the organization. Overall, the balanced scorecard is a useful management tool for organizations now that we are in the information age.

Getting Further Out of the Box!

Change is occurring very fast these days. It is important to stay open to new information and to new ways of doing things to stay relevant. Our perspective is very important as we forge ahead. Thus we need to consider some other information.

Quantum Physics

> *Quantum* is defined as a 'discrete quantity of electromagnetic radiation.'... The science of quantum physics has demonstrated that our world actually occurs in very short, rapid bursts of light. What we believe we see as the swing of a baseball batter on home plate, for example, in quantum terms is actually a series of individual events that happen very fast and very close together. Similar to the many still images that make up a moving film, these events are actually tiny pulses of light called *quanta*. The quanta of our world occur so rapidly that although our eyes are capable of doing so, our minds do not discern individual bursts. Instead, the pulses are averaged together into what we see as one continuous event.... Quantum physics is the study of these minute units of radiating waves, *nonphysical* forces whose movements create our physical world (Braden, 2000, p. 96).

If it seems like this is getting *way out there*, this is really fairly old information that goes back to Albert Einstein's research leading the way into our present reality. And the research continues to identify more about our world.

So if our world is actually a series of energy fields, let's look at the world around us. It is, "A vast porridge of being where nothing is fixed or measurable…. [There are] dynamic patterns continually changing into one another—the continuous dance of energy…. The universe begins to look more like a great thought than like a great machine" (Wheatley, 1992, pp. 31–32).

This means that the energy fields can be affected by our thoughts. *Our thoughts create our reality*. This quantum physics research aligns with another source:

> That which is, already has been;
> That which is to be, already is.

> *Ecclesiastes 3:15*

Both sources present us with a different way of viewing our world. Going on with the idea that *our thoughts create our reality*, "that which is" was caused by the thought we previously had. "That which is to be," our present thought, "already is" because we are thinking it, and it will be what happens next.

So using this concept, what thoughts preceded our present reality? Do we actually have choices in our reality? How does this work? Let's go on with some additional research results:

> Under the right conditions, two atoms were occupying exactly the same place at precisely the same time! Until these studies were verified, such a phenomenon has been believed to be impossible. Now we know that it is not. The outcomes of our world at any given moment in time is made of people, machines, earth, and nature. At their most fundamental level, our outcomes are made of atoms. If two of the basic building blocks of our world *may coexist at the same instant*, [our emphasis] then the doorway has been opened for many atoms, resulting in many outcomes, to do the same…. Through our refined language of quantum science, we now have the vocabulary to describe precisely how we participate in determining the outcome of our future…. Quantum physics suggests that by redirecting our focus—where we place our attention—we bring a new course of events into focus while at the same time releasing an existing course of events that may no longer serve us (Braden, 2000, p. 26).

This means that our thoughts create our reality, and at each moment there *are several possibilities* all present that we can choose from.

If this is the case, we need to really be careful what we think about. For example, many of us worry, worry, worry. Worry—giving thought to bad or awful events—gives energy to the awful event, which then could become our reality. Conversely, when we think about some positive event, we give energy to the positive event becoming reality. Let's take this a step further.

What thoughts resulted in the monetary cutbacks we are experiencing in health care today? Are we so caught up in *scarcity* of resources (our thought) that we have created that reality? How often are we saying, "There is not enough money for health care?" Should we change this thought?

> Accounting and finance are applied areas of microeconomics. The theory of economics forms the foundations upon which all financial management is ultimately built. The essence of economics is that society has *a limited amount of resources*, [our emphasis] with competing demands for them. The economic system attempts to allocate those resources in an optimal fashion (Finkler and Kovner, 2000, p. 4).

Microeconomic theory encourages us to think our resources are limited. If we choose to believe this, our present reality is formed. So the question is, is this the reality that we want to create? ***Do we want to continue, like the ostrich with his head in the sand, with our present view of reality??*** It is something to ponder.

Let's consider another possible scenario for our present picture of health care. What if we substituted the word, *abundance*, for *scarcity*? Then our thoughts should create a different reality. We would have an abundance of resources, and would not have to compete for those resources. We would have an abundance of nurses or other health care givers. We can shun this idea… but what if it is true? We might be able to create a different, better reality. This might really result in better services for our patients/residents/clients, as well as a more satisfied workforce.

So, going on with our scenario, recently we have been involved with making budget cuts. What if we instead pictured that *there is enough money and enough staff to give the services needed*. Isn't that the reality that we would rather create?

Or take the argument that we cannot achieve quality when we have to make budget cuts. This thought means that we will get lowered quality (our patients will suffer) along with budget cuts. Is this what we really want? Are we stuck in that box too?

We can change this thought to thinking about how much fun it is to work toward achieving quality, and how rewarding it is when we feel we have achieved quality work. The choice is ours—and, according to quantum physics research—the outcome we think about happens.

Continuing this idea, we can choose to see our reality as a *difficult challenge*, or as an *opportunity* to create our future. The choice is ours.

It is interesting that positive affirmations have become a common occurrence in our present reality. Things such as, *I am in perfect health*, or *I accomplish _____ easily and effortlessly*. There are entire books (Hay, 1988) written on this subject. If one believes in affirmations, it is important to remember the "*do no harm*" clause in our nursing and medical professions as we live in a world of duality, i.e., good and evil, male and female, yin and yang, and so forth. After all, we need to be ethical about this.

Perhaps this further explains the mind-body connection discussed previously in this chapter.

Chaos Theory

> Chaos is an essential constituent of all change. It works to unbundle attachment to whatever is impeding movement. Chaos challenges us to simultaneously let go and to take on. It reminds us that life is a journey of constant creation (Porter-O'Grady and Malloch, 2003, p. 2).

Another scientific field of thought presently is *chaos theory*. Chaos theory offers hope for our future. In this theory the world seems chaotic all around us. However, when all this seeming chaos "is plotted over millions of iterations," it plots out a perfectly proportioned picture (see **Exhibit 2–5**). This offers great hope for us. Even when it seems like total chaos surrounds us, if we could rise above our present chaos and look down at it, there is order and perfection.

Sometimes when unexpected things happen, or when we have setbacks or experience difficult situations, it can be comforting to know that these experiences accomplish good things for us as well. We can learn from such situations and become better persons. In addition, these experiences can lead us to something different or new, that we probably would never have tried if the difficulties had not occurred.

When we think about planning change, chaos theory tells us that we cannot possibly plan, or map out, all the details of the plan because of chaotic occurrences. As these occurrences happen, they will necessitate a change in the plan. This is why all staff need to be

---

Exhibit 2–5 Three-Winged Bird: A Chaotic Strange Attractor

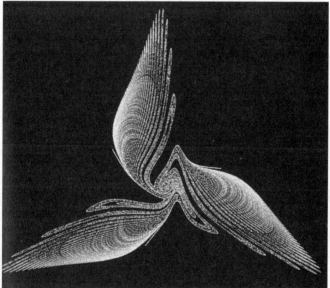

This is a self-portrait drawn by a chaotic system. The system's behavior is plotted over millions of iterations. The system appears to be wandering chaotically, always displaying new and different behavior. But over time, a deeper order—a shape—is revealed. This order is inherent to the system. It was always there, but not revealed until its chaotic movements were plotted in multiple dimensions over time.

From the work of Mario Markus and Bruno Hess, Max-Planck Institute, Dortmund, Germany. Used with permission.

From: Wheatley, M. (1999). *Leadership and the New Science: Discovering Order in a Chaotic World*, 2nd ed. San Francisco: Berrett-Koehler

involved in understanding the plan, and have to be empowered to accomplish it—because
the final product, or components of the final product, will ultimately be different in the
end. And really, there is no final product. Chaos will continue to change what was implemented. So we cannot rest on our laurels but need to continually move on into uncharted
territory.

Many of us (administrative leaders) do not understand this concept of constant change.
Instead we still buy into the Industrial Age idea that everything is rational and can be
planned out in minute detail, and that we can just order others to follow through on our
plan—and then get frustrated when people don't follow this to the letter. This is not reality. If we continue to believe this, we open ourselves up for a lot of unnecessary frustration, and the people that we supervise will be frustrated as well.

Instead, all of us need to be open to the reality around us, see the changes that are occurring, and help to interpret this for one another. For although we are all in our boxes (our
views of reality), if we do not pay attention to the chaotic reality that actually happens, the
changes will occur and leave us behind. We will become obsolete and unfulfilled.

> Leaders now must incorporate the vagaries of complexity and chaos into
> the process of anticipating and planning for the future. Detailing the
> specifics of some future state is no longer a viable means of planning.
> Discernment and signpost reading are better skills to have than are those
> related to defining and direction setting. Leaders must realize that no
> real-time insight is sustainable, nor is it entirely accurate. It is simply a
> reflection of the particular point a person or organization is at in their
> continuous and relentless unfolding and becoming.
>
> A good leader is one who can read the signposts suggesting that a
> change is imminent and can discern the direction of the change and the
> elements indicating its fabric. The good leader synthesizes rather than
> analyzes and views the change thematically and/or relationally, drawing
> out of it what kind of action or strategy should be applied—the response,
> that is, that best positions the organization to thrive in the coming cir-
> cumstances.
>
> For a leader to act as a strategist nowadays means not detailing the orga-
> nization's future actions, but translating the signposts of change into lan-
> guage that has meaning for those who must do the work of the organi-
> zation. Translating the signposts into understandable and inspiring lan-
> guage is more critical than almost any other strategic task. It is vital that
> a change have implications for those who are doing the work. Another
> way of saying this is that it must have meaning to them within the frame-
> work of their work activities so that they can commit to it, which they
> must do if they and the organization are to adapt to the change success-
> fully.
>
> In this new era, leaders need insights about contextual themes rather
> than step-by-step guidance on how to implement a minutely defined
> vision. They must understand that their organization is on a journey and

that they need to continuously peruse the landscape for guidance rather than create a list of steps through which the organization will move on its way to a preset future. Becoming aware of the themes and undercurrents and reading the contextual signposts regularly is a wiser and more effective strategy for the new age leader than laying out a itemized plan that may or may not correspond with future conditions (Porter-O'Grady and Malloch, 2003, pp. 23–24). (See **Exhibit 2–6**.)

Exhibit 2–6 Interdependence

In nature everything is interdependent. There is an ebb and flow between all the elements of life. Leaders must see their role from this perspective. Most of the work of leadership will be managing the interactions and connections between people and processes. Leaders must keep aware of these truths:

- Action in one place has an effect in other places.
- Fluctuation of mutuality means authority moves between people.
- Interacting properties in systems make outcomes mobile and fluid.
- Relationship building is the primary work of leadership.
- Trusting feeling is as important as valuing thinking.
- Acknowledging in others what is unique in their contribution is vital.
- Supporting, stretching, challenging, pushing, and helping are part of being present to the process, to the players, and to the outcome.

From: Porter-O'Grady, T., and Malloch, K. (2003). *Quantum Leadership: A Textbook of New Leadership*. Sudbury, MA: Jones and Bartlett, p. 22.

References

_____. (2000). Patient satisfaction: Survey profiles & demographics. *Hospitals & Health Services*.

Agency for Health Care Research and Quality. (1998, June 17). *The challenge and potential for assuring quality health care for the 21st century*. Retrieved October 27, 2002 from http://www.ahrq.gov/qual/21stcenc.htm.

Al-Assaf, A., & Schmele, J. (1993). *The textbook of total quality in healthcare*. Delray Beach, FL: St. Lucie Press.

Alexander, R. (October 2002). A mind for multicultural management: Foster an environment that celebrates patient diversity. *Nursing Management*, 30–34.

Baker, L., Reifsteck, S., & Mann, W. (March–April 2003). Connected: Communication skills for nurses using the electronic medical record. *Nursing Economic$, 21*(2), 85–88.

Bantz, D., Wieseke, A., & Horowitz, J. (March–April 1999). Perspectives of nursing executives regarding ethical-economic issues. *Nursing Economic$, 17*(2), 85–90.

Barnsteiner, J., & Prevost, S. (Second Quarter 2002). How to implement evidence-based practice: Some tried and true pointers. *Reflections on Nursing LEADERSHIP*, 18–21.

Barnum, B. (2003). *Spirituality in nursing: From traditional to new age*. 2nd ed. New York: Springer.

Brooke, P. (Winter 2002). Why incident reports are a must. *NSO Risk Advisor*, 4–5.

Bruck, J. (Jan. 1997). Eden. *Nursing Homes*, January 1997, pp. 29–32.

Buerhaus, P. (Third Quarter 1999). Lucian Leape on the causes and prevention of errors and adverse events in health care. *Image: Journal of Nursing Scholarship, 31*(3), 281–286.

The Business Roundtable. (1997, September). *Quality health care is good business: A survey of health care quality initiatives by members of The Business Roundtable.* Retrieved November 6, 2002 from http://www.businessroundtable.com.

Carpenter, D. (January 2003). Not-so-loony tunes. *Hospitals and Health Services Networks*, 24–25.

Chaiken, B. (May–June 2001). Enhancing patient safety with clinically intelligent physician order entry. *Nursing Economic$, 19*(3), 119–120.

Chapman, E. (2004). *Radical loving care: Building the healing hospital in America.* Nashville, TN: Baptist Healing Hospital Trust.

Collins, J., & Porras, J. (1994). *Built to last: Successful habits of visionary companies.* New York: Harper Business.

Committee on Quality of Health Care in America. (2001). *Crossing the quality chasm: A new health system for the 21st century.* Institute of Medicine.

Culhane-Pera, K., Vawter, D., Xiong, P., Babbitt, B., & Solberg, M. (2003). *Healing by heart: Clinical and ethical case stories of among families and western providers.* Nashville, TN: Vanderbilt University Press.

Dienemann, J., Ed. (1993). *Continuous quality improvement in nursing.* Washington, DC: American Nurses Publishing.

Dunham-Taylor, J., & Pinczuk, J. (2006). *Health care financial management for nurse managers: Applications from hospitals, long-term care, home care, and ambulatory care.* Sudbury, MA: Jones and Bartlett.

Edlich, R. (1997). *Medicine's deadly dust: A surgeon's wake-up call to society.* Clearwater, FL: Vandamere.

Finkler, S. (2001). Accountability and control. In *Financial Management for Public, Health, and Not-For-Profit Organizations* (pp. 221–226), Upper Saddle River, NJ: Prentice-Hall.

Finkler, S., & Kovner, C. (2000). *Financial management for nurse managers and executives.* 2nd ed. Philadelphia: W. B. Saunders.

Gerteis, M., Edgman-Levitan, S., Daley, J., & Delbanco, T. (1993). *Through the patients' eyes: Understanding and promoting patient-centered care.* San Francisco: Jossey-Bass.

Giger, J., & Davidhizar, E. (2004). *Transcultural nursing: Assessment and intervention.* 4th ed. New York: Mosby.

Goldsmith, S. (1994). *Essentials of long-term care administration.* Gaithersburg, MD: Aspen.

Gray, J. (1992). *Men are from mars, women are from venus.* New York: HarperCollins.

Grayson, M. (October 2002). Forward motion. *Hospital and Health Services Networks*, 34–38.

Guidelines on Reporting Incompetent, Unethical, or Illegal Practice. (1994). Washington, DC: American Nurses Publishing.

Guide to Clinical Preventive Services. 2nd ed. (1996). Washington, DC: American Nurses Publishing.

Hansten, R., & Washburn, M. (July 1999). Seven steps to shift from tasks to outcomes. *Nursing Management*, 25–27.

Harris, M. (1997). *Handbook of home health care administration*. 2nd ed. Gaithersburg, MD: Aspen.

Haugh, R. (April 2000). To the rescue: New tools to prevent medical errors are on the market. Why aren't more hospitals buying it? *Hospital & Health Networks*, 44–48.

Hay, L. (1988). *Heal your body*. Carson, CA: Hay House, Inc.

Health Care Advisory Board. (1999 August). *Balanced scorecards*. Retrieved November 9, 2002 from http://www.advisory.com.

Health Care Advisory Board. (2000 December). *Harvard business review: Corporate scorecard model helped Duke Children's Hospital reverse fortunes*. Retrieved November 9, 2002 from http://www.advisory.com.

Health Care Advisory Board. (2001 August). *Balanced scorecard guides Duke Children's Hospital to financial turnaround*. Retrieved November 9, 2002 from http://www.advisory.com.

Health Care Advisory Board. (2002). *Current conditions require vigilant performance monitoring*. Retrieved November 9, 2002 from http://www.advisory.com.

Health Care Advisory Board. (2002). *#1 metric balance avoids the vulnerability of narrow focus*. Retrieved November 9, 2002 from http://www.advisory.com.

Health Care Advisory Board. (2002). *#2 'metric austerity' ensures big picture awareness*. Retrieved November 9, 2002 from http://www.advisory.com.

Health Care Advisory Board. (2002). *#3 Graphic display facilitates prompt recognition of trends*. Retrieved November 9, 2002 from http://www.advisory.com.

Health Care Advisory Board. (2002). *Poor performance measurement can drive financial crisis*. Retrieved November 9, 2002 from http://www.advisory.com.

Heim, P. (1996). *Gender Differences in the Workplace Series*. Videotapes produced by Cynosure Productions, LTD. and KTEH, Channel 54, San Jose, California.
  • The Power Dead Even Rule
  • Invisible Rules: Men, Women and Teams
  • Conflict: the Rules of Engagement
  • Changing The Rules

Herzlinger, R. E., & Nitterhouse, D. (1994). *Financial accounting and managerial control for nonprofit organizations*. Cincinnati, OH: South-Western Publishing.

Hill, P., Lipson, J., & Meleis, A. (2003). *Caring for women cross-culturally*. Philadelphia: F.A. Davis.

Hoppszallern, S. (2001). Patient satisfaction survey. *Hospitals and Health Networks*.

Hunt, V. (1993). *The Human Energy Field and Health*. Videotape produced by Malibu Publishing Company, P.O. Box 4234, Malibu, CA 90264.

Hypnar, L., & Anderson, L. (November 2001). Attaining superior outcomes with joint replacement patients. *JONA, 31*(11), 544–549.

Implementing Nursing's Report Card: A Study of RN Staffing, Length of Stay and Patient Outcomes. (1997). Washington DC: American Nurses Publishing.

_____. (July 12, 2000). Fatal falls: Lessons for the Future. *JCAHO Sentinel Event ALERT*, 14.

Jennings, B., & Staggers, N. (Fall 1999). A provocative look at performance measurement. *Nursing Administration Quarterly*, *24*(1), 17–30.

Johnson, C. (April 2000). We made a mistake: Caregivers and administrators bring medication errors out in the open—especially with patients. *Nursing Management, 31*(4), 22–24.

Kaplan, R. S., & Norton, D. P. (1996). *Translating strategy into action: The balanced scorecard*. Boston: Harvard Business School.

Kelly, J. (October 2002). Equal Access for All. *Hospitals and Health Services Networks*, 24.

Knollmueller, R. (1994). *Prevention Across the Life Span*. Washington, DC: American Nurses Publishing.

Kohn, L., Corrigan, J., & Donaldson, M. (2000). *To err is human: Building a safer health system*. National Academy Press.

Lighter, D., & Fair, D. (2000). *Principles and methods of quality management in health care*. Gaithersburg, MD: Aspen.

Lopez-Bushnell, K. (November 2002). Get research-ready. *Nursing Management*, 41–44.

Maddox, P. (May–June 2001). Update on national quality of care initiatives. *Nursing Economic$, 19*(3), 121–124.

Marino, G., Reinhardt, K., Eichelberger, W., & Steingard, R. (2000). Prevalence of errors in a pediatric hospital medication system: Implications for error proofing. *Outcomes Management for Nursing Practice, 4*(3), 129–135.

Marino, B., & Ganser, C. (April 1997). Sensitivity of patient report of care to organizational change. *JONA*, *27*(4), 32–36.

Markey, D., & Brown, R. (2002). An interdisciplinary approach to addressing patient activity and mobility in medical-surgical patient. *Journal of Nursing Care Quality, 16*(4), 1–12.

McCue, M., Mark, B., & Harless, D. (Summer 2003). Nurse staffing, quality, and financial performance. *Journal of Health Care Finance, 29*(4), 54–76.

Meisenheimer, C. (1997). *Improving quality: A guide to effective programs*. 2nd ed. Gaithersburg, MD: Aspen.

Moyers, B. (1993). *Healing and the Mind*. (Five Videocassettes). WNET of New York.

Murphy, E. (March 2000). The patient room of the future. *Hospitals and Health Services Networks*, 38–39.

Murray, M. (January–February 2001). Outcomes of concurrent utilization review. *Nursing Economic$*, 19(1), 17–23.

Nance, J. (March 19, 2001). *Enhancing Patient Safety Through Teamwork Solutions!* American Organization of Nurse Executives Annual Meeting. (Audiotape available from National Nursing Network, 4465 Washington Street, Denver, CO 80216.)

The National Academy of Sciences, Institute of Medicine. (1990). *Medicare: A strategy for quality assurance, volume 1*. Retrieved November 4, 2002 from http://nap.edu/openbook/0309042305/html/1.html.

Nooner, K. (May 2004). Bouncing patients? Capacity issues and diversion status toy with efficient throughput. *Nursing Management, 35*(5), 39–44.

Nurse Staffing and Patient Outcomes in the Inpatient Hospital Setting. (2000). Washington, DC: American Nurses Publishing.

Nursing Quality Indicators: Guide for Implementation. 2nd ed. (1999). Washington, DC: American Nurses Publishing.

Nursing Quality Indicators Beyond Acute Care: Literature Review. (2000). Washington, DC: American Nurses Publishing.

Nursing Quality Indicators Beyond Acute Care: Measurement Instruments. (2000). Washington, DC: American Nurses Publishing.

Ohio Hospital Statewide Financial Performance. (2003). *Vital $igns: Indicators of Ohio hospital financial viability.* Columbus, OH: Ohio Hospital Association.

_____. (March–April 2000). "Patient Compliance." *Nursing Economic$, 18*(2), 90.

Pointe, P., Conlin, G., Conway, J., Grant, S., Medeiros, C., Nies, J., Shulman, L., Branowicki, P., & Conley, K. (February 2003). Making patient-centered care come alive: Achieving full integration of the patient's perspective. *JONA, 33*(2), 82–90.

Porter-O'Grady, T. (March–April 2003). Of hubris and hope: Tralnsforming nursing for a new age. *Nursing Economic$, 21*(2), 59–64.

Porter-O'Grady, T., & Malloch, K. (2003). *Quantum leadership: A textbook of new leadership.* Sudbury, MA: Jones and Bartlett Publishers.

Powell, S. K. (2000). *Case management: A practical guide to success in managed care.* 2nd ed. Baltimore: Lippincott.

Public Health Nursing: A Partner for Healthy Populations. (2000). Washington, DC: American Nurses Publishing.

Pugliese, G., & Salahuddin, M. Ed. (1999). *Sharps injury prevention program: A step-by-step guide.* Chicago: American Hospital Association.

Purnell, L., & Paulanka, B. (2003). *Transcultural health care: A culturally competent approach.* 2nd ed. Philadelphia: F.A.Davis.

Quantifying the Conventional Wisdom: Rank Ordering the Cost of Complications. (2000). The Advisory Board Company.

Rantz, M. (1995). *Nursing quality measurement: A review of nursing studies.* Washington, DC: American Nurses Publishing.

Robbins, D. (1996). *Ethical and legal issues in home health and long-term care.* Gaithersburg, MD: Aspen.

Rudy, E., Lucke, J., Whitman, G., & Davidson, L. (Second Quarter 2001). Benchmarking patient outcomes. *Journal of Nursing Scholarship, 33*(2), 185–189.

Sarudi, D. (April 2001). Keeping patients safe. *Hospitals & Health Networks*, 42–46.

Sarudi, D. (May 2001). The leapfrog effect. *Hospitals & Health Networks*, 32–36.

Scope and Standards of Home Health Nursing Practice. (1999). Washington, DC: American Nurses Publishing.

Scope and Standards for Nurse Administrators. (1996). Washington, DC: American Nurses Publishing.

Scope and Standards of Advanced Practice Registered Nursing. (1996). Washington, DC: American Nurses Publishing.

Scope and Standards of College Health Nursing Practice. (1997). Washington, DC: American Nurses Publishing.

Scope and Standards of Diabetes Nursing (written in collaboration with the American Association of Diabetes Educators). (1998). Washington, DC: American Nurses Publishing.

Scope and Standards of Forensic Nursing Practice (written in collaboration with the International Association of Forensic Nurses). (1997). Washington, DC: American Nurses Publishing.

Scope and Standards of Nursing Practice in Correctional Facilities. (1995). Washington, DC: American Nurses Publishing.

Scope and Standards of Parish Nursing Practice (written in collaboration with Health Ministries Association, Inc. (1998). Washington, DC: American Nurses Publishing.

Scope and Standards of Pediatric Oncology Nursing (Written in collaboration with the Association of Pediatric Oncology Nurses). (2000). Washington, DC: American Nurses Publishing.

Scope and Standards of Practice for Nursing Professional Development. (2000). Washington, DC: American Nurses Publishing.

Scope and Standards of Psychiatric-Mental Health Nursing Practice (written in collaboration with the American Psychiatric Nurses Association and the International Society of Psychiatric-Mental Health Nurses). (2000). Washington, DC: American Nurses Publishing.

Scope of Practice for Nursing Informatics. (1994). Washington, DC: American Nurses Publishing.

Shindul-Rothschild, J., Berry, D., & Long-Middleton, E. (November 1996). Where have all the nurses gone? Final results of our patient care survey. *American Journal of Nurses, 96*(11), 25–39.

Silva, M. (1995). *Annotated bibliography for ethical guidelines.* Washington, DC: American Nurses Publishing.

Silva, M. (1995). *Ethical guidelines in the conduct, dissemination, and implementation of nursing research.* Washington, DC: American Nurses Publishing.

Simpson, R. (June 2000). Medical errors, airplanes, and information technology. *Nursing Management, 31*(6), 14–15.

St. Hill, P., Lipson, J., & Neleis, A. (2003). *Caring for women cross-culturally.* Philadelphia, PA: F.A. Davis.

Standards of Addictions Nursing Practice with Selected Diagnoses and Criteria. (1987). Washington, DC: American Nurses Publishing.

Standards of Clinical Nursing Practice. 2nd ed. (1998). Washington, DC: American Nurses Publishing.

Standards of Clinical Practice and Scope of Practice for the Acute Care Nurse Practitioner (written in collaboration with the American Association of Critical-Care Nurses). (1995). Washington, DC: American Nurses Publishing.

Statement on the Scope and Standards for the Nurse Who Specializes in Developmental Disabilities and/or Mental Retardation (written in collaboration with the Nursing Division of the American Association on Mental Retardation). (1998). Washington, DC: American Nurses Publishing.

Statement on the Scope and Standards of Genetics Clinical Nursing Practice. (1998). Washington, DC: American Nurses Publishing.

Statement on the Scope and Standards of Oncology Nursing Practice (written in collaboration with the Oncology Nursing Association). (1996). Washington, DC: American Nurses Publishing.

Statement on the Scope and Standards of Otorhinolaryngology Clinical Nursing Practice (written in collaboration with the Society of Otorhinolaryngology and Head-Neck Nurses, Inc.). (1994). Washington, DC: American Nurses Publishing.

Statement on the Scope and Standards of Pediatric Clinical Nursing Practice (written in collaboration with the Society of Pediatric Nurses). (1996). Washington, DC: American Nurses Publishing.

Statement on the Scope and Standards of Respiratory Nursing Practice. (1994). Washington, DC: American Nurses Publishing.

Stone, P., Curran, C., & Bakken, S. (Third Quarter 2002). Economic evidence for evidence-based practice. *Journal of Nursing Scholarship, 34*(3), 277–282.

Stutts, A. (June 2001). Developing innovative care models: The use of customer satisfaction scores. *JONA, 31*(6), 293–300.

Take Control: A Guide to Risk Management. (1998). Washington, DC: American Nurses Publishing.

The Scope and Standards of Public Health Nursing Practice. (1999). Washington, DC: American Nurses Publishing.

Tannen, D. (1990). *You just don't understand: Women and men in conversation*. New York: Ballantine Books.

Targ, R., & Katra, J. (1998). *Miracles of mind: Exploring nonlocal vonsciousness and spiritual healing*. Novato, CA: New World Library.

Thomas, W. (1996). *Life worth living. How someone you love can still enjoy life in a nursing home: The eden alternative in action*. Acton, MA: VanDerWyk & Burnham.

Ubel, P., Dekay, M., Baron, J., & Asch, D. (May 2, 1996). Cost-effectiveness analysis in a setting of budget constraints: Is it equitable? *The New England Journal of Medicine*, 1174–1177.

Uustal, D. (1993). *Clinical ethics and values: Issues and insights*. Jamestown, RI: Educational Resources In HealthCare, Inc.

Van Servellen, G., & Schultz, M. (April 1999). Demystifying the influence of hospital characteristics on inpatient mortality rates. *JONA, 29*(4), 39–47.

Veatch, R., & Fry, S. (1987). *Case studies in nursing ethics*. Philadephia: Lippincott.

Wakefield, M., & Maddox, P. (March–April 2000). Patient quality and safety problems in the US health care system: Challenges for nursing. *Nursing Economic$, 18*(2), 58–62.

Walton, M. (1986). *The deming management method*. New York: Perigee Books.

Watson, J. (2004). *Postmodern nursing and beyond*. New York: Elsevier.

White, G. (1993). *Ethical dilemmas in contemporary nursing practice*. Washington, DC: American Nurses Publishing.

Wheatley, M. (1992). *Leadership and the new science*. San Francisco: Berrett-Koehler.

Windemuth, D. S. (1994). *Total quality management: Using cost accounting techniques in the total quality-management framework*. In S. Finkler (Ed.), Issues in cost accounting for health care organizations (pp. 269–274), Gaithersburg, MD: Aspen.

Woods, A., & Doan-Johnson, S. (October 2002). Executive summary: Toward a taxonomy of nursing practice errors. *Nursing Management*, 45–48.

Wroblewski, M., Werrbach, K., & Fattuso, M. (September 1999). Nurses gain more time with patients. *Nursing Management, 30*(9), 35–36.

CHAPTER 3

Quantum Leadership: Love One Another

Janne Dunham-Taylor, PhD, RN

Why have a chapter on leadership in a financial book? Because if there is poor leadership at any level of the organization, it will cost the organization extra money—and it can be CONSIDERABLE budget dollars. Direct financial effects of poor leadership include decreased satisfaction levels from patients and their families, staff, physicians, and from other interdisciplinary team members. This results in fewer patients wanting to come back, higher staff turnover, and disgruntled physicians. Then there are the indirect effects—more unsafe situations, more patient complications, and more legal issues. All this DRAMATI-CALLY effects the bottom line. Thus it is very important to pay attention to the quality of the leadership at all levels in an organization.

> Leadership is a journey. It is not a trip, with an identifiable destination and triptiks to keep you on the right road. A journey unfolds gradually. It meanders. You stop and start, take side roads, get bogged down. You meet travel companions and sometimes stay with friends for a while. A journey is not predictable, even though there may be an end goal. On a journey, the process of getting there is part of the overall goal.... Our leadership journeys are only at midpoint when we have achieved a position of power. The second half of the leadership journey comes once we pass age thirty-five; it is then that we have the opportunity to lead from our souls... Soul leadership begins to emerge when we find our existing leadership style less rewarding, less satisfying than it was; when we must either shift to the inner leadership journey or recycle to an earlier leadership style which is more comfortable and predictable.
>
> [Soul leadership] is not about skill development, it is about facing fear, letting go of control, gaining self-worth and inner strength, finding inner freedom and moral passion—the things you learn only after you think you know it all. This journey takes you to your core, including your dark core (shame, fear of abandonment, rage), wherein lies the raw power of transformation. It is not an easy journey, and the goal is not to be successful in the traditional sense; it is to be faithful to the journey itself. The only requirement is courage (Hagberg, 1994, p. 227).

So What Is Good Leadership Anyway?

Love one another.

This is such a simple concept, yet is something that we may work at for a lifetime and still be able to do it better! This is what soul leadership is all about, for *love* needs to permeate everything we do. Love dissolves conflicts. We feel better when we are loved and when we are loving. Victor Frankl discusses this in his book, *Man's Search for Meaning*, written as he experienced a concentration camp during World War II: "Then I grasped the meaning of the greatest secret that human poetry and human thought and belief have to impart: The salvation of man is through love and in love" (p. 57).

It is such a simple statement yet so complex to implement every moment of our lives.

The word, *love*, has different meanings for different people. The way we mean it here is defined as follows:

> Far from being irrelevant or impractical, the intention to express love is fundamental for effective leadership. This is so because in the final analysis, a leader's motivation is communicated to others in countless subtle ways. Leaders whose actions are perceived as self-serving often create disharmony, resentment, and disloyalty. On the other hand, those who base their behavior upon a genuine empathy and concern for others can gain loyalty and support that make the attainment of even difficult goals possible.
>
> Actually, although love occupies such an important place in everyone's thoughts, it is often misunderstood. Love is more than an agreeable feeling or a pleasurable sensation derived from the contact of physical bodies. Frequently, what people call love is either sentimentality or the pursuit of carnal pleasures. This means that for many, what passes for love may actually be nothing other than self-centeredness or lust....
>
> This does not necessarily mean that events proceed gently and smoothly. Activities that manifest mature love are performed in a spirit of truthfulness and knowledge. Although truth can be painful, sometimes the desire to attain a higher good will require leaders to face unpleasant realities and act forcefully. Indeed, love is merely sentimental unless it is based on honesty. Leaders need a high level of knowledge, skill and discernment to express their love appropriately according to the circumstances.
>
> Therefore, although love is sometimes soft, it can also be harsh. At times, a leader may demand difficult sacrifices from others for their own well-being. In either case—whether one's actions appear gentle or brutal—the important factor is always the motivation. A leader whose behavior is inspired by selflessness acts just like a mother who sometimes shows love by punishing her children in order to help them develop properly. Leaders must deliberately choose to maintain a level of consciousness that gives priority to what is best for others regardless of outward appearances....

One way to develop mature love is to see each person as a part of God, dear to Him and under His watchful eye....

You cannot love others if you do not sufficiently love yourself, because azit is impossible to give or share what you do not possess.... Love of self does not mean love of the body or of the mind, but of the soul.

Loving activities are in harmonoy with the universe. Those who are out of harmony with the universe draw negativity to themselves, whereas those who are in harmony act in constructive and fruitful ways, protected from harm.

In the course of your duties as a leader, you constantly fact pitfalls and dangers. To ensure your success, you can learn to protect yourself against the onslaughts of negative thoughts and actions. Not only is it important for you to think and act in a dynamic, positive way, but you should also be conscious of potentially harmful people and situations in order to avoid their invasive negative energy. Your most powerful shield of protection in these circumstances will come from a strong sense of love and compassion.

... You should remember that you are called to love your neighbor as well. All of the major religions of the world emphasize this point:

- Brahmanism: Do not do unto others that which would cause you pain if done to yourself.
- Buddhism: Hurt not others in ways that you yourself would possibly find hurtful.
- Christianity: Do unto others as you would have them do unto you.
- Islam: Not one of you is a true believer until he desires for his brother that which he desires for himself.
- Judaism: Whatever is hateful to you, do not do to your fellow man.
- Zoroastrianism: That nature alone is good which refrains from doing unto another anything that is not good for itself.
- Taoism: Always regard your neighbor's gain as your gain, and your neighbor's loss as your own loss.

... As you use what you have wisely, committing your leadership to the service of others, you will surely benefit. However, the converse is also true. If you do not properly use the resources and position that you have, then even if you temporarily live "well," eventually you will be brought down by those you lead as they realize that you do not have their best interests at heart.

... Learn to love everybody dearly and allow this love for others to radiate through you. As you let the energy of love vibrate around you, all who align themselves with you will contract this contagious, sublime state, and spread it enthusiastically to others (Krishnapada, pp. 17–24).

Our present research gives us some other clues about love. Based on a quantum perspective, we are all interconnected. Each small effort we make is linked with the whole global system. As a nurse administrator provides effective leadership, the quantum view is that this energy combines with the energy of other leaders around the globe—all contributing to an improvement of man's condition and the earth as a whole.

Although this may sound rather far-fetched, it is actually based upon 20th century research that Margaret Wheatley describes in her book, *Leadership and The New Science*. Wheatley presents current scientific thought in an understandable way, and applies this to leadership and organizations:

> Changes in small places... affect the global system... because every small system participates in an unbroken wholeness. Activities in one part of the whole create effects that appear in distant places. Because of these unseen connections, there is potential value in working anywhere in the system. We never know how our small activities will affect others through the invisible fabric of our connectedness (Wheatley, p. 45).

One example of the quantum view is exemplified by the Berlin wall. It came down even though the powers that be did not want this to occur. Local efforts—and other similar energies around the world—combined until they were finally strong enough to tumble the wall, even though the government officials wanted the wall to remain. Think of the possibilities that confront us; think of what we could do to improve our world as we know and experience it.

Our interconnectedness also affects each of us. It is reflected in energy fields flowing both through us and all around us. Each of us bumps into and merges with others' energy fields:

> Human beings live in a cosmic river of flowing energy. Everything is energy. All energy is in motion, whether or not that motion is perceptible to the lower, gross human senses of sight, smell, touch, taste, or hearing. The rate at which the energy moves determines one's ability to perceive it: The slower the movement, the more it is perceptible to the physical senses.
>
> Energy is composed of light—the light that emanates from God. Light is at the heart of matter, residing inside every atom. When modern scientists were finally able to split the atom, what they unleashed was the tremendous power of light. As particles of light, atoms vibrate at different speeds, creating electrical charges that cause them to bind together into molecules. Among these molecules, those moving at slower rates of speed join with one another to form what people perceive as the material world....
>
> This energetic composition of reality helps explain how everything is one. For example, the cosmic river of flowing energy is what allows the thoughts of one person to be transmitted to someone in another location... It enables a loving mother to "know" that her child is in danger, even when the two of them are apart.

Because this energy—also known as prana, mana, chi, or ki—encompasses everything that exists, it is inexhaustible. The very air people breathe is filled with it, and the entire universe can be considered an electrical energy grid that conducts these energies. In this view, a person's energies travel across this grid like sound waves, having an effect on various other energies as they move, and then "bouncing back" in kind....

Much of this energy takes the form of thoughts, words, and deeds. Although people can easily perceive their words and actions and frequently observe their impact, they may be tempted to believe that their thoughts have no effect. However, they would be mistaken. Although invisible to the naked eye, thoughts are things. They are individual electrical entities that group themselves with similar energy to form clusters. They are real; they are substantive; and they are a force that everyone can learn to balance and control.

In addition to these fundamental forms of energy, people generate less obvious types of energy that are nonetheless major influences upon the world around them. These include: emotional energy, such as guilt, anger, fear, hate, jealousy or envy; sexual energy, which is so powerful that one must use it extremely carefully; physical energy, the force that enables people "to move mountains;" and love energy which, in its pure and selfless state, is the most powerful force in the universe. Human beings may also be influenced by other energies that many consider to be "concepts," including, for example, truth, justice or compassion. These energies vibrate at extremely high rates because they are derived from divine principles....

Energy has two important characteristics that make it possible for people to direct and control it effectively. First, energy is impartial, nonresistant and totally malleable to individual desires.... The intent,... is what determines this vibratory level, rather than the ultimate outcome of one's actions.... A second characteristic of energy is that it cannot be destroyed, only transformed. When a skyscraper burns to the ground, apparently destroyed, in reality the fire has simply returned the building's materials to their original elements—such as carbon or hydrogen—or changed them into newly formed substances called soot and ashes. Any remaining energy has either recombined with energies existing in the surrounding air, water or land, or returned to the universal energy pool as uncombined energy. Energy can also be accumulated, moved, gathered and stored, transmitted, dissipated, shattered, released, transmuted or balanced.

Nothing exists unless it is sustained by thought. Therefore, the easiest way to control and manipulate energies is by thought processes. People can control their words and actions simply by changing the way they think, recognizing that "as a man thinketh, so shall he be." The biblical story of Job is an excellent example of the law of thought in operation. Unfortunately, Job worked the law against himself, not realizing that each calamity he worried about manifested because he had created it in his mind.

Worry is a prayer for something one does not want. To avoid an undesirable outcome, people can learn to control their thoughts, especially when they are under stress and have an emotional investment in a desired outcome. At such times, stress and emotions represent thought energy fueling the creation of the image being held in their minds. Instead of worrying, one can replace the negative thought with a visual image of the desired outcome, and then help that image manifest rather than the unwanted one. As people get into the habit of energizing only the positive, their thoughts, words, and actions will automatically reflect this higher state of mind....

One of the most obvious, but perhaps least recognized, ways that people handle energy is to accumulate it in their physical bodies instead of releasing it. Stagnant, unreleased emotional energy can eventually have a harmful effect. These energies are dense, vibrating at a level too low to be processed by the highly efficient physical body. As a result, they become blocked and crystallized, manifesting at best as diminished stamina or decreased mobility, and at worst as disease. Such energies can be released through methods such as forgiveness, prayer, or meditation, or through conscious transmutation [To transmute simply means "to change or alter in form, appearance or nature"] (Krishnapada, pp. 47–51).

This concept is introduced in a wonderful, entertaining book, *Zapp! Empowerment in Health Care* (Byham, 1996). In this book—written as a novel—as certain events occur, a nurse manager begins to realize that specific interactions sap the energy of the people involved, while people become energized by other interactions (zapp). It provides an actual example of true empowerment, which is described later in this chapter.

The quantum view of leadership is a dynamic process that varies with different groups of people. No leader is the same. No group is the same. What works well with one group will fail abysmally in another. However, there are certain landmarks, such as *Love one another*, that every leader needs to observe to be effective, regardless of how each person implements leadership or love.

Dynamic leadership involves seeing the whole and understanding how we fit in it. For instance, in quantum leadership the organization is a flexible whole, ever changing, both internally and externally. The people we serve—and their needs—change; we change, our work group changes; the community changes; and societal expectations change. Our work is fluid and ever-changing. *Everyone we come in contact with is a valuable resource, necessitating our need to change to accomplish the best outcomes*. There is always more to do to make things better. Staff, physicians, and patients are equitable and accountable partners with administrators. They can think of better ways to do things, or have new ideas that never occurred to the administrator. All are leaders. Each has definite things to do that benefit everyone else—and that will not be done by anyone else. All need to be empowered to go ahead with the work, while supporting the core values (as discussed in the next section).

In fact, *dynamic leadership is needed from every person on earth*. Leadership occurs at all levels in an organization—from the patient or housekeeper to the board chairperson. Patients and their families are leaders as they make decisions about what they need and want. Housekeepers are leaders as they perform various cleaning activities. Staff nurses are leaders as they determine priorities and provide care to patients.

We have many practices in health care that do not encourage patient leadership, such as having to wear hospital gowns, setting visiting hour limitations, or automatically putting heavy patients on 800 calorie diets at a time when they are experiencing a health crisis and have not chosen to lose weight. It is important to think about how our decisions and policies either limit or enhance patient autonomy, and thus, patient leadership.

Leadership Fallacies

Leadership fallacies can negatively affect leadership effectiveness. Fallacies, as shown in **Exhibit 3–1**, are traps that cause us to get derailed or become less effective. Once understood, fallacies can be overcome and our leadership will improve.

Perhaps it is best to start with our language, which can enhance or detract from our leadership effectiveness. There are a few words—popular in current business journals—that do not support quantum leadership. The terms *"subordinate"* and *"superior"* indicate that one person is better than another. The authors recommend that an effective leader never use such terms. Each person in an organization has gifts and abilities that will benefit everyone else. The housekeeper is just as important as the CEO. After all, if the wastebaskets are not emptied and the bathrooms not cleaned properly, we all suffer. Everyone uses leadership to more effectively accomplish their work. In this book, even when quoting other authors from the business journals that use these terms, we have substituted the terms *"staff"* and *"supervisor, administrator, or boss"* for *subordinate* and *superior*.

Another example of problematic language is to call everyone *my* staff, or *girls/boys/kids*. In the first case, although we all might be in the same work group, no one belongs to anyone else, including the leader. In the second case, it is demeaning to call someone by a child title. This indicates that we do not think they are capable adults. We enhance this concept in the nursing profession when we use such expressions as "girls" implying that staff are little children, have not yet grown up, and need parenting. However, in an effective organization staff at all levels are leaders.

Another word commonly used in business literature is *"control,"* such as the span of control of a manager. In fact, according to some of the management literature, a managerial function is "control." Control is a myth. We suggest not using this term. After all, controlling ourselves is hard enough! Think of our inability to turn down a wonderful dessert full of sugar and lots of calories. How well do we *really* control *ourselves*? It is a fallacy

Exhibit 3–1 Leadership Fallacies

Leadership Fallacies	Replace By
Subordinate and *superior* are appropriate labels for people within organizations, as are *my* staff and *girls*, *boys*, *kids*.	Language can enhance effectiveness. Use the words *staff; supervisor or administrator;* and *women* or *men*.
Control is a component of effective leadership.	Control of others is impossible. Staff are equitable and accountable partners in the work.
Patients are described as being *noncompliant*.	What about the patient's point of view?
The administrators are the leaders while other staff are followers.	Everyone is a leader.
Leaders have inborn qualities. It cannot be learned.	Leadership can be learned by anyone. It has more to do with our gifts and life purpose.
Leadership is better than management.	Actually we need a combination to effectively accomplish work. The problem occurs when someone is predominantly transactional, not taking into account other's perceptions, ideas, knowledge, and relationships.
The leader, or CEO, has all the answers.	We have some of the answers, but other answers will come from other people around us—including those reporting to the leader.
When everyone is empowered and there is effective leadership, the result is peace and harmony.	Actually the result is that not everyone agrees. Conflicts occur necessitating dialogue to work through issues. Better solutions result.
There is one right way to do the work.	There are many ways that are effective.
What works well in one group will work well in another.	People are different and thus groups of people differ as well. What could work effectively with one group might not work with another.
Administrators strive to have everyone like them.	This is not possible. A better goal is that everyone *respects* the administrator because the administrator consistently supports the core value.
Effective leaders always use a participative leadership style, involving staff in every decision.	There are times, such as in an emergency, when being participative is not an effective method. In this case someone must make a decision quickly.
A leader must always win.	This is not humanly possible.
Claim another person's idea or work as one's own.	Integrity is important. Give credit where credit is due.
Do not want staff to outshine oneself or are threatened by more competent people.	Competent staff increase a leader's effectiveness, and make the work group look more effective.

Leaders do not fear anything.	It is important to recognize our fears and deal with them.
Charisma is an essential aspect of leadership.	The core values are the essential part of leadership.
Our leadership is perfect; the problems are caused by everyone else's behaviors.	Our actions may be causing the problem. Thus we always need to examine whether we are contributing to the problem.
We have always done it this way.	The only constant is change.
We think we are better than others because of our administrative title or our degree.	Everyone is equally important.
Pursue one's own selfish agendas.	Think about how each action affects others.
Gender or race bias issues can contribute to erroneous decisions.	It is better to base our assessment of others based on their gifts and contributions.
Successful managers/people are promoted before effective managers/people.	Effective managers/people do a better job.
A manager who politicks regularly with the supervisor is effective.	The supervisor needs to always do regular rounds to determine manager effectiveness.

to think that we control others. Dictators have tried—and continue to try—but no one has achieved it. After all, a controlling manager is an ineffective one. We suggest a better word for control is the word *responsibilities*. We could list a manager's responsibilities rather than saying span of control.

Another problematic term used in health care in "*noncompliance*." Most often we say that patients are noncompliant, meaning that the patient did not follow our treatment regimen. This can be a serious problem, especially when a patient starts an antibiotic, feels better, and stops taking it before the prescribed time is completed. But the use of this term also smacks of saying, "Do this *my* way." What about the patient's point of view? Was this considered before deciding what treatment regimen to use?

Another misconception people can get from the business literature is the implication that the administrators (especially CEOs) are the leaders, all others being followers. In reality staff need to be leaders as well.

There is a question by some as to whether leadership can be learned. Some say that leaders have inborn qualities that cannot be taught to others. However, leadership can be learned, and we can always improve our leadership, regardless of inborn leadership qualities. This learning can happen serendipitiously but can happen in infinite ways as we experience life. Mentoring has become so popular because we can learn from effective leaders who feel a special affinity to help us learn more about the role. The more important point here is that each of us has certain gifts. If we pay attention to the gifts, we can be leaders in those areas. This is not to say that everyone should be an administrator. There are some people who are very unhappy in the administrative role because it is not a match with their gifts.

Another issue is that leadership is more important than managing day-to-day activities. Both are important, and an effective leader knows when to do each. In fact, the work needs to be done. We need a combination of both to achieve this work being done most effectively. The problem occurs when someone is predominantly managing because this means that this person is not tuning into others perceptions, ideas, and knowledge. The ideal is to more predominantly lead.

Along the same lines, another fallacy is that the leader has all the answers. Since we are human, we will never achieve this. In administration there is always a new or different twist to situations that must be taken into account. Many times the best answer will come from another person, or some event that triggers us to think about the problem differently. It is OK for a leader not to know what to do. It is OK to say, "I do not know what I will do yet. I need to think about this and get back to you." Or, "Do you have any suggestions or solutions to this problem?" This is all part of the dialogue that produces more effective solutions to problems. Creative thinking, discussed later in this chapter, is so important to effective leadership.

Another fallacy is to assume that when all in the work group are empowered, *the result will always be peace and harmony!* Instead, at times, there will be conflict. Dialogue with each other on the conflicts. Disagreement and healthy argument on issues provide different perspectives and helps a group move to better outcomes that would not have occurred without the disagreement. Thus continuous improvement is achieved.

Another erroneous leadership expectation is that *there is one right way to do the work.* Expecting others to "do it my way" does not necessarily achieve the best possible result. People differ. Work groups are never the same.

It is a mistake for a leader to think that what works well with one group will work equally well with another. *What might work effectively with one group could bomb with another.* It is important for an effective leader to know each person in the work group as well as to know how group members work together. Then the leader can better anticipate what might work effectively with that group.

Some administrators *want everyone to like them.* This can be very dangerous because, realistically, everyone will not. It may be as simple as we resemble Aunt Alice or Grandpa Mike, who treated the person badly in the past. If an administrator wants everyone to like him/her, then the administrator may change decisions depending upon what the current individual or group wants. There will be a lack of consistency in the administrator's actions. People will see this. The administrator will be ineffective. This is a trap. A better option is to have staff respect making decisions that support the core value, what is best for the patient. Sometimes staff will disagree with the administrator's decisions. Such is life. This is OK. Even though they may disagree, staff will respect the administrator because they know that the administrator consistently supports the core value.

Another fallacy is that *effective leaders always use a participative leadership style,* involving staff in every decision. If an administrator never makes a decision without having staff discussion and getting a staff vote, this is not effective leadership. There are times, such as an emergency situation, when the administrator needs to make decisions and proceed without participation; or to make decisions based on current data. The key here is that the administrator knows when it is best to just make the decision, when it is best to have dialogue about a situation, and when it is best to have staff decide what to do (see the decision making section later in this chapter).

Another trap is that *one must always win*. First, this does not represent life very accurately. How important is the incident? Is it something that we will even remember ten years from now? Invariably there will be conflicts at the work place. It is not humanly possible to resolve every conflict. If some issue is really important, such as not following the core values (discussed in the next section), it is important that it becomes an issue. However, if it is a trivial issue, it may be best to just overlook the situation. Second, how do we know that we have the best solution? Maybe someone else has a better one. Third, as people share ideas with us it may be better to encourage them to try their ideas—and not add how we might do it. If people interpret the leader's comments as saying that their idea really isn't very good, people will not be as committed to the idea as they were at the beginning of the conversation. Fourth, as we lose, it can teach us a lot—things like humility, or not doing something a certain way again.

Sometimes, a manager takes another person's idea or work and claims the success as her/his own. This selfish action does not demonstrate integrity. Generally word will get out, the manager will be "found out," and others will lose respect for the manager. When we do not give another person credit for work, we are not effective as leaders. Integrity, discussed later in this chapter, is important. We must always give credit where credit is due.

Some administrators do not want staff to shine, or to look better than the leader. Usually this happens when the administrator is threatened by someone who seems very competent. The administrator is ruled by *fear* because the competent person looks better than the administrator, or might even upstage the administrator. In this case, the administrator will be drawn to, and hire, incompetent people. Is it any wonder that their work group will usually have problems, being mediocre at best? This administrator may need to be replaced, or will need to do a lot of work to change such behavior.

Another fallacy is that the leader does not fear anything. Fear is a human trait. Fear of any kind will interfere with our leadership effectiveness. When we fear anything, we must stop and catch ourselves. Fear causes a downward spiral in our choices of actions, and only worsens with time. The best way to deal with the fear is to realize that feeling and then find a way to deal with the fear. For instance, in the Judeo-Christian tradition, one comforting place to turn is Psalm 91:

> He who dwells in the shelter of the Most High,
> Who abides in the shadow of the Almighty,
> Will say to the Lord, "My refuge and my fortress;
> My God, in whom I trust."
> For he will deliver you from the
> snare of the fowler and from the deadly pestilence;
> he will cover you with his pinions,
> and under his wings you will find refuge;
> his faithlessness is a shield and buckler.
> You will not fear the terror of the night,
> nor the arrow that flies by day,
> nor the pestilence that stalks in darkness,
> nor the destruction that wastes at noonday.

A thousand may fall at your side,
ten thousand at your right hand;
but it will not come near you.
You will only look with your eyes
and see the recompense of the wicked.

Because you have made the Lord your refuge,
the Most High your habitation,
no evil shall befall you,
no scourge come near your tent.

For he will give his angels charge of you to guard you in all your ways.
On their hands they will bear you up,
lest you dash your foot against a stone.
You will tread on the lion and the adder,
the young lion and the serpent you will trample under foot.

Because he cleaves to me in love,
I will deliver him; I will protect him, because he knows my name.
When he called to me, I will answer him;
I will be with him in trouble,
I will rescue him and honor him.
With long life I will satisfy him,
And show him my salvation.

Charisma has been identified by some people as being an important component of effective leadership. There has been a lot of research measuring charisma. Some confuse charisma with convincing others to do what we want them to do. Instead we need to ask: "How do we know that what we want to do is best? What harmful side effects might be caused by this? What will people do when we are not around?" This is like control—we cannot control others. In actuality, many researchers have concluded that being charismatic is not an essential part of effective leadership and can, in fact, be detrimental to a company (Collins and Porras, 1994; Khurana, 2002). Instead, the important factor is really the commitment of the leader to the mission and values, and that the leader is living the values consistently and humbly. This then inspires and motivates others.

We must never consider *our leadership to be perfect*, or assume problems are caused by everyone else's behaviors. Sometimes, administrators do not realize that they operate using this fallacy, which can be very dangerous. As discussed previously in this chapter, we always must first examine how *we* might have contributed to the problem. We all have "Achilles' heels". Our own actions may actually be causing the problem. Others may do those things better, or think of better ways to handle situations. See a wonderful book, *Leadership and Self Deception* (2002), which discusses how, in the midst of tensions, conflicts, and problems; the first thing we need to look at is *ourselves*. We need to determine if we are the cause of, or contributing to, the problem. The people around us every day— staff, colleagues, family members—can give us the best feedback on our issues for improvement. For example, say one realizes that one does not listen to customers enough. One could go to seminars on customer improvement. However, isn't the best way just to make it a point to talk directly to customers? Aren't they the best source of information on customer needs? Or perhaps one decides to change some behavior. After accomplishing this, feedback from colleagues as to their perception about the change can help. Have they noticed that we have made the change? This is the real test as to how effective we have actually been in the change.

Another fallacy is that *we have always done it this way*. While it is best to get to know the history behind certain actions, this perspective means that the person or group saying it is probably ineffective, as the only constant is change.

Falling into the importance of the title—such as vice president or manager—or degree—such as getting a master's degree—and thinking we are better than others is another fallacy. Actually, everyone is equally important.

Along this line, it can be tempting to pursue our own selfish agendas, not thinking of how this may affect others (this will be discussed later in the chapter under *Developmental Levels of Leadership*). People do not thrive under dictators unless they support the dictator's views. And even then, they must be careful not to say or do something unacceptable to the dictator, so even the supporters do not really thrive.

Another fallacy can revolve around *gender or race bias issues*. Some people do not think women or people of a certain race can lead effectively. Or people feel more comfortable dealing with others who are like them. For example, within nursing we have some amongst us who discriminate against male nurses. Female applicants for an administrative position may not be considered, with preference given to the male applicant. In non-leadership research, it has been shown that when resumes are reviewed, if one can tell whether the person is male or female, the female is rated lower than the male, by both men and women. Unfortunately this is equally true in racial situations. All this creates unnecessary conflicts but, unfortunately, is a fact of life. We have not yet achieved perfection societally. Biases still exist. The place to start is changing ourselves. It is a better policy to treat everyone with respect and to give all equal treatment based upon each person's gifts, abilities, and experiences.

At times research on administrator effectiveness shows differences in leadership styles based on gender. For instance, in business research, studies consistently show that women are more transformational (transformational leadership is explained in the next section of this chapter) than men (Sharpe, 2000; Gogoi, 2000). However, in studies examining nurse executive leadership, the results consistently show that it does not matter whether one is male or female, nor is effective leadership determined by one's race. When one looks at who is most effective in these studies, it can be any of the above. Somehow, there is a factor in nursing that makes both men and women equally transformational in their leadership style.

Another issue with leadership is identified by Luthans (1988). In an observational study, Luthans discovered that there was a distinct difference between what he labeled "*successful*" versus "*effective*" managers. Some managers were able to achieve both, but more often managers exhibited one trait more predominantly:

> *Successful managers* give relatively more attention to networking (socializing, politicking, and interacting with outsiders)… and give rel-

atively little attention to human resource management activities (motivating/reinforcing, managing conflict, staffing, and training/development) (p. 127).

Yet *"effective"* managers have a very different work style:

> *Effective managers* give by far the most relative attention and effort to communicating (exchanging information and processing paperwork) and human resource management activities and the least to networking (p. 127).

According to this study a *"successful" manager* is promoted relatively quickly while the *"effective" manager* may not be promoted quickly, but has "satisfied and committed" staff who achieve higher quantity and quality in their work performance. So if there is a leadership problem, the manager may be more like the *"successful"* manager Luthans identified. If so, it might be helpful to coach this person to pay more attention to *"effective"* management activities.

There is another pitfall for supervisors. A successful manager, by politicking with the supervisor, may be perceived to be a better nurse manager than is actually the case. This is where it is so important for administrators *at all levels* to *regularly do rounds*. In doing rounds effectively, it can become readily apparent that there is a leadership problem, whereas one might not recognize this problem if only hearing what the manager has to say.

Another way to determine an administrator's effectiveness is evaluative feedback on a yearly basis from the individuals who report to that administrator (a 360 evaluation). To be most effective this needs to be handled confidentially. This feedback can provide helpful information for an administrator to improve certain areas as well as provide confirmation that her/his leadership is effective. If the feedback identifies real problems, the administrator's supervisor must take action.

By understanding leadership fallacies, we can avoid possible traps that will make us less effective. Now we will turn to leadership excellence.

Quantum Leadership Excellence

> All the results of good nursing may be spoiled or utterly negated by one defect—petty management—or, in other words, by not knowing how to manage so that what you do when you are there is done when you are not.
>
> *–Florence Nightingale, 1869.*

Excellent nursing leadership is orchestrating your professional practice climate in such a way that the system moves effectively in the caring of patients, and is cost effective, yet your hand is hardly noticed.

—(This quote is from a nurse executive interview as part of a research project. Confidentiality was promised so the person cannot be named here.)

Quantum leadership is dynamic. It changes as we grow both individually and societally. Because leadership is a dynamic process, it is hard to capture it on a two-dimensional page. What is here represents where we are currently. We learn from what is. We are in various stages of learning because a whole range of leadership styles exist. (Actually, some of the styles, such as dictatorships, are not effective, and one hesitates to call them leadership.) Our leadership knowledge base is expanding and ever changing as we all learn and contribute to it. We are in a time of discovery and we need more research to provide us with better answers.

The *dynamic* role of leadership also means that various components of leadership need to be *integrated* into a dynamic whole. For a while leadership research focused on leadership traits. The problem with this research was that initially no one realized the connections between all these traits; the individual personality traits of the leaders were not accounted for. Then the connections began to be identified and linked with outcomes.

Now, in quantum leadership, we realize that if any one leadership component is weak or missing, the entire process is affected. The same is true when certain leadership components are used too much or at the wrong time. In interviews with "excellent" nurse executives,

> they described their leadership style as a dynamic process. Their leadership style was rather amorphous having no regular structure, yet having a number of leadership characteristics that must all be present and intermesh with one another. For example, while making a difficult decision that supported their vision, their integrity was always intact. They were 'deadly serious' about the various aspects of leadership. If a characteristic was missing or overused, a leader would not be effective.... All characteristics were required together and all needed to be used at appropriate times (Dunham-Taylor, p. 15).

Research began to reflect this dynamic quality of leadership, calling it transformational, as opposed to transactional, leadership. Transformational leadership was more concerned with the process an effective leader used to achieve a positive outcome. A transformational leader:

- Had integrity,
- Was committed to end values that the people following that leader also were committed to,
- Established trust,
- Identified a vision of where the group wanted, or needed, to go next,

- Intellectually stimulated followers,
- Gave individualized consideration to followers,
- Was a role model for followers,
- Provided meaning and challenge for followers' work,
- Empowered followers, and
- Approached situations using appropriate first or second order change (Watzlawwick, Weakland, and Fisch, 1974; Burns, 1978; Bennis, 1985; Bass, 1998).

Transactional leaders, on the other hand, were more like the traditional manager. They might use contingent reward, only give feedback to others when things go wrong, or even provide laissez-faire leadership rather than having the transformational qualities. A leader would tend to exhibit both types of leadership, transformational and transactional, but have an overall leadership style that was more like one of the styles. Transformational qualities are preferable, but both qualities are needed to get the work accomplished.

Research began to show that transformational leadership, or dynamic leadership, *leads to a better bottom line* (Bass, 1998). For instance, Simons' (2002) research, which examined managers' behavioral integrity discussed later in this chapter, found that:

> The ripple effect we saw was stunning. Hotels where employees strongly believed their managers followed through on promises and demonstrated the values they preached, [the hotels] were substantially more profitable than those whose managers scored average or lower. So strong was the link, in fact, that... a profit increase of more than $250,000 per year [was noted.] No other single aspect of manager behavior that we measured had as large an impact on profits (p. 18).

The research on effective leadership then continued to add to this knowledge base. For example, organizationally, the magazine *Fortune* provided survey results from their "Most Admired Companies" survey. These companies:

- Are far more satisfied with the quality and breadth of leadership at both their executive and senior management levels;
- Are less tolerant of inappropriate leadership behavior to meet their numbers;
- Place more value on leadership development, and put more emphasis on ongoing development efforts that are linked closely to strategic business goals and supported by formal rewards programs;
- More frequently use competency models and various developmental programs in selecting and advancing their leaders; and
- Have leaders who are perceived as demonstrating more emotional intelligence (Stein, 2000).

In another study McClelland found that, "when senior managers had a critical mass of emotional intelligence capabilities their divisions outperformed yearly earnings goals by 20%" (Snow, 2001).

So what is emotional intelligence? "Emotional intelligence is the capacity for recognizing our own feelings and those of others, for motivating ourselves, for managing emotions well in ourselves and in our relationships" (Snow, p. 441). Goleman's (1998) book, *Emotional Intelligence and Working with Emotional Intelligence*, outlines four capabilities that are present when one has emotional intelligence. This is further discussed by Vitello-Cicciu (2002). See **Exhibit 3–2**.

> Emotional intelligence is the ability to manage ourselves and our relationships effectively. Each capability is composed of a set of competencies. Emotional intelligence skills and cognitive skills are synergistic; top performers have both. The more complex the job, the more emotional intelligence matters.… Emotional competencies cluster into groups…; each is based on a common underlying emotional intelligence capacity. The underlying emotional intelligence capacities are vital if people are to successfully learn the competencies necessary to succeed in the workplace. [For example,] if they are deficient in social skills,… they will be inept at persuading or inspiring others, at leading teams, or catalyzing change. If they have little self-awareness, they will be oblivious to their own weaknesses and lack the self confidence that comes

Exhibit 3–2 Emotional Intelligence Framework. Copyright Hay Group 2001.

	SELF	**OTHERS**
AWARENESS	**Self-Awareness** • *Self Confidence*: Certain of one's own expertise • *Accurate Self-Assessment*: Conscious of one's limitations • *Emotional Self-Awareness*: Cognizant of one's positive and negative biases	**Social Awareness** • *Empathy*: Learning from other people's experiences, expertise • *Organizational Awareness*: Remaining cognizant of organizational life, politics
ACTIONS	**Self-Management** • *Self Control*: Remaining poised even when under pressure • *Adaptability*: Welcoming new ideas • *Trustworthiness*: Displaying honesty/integrity	**[Relationship Management]*** • *Visionary Leadership*: Inspiring and executing effective tactics • *Communication*: Establishing positive relationships and managing expectations • *Conflict Management*: Developing consensus and mitigating conflicts

* Snow called Relationship Management *Social Skills*. The authors prefer Relationship Management because the social skills are used within relationships established with others.

Source: Snow, J. (September 2001). Looking beyond nursing for clues to effective leadership. *JONA*, 3(9), 442.

> from certainty about their strengths. None of us is perfect in using all of the emotional competencies; we inevitably have a profile of strengths and limits. However, *the ingredients for outstanding performance require only that we have strengths in a given number of these competencies (at least six or so), and that the strengths are spread across all four areas of emotional intelligence* (pp. 441–442).

Goleman's and McClelland's (1973) research shows that there is a "strong link between an organization's success and the emotional intelligence of its leaders. The research also demonstrates that if people take the right approach, they can develop their emotional intelligence. The research supports the idea that leaders are not born but that people can learn how to manage their emotions and how to motivate people they lead" (Snow, p. 441). This research has helped to explain how leaders who are very different can be very effective.

> Emotionally intelligent nursing leaders will help their organizations create competitive advantage through the following:
>
> 1. Improved performance of nursing personnel, leading to more satisfied patients, physicians, and families;
> 2. Improved retention of top talent;
> 3. Improved teamwork among nurses;
> 4. Increased motivation by team members;
> 5. Enhanced innovation in the nursing group;
> 6. Enhanced use of time and resources;
> 7. Restored trust between nurses and their leaders (Snow, 2001, 443).
>
> Recent neurobehavioral research on the limbic system indicates the emotional intelligence can be learned through motivation, extended practice, and feedback. Goleman contends to enhance emotional intelligence, one must break old behavioral habits and establish new ones through an individualized approach. He also states that "building one's emotional intelligence will not happen without a sincere desire or concerted effort on the part of an individual. A brief seminar won't help or a how-to manual. Learning to internally empathize as a natural response to people is much harder to learn than regression analysis" (Vitello-Cicciu, 2002, 207).

New aspects about effective leadership are continually identified. Meanwhile, all of us must stay in touch with our intuitive, inner core to achieve more effective leadership. This can be difficult in the frantic pace of the workplace. Each of us needs to find our way to stay in touch with this core. Tall order, isn't it?

> With a quantum sensibility, there are new possibilities for how to create order. Organizational behavior is influenced by the invisible. If we attend to the fields we create, if we help them shine clear with coherence, then we can clean up some of the waste of organizational life.... In a field

view of organizations, we attend first to clarity. We must say what we mean and seek for a much deeper level of integrity in our words and acts than ever before. And then we must make certain that everyone has access to this field, that the information is available everywhere. Vision statements move off the walls and into the corridors, seeking out every employee, every recess in the organization.… We need to imagine ourselves as beacon towers of information, standing tall in the integrity of what we say, pulsing out congruent messages everywhere. We need all of us out there, stating, clarifying, reflecting, modeling, filling all of space with the messages we care about. If we do that, a powerful field develops—and with it, the wondrous capacity to organize into coherent, capable form. Let us remember that space is never empty. If it is filled with harmonious voices, a song arises that is strong and potent. If it is filled with conflict, the dissonance drives us away and we don't want to be there. When we pretend that it doesn't matter whether there is harmony, when we believe we don't have to 'walk our talk,' we lose far more than personal integrity. We lose the partnership of a field-rich space that can help bring order to our lives (Wheatley, pp. 56–57).

Effective leadership is like quality. No matter how effective we become, we can always improve. Good leadership can be taught and learned. So do not become discouraged when we stray from the path once in a while; it's human. When we realize this has happened, start back on the path being open to new ideas and new ways of doing things.

Our present model of dynamic leadership is all of the above plus listening to our intuitive center. The emotional intelligence research suggests that effective leadership starts with work we accomplish within ourselves. As Snow pointed out, none of us achieve perfection, but we can improve our own personal mastery. We further learn when we *work with others*, the social awareness and relationship management skills defined in the emotional intelligence research occurs.

Developmental Levels of Leadership

Kuhnert and Lewis (1987) identified several developmental levels of leadership. At the first level leaders are only concerned with their "personal goals and agendas" (p. 652). This approach is a selfish one. The second developmental level occurs when the leader is able to see that joining a group and having mutual goals and partnerships is more advantageous than the selfish goals present at the first stage. The problem with the second stage is that sooner or later one is torn between two groups. For example, a nurse manager might realize that staff wants something that is the antithesis of what the higher level administrative group wants. The third stage of leadership resolves this dilemma. At the third stage the leader has developed end values— doing what is best for the patient—that "transcends" the leader's own goals and agendas. Even though the staff and the higher level administration groups do not agree on a goal, the leader makes a decision based on the end value of what is best for the patient.

Dunham-Taylor (1995) identified four stages of leadership among nurse executives. The *first group* "influences others on a situational basis, is action oriented, is still learning, experiences emotional discomfort, and is working on personal change" (p. 31). At the *next stage* the nurse executives "used common sense; were not afraid to fail and admit mistakes; lacked a leadership definition; thought leaders were born, not made; had difficulty with balance; were aware of strengths and weaknesses; and were inconsistent" (p. 30). The *third stage*, which is highly transformational, "enjoy 'cleaning up' difficulties; underestimate their own abilities; are not maintenance people [meaning that they will not stay in the same position for years]; hire the best staff possible; work to develop staff; have people skills; are visionary; have perseverance; enjoy analyzing problems with staff, discussing alternatives, and then have staff decide what to do; want staff to let them know when something goes wrong; are not as balanced; personalize issues; and can become easily frustrated if standards are not met" (pp. 26–27). The *fourth, or highest, stage* achieved more balance, were always striving for higher quality—both organizationally and personally, possessed humility, had a dynamic leadership definition and style, were deadly serious about their work, felt that their work mattered, were comfortable with change, had integrity, identified values, experienced intuitive decision making, were a coach and mentor to others, were humanistic, had humor, had charisma, were visionary, and were aware of their own humanity." [They often were in executive positions for years and always felt that there was more that needed to be accomplished] (p. 29).

The Only Constant Is Change

> As we discuss leadership excellence, there is a theme that we consider a given in life. Change is not a thing or an event; it is instead a dynamic, the major element of a universe that is still unfolding.... Change is the major motivator of life and movement in the universe. People have no control over the condition of change but do influence its circumstances and actions. In short, people don't make change they simply give it form. Change is not something we define; it is more something we discern... The direction change takes, its application in human experience, and its impact are what humans can influence and affect (Porter-O'Grady, 2003, p. 59).

All through this book, it is evident that the only constant in life is change. As we work to take on the administrative role, we realize that everything, including ourselves, changes, with the possible exception of the core values and the need for integrity and love. Even with core values, we may add to the list; hopefully, one's integrity and love grows over time. We all change—whether we want to or not—and the environment around us changes. Even when we specifically do not want to change, we change by becoming more rigid.

When we flow with change that seems right for the moment, we are more balanced and in tune with the world. This dynamic permeates everything. In fact, in a leadership role, we even become catalysts, either initiating or managing, change. Since we have said that everyone in an organization needs to be a leader, this is a tall order. The goals we are working to achieve will change; both success and failure will result from change; our relationships with people change; the people around us change; our leadership changes; our work environment changes; and we can always improve ourselves or our environment—another change.

> Schrodinger, a famous middle 20th century physicist, proved with his famous "Schrodinger's Box" analogy that there are two prevailing realities that operate at any given time: actual reality and potential reality… The former is the reality that currently occupies our immediate experience and moments; the reality in which our senses and awareness are presently engaged. Potential reality is inevitable, on the other hand, is current and present to us at any given moment but, while present, is not yet experienced. Potential reality is inevitable and just as current and applicable as actual reality; it is just not yet experienced. Until applied, it is still potential; present but waiting for the right moment of its expression when it will then become actual much like a stop sign in the street can be seen long before it is responded to by a driver.…
>
> It is in this arena of potential reality that leadership takes its form. The leader is differentiated from the follower in that the leader derives the preponderance of his or her role within the scope of potential reality. It is the leader's role to engage unfolding reality in advance of others experiencing it; to see it, note its demands and implications, translate it for others, and then guide others into processes that will act in concert with the demands of a reality that is not yet present but inexorably and continuously becoming (Porter-O'Grady, p. 59).

Our leadership role means that we need to keep abreast with this unfolding reality, bringing it out for others to see, hear, and experience, lifting all of us to new levels not yet achieved. When we are in the middle of experiencing unfolding reality, it can be very difficult to discern where we are headed. Some big changes that we are facing include:

- The Internet is the fastest growing primary business tool of the time, shifting much of how information is managed to an entirely different formula for its application. It is predicted it will be the primary source of reference, education, and application within the next two decades.
- Fiber optics has connected the world together in a seamless communication network that transmits instantly from one end of the world to the other. In conjunction with satellite technology, there is no place on the globe where one cannot communicate with another place in an instant in time…
- Access is highly portable allowing consumers to get anything they want or need anywhere in the world with corollary shipping and transporting capabilities.…
- The consumer/user now has control over almost any relationship, whether personal or business, and now can personalize any interaction within any context he or she provides at any time and in any way. The consumer is not concerned with what nurses

have to give them, rather they are interested in what they get from nurses (from a process orientation to an outcome perspective.)

- Microprocessing increases the mobility of persons while still keeping them connected to everything. Furthermore, such micro-technology makes innovations in service, telecommunication, information, and health care intervention quicker, easier, and less expensive than ever before....
- Portability is now making it possible to provide health services in a wider variety of places and in so brief a timeframe that it is no longer necessary to go to the hospital and stay long periods of time for clinical care (Porter-O'Grady, pp. 60–61).

This list is by no means complete. As we have noted elsewhere, other clues include less invasive treatment modalities, a wealth of outcome research data becoming readily available, and information barraging us at every turn. All these changes are forcing us to change the way we work and communicate with one another. This translates into an adaptation of both how we care for patients, and how we communicate with others. For example, tele-health is a reality.

This high level of change can be overwhelming. I am reminded of my grandmother who first experienced electricity (for lighting, appliances, and so forth) and a motorized car rather than a horse and buggy. Our ancestors came through rapid changes just fine, and we can too. The main point is to remain open to what is in that potential reality. One change within nursing is that our patients are generally not with us for long amounts of time. So we do not know them as well as we did. Someone can come in for an operation and go home the same day. Nurses, and other interdisciplinary workers, come and visit us in our homes to follow up on the surgery or treatment needed. This is an enormous change in the way we care for patients. As leaders, we need to help staff understand these changes and work out new work expectations and new ways of working with patients who will not be with us as long. An excellent reference about all this is the book, *Quantum Leadership: A Textbook of New Leadership*, by Tim Porter-O'Grady and Kathy Malloch (2003).

In this chapter we discuss several aspects of leadership that are part of the fluid experience of change. One way of thinking about change is to examine first- and second-order change (Watzlawick, Weakland, and Fisch, 1974). In *first-order change*, a method or person changes. Here, when one asks the question *Why?* the solution is based on common sense. Many changes are actually first-order changes. For example, if there is not enough light in the room so I can read. I can ask, "Why isn't there enough light?" I then decide to add a lamp to supply the needed light and the problem is solved.

At times though, first-order change does not accomplish anything. Asking, "Why?" does not solve the problem. For instance, during layoffs, some employees in an outpatient department were asked to describe an outpatient role they would like to do, to decide upon what they would charge to do the role, and to give all these details to the administrator by a certain date. Otherwise they would be laid off. Being told this, several employees asked, "*Why* are you doing this to us?". They became stuck in first order change and could not get beyond the question, *why?* Eventually, they were laid off.

Instead, a few employees realized that asking *Why?* did not result in their keeping their jobs. They turned to the question, *What?*—"What do we need to do?" When using the question, *What?*, they turned to *second-order change* and reframed the situation. *Reframing* (Watzlawick, Weakland, and Fisch, 1974) demands creativity and getting out of the box. Reframing involves looking at a situation differently than we usually do. An example would be if we look into a house through one window and get one perspective, then we look in another window to get a different perspective. The employees who turned to second-order change began to imagine their work roles in a different way, a way that they had not imagined before. They began to devise the role, develop costs for their services, and give it in writing to the administrator by a certain date. The employees choosing to use second-order change still had jobs and were not laid off.

Second order change often means we need to get out of the box for the solution. For example, during Nazi occupation of Denmark in World War II, King Christian was told to issue a decree that all his countrymen should wear the Star of David armband if they were Jewish. King Christian did not want to do this, yet the Nazis in occupation would enforce it even if he refused—a dilemma. Instead, King Christian used second-order change by very effectively getting out of the box. He issued a decree that all countrymen would wear the Star of David armband. The Nazis soon rescinded the order.

Using a health care example, a nurse administrator was working with a medical chief of a service. He was wonderful with patients and really cared about their receiving good treatment. However, he had a flaw that could sometimes cause a problem. When a nurse had not made appropriate decisions, thus causing a problem with a patient, or the nurse's decisions had made a bad situation worse, this medical chief would lose his temper in the nurse's station, saying in a loud, angry voice that the nurse should be fired. Thus the nursing staff had decided that they did not like this medical chief and wanted the administrator to do something about it. This situation has a couple of dilemmas for the nurse administrator. First, the physician behavior was a problem. Staff observed consistency in the behavior when difficult situations occurred. Second, staff wanted the administrator to be the parent and take care of the problem—with staff not assuming any responsibility to work out a solution to the problem.

The nurse administrator realized that the staff picture of this physician was negative because of his angry behavior. It would be necessary to help staff reframe the situation. The physician was not a bad person, in fact the physician really cared about giving good care to patients. The problem was the physician's behavior in these difficult situations. The administrator decided to try a potential solution, asking staff to call the administrator the next time such an incident occurred. At this point, the administrator located the medical chief in his office, and broke the news to him there. The medical chief was able to rant and rave in the administrator's presence, but no one else heard what was said. When the physician had calmed down a bit, the administrator began to discuss what could be done to deal with the incident. After some dialogue, the two could go together to the unit and discuss what to do with the staff and with the patient and/or family. This worked.

After that success, the administrator encouraged the nurse manager to use this approach with the medical chief if and when the next incident occurred. Then, the nurse administrator and nurse manager discussed this physician with staff who had labeled him to be a "bad" physician. The process of reframing was discussed with staff. They agreed that he did give really good care to patients and really cared about the patient. They also noticed the difference in the physician's behavior. After several incidents, even the staff were able to take the physician aside when an incident occurred, so the incident would be discussed in a private area. Eventually, the nurse administrator could bring up this approach with the physician, asking the physician if he realized how his behavior had affected everyone. The physician was able to change.

Personal Mastery

Know thyself.

We change as we begin to know ourselves better. This internal process is called *personal mastery*. Personal mastery does not occur immediately in life, but follows a great deal of personal work. And even then, we are continually working to better our personal mastery if we choose to increase our effectiveness. This continual work can occur as we work internally to improve ourselves, or can occur as we experience various difficulties we encounter in our environment. Sometimes hard environmental lessons, or personal crises, bring about a change within us even when we did not plan to change, or try to achieve personal mastery.

Personal mastery may not mean what is perceived as success in our society. It is not having a title, getting rich, being popular, achieving physical beauty, or getting an advanced educational degree. Instead personal mastery is what is present inside us—what is there, despite what is going on around us.

How Does One Achieve Personal Mastery?

Since each of us is different with different gifts, personal mastery is an individual process. We are most effective if we can be brutally honest with ourselves about *our life purpose, our gifts, and our personal strengths and weaknesses*. As we realize that we are not perfect and that there is always more to learn, our personal mastery and leadership improves. Personal mastery is something that we can get closer to, but never totally achieve in our lifetime. It is elusive, just like continuous improvement. As we become more and more effective and closer to personal mastery, there are new nuances and directions that we realize we need to master. Our cues come from all over. It is amazing how *what one needs at any point in time will suddenly emerge* when one needs it.

Self Awareness

Although we never know ourselves completely, we must be able to accurately assess our strengths and weaknesses, know how we respond to certain situations, and be aware of our internal states and resources, our emotional awareness, our spiritual beliefs, our preferences, our biases, and our intuitive capabilities. If we do not realize what our weaknesses are, our judgment could be faulty, our interpersonal relationships may suffer, and we will not achieve our life purpose as well, or at all:

> Goleman (1998) found that people who are competent at self-assessment
> are: (a) aware of their strengths and weaknesses; (b) reflective, learning
> from experience; and (c) open to candid feedback, new perspectives,

Exhibit 3–3 Johari Window

1 Known to self and others	Blind 2 Known only to others
Hidden 3 Known only to self	Unknown 4 Known neither to self nor to others

From: Sundeen, S. J., Stuart, G. W., Rankin, E. D., & Cohen, S. A. (1985). *Nurse-Client Interaction, Implementing the Nursing Process* (3rd Edition). The C.V. Mosby Company.

continuous learning, and self-development. Honest self-awareness may be a challenge for some leaders to achieve. Howlin and Hickok (1992) identified several factors that may discourage executives' self-awareness:

- The power of their position may isolate them from criticism.

- Expectations of high performance may cause executives to continue to do what they've done well in the past.

- The nature of many executive jobs leaves little time and provides few rewards for introspection.

- Successful executives learn to focus and build on strengths and may be unaware of their own weaknesses.

… In a study of top executives who failed,… the two most common traits… were:

1. *Rigidity*—an inability to adapt to changes in organizational culture or to respond to feedback about traits that need to be changed or improved.

2. *Poor relationships*—being too harshly critical, insensitive, or demanding; ultimately alienating those they work with.

Other characteristics identified… include poor self-control, reacting defensively to criticism, being ready to get ahead at the expense of others, and poor social skills (especially lacking empathy and sensitivity)

Exhibit 3–4 Johari Window

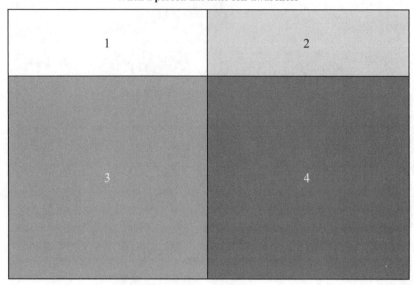

From: Sundeen, S. J., Stuart, G. W., Rankin, E. D., & Cohen, S. A. (1985). *Nurse-Client Interaction, Implementing the Nursing Process* (3rd Edition). The C.V. Mosby Company.

Exhibit 3–5 Johari Window

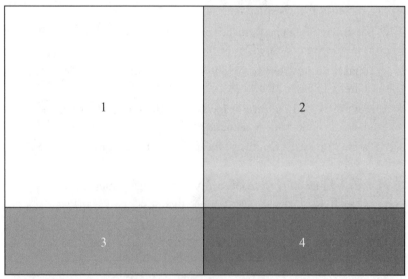

From: Sundeen, S. J., Stuart, G. W., Rankin, E. D., & Cohen, S. A. (1985). *Nurse-Client Interaction, Implementing the Nursing Process* (3rd Edition). The C.V. Mosby Company.

Kerfoot (1997) describes three situations that can cause good leaders to stumble:

1. Interpreting present day events in terms of past successes.
2. Not being open to new ways of filtering information; processing information through old paradigms.
3. "Egotistical invincibility;" resting comfortable on one's past success (Chaffee and Arthur, pp. 226–227).

The Johari Window provides a nice depiction that can be used in self assessment and is displayed in **Exhibit 3–3**. Quadrant 1 consists of the information that we know about ourselves that others also know about us. Quadrant 2 contains aspects about ourselves that are unknown to us (we are blind to them), but that others know about us. Quadrant 3 encompasses hidden information that we know about ourselves that others are not aware of. Many of our beliefs and assumptions are in this quadrant. Opening these up to others can help one examine, and possibly be challenged, by others. But it keeps us from being blindsided by others when we are able to more clearly define these beliefs even under fire. Sometimes we can be blinded by our own perceptions that will cause us to respond to situations in a certain way. Quadrant 4, the unknown area, is the part that no one knows about.

> Three principles may help one understand how the self functions in this representation:
>
> 1. A change in any one quadrant will affect all other quadrants.
>
> 2. The smaller the first quadrant, the poorer the communication.
>
> 3. Interpersonal learning means that a change has taken place so that quadrant 1 is larger, and one or more of the other quadrants are smaller (Sundeen, Stuart, Rankin, and Cohen, 1985, pp. 62-63).

As you can see in **Exhibit 3–4**, Quadrant 1 is smaller when we lack self awareness; in **Exhibit 3–5**, Quadrant 1 gets larger when we are more self-aware and have achieved better personal mastery. When we remain blind to information in either Quadrant 2 or 4, we cannot grow.

Additional personal feedback can be gained by taking work style inventories, such as the Myers-Briggs[1] or the *Life-Styles Inventory (LSI 1)* from Human Synergistics.[2] These inventories can be used to identify what styles one uses when approaching life or work. Then one can determine how he or she works, how this differs from other styles, and how people with this style interact with other styles. This gives us a better understanding of ourselves. This data can be used to change how we respond to situations. The *LSI 1* can also be used by staff directly reporting to a manager. Here staff members rate their perception of their manager's leadership. This provides a "360 evaluation." This view can help supervisors who may not perceive that there are leadership problems and provide the manager with ways to improve effectiveness.

---

[1] This is widely available. One source: Keirsey, D., & Bates, M. (1984). Please Understand Me: Character & Temperament Types. 5th ed. Del Mar, CA: Prometheus Nemesis.

[2] This is available from Human Synergistics International, 39819 Plymouth Road, C-8020, Plymouth, MI 48170. (1-800-622-7584) (313-459-1030) (Fax: 313-459-5557) e-mail: info@humansyn.com or http://www.humansyn.com on the internet.

Once we possess self-awareness and expand our capabilities, our self-confidence and self-worth increases. We begin to be able to regulate our internal states, our impulses, our internal resources. We have more self-control, keeping disruptive emotions and impulses in check. We strive to improve. We handle change better because we are more adaptable and flexible. We can become more comfortable with new information, different approaches, or novel ideas that help us to be more innovative. We can experience optimism—that "can do" attitude. A growing awareness of our gifts and our life purpose develops. We then can start to manifest these gifts. We can become more persistent in pursuing our goals even when obstacles cross our path or when we experience setbacks. This knowledge increases our ability to better relate to the world at large.

All of this is an individual choice; it is like a spiral. The spiral can move upward toward personal mastery, or downward in a more negative direction where we become more rigid and entrenched in our beliefs, lose integrity, and become a dictator. Pessimism and depression can result. However, at any point we have a choice and can change the direction of the spiral.

As we identify bad or destructive habits in ourselves it is important to stop these behaviors as well as to be vigilant in identifying bad habits as we move through life:

> Just say no to them. It is the strength to shift behavior and refuse to participate in actions that do not serve us well. This shortcoming could be anything that doesn't work, such as an uncontrolled temper, failure to meet deadlines, an unwillingness to work with others, or being "too busy" to make patient care rounds or spend time with faculty and students. Any of these habits may violate professional standards, and curtailing or stopping these habits creates an opportunity to strengthen character (Kowalski and Yoder-Wise, p. 27).

As we work on problems, forgiveness of both ourselves and others is important. If we do not do this, we may become so bogged down in our thoughts that we do not deal with the problem areas effectively. Forgiveness in a larger sense is also important in personal mastery:

> There are times when each of us are hurt by others or hurt others. If we respond with resentment and the desire for revenge in the first instance or smugness and glee in the second instance, weakened character results, and we are less human than we could be. Forgiving those who hurt us is paramount. At the same time, asking for forgiveness when we hurt someone is equally important. Another aspect of forgiveness, forgiving ourselves, after committing a hurtful act toward another or making a grievous error of omission or commission is critical to personal growth in the leadership role. It is difficult to let go of self-condemnation, yet it is essential to continuing development as a leader (Kowalski and Yoder-Wise, p. 27).

A positive belief in self is essential when pursuing personal mastery. In the emotional intelligence research, *self-confidence*, being certain of one's own expertise (Snow, 2001), is part of personal mastery. We achieve success in meeting our life's goals when we believe we have the capability to succeed, are able to seize the opportunities, act on them, and work with or around the obstacles. When we can picture the outcome, we are more likely to achieve it. One effective nurse executive said, "There's nothing I can't do if I don't want to, except sleep."

Our self-confidence can also be enhanced by our environment and by our own presentation. If we find comfort being around water, perhaps living somewhere where there is a view of water will be helpful. How we dress or fix our hair can enhance or detract from our self-confidence as well as give out a message to others. Presentation is also important in our work. As we write a report, if it is clear, succinct, and well-presented, chances are it will be more favorably received, as opposed to one having a sloppy appearance or having a less coherent approach.

Finding Our Life Purpose

Part of self-awareness is identifying our life purpose. The problem is that we often do not have a clear idea about our life purpose until we are well into our thirties—and sometimes it can occur much later. In our younger years, our picture is still clouded and as we experience life a clearer picture begins to emerge. At times we may think that we have a clear picture, and learn that we did not fully understand the picture, or even that we need to go in an entirely different direction.

The best answer always lies within. What feels right? When things are clouded, then it is not yet time to understand. Once we understand, we have a choice. Do we follow what our inner core tells us? Or do we ignore it? If and when we do follow that inner guidance, the world becomes more clear, and more opportunities, including the challenges, occur to enhance our achievement of our life's purpose. Brooks (1966) suggests that through stillness we can find the answers:

> The cultivation of inner quiet, so that in a true sense one can become all eyes, as one sometimes calls a heightened receptivity. ... As long as the head is still busy, full sensory receptivity is impossible, while with increasing stillness in the head, all perception, traveling unimpeded through the organism, automatically becomes sharper and more in context. In this new stage of more awareness and permissiveness the self-directive powers of the organism reveal themselves ever clearer, and we experience on a deeper level the unexpected transformations we can undergo.... [When] one reaches a state of relative balance, simultaneous changes happen throughout the whole person. The closer we come to such a state of greater balance in the head, the quieter we become, the more our head 'clears', the lighter and more potent we feel. Energy formerly bound is now more and more at our disposal.... We find ourselves being more one with the world where we formerly had to cross barriers. Thoughts and ideas 'come' in lucidity instead of being produced. We

don't have to try to express ourselves... but utterances become just part of natural functioning. Experiences can be allowed to be more fully received and to mature in us. As Heinrich Jacoby once remarked: 'Through becoming conscious we have been driven out of paradise, through consciousness we can come back to paradise' (pp. 502–503).

Claxton (2000) makes the observation that in the West we do not value contemplation which he calls *slow knowing*:

> As a culture we have lost our sense of the unconscious intelligence to which these more patient modes of mind give access.... Modern Western culture has so neglected the intelligent unconscious—the undermind, I shall sometimes call it—that we no longer know that we have it, do not remember what it is for, and so cannot find it when we need it.... Instead, we give exclusive credence to conscious, deliberate, purposeful thinking.... At its most basic, [contemplation] enables an organism to pursue its goals and interests as successfully as possible in the whole intricate predicament in which it finds itself (pp. 5–16).

In addition to listening to our inner core, we can turn to many helpful people—significant relatives, mentors, teachers as well as other references concerned with personal mastery. For example, one wonderful reference, among so many possibilities on personal mastery, is a book written by Morris (1995) called *True Success: A New Philosophy of Excellence*. Morris has organized the mastery process as having seven elements: a conception of what we want, a confidence to see us through, a concentration on what it takes, a consistency in what we do, a commitment of emotion, a character of high quality, and a capacity to enjoy:

> Realizing that he or she cannot be totally knowledgeable in all fields and that what is best in any given situation is not always apparent (and probably wasn't covered in the textbook), the effective leader seeks out and heeds wise counsel. The best mentors may be the modest warriors who have been in the trenches, lost a few battles along the way, and learned from years of experience what works and what does not work. Learning from failure often breeds success! (Lysaught, p. 26)

Balance

Inner quiet is intertwined with balance, another aspect of personal mastery. When balance is achieved, we are calm yet have energy for whatever we feel is important at that moment. When we are not balanced we experience stress and anxiety and our performance suffers. In fact, a popular phrase, *living in the moment*, is useful for achieving balance and personal mastery. Living in the moment means just what it says: giving our attention to what is happening at that moment, leaving other cares or worries elsewhere. It is not remembering the past—that has already happened and we cannot change it. It is not thinking of the future—that has not happened and is yet to be.

Balance can be maintained only as a dynamic equilibrium. The road to mental health and to high-level wellness both for the individual and for society, depends largely upon striving to attain and maintain a balanced position within the reality of change, guided by purpose sufficient to light the way (Dunn, pp. 61–62).

Achieving balance at all times is the ultimate goal. Some helpful hints:

- Accept that administration is generally a multi-tasked job—we handle multiple inputs and tasks simultaneously. We start one thing, get interrupted by another, and so forth.
- We achieve our goals but it may not happen when we think it *should* occur. *Shoulds* do not "go with the flow." It may not be the divine plan to achieve something at the moment when we have decided it should be achieved.
- Part of the leadership role is learning to respond to what seems to be the most important issue in that moment. There are days when personal goals may not be achieved at all because one is so busy responding to other's issues or crises. Balance is when we are not bothered by such unexpected events but go with the flow.
- Balance is when we choose to take care of something because our intuition tells us to do it, and vice versa.
- Balance *keeps things in perspective*. When something goes wrong, it can be helpful to think ahead five years. How important will this issue be then? Perhaps we will not even remember the incident.

As we discuss balance, we cannot avoid the issue of what causes stress. This varies for different people. Actually, there is eustress—which is wonderful, and there is distress—which is not desirable. Stress is useful when it mobilizes us to take action. It is harmful when it has more negative outcomes. When negative, stress can affect our immune system and create dis-ease. What causes stress in one person may not in another. Why is that? It depends upon our perspective about issues confronting us. I am reminded of a woman who suddenly lost her son in a tragic accident. She said, "It's amazing to think about what used to cause me stress. It was little things that I won't even remember tomorrow. Those things are not important in the scheme of life. Now I realize that only the far more important matters are stressful issues."

So we have a *choice* whether to become stressed; it is a personal experience. How empowering. I can choose whether to be stressed; I can choose detachment and calmness—it is up to me.

Stress can also be caused by fear and worry. Fear is very negative and hurts us. People's fears vary greatly. One commonality among people's fears is that many of their fears are of things that may never happen but we put energy into them, which is more likely to make them occur. *So the question is, do we want to put energy into such negative things??*

Various coping mechanisms can help one keep in balance. It differs for each person ranging from swimming, walking, or running, to meditation and prayer, to sitting on a mountain looking at the view, to regulating breathing. It is best if this can occur on a regular basis. In fact, to decrease stress and encourage health in employees, some companies encourage staff to exercise in facilities provided by the employer, to not take work home in the evening, to engage in counseling made available for employees, to provide massage therapy for employees, and to have better health habits such as eating more nutritious foods, not smoking, and so forth.

Balance harmonizes left brain/masculine/yang and right brain/feminine/yin. **Exhibit 3–6** illustrates these attributes. This is a subtle process where we need to choose the appropriate characteristic for each moment. Each trait is wonderful when used at the right time and is inappropriate when used at the wrong time. This supposes that we have the capability to access both sides at all times. Have you noticed how certain people seem to be dominant on one side or the other? This is not balanced, as these people are not using a good part of the energy within themselves. These traits are not determined by our biological sex. The attributes are all present in each of us. It is up to each of us whether we use them or not. The knowledge of which attribute to use at what time is deep within ourselves if we choose to tune in to it.

Balance also involves a recognition that, because everything is constantly changing, a bad situation will change. It will not last forever; happiness will not last forever either. In this world there is duality. Sometimes we will experience sadness and sometimes happiness. Neither will last forever. Actually, balance often is the area in between the extreme high and the extreme low. Balance is when we experience calmness.

Balance not only occurs internally—with feminine and masculine traits, or with the analytic/cognitive and emotional/feeling parts—but includes balancing life issues. Balance includes such things as balancing the personal life with the professional life; balancing different groups that we are a part of; and balancing personal, organizational, professional,

---

Exhibit 3–6 Left-Brain and Right-Brain Attributes

Left Brain (Masculine)	Right Brain (Feminine)
Conscious mind	Subconscious mind
Aggressive/Assertive	Passive/Receptive
Logical/Analytical	Emotional/Sensitive
Intellectual	Intuitive
Mental	Psychic
Objective	Subjective
Giving	Receiving
Will	Creation
Force	Power
Knowledge	Wisdom
Voluntary systems	Involuntary Systems
Separate/Individualized	Inclusive/Unifying
Sun	Moon
Yang	Yin

From: Krishnapada, S. (1996). *Leadership for an Age of Higher Consciousness*. NY: David McKay/Random House, p. 57.

and societal commitments (Dunham-Taylor, p. 25). Specific ways to achieve balance, as well as encouraging others to achieve balance, are infinite.[3]

Achieving balance is most often a process of becoming. At times we are better with achieving it; at other times we relapse. The goal is to become balanced as we experience each moment, and not think about the past or future.

Fulfillment—Achieving One's Potential

Contemplation and balance can be helpful in bringing about life purpose awareness. Once we understand our life purpose, it becomes a powerful motivator as we proceed through life. We can then more fully use our talents, capacities, or potentialities. Life purpose provides a powerful work ethic. This is what Maslow called *self-actualization.* "There is increasing agreement among psychologists that the greatest satisfaction and experience of fulfillment in life is reached by bringing one's best potentials to materialization" (Buhler, p. 19). At first in life we may be unaware of our full potential, and it may remain latent throughout life. However, when activated, our imagination lights up, releases creative energy, and new ideas result. We become enthusiastic about it. Thus fulfillment is achieved by maximizing our potential, realizing and using our gifts. Fulfillment can be that wonderful feeling when we achieve something we have worked hard to bring to fruition; it also can involve very difficult, life-threatening goals, such as sacrificing one's life to save another's. Our actualized gifts contribute to our society.

As we begin to understand our full potential we become more creative. We experience a passion for our life's work. We appreciate new ideas, concepts, feelings, and spiritual beliefs that can change our perception of life and the way we interact with the world. This awakening helps us to understand what we need to create. In the popular phrase, this helps us "to get out of the box." We trouble shoot more effectively. We pay more attention to our intuition and know what is right or what to do next. We become more aware of other areas to explore. We learn how others might fit into this dynamic process.

Sometimes difficulties we face lead us in creative directions we never would have considered otherwise. When we experience failures, we can develop humility. Maybe we are going to need to try again and see if we can do it better. Occasionally obstacles are significant crucible events:

> Our recent research has led us to conclude that one of the most reliable indicators and predictors of true leadership is an individual's ability to find meaning in negative events and to learn from even the most trying circumstances. Put another way, the skills required to conquer adversity and emerge stronger and more committed than ever are the same ones that make for extraordinary leaders....
>
> For the leaders we interviewed, the crucible experience was a trial and a test, a point of deep self-reflection that forced them to question who they were and what mattered to them. It required them to examine their values, question their assumptions, hone their judgment. And, invariably,

---

[3] For a perspective on balance in nursing leadership, see Distefani and Bledsoe's article, "A balanced approach to leadership" (2003).

they emerged from the crucible stronger and more sure of themselves and their purpose—changed in some fundamental way. Leadership crucibles can take many forms. Some are violent, life-threatening events. Others are more prosaic episodes of self-doubt.... A crucible is, by definition, a transformative experience through which an individual comes to a new or an altered sense of identity. It is perhaps not surprising then that one of the most common types of crucibles we documented involves the experience of prejudice.... Some crucible experiences illuminate a hidden and suppressed area of the soul. These are often among the harshest of crucibles, involving, for instance, episodes of illness or violence.... Fortunately, not all crucible experiences are traumatic. In fact, they can involve a positive, if deeply challenging, experience such as having a demanding boss or mentor....

So, what allowed these people to not only cope with these difficult situations but also learn from them? We believe that great leaders possess four essential skills, and, we were surprised to learn, these happen to be the same skills that allow a person to find meaning in what could be a debilitating experience. First is the ability to engage others in shared meaning.... Second is a distinctive and compelling voice.... But by far the most critical skill of the four is what we call "adaptive capacity." This is, in essence, applied creativity—an almost magical ability to transcend adversity, with all its attendant stresses, and to emerge stronger than before. It's composed of two primary qualities: the ability to grasp context, and hardiness. The ability to grasp context implied an ability to weigh a welter of factors, ranging from how very different groups of people will interpret a gesture to being able to put a situation in perspective. Without this, leaders are utterly lost, because they cannot connect with their constituents.... Hardiness is just what it sounds like—the perseverance and toughness that enable people to emerge from devastating circumstances without losing hope.... It is the combination of hardiness and ability to grasp context that, above all, allows a person to not only survive an ordeal, but to learn from it, and to emerge stronger, more engaged, and more committed than ever. These attributes allow leaders to grow from their crucibles, instead of being destroyed by them—to find opportunity where others might find only despair. This is the stuff of true leadership (Bennis and Thomas, pp. 39–45).

Competence

Personal Competence. Personal competence is necessary to achieve effective leadership. This includes such capabilities as a good memory, and being able to have good concentration as one accomplishes work. It is being goal-oriented and losing our sense of self in the accomplishment of something. It is being completely serious, or motivated, about our work, and keeping a sense of humor. Research has shown over and over again that humor, and laughing, relieve stress. When we are fulfilling our life purpose—at home or at work—we are more likely to be happy, motivated, enthusiastic, optimistic, and enjoy life. Life flows more freely.

It is seeing opportunities and challenges as stimulating, or at least, as something that we can successfully deal with. (A world view of abundance is preferable to one of scarcity.) Personal competence also involves knowing when it is time to leave a position, such as when issues cease to be challenges, when we are tired of dealing with issues, and when we have grown stagnant on the job; or when we physically can no longer do the work.

Clinical Competence. In the nursing profession, fulfillment comes from interacting with the people we serve, thus developing our clinical competence. The more we understand about our customer—patient, resident, client—the more effective we will be in delivering appropriate care to that customer. This means that we must dialogue with our customer whenever possible, and it is important to encourage all staff to do so. In this way, we are aware of what the customer actually wants. In health care, we often see our customers when they are in crisis so this clinical competence concept also means that we are effective in helping our clients to better manage their crises. In Benner's (1984) work, she identifies how we start as a novice and gradually, as we get more experience, become an expert.

When we are in an administrative role, having an understanding of the patient experience enables us to be more effective. In fact, one problem that occurs regularly with health care administrators is that those who do not have a health care background, cannot understand the service side—what patients experience—of the health care business. Unfortunately, that is why at the executive level it is often only the CNO (chief nurse officer) asking about what is best for the patient. When administrators are clinical professionals, they have the added patient-care dimension that makes them more effective in health care administration. They understand the "care" side of our business. Hospital administrators who lack this dimension can have an eye-opening experience when they experience a life-threatening illness, and suddenly experience the service side from the patient perspective. They often become more effective administrators after having had this experience. (Actually, this is often the case for nurses and physicians as well!!)

This clinical competence expertise, along with regular dialogue with patients and families, gives us many clues for ways we can improve our clinical effectiveness as well as ways we can improve the health care environment. Too often our goals for the customer do not fully match theirs. For instance, *we make people wait to see us.* (Do you remember how frustrating it is to have a 2 PM appointment at a clinic, having taken off time at work, and to still be waiting to see a health care professional at 3 PM?) Or *we do not treat people with dignity.* (Have you ever worn a hospital gown that might flap open in back as you are walking down the hall?) And *we do painful invasive procedures* (It is not fun being poked and prodded.) *We may make choices the patient does not want*, such as not recording their wishes about how extensive to be in life-threatening situations.

Clinical expertise also ties in with customer service, which is essential to achieving our mission in health care delivery regardless of setting. When we understand this, we become customer-focused in all that we do. We model commitment to customer service and encourage others to model this as well.

From a marketing perspective, most of our customers are not saving their dollars because they are looking forward to buying hip replacement surgery. They may be saving for a new car, or saving in case they experience catastrophic illness, but it is more of a worry that illness will deplete their funds, rather than something they look forward to with anticipation. Yet when experiencing a health crisis, suddenly people want our help.

Having clinical skills enhances our ability to anticipate patient needs and to understand why there is no one best practice for a patient with a certain diagnosis. After all, we treat the whole patient with all the baggage they bring to us. The baggage differs, as does the patient response to certain treatments. Clinical competence is necessary to understand processes, procedures, standards, methods of treatment, and technologies related to the care, and then to choose the best options for each patient's needs and individual differences.

Clinical competence is always changing. It is easy to give outdated care simply because we do not realize there is a better way. For this reason we included the Information Chapter in this book, as there are readily available resources that we can use to ensure that we remain clinically competent and aware of treatment differences brought about by changes in technology, research, medications, and procedures.

When in administrative roles, clinical competency enables us to be more effective managers. When we can pitch in and help with patients when the going gets rough, we earn staff respect and trust because staff can see that the nurse manager can provide safe, competent patient or resident care. As one moves up the ladder in administrative positions being clinically competent in all the areas that we may supervise becomes impossible. At this point, we must continue to learn and enhance our clinical competence, but also trust other's expertise to best manage patient care.

Organizational Awareness. A nurse administrator must have another competency necessary for leadership effectiveness. One needs to possess a dynamic picture of the organization as a whole, to know how different departments and people work together. With this knowledge one can often guess, with fair accuracy, how people in the organization respond to different situations. This is a critical thinking aspect of administration. The dynamic part is that nothing remains the same. Our picture yesterday is not totally accurate today.

This assessment capability enables an administrator to walk into a work area and sense when things are going well, or when something is wrong. This has been called the unit atmosphere, but it is just as true for a department or home care office. Having this capability, the administrator can help staff when needed. This awareness accomplishes several things: first, staff realize that the administrator has sensed that something is wrong and wants to help out; second, it enhances better teamwork when staff members realize that the administrator cares and pitches in when needed; and third, the work group is more likely to formulate flexible strategies or plans that can be used another time when something goes wrong again.

Organizational awareness is one of the emotional intelligence competencies, defined as being cognizant of organizational life and politics (Snow, 2001). Actually organizational awareness extends beyond the organization. It includes a picture of how the organization fits into the community, and how larger societal issues impact the organization. No organization exists in a vacuum but is always part of a larger whole. In fact, organizations have obligations to the community as a synergy is needed between the organization and the community for the continued survival of both. Although we never have the total picture, our picture is dynamic and ever changing; we are more effective when we can take what we know, or sense, into account both when interacting on the day-to-day issues and when doing strategic planning for the future.

Continual Learning. Every moment in our lives provides the teaching most needed. It gives us the opportunity to constantly grow and learn. Our choice: to trust the process and allow the lesson to seep in, or to fight it/ignore it. Learning is dynamic. Our learning changes too. What may interest us at one point in our lives may not later. Then we can learn about something new or different, or we can appreciate certain nuances that we were unaware of before. Chances are we will continue to learn until we die. As we learn we acquire more wisdom, accomplish our work more effectively, and become more proficient in life. There can be joy in learning new things—exploring new vistas—especially when our explorations match our gifts and interests. Having personal goals stimulates our learning as we need to learn more about issues related to those goals.

This is also true on an organizational level. In a study with nurse executives identified as "excellent," interviews revealed that, "No matter how much things improved, there always was more that could be achieved. This did not produce frustration, but provided an ongoing commitment. These executives were highly satisfied personally and professionally—yet they balanced this with more to be accomplished" (Dunham-Taylor, p. 25). Research has found that people like to have something different to do in their work or they get bored. Therefore, remember that no matter how much things improve, there is always more that can be achieved. Status quo is the kiss of death. Change keeps us alive. There is no single best way to do anything. Each of us responds differently to situations. Creativity is part of the process as constant improvement has to be improvisational. (This is not to say that some consistency is helpful, as too much change all at once can be overwhelming.)

Learning can challenge and stretch us. It can offer new opportunities. We can strengthen areas that have been weaknesses. However, the joy of learning can be extinguished by life circumstances, illnesses, or even past educational experiences. Sometimes the most profound learning happens when we experience difficulties, or make mistakes; it is the conflicts we face, and the people that we have conflicts with, that teach us the most. These challenges can be reframed and are wonderful opportunities for further learning. No matter what we have done, or have not done, there is always hope, for anyone can learn and improve.

We learn in many ways—from those around us, from life experiences, from reading, from attending a conference, from watching the media or the Internet. But learning is more than just passively being a sponge. It involves listening, asking questions, processing information, identifying patterns of similarity, and reflecting on events, processes, issues, or other things that have presented themselves to us. It is actually trying things and learning from the experience. Learning also brings us a broader transfer of knowledge from one context to another. For instance, as we learn about gardening we can apply the knowledge about nurturing plants to nurturing our patients or people in the work group. Learning involves being aware of history and its impact on our present situation; history helps us to understand why current problems occur. Then we can respond more appropriately to new or changing situations, or, if we choose not to change, the changed situation may bring about our learning. Learning, and the wisdom that results, provides us with a more adaptable or flexible approach to life that enhances our being.

At some point(s) in our life there will be significant teachers, or mentors, or masters, (titles vary for these significant people) who will help us to achieve profound learning. This gift always occurs at just the right time. It is then up to us to decide whether to make use of this relationship, and the potential learning contained in it.

Our work life contributes to our learning. Our personal gifts flourish when work enhances them. Bass (1998) explains that we all need intellectual stimulation in our work. What will stimulate one person can be very boring to the next because people have different gifts. But all of us need sources for intellectual stimulation as we pass through life. It provides grist for our creativity, giving us new ideas and providing new connections with others. Being able to imagine and create is fun.

In fact, in the administrative role our leadership, when effective, enhances the learning possibilities for both ourselves and others, as all of us have more to learn. One could ask, "Am I open to continued growth and learning? Am I providing opportunities for continued growth and learning for all in the work group?" Providing mentorship for all in a work group can be very positive. In fact, having several mentors is wonderful so we can be exposed to different perspectives and ways of thinking. This assumes the true meaning of mentorship, that there is good chemistry between the mentor and the mentee. Each person in the work group can potentially be a good mentor, so it is important for all of us to encourage exploration, learning, and creativity.

As we talk about continual learning, we need to consider our mind and its potential. According to various research studies, we only use five to ten percent of our brains. Think of this untapped resource within each of us. We have so much more potential that could be used as we live our lives! Our minds are capable of things like superlearning where one listens to certain music, i.e., the Mozart effect, and in this relaxed state, one has the potential to learn more effectively. In health care where we deal with dis-ease, the mind is working too, along with our emotions. The words dis-ease sounds as though we are not in a balanced, relaxed state. Instead, our mind is tuning into emotions that disturb us. All this, when continued over time, builds into dis-ease.

Our minds lead us into our future. For instance, when we positively picture something, it is more likely to happen; and vice versa, as we worry about something, we put energy into it so it is more likely to happen. Since this was covered in more detail in Chapter 2, it will not be repeated here.

There are many opportunities for learning in our work life. This starts with self-evaluation. For example, we could answer the question, *why do we do things the way we do them*? Since we all wear our blinders that keep us "in the box," we need to question our basic assumptions. For instance, a nurse administrator could ask such questions as:

- Why do I procrastinate and wait until the last minute to complete something?
- Why do we need shifts? Why does everyone have to work an eight or twelve-hour day?

- Why do we need a policy and procedure for everything—do nurses really use them? Aren't nurses professionals? If so, why do we need more policies and procedures for the RNs than we do for the aides?
- Why do we teach using only a lecture format? What is the best method for us to learn about something new?

Often our own self-evaluation can provide us with a starting point for the continual improvement process. We may realize that there are certain things about ourselves that we want to improve, or we may dream about something that gives us a message that we need to deal with an issue.

Sometimes we may decide not to work on the flaw but to compensate for it in some other way. For example, in the author's research with nurse executives, most identified a personal weakness, in that they were not "detail people." They dealt with that weakness by making sure that there was someone reporting to them that was very good with details. Actually this "flaw" might be a blessing in the nurse executive role as this person needs to see the big picture and delegate effectively.

Our leadership needs to continually change; it's dynamic. No matter how wonderful our leadership, there are always ways that it can be improved. It is a lifelong process. An effective leader is always thinking, "How can I improve my leadership?" Isn't it wonderful that there is always more to learn? Boredom remains at bay as the world continues to offer so much for us to learn.

As we help others in the work group to achieve better leadership in their work roles, remember they need opportunities for learning, just as we do. I continue to be amazed to hear wonderful staff nurses say that they are not leaders and that leadership content does not apply to them. This seems to be a common misconception engrained in our profession. We need to work to change this because staff nurses, in actuality, are leaders as they go about their work each day. For that matter, there are wonderful aides that provide the backbone of the day-to-day care that would not describe themselves as leaders either. Yet they, or the housekeepers, are often the person who is the most significant to an inpatient or resident.

Wisdom

Wisdom is the result of much learning, often enhanced by such things as encountering a crucible experience, or achieving a quietness within, that helps us to lose our sense of self (as contained in selfish), gaining our sense of selflessness, and realizing our interdependence with the world.

> The wisdom of a learned man cometh by opportunity of leisure; and he
> that hath little business shall become wise
>
> –*Ecclesiastes 38:34.*

One bonus of the quest for personal mastery is that it leads to wisdom. Interestingly, as we become wise and possess wisdom in some areas, chances are we are beginning learners in other areas. After all, there are so many things to explore in this world. Wisdom is enhanced when we have developed a broad knowledge base and possess practical knowl-edge based on life experience, yet have insights about situations or people, or can perceive the motivations of others. It is a road that spirals ever upward if we are paying attention to what is within.

> Ultimately we have just one moral duty: to reclaim large areas of peace in ourselves, more and more peace, and to reflect it towards others. And the more peace there is in us, the more peace there will also be in our troubled world.
>
> Etty Hillesum, Holocaust Victim, *An Interrupted Life*, Hagberg, p. 227.

Humility

As one approaches personal mastery, one becomes more influential within the world and yet still understands that one is only a very small part of it. Part of humility is assuming responsibility for our personal performance; having high standards; being conscientious. We are harder on ourselves than others will be. We are brutally honest about our motiva-tions. We are committed to our life purpose. At the same time we begin to see in the scheme of things how insignificant we are.

> Leaders with strong character do not need public recognition such as awards or tributes. They don't need to talk about or parade all their virtues (what a great boss they are, what respectful physicians they are, how staff appreciate everything they do, etc.). Rather, leaders know they are most effective when the followers say, "We did it ourselves" (Kowalski and Yoder-Wise, p. 27).

We have a greater awareness of our gifts, of ways we can make the world better, of what we need to do next. The amazing thing is that if each of us explore our special gifts, every-thing fits together beautifully. One person's gifts will make a contribution because no one else is meeting that particular need. Thus if we all can stay in tune with our gifts and cre-ativity, all fits together so that we have all we need to live full, productive lives. "It means to act according to one's conscious conviction, but still always having the humility to keep the door open and be proved wrong" (von Franz, p. 145).

> Eisenhower never fell into the trap,... believing the rules no longer applied to him or that he was better than anyone else.... He was never arrogant or condescending, and he was thoroughly honest.... Humility like Ike's, which conveys absolute assurance but at the same time acknowledges a leader's equality with followers, can be truly inspiring (Gergen, p. 21).

We remain aware of our vulnerabilities and weaknesses during personal mastery. We are aware there is still so much more to learn and improve about ourselves. This self-aware-ness in the emotional intelligence research would include *accurate self-assessment*, being aware of one's limitations (Snow, 2001), and *emotional self-awareness*, where one accu-rately knows one's positive and negative biases (Snow, 2001). As this awareness grows, we become more humble.

In past research interviews with "excellent" nurse executives, they were comfortable with themselves, but ego was not a part of this process. In fact a quality of humility… was evident. Perhaps this is why their own transformational scores were lower than staff ratings of them. They did not see themselves at the top of a pyramid in power positions but saw staff members as pivotal to organizational success. Their role was to support and facilitate staff members within the organization. They also freely admitted and owned their mistakes (Dunham-Taylor, p. 25).

Integrity

The bedrock of both personal mastery, and of effective leadership, is *integrity*—remaining true to oneself while doing what is best for everyone concerned. Integrity is morality, or what is good or right for people as they interact together. Integrity respects everyone. It occurs when one can be empathetic with another person and understand why they are doing what they are doing. One can separate the behavior from the person. (It does not mean that we judge others because we have not walked in their shoes.) We understand their position or their choices—even when we may not agree. We are compassionate. It represents justice and fairness. It does not violate anyone's rights or personal welfare.

Integrity results in a shared resonance of feelings with others, an appreciation of both one's own and other's needs; it supports both the fulfillment of self and of others. This is a tall order. It is incremental. When we live it we are strong and balanced. We are *tuned in to that inner core* that lets us know what is right in a situation. There is a oneness within ourselves. As we work toward this wholeness, every situation we encounter helps us to better understand and reach toward this wholeness:

> *It did not really matter what we expected from life, but rather what life expected from us.* We needed to stop asking about the meaning of life, and instead to think of ourselves as those who were being questioned by life—daily and hourly. Our answer must consist, not in talk and meditation, but in right action and in right conduct. Life ultimately means taking the responsibility to find the right answer to its problems and to fulfill the tasks which it constantly sets for each individual (Frankl, p. 98).

Integrity becomes our choice each moment in our lives. It's a series of choices, each adding to the other. It is incremental. It spirals. In a previous leadership study with "excellent" nurse executives, they stressed the importance of having very high professional, moral, and ethical standards—and stressed the importance of *not compromising* these standards. In other words, they stressed integrity.

A wonderful book, written as a story, further explores leadership and integrity. It is called *Leading with Soul: An Uncommon Journey of Spirit* (2001) by Bolman and Deal. It states:

> Our approach is ecumenical, embracing many spiritual sources: some secular, others religious. Our purpose is to apply wisdom and insights from diverse sources to the deeper, spiritual concerns of the modern

manager. Though everyone needs a personal road to faith, the world needs a spirituality that transcends sectarian boundaries. Living in the global village inevitably means that cultures and faiths meet and interpenetrate at a dizzying pace. All too often, the tragic outcome is a collision of hatred and murder. Yet the basic spiritual teachings and moral precepts of the world's great religions are remarkably similar. Mahatma Gandhi said that he believed in the truths of all of them and that "there will be no lasting peace on earth unless we learn not merely to tolerate but even to respect the other faiths as our own."

In the workplace, all of us need a language of moral discourse that permits discussions of ethical and spiritual issues, connecting them to images of leadership. As management expert Elsa Porter puts it, "in a seminar with seventeen executives from nine corporations, we learned how the privatization of moral discourse in our society has created a deep sense of moral loneliness and moral illiteracy; how the absence of a common language prevents people from talking about and reading the moral issues they face. We learned how the isolation of individuals—the taboo against talking about spiritual matters in the public sphere—robs people of courage, of the strength of heart to do what deep down they believe to be right. They think they are alone in facing these issues" (p. 2).

Behavioral Integrity. If we have integrity, it extends to our behavior. Simons (2002) conducted research measuring managers' behavioral integrity with 6,500 employees at 76 United States and Canadian Holiday Inns. Employees were asked questions about their manager's behavior that included statements like: "My manager delivers on promises." "My manager practices what he preaches." "I am proud to tell others I am part of this hotel." "My coworkers go out of their way to accommodate guests' special requests." When employees felt this to be the case, the satisfaction level was higher, and the financial performance of the hotel was considerably higher. Responses to these items were correlated with customer satisfaction surveys, personnel records, and financial records. "No other single aspect of manager behavior that we measured had as large an impact on profits" (p. 18).

Intuition—Paying Attention To Our Inner Core

Intuition (listening to our inner core) is another capability that we can enhance. We can start by just paying attention to our gut level and the direction it leads us. Have you ever had the experience where you wake up in the morning and suddenly you know what to do about a certain problem or situation? Or had a dream where you know that your child is in danger while on his bike? Or suddenly you start thinking about someone and then they call you; or you know that you need to call them? Or you know that you will be safe in some scheduled surgery? Or you know that a patient is "going bad?" All this information comes from our intuition.

In nursing, we have been more aware of our intuitive capabilities because we are involved with so many people experiencing life-threatening events. Intuition is what helps us deal more effectively with ambiguity, with situations where we do not have all the facts, when there is uncertainty, or when there is complexity. Intuition can also lead us to have better timing in our actions. Our "gut level" tells us what is right and when the right time is to do something.

Our intuition, or inner core, (if we tune in to it) is a wonderful gift. Our "gut level" signals us, if we listen to it, and tells us what is right in each life situation. Some situations are rather mundane so following our inner core is quite easy; at other times we are really tested. For example, in interviews with nurse executives, many of them said that in our present volatile work situations, they knew that they might lose their job at any moment. When something happens that is ethically wrong, they face a choice. What should they do? Confront it or overlook it? If one decides to confront it, one may need to go against a powerful physician, or one may not have the support of the CEO or COO. Several executives discussed confronting such situations and leaving their positions because they could not get support to do what was ethically correct. In other situations, both the executive team and physician group rallied around, doing what was right, with the nurse executive continuing to work there. Health care is fraught with such ethical dilemmas.

The bottom line is always, "Can I live with my decision?". Ironically, even when something awful happens to us (like suddenly losing our job or resigning unexpectedly), if we have followed our inner core, it will always lead us to something better—something we may never have found if this situation had not happened. So in the midst of difficulties and crises, there is *hope*. Our choice at each step is whether to pay attention and to support our inner core or to ignore it. A helpful resource on developing, or tuning into, our intuition can be found in Schultz (1965) *Awakening Intuition: Using Your Mind-Body Network for Insight and Healing*. This book discusses research on intuition, and gives personal stories as well:

> Most people don't have any striking syndromes or atypical brain organization. Most people in our culture, men as well as women, tend to be left hemisphere-dominant, with strong, well-developed frontal lobes. Left-hemisphere people, as you know, put all their faith in intellect. They are very rational, linear, well organized, and verbal. They're the librarians [the financial personnel or critical care nurses], the William Safires of the world, to whom precision of language is important. They may not look like a whole lot of fun, but, boy, do they know language. If they see a leaf falling from a tree, they can go into rhapsodies describing that leaf, its color, the way it's falling, the swirls and spirals and eddies it makes in the air. They'd compose an ode to that leaf, because that's how they think—very precisely, in great detail, with the feeling submerged in verbiage. A right-hemisphere person, by contrast, would look at that leaf and say, "Wow, what a leaf."
>
> The right hemisphere, you'll recall, provides a feeling, an instinct, an impression, or a general outline of a thought or an image—the gestalt of a situation. Intuition tends to come to us initially through the right hemisphere and the temporal lobe. The left hemisphere is very detail-oriented and focused: it has to fill in the details of the intuition we're getting. If

we were making a cookie, the right hemisphere would provide the cookie-cutter configuration, while the left hemisphere supplied the sprinkles on the icing. Or it would work like something I saw in the news after Mother Teresa died. One of her nuns in India made a huge mosaic of Mother Teresa's face on the grass. From a distance, you could see the outline of the nun's face and features; but when you went in closer, you realized that the details were created by thousands of individual flower petals. The two together, the outline and the individual flower petals, made the portrait distinctive. In the same way, it takes both the right hemisphere and the left hemisphere working together to make our intuition intelligible to us (p. 336).

Ideally, we are balanced between both hemispheres. However, in reality many people are not. Instead a person leans toward one hemisphere. Currently in our society, there is a left-hemisphere dominance that can interfere with our ability to tune in to our intuitive processes:

This is the problem for people who live too much in the left hemisphere. Their powerful frontal lobes are always telling them to ignore what's coming from the right hemisphere. As they drown out any input from the right brain and the temporal lobe, these frontal lobes repeat, "You don't know that. You can't know that. That can't be." They thus inhibit the input of emotion, intuition, and body connection from the right hemisphere. Consequently, left-brain people believe they're not intuitive. The fact is that they simply have determined their intuitive strengths and learned how to use them to help overcome and shore up their intuitive weaknesses.... Left-hemisphere people, for instance, tend to think very symbolically, and they may get strong intuition through dreams.

Right-hemisphere people, meanwhile, have their own weaknesses. They may get strong intuitive images, but they're all cookie-cutter configuration and no detail. A right hemisphere doing a reading of someone would be able mainly to describe a scene: "Oh, this person looks like a real mother. She's ethereal and dreamlike. She loves pastels. Her work involves gardening and flowers." This is nice pictorial information, but it's not very analytical. It doesn't give you a lot of context. It requires a left hemisphere to come in and say, "She's about 5 feet 5, her left eye points in, and boy, does she have a pain in her left wrist." The left hemisphere puts a name to what you see or hear intuitively or to the emotions that you're feeling. It tells you, "That person is depressed," or "That person is lonely." Someone who's all right brain tends to express his or her intuition too impressionistically. This doesn't give you anything to sink your teeth into....

Both the left hemisphere and the right hemisphere play an important role in intuition. Where people might have gifts in one versus the other, both are needed to make your intuition useful and available for you to act upon (Schultz, pp. 336–337).

Persistence

When something is important, yet we are not able to achieve it easily, it becomes important to have persistence. We are like a river that flows along and when there is an obstruction, the water tries to find a way around the obstruction—or flow under or over the obstruction, causing its meandering course. Life is like a river. As we are obstructed in pursuing our life purpose, persistence is needed as we meander around the obstruction, or overcome the obstacle. Sometimes we find that we have created the obstruction within ourselves. In this case, persistence means working through our own obstruction. Occasionally, there is a large enough obstruction that we cannot find a way around it. At this point, we must accept what is and move on from there. It does not make sense to continue to knock our heads against the obstruction. However, if something is really important, persistence may well be necessary before one can achieve one's objective.

A wonderful, easy-to-read book about such issues is Johnson's (1998) *Who Moved My Cheese*, written about how we respond to change. This book shows how persistence under the wrong circumstances does not change the present circumstances. The theme of the book is: "change happens (they keep moving the cheese); anticipate change (get ready for the cheese to move); monitor change (smell the cheese often so you know when it is getting old); adapt to change quickly (the quicker you let go of old cheese, the sooner you can enjoy new cheese); change (move with the cheese); enjoy change (savor the adventure and the taste of the cheese); and be ready to quickly change again and again (they keep moving the cheese)" (p. 74).

> Persistence is needed with our commitments we make, and keep, to ourselves and to others. When we make a commitment, we are bound to that specific outcome by a promise or a pledge. In the process we carry this pledge or promise to some kind of action. Many of us, in the heat of the moment, make promises or commit to an action but are unable to flow through to the end. Maxwell believes that commitment is the will of the mind to finish what the heart has begun long after the emotion in which that promise was made has passed. This means that, when the high levels of excitement that occur in the initial phases of an idea or project give way to the long hours of focused detail and plain hard work, we remain committed to the promise (Kowalski and Yoder-Wise, pp. 27–28).

Relationship Effectiveness

Now that we have discussed internal personal mastery issues, we can turn to the way we interact with the world around us. Leadership involves working closely with people in the external environment. We recognize the connectedness between all of us. This external capability allows us to be able to effectively work with, and build relationships with, people and groups with various personalities or characteristics. This is *relationship effectiveness*. Emotional intelligence research has labeled this external function as involving social awareness and relationship management. Certainly this interpersonal effectiveness component is an important part of dynamic leadership. *As with personal mastery, this external leadership capability can be learned and improved.*

Social awareness and relationship management develop as we mature. We exist in interdependent relationships where each person influences others. Close relationships are important for human survival; thus we build bonds, nurturing instrumental, authentic relationships. These relationships are strengthened when we have empathy for each other, and understand each other and the predicaments that we all face. As we experience relationships, it is helpful if we have some social competence and political awareness and have a certain adeptness at knowing when to accept the course others are taking. We need to know when to inspire or persuade others to take a different approach or respond differently to something, reading a group's emotional currents and power relationships.

An effective leader exhibits good interpersonal skills with others, both individually and in groups, recognizing that we have different personalities and come from different backgrounds. This means that we are effective communicators—in expressing ourselves, in listening openly and intently, in actively seeking feedback from others, and in wanting to better understand others. Communication is one of the competencies identified in emotional intelligence research. This is defined as establishing positive relationships and managing expectations (Snow, 2001). "If your words don't stick, you haven't spoken" (Useem, p. 56) Effective leadership involves constant dialogue both written and verbal, coupled with good interpersonal skills.

The word *dialogue* is used consistently in this book to mean the process of communication where everyone discusses their ideas with one another *as well as respects and listens to one another*. It is a two-way process that is a very important component of effective leadership. This form of dialogue, or the Socratic method, so called because it came from Socrates in ancient Greece, is very important, not only to leadership effectiveness but to an organization or work group.

Sometimes communication is most effective when stories are shared. Some people learn by experience, some by hearing, and some by seeing. Stories can achieve learning for each of these learning styles, and thus may be the most effective way to communicate what is important. People may remember the story, and the meaning of the story, for a long time, long after a discussion of just the principles involved within the story would have been forgotten. Stories can also enhance our relationships with others.

When all from the top down use this method, there is better communication and fewer *roads to Abilene*. This concept is explained in a classic article by Harvey (1988). This article discusses how no one really wants to go to Abilene for dinner, but all are afraid to speak out and say so when one person suggests they go. Thus all go to Abilene, and come to find out, if they had honestly discussed the question, none would have chosen to go.

As we discuss issues together honestly, we come up with better ideas and better methods of doing things. As we know each other better, we work together better, so teamwork improves. We tend to know each other's gifts and preferences, and divide the work accordingly. No matter how much or how well we communicate, we have never communicated enough. Communication should be direct and stay in the present. No one, including the leader, should play games. Good communication is knowing when to say something, when to be silent, and when to listen. It is authenticity.

Now that we are in the information age, our communication ability has been both greatly enhanced and yet very impersonal, causing misunderstandings if clarification or dialogue does not occur. First, we need to have skill at various types of information technology— everything from the cell phone, to the Personal Data Assistant (PDA), to the computer, to the Internet:

> The ability to communicate well... actually grows difficult as technol-
> ogy makes communication instantaneous, impersonal, and overwhelm-
> ing. No longer needed to merely pass on information, this century's
> leader needs to help followers understand, frame, and manage the flood
> of information bombarding them, and listen to their concerns and issues.
> In today's email society, communication of meaning, previously done by
> gesture, tone, inflection, body language, and eye contact, is attempted by
> :), J, L, :-o, :-Q, :&, etc., and often is misunderstood. (Remember that
> capital letters mean you are shouting at the recipient.) Future leaders
> need opportunities to develop skill in all forms of electronic communi-
> cation and encouragement to embrace new communication technologies
> (Nauright, p. 26).

Relationship effectiveness is actually a humanistic approach where we are authentic and appreciate authenticity in others. We put people first, and often get recharged by people. This way we are able to accept, and even delight in, other's differences and successes; we also have empathy for problems that others face. This calls for sensitivity—accuracy in interpreting social cues, recognition of all the interconnections between us, treating every-one with dignity, and knowing that we need to build links between individuals, groups, the community, and society. "Interpersonal ineptitude in leaders lowers everyone's perform-ance. It wastes time, creates acrimony, corrodes motivation and commitment, and builds hostility and apathy" (Snow, pp. 442–443).

Relationship effectiveness is not humorless. Relationships can be enhanced by encour-aging everyone's humor. Humor can make the world a better place because it relieves ten-sion. When we enjoy our work and those we work with, life is so much more fun. All can enjoy life, work and the workplace, when everyone can express their lighter side.

Building relationships is an important administrative competence. Collaboration increases as relationships deepen. As one builds relationships, it is inevitable that conflicts occur. This occurrence does not mean that we have been ineffective leaders, but does require us to respond to the conflicting issues that result from differences. When negotiat-ing conflict, effective leaders create an environment where people respect each other, and can openly discuss their differences, ideas, and perceptions. This can lead to finding ways to resolve conflicts, or to at least better understand where others are coming from in their relationships with us:

> This role competence requires the leader to communicate effectively
> with others in a way that anticipates and, as necessary, disarms the

potential for conflict. This leader focuses on establishing relational and emotional bonds in the team that develop the emotional maturity of team members and facilitate the stability of positive and effective relationships. The enthusiastic, caring, and supportive leader generates those same feelings throughout the team. This individual supports the power of humor, kindness, communication, and availability to others in a way that creates a context of inclusion and caring (O'Grady, p. 109).

It is important to note here that both the external and internal components of leadership have to be integrated together. Thus we continue to respect each person, be honest, possess integrity, and be trustworthy. In our relationships, we encourage everyone to find meaning in her/his life and work—even when this may cause us some difficulties as leaders. For instance, it may be best to encourage a staff member to take another job more suitable to their gifts and life purpose, even when this means we will have to find someone to replace them.

CORE VALUES

As we further explore social awareness and relationship management, there are some important cornerstones that can enhance our effectiveness. One cornerstone, already discussed within personal mastery, is integrity. In relationship management, another cornerstone involves the *identification of core values*—such as doing what is best for the patient, honesty, fairness, excellence, high quality, integrity, credibility, trust, caring, justice, commitment, compassion, loyalty, generosity, reciprocity, dignity, sympathy, caring, mercy—and *constantly living the values. If one skips over this, the result is ineffective leadership.* In fact, the core values are SO important, every decision and the timing of the decision needs to support the identified core values. (Even not making a decision is a decision!)

Identifying and living by core values suddenly became popular in organizations when Collins and Porras' book, *Built to Last*, came out in 1994. In the book they identified visionary companies that met the following criteria:

- Premier institution in its industry,
- Widely admired by knowledgeable business people,
- Made an indelible imprint on the world in which we live,
- Had multiple generations of chief executives,
- Been through multiple product (or service) life cycles, and
- Founded before 1950 (p. 2).

They found that each of the visionary companies had identified and lived by core values. The identified core values differed among the visionary companies, but all deeply believed and consistently lived the identified value:

> A visionary company almost religiously preserves its core ideology—changing it seldom, if ever. Core values in a visionary company form a rock-solid foundation and do not drift with the trends and fashions of the day; in some cases, the core values have remained intact for well over

one hundred years. And the basic purpose of a visionary company—its reason for being—can serve as a guiding beacon for centuries, like an enduring star on the horizon. Yet, while keeping their core ideologies tightly fixed, visionary companies display a powerful drive for progress that enables them to change and adapt without compromising their cherished core ideals (pp. 8–9).

Examples of core values identified by the visionary companies included:

- Hewlett Packard: "Respect and concern for individual employees,"
- Wal-Mart: "Exceed customer expectations,"
- Boeing: "Being on the leading edge of aviation; being pioneers,"
- 3M: "Respect for individual initiative,"
- Nordstrom: "Service to the customer above all else," and
- Merck: "We are in the business of preserving and improving human life" (pp. 81–82).

Collins and Porras stressed that "ultimately, the *only* thing a company should not change over time is its core ideology.... Over time, cultural norms must change; strategy must change; product lines must change; goals must change; competencies must change; administrative policies must change; organization structure must change; reward systems must change" (p. 82).

Core values are so important, that, in a way, it is too bad this gained popularity prompted by *Built to Last* being published. So often, the "in thing" quickly passes as everyone tries to copy it, some succeed in achieving it, most do not, and the fad changes to the next thing that gains popularity. Having core values, and living them, *cannot* be a fad. It is a very difficult endeavor, but one well worth the effort if one wants to be effective as an individual, as a leader, and as a work group or organization.

Identification Of Core Values

How do we identify our core values? Or, if they already exist, how do we re-evaluate them occasionally? As a leader, think of what is important for yourself. For instance, perhaps one identifies with the value, "I want patients to receive the same care I want my family member to receive."

Once the leader has given this some thought, dialogue with staff about it. Is this value important to staff? Are other values important to staff?

The next step after discussion is for both leader and staff to agree to constantly live by these values. All their decisions and actions support the values. Can all agree to make this commitment? This step to achieve value congruence is very important. If this is skipped, staff commitment to the core value(s) may not occur.

Executive groups in organizations often identify a core value(s) within a philosophy statement. It is most helpful if the philosophy or mission statement can be simply stated. After all, no one can remember ponderous mission statements that go on for pages! Sometimes this statement is posted near the health care organization entrance, or posted in the hall or elevator. Another common place to find it is on the back of employee name badges. An organization is healthiest when all have agreed to live by these core values.

Collins and Porras (1991) have written an excellent, thoughtful article on developing organizational mission statements, "Organizational Vision and Visionary Organizations," in the *California Management Review*. Another thoughtful article, "Make Your Values Mean Something" (Lencioni, 2002), identifies additional issues with ensuring the values identified are appropriate and authentic.

Living By The Core Values

Identification of core values is the first step in effective leadership. Then the hard part begins—actually living by the identified core values. As situations occur, both the administrators and staff need to constantly ask, "Is this the care I would want my family member to receive?" Or, "Was I respectful as I did this action?". Encourage everyone to critique each situation by asking the core value question. When someone, *including ourselves*, is not supporting the core values in an action, explore why and how this situation could have been handled differently to more effectively support the core value.

One very important component of administrative competence is generating trust. We achieve this by exhibiting consistent behaviors. What we say is what we do. Our actions match our words. For instance, if the administrator says that there will be no layoffs during a budget cut, then no layoffs occur. Or if the administrator doesn't know what will happen, it is best to say so to staff. In the emotional intelligence, research trustworthiness includes displaying honesty and integrity (Snow, 2001). Every action the administrator takes, every word out of the administrator's mouth, needs to support the core value(s).

Core values may be directly identified as such, be a mission statement, or may be buried in philosophy statements. If the statement is too long, it is easy to ignore it. It is also easy to ignore it when actions taken by the board and executive group do not seem to support core values. *Actions speak louder than words.* Administrators may think that all they have to do is give lip service to the values. Instead, staff will look at the leader's actions and quickly see whether or not the administrator actually means and lives by the values. And if the organizational leadership does not support the core values, this has a downward spiral effect organizationally. *"A fish starts to rot from the head."*

Because core values are the cornerstone of leadership integrity, when the fish starts rotting at the top, the downward spiral from the top continues as other organizational groups ignore values and become dysfunctional. When dysfunctional groups abound throughout the organization, chances are the organization will start to experience financial difficulties. There is a direct correlation between poor leadership and financial statements:

> Empty values statements create cynical and dispirited employees, alienate customers, and undermine managerial credibility.... The debasement of values is a shame, not only because the resulting cynicism poisons the cultural well but also because it wastes a good opportunity. Values can set a company apart from the competition by clarifying its identity and serving as a rallying point for employees. But coming up with strong values—and sticking with them—requires real guts. Indeed, an organization considering a values initiative must first come to terms with the fact that, when properly practiced, values inflict pain. They make some

employees feel like outcasts. They limit an organization's strategic and operational freedom and constrain the behavior of its people. They leave executives open to heavy criticism for even minor violations. And they demand constant vigilance (Lencioni, p. 114).

Healthier bottom lines result from effective leadership. It saves A LOT of money when a leadership problem is fixed; besides the bottom line there will be lower turnover rates, and a more committed staff giving better care to patients and their families. The leadership problem may have to be fixed by improving or changing unit leadership, or it may be a much larger systems problem. "Rotten to the core" does not just refer to fruit! In this case, *fixing the leadership problem may extend to those above the nurse administrator—including the CEO and the board.* When poor leadership is not recognized, or is allowed to continue, the message to staff, physicians, patients, and families is that poor job performance is acceptable behavior. Employee retention becomes a problem as qualified, high performing staff find another workplace that supports core values.

If you find that the top leadership does not support and exemplify the values, one needs to ask, "Can I live with this?" The question is, is the situation better somewhere else? Or, is it best to remain and work to make things better within the realm of current responsibilities? In either case, it is important to stay tuned into our inner self, our gut level, which provides us with the answer to this dilemma. This intuitive knowledge source always leads us in the appropriate direction. Whereas one person may leave, another may stay. My life purpose may be to work to make a place better within an organization, while another person's purpose is to go somewhere else and work there. If it "feels right," do it. Going against this inner core generally results in more difficulties.

If a person decides to stay, it will be important to start with the identification and verbal commitment to core values within the work group, and then to live the core values, expecting all in the work group—including the top administrator and board—to support the core values through their actions. After all, our small efforts, if combined with enough other such efforts, can improve things, not only within the work group but at other levels as well. Remember, the Berlin wall did come down! The challenge, or rather opportunity, is for all of us, in our small way, to make a difference. Then we can look in the mirror each morning and feel good about what we have done. When enough of us achieve this, the Berlin wall—dysfunctional work groups, administrators, and boards—will come down, even when the powers that be want it to remain. There will be an improvement in the way health care is delivered, and we personally will be happier with ourselves and with our work.

Thus within organizations, leadership is most effective when all are working to support the core values in every action. This is essential throughout the organization for overall organizational success. The effects of living the core values has a reverberation effect. The crazy, but wonderful, result: *Living by core values achieves both quality care and dedicated employees, as well as cost effectiveness.* What a powerful statement!

When an administrator lives by the core values, the administrator gains staff respect, even when staff members do not agree with the leader's decision(s). The way leaders treat staff is the way staff treats patients. If we have satisfied staff, we have satisfied patients.

Satisfaction follows effective leadership. So does higher productivity; fewer expenses; more satisfied staff, physicians, and patients; and, most importantly, better patient outcomes. Effective leadership, starting with the core values, has a spiral effect upward. This is such an important concept that many leaders and authors have spent their entire career further developing and sharing their leadership experiences, (i.e., DePree in *Leadership is an Art*; Bennis and Nanus in *Leaders: The Strategies for Taking Charge*; and Lencioni in *The Five Temptations of a CEO*, to name a few).

VISION OR STRATEGIC DIRECTION

> Reagan recognized that to stir people, you must give voice to their own deep desires, inspiring them to believe they can climb mountains they always thought were too high.
>
> *–Gergen, p. 20.*

Once an organization agrees on core values, it must then determine its strategic direction. Having a vision became a popular fad a few years ago. Actually, the vision is the present strategic direction, while remaining dynamic and ever changing as the environment changes. After all, if we don't have goals, how do we know where we are going ? It is a fallacy to believe that the leader or president or executive group knows and sets the vision—or strategic direction—alone. Bits of the vision emerge from everyone. The administrators dialogue with staff, patients, families, physicians, suppliers, and others. From this the administrator pulls the strategic direction together. Then each person must committ to work to make the plan a reality, continuing to tweek it as changes become evident.

When staff sees a meaningful relationship between the strategic direction and staff work, and understands how such work contributes to the successful accomplishment of the vision, staff members become committed to supporting the strategic direction. A synergy happens. In fact, staff members know what needs to be done, and when they are committed to the strategic direction, they work harder and accomplish more. This commitment is strengthened when leader and staff are both willing to transcend their own agendas to accomplish these goals. And, of course, the strategic direction must support the core values that both leader and staff have agreed to previously.

As everyone works toward the vision, some things succeed or work fairly well. Other things fail or do not work as well. People make mistakes or get off track. The leader may need to follow up on the important aspects of the vision to ensure the strategic direction can become a reality. All this is part of the dynamic process. The vision is not a road map, it is a journey we take together. As the vision changes, it is as though we started by looking into one or two windows in a house; then, as we look into more windows, our view, or vision, changes. Everyone adds to, or changes, parts of the vision. At times a whole new house is built. Hopefully, the strategic plan, as well as everyone's goals within the organization, mirrors the dynamic, changing vision. Being able to "change on a dime" has become a popular term meaning the work group needs to be flexible. Things can always be improved. Goals, and thus the strategic direction, changes and need to be better than they were previously. The bottom line, when living the vision, is that we always support the core value—*what is best for the patient?*—and make the necessary changes to achieve this value as well as to improve or change the vision.

A vision should stretch everyone yet seem possible to accomplish. As the administrator you may see further ahead than some in the group; conversely some other group members may be ahead of you. We all learn from each other. We all need to be open to everything and everyone around us to bring more coherence to the vision. Visionary leadership is one competency of an effective leader, identified in both transformational leadership and emotional intelligence research.

THE PYGMALION EFFECT

Within the interpersonal environment, the *pygmalion effect* is something very important for administrators to consider. This concept is discussed in detail in a classic *Harvard Business Review* article, "Pygmalion in Management" (Livingston, 2003). Research has shown that the supervisor's beliefs about the person being supervised becomes a self-fulfilling prophecy—even when the person may believe the opposite. In other words, if the nurse executive believes that a nurse manager is doing a poor job, even a high achiever will eventually be doing poor work. The same is true for a nurse manager. If the nurse manager believes that a staff member is a wonderful employee—this will become a self-fulfilling prophecy. And conversely, as in the movie *My Fair Lady*, even when the staff member believes s/he can not do the job, *as long as the supervisor believes the staff member can do the job, the staff member will successfully accomplish the work*. This is why it is important to have good chemistry with your supervisor, as well as with those who report to you. When this occurs, anyone can succeed given the values, support, and opportunity.

If an employee is having problems, the first thing we supervisors need to do is to examine our own beliefs about the person who is not performing adequately—a powerful message for any supervisory person! "Do I believe this person is doing well, or is capable of doing well, on the job? Do I believe this person can improve?" Self examination about one's own likes and dislikes, as well as personal biases, about each staff member is the first step one must take when in the supervisory role. The Pygmalion article finds that effective leaders provide "high performance expectations that [staff members] fulfill," while ineffective leaders "fail to develop similar expectations, and as a consequence, the productivity of their [staff] suffers" (p. 122). Do we administrators set high performance expectations for staff—and expect that staff will accomplish these? An administrator must be fair to each employee. Then anyone can succeed given the support and opportunity.

After all this self-exploration on the part of the supervisor, if the employee still is having a performance problem, then it is important to discuss the specific problem with the employee. As we previously discussed, if the employee is in a job that does not fulfill her/his gifts, it may be that a change in responsibilities or jobs would help. If the problem persists and is serious enough, it then is time to begin the counseling process. We recommend involving the employee in the counseling process as described in another classic *Harvard Business Review* article by Campbell, Fleming, and Grote (1985) "Discipline Without Punishment—At Last." Here the goal is to involve the problem employee in solving the problem, to issue "reminders" instead of "warnings," and to use a decision-making short leave day for the employee to decide whether to change and stay, or to submit their resignation.

> When we care for the care giver, the care giver will then care for the patients.

Exhibit 3–7 Hagberg's Model of Personal Power

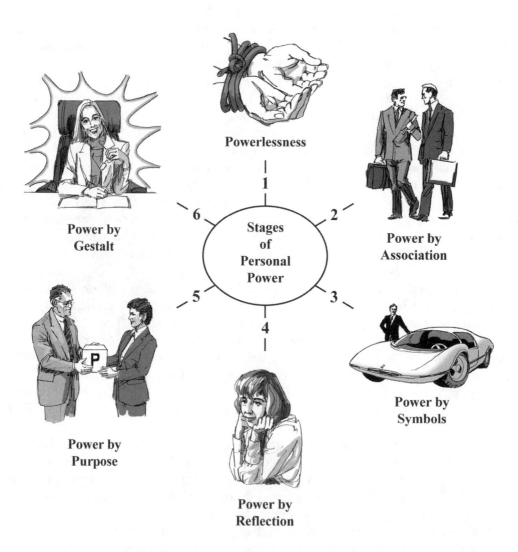

EMPOWERMENT

The pygmalion effect influences how effectively we are able to empower others. Empowerment is an important factor in quantum leadership. It is important that everyone be empowered to go ahead with their work in ways that support the core values. After all, everyone has something unique to offer based on their gifts. The word "empowerment" has been a popular fad, yet many different definitions of empowerment abound. Two people using this term may mean very different things. Some administrators will say, "I empower staff. I let them do the work." This really says, "I delegate the work but make sure you do it my way." In actuality, empowerment has a very different definition in quantum leadership.

Power

In order to define empowerment, let's examine our definition of power. Do you think power is finite? If so, there is only so much of it. This means that for me to get more power, I must take it away from someone. The quantum view would say that power is *infinite*, that there is always more power available. So if I give it away by empowering others, there is still plenty left for myself. In fact, if I encourage others' leadership, I will be enhancing my own leadership. The idea here is that the more I give away, the more power I create for myself. After all, continuing with the quantum view, we are all in this together. (Just as an effective leader possesses all aspects of leadership integrated within oneself, so are we all interrelated in this world of ours.)

This is why such wonderful energy can result when a group works together to accomplish a certain objective. All come with different perspectives which, when empowered, can lead the group as a whole to develop shared visions of the past, the present, and the future. The future vision will be better than what any one of the persons involved could have come up with alone, and all will have a more accurate picture of what this vision is because they participated in creating it.

Stages of Power

A wonderful resource on power representing the quantum perspective is Janet Hagberg's book (1994), *Real Power: Stages of Personal Power in Organizations*. It states that: "Personal power is the extent to which one is able to link the outer capacity for action (external power) with the inner capacity for reflection (internal power)" (p. xxi).

Using that power definition Hagberg identifies six developmental stages of personal power (see **Exhibit 3–7**). The first three stages reflect the external power perspective while the last three stages become internally oriented. The definition of power changes at each stage, and has resultant positive and negative aspects that cause developmental dilemmas a person needs to resolve before moving on successfully to the next stage. One can manifest different stages of power when we experience different situations and people, yet we have a "home" stage where we tend to be most often.

Stage One, Powerlessness. When in Stage One, *Powerlessness*, people do not think they possess much power. Because of this world view, they deal with the world *using manipulation*:

> Powerless people feel they are constantly being *manipulated by others*, pushed around, helped, controlled, duped, or taken care of, but they also find they depend upon *manipulating others* to get things done or to acquire things for themselves (p. 2).

The struggle at this stage is to overcome dependence. Resolution begins when people start to feel good about themselves, develop self-esteem, and begin to use other more effective skills to deal with the world. In Stage One a person's most consistent deterrent is fear. When fear rules, a person will divert back to manipulation again.

Stage Two, Power by Association. When her/his skills increase, a person moves on to Stage Two, *Power by Association.* "People at Stage Two usually want to be like someone else. They frequently have a role model or at least identify themselves with other more powerful people" (p. 19). Within an organization, people at this stage identifiy the people with the power and hope that maybe some of the power will rub off on them. Magic—their description of power—is expected. "They are apprentices to power [but] . . .can't grasp it" (p. 20). This is the stage where bosses take on the most significance. These people love to be mentored. To move on to Stage Three, one needs to further develop self-esteem and learn to have self-confidence—not have a need for the confidence or security gleaned from others.

Stage Three, Power by Symbols.

> As people gain self-confidence [and self-esteem], they will progress on to Stage Three, *Power by Symbols.* This is the dynamo stage.... They are learning or have learned to play the game, and for the most part they are rewarded for it.... Thousands of people at Stage Three have been led to believe all their lives that 'this is it!' (p. 45).

At this stage a person strives for something—a degree, a position, a special car, a fancy home—and when attained, think that one has "made it." These things become symbols of success. Threes enjoy showing off these symbols. Their description of power is *control.* They can become stuck at this stage because they like it. Often a crisis moves a person on to Stage Four. The crisis—whether internal or external—prompts the person to question how important these things *really* are. Then confusion begins. Up to this point their power definition has been provided *externally* by others. This confusion begins an *internal* search where one eventually arrives at Stage Four. Note that in the first three stages empowerment has not occurred.

Stage Four, Power by Reflection. In Stage Four, *Power by Reflection*, a person is competent and has developed her/his own leadership style. This style may or may not fit with organizational norms. These persons have integrity. "Fours have a solid reputation of honesty, fairness, sound judgment, and follow-through" (p. 73). Yet they have inner unresolved dilemmas that may not be apparent to others. Thus it is a time for reflection. What is really important? Here true leadership begins—leadership that is based on values, not on symbols or positions. At this stage "they can admit their mistakes without having to be found out first" (p. 83). They also are better risk-takers and are more courageous. *True empowerment does not happen until one is at this stage.*

When we empower others, it means that we trust them to accomplish the goal(s)/tasks. Here a leader realizes that *leaders succeed through the successes of others.* Empowering others can involve several processes: mentoring and coaching others in their learning and development; fostering staff creativity, encouraging growth, determining and trying out new solutions; enhancing and recognizing staff successes; protecting staff from unnecessary work; and respecting and valuing staff contributions. Since each staff member has different gifts, this process varies with each person. Empowerment also occurs in times of trouble. Giving staff support and help when overwhelmed or experiencing a problem; discussing possible alternatives in a difficult situation; or even recognizing mistakes but making sure that someone is not devastated by what they have done, are all examples of empowerment.

In Stage Four there are two traps—both coming from the ego. One can gain influence and enjoy the power one has amassed and become stuck, or one can develop some thing—develop a program or building—that represents oneself and carries on one's memory after one has gone. At this stage the only way to overcome the ego is to go within. One needs to discover a meaningful life purpose. This process is different for everyone. There is no cookie cutter approach or one size fits all. The answer is found within.

Stage Five, Power by Purpose.

> When a meaningful life purpose has been discovered, people move on to Stage Five, *Power by Purpose*. Stage Five is unlike all of the preceding stages. Its uniqueness lies in the strength of the inner person relative to the strength of the organizational hold on that person. The guide for behavior in Fives is the inner intuitive voice. They trust it more than they trust the rules. Stage Fives are different internally and externally now. They are more congruent because they no longer have to live two separate lives as Stage Fours do. And it is even harder to spot Fives because they don't care if they're ever spotted. In fact, they may even hide a bit. Fives have a life purpose that extends beyond themselves (p. 103).

Here is where the infinite power definition comes in. "Power is like love. You can't have it truly until you give it away or let it go, and the more of it you give unselfishly, the more it multiplies" (p. 104) and comes back to you in different ways. Fives let others lead. They believe that power is based on the values—not on organizational norms or positions—and make decisions accordingly. "They do not attempt to gain or accumulate power because they find the other forms in which it reappears, like caring, appreciation, and friendship, more rewarding" (p. 104). They are humble and possess inner vision. "They see themselves paradoxically for the first time: On the one hand, they are insignificant and, on the other hand, tremendously important in the larger scheme of things" (pp. 104–105). They concentrate on the things that give meaning—both to them and to others. Their ultimate objective is to empower others. They do not need to be in charge, preferring to work behind the scenes.

> The crisis that people experience in moving from Stage Five to Stage Six is that of understanding the cosmos. No longer does the individual matter in the larger scheme of things, and yet the individual is all that matters. That paradox, once understood, accepted, and humbly loved, moves one toward wisdom. In fact, coming to understand paradox as a guiding force in life is one of the clues that a Five is moving to Stage Six. A par-

adox in the move itself is that Fives do not seek to move anywhere; they just love and may or may not emerge as Sixes. It doesn't really matter. And that may be why they become Sixes (pp. 124–125).

Stage Six, Power by Gestalt. Stage Sixes, *Power by Gestalt*, possess wisdom. "Gestalt means more than the sum of the parts" (p. 130). They often spend a lot of time alone and gain strength from higher sources. They possess an inner calm and have quiet strength. These individuals often go unrecognized because they choose not to take prominent positions. Instead they prefer to be alone tuning into higher sources.

Using Hagberg's definitions of power, it becomes more obvious how to define effective leadership. "People can be leaders at any stage of personal power, but they cannot be TRUE leaders until they reach Stage Four—Power by Reflection" (p. 149).

Empowering Based on Gifts

> By allowing others to shine that light will end up somehow reflecting back to you.
>
> *(This quote is from a nurse executive interview.*
> *Confidentiality was promised so the person*
> *cannot be named here.)*

From Hagberg's stages then, we can see that effective leadership involves empowering staff to do work that is a match with their gifts; and that a leader must be at least at Stage Four to begin to achieve empowerment. In fact, "Maxwell hypothesized that being immensely secure in yourself is at the heart of serving people" (Kowalski and Yoder-Wise, p. 30). How wonderful it would be if all we nurses, not to mention every other person working in health care organizations, were at least in Stage Four.

Bass (1998) has called this kind of empowerment *individualized consideration*. Individualized consideration is needed because people are in different places with different abilities and gifts. A leader delegates differently to different individuals. Leaders empower others by giving as much responsibility to staff and patients at all levels to make the most of whatever talents and experience staff have. It is best if abilities are stretched in an empowering environment. When we empower, or delegate, we trust. Our message is that we know they can accomplish the work successfully. (Remember The Pygmalion Effect?)

Empowering is effective because people want to make a difference. We want our lives to have meaning. Each of us comes to this world to accomplish something special that no one else will do. This serves a larger purpose, making this a better world. We reach our highest potential when we pursue and use our gifts. Identification of our personal gifts starts us on the road to achieving our life purpose.

> Man's search for meaning is the primary motivation in his life and not a "secondary rationalization" of instinctual drives. This meaning is unique and specific in that it must and can be fulfilled by him alone; only then does it achieve a significance which will satisfy his own *will* to meaning (Frankl, p. 121).

At times people are in the jobs that are not a match with their gifts. They may not be performing well because they are not *engaged* in the work; the work does not tie in with their life purpose and their gifts. They are probably unhappy, and are in the wrong place. As a leader, you may need to talk to a person when you perceive a mismatch with her/his work and gifts, and then encourage a change in jobs to better achieve her/his life purpose.

Empowerment, at times, can achieve magical results. In past research conducted by the author, one hospital nurse executive described how the wheelchairs kept disappearing and were not in the locations where they were needed. An orderly approached the nurse executive and said that he would like to be put in charge of the wheelchairs. The nurse executive said, "Go to it," and put him in charge—announcing that the orderly was in charge of wheelchairs at the next set of meetings she had with staff on all shifts. Her comment to the researcher was, "I didn't know how to fix this problem and I didn't have the time to deal with it!" The orderly was proud of his responsibility, felt empowered, fixed the problem, and there were always wheelchairs where they were needed.

Just think of what could be accomplished if more empowerment occurred! When someone wants to try to improve something, why not encourage them, and give them the time and the authority to do it? It is easy with circumstances that seem limiting—such as the nursing shortage—to say that there is no way this person can be given extra time. Somehow, if we really believe there is a solution to finding the time, there will be one! Job satisfaction studies show that people are more satisfied with their jobs when they do not consistently do the same things everyday. All of us need challenges. In fact, challenges result in retention—a reason the person stays rather than moving on.

COLLABORATION

Collaboration is another component of relationship effectiveness. Relationship building, or effectively functioning as a team, is enhanced when collaboration occurs. In quantum leadership, building teams based on collaboration is extremely important. When we collaborate, we are working with others to achieve shared goals. We are cooperating. We are sharing knowledge with each other. There is an element of shared meaning within the group. We are creating group synergy in the pursuit of collective goals. We are making sacrifices to achieve the goals. Invariably conflicts will occur. We are most apt to experience success if we forget about winning and losing. After all, if the goal is not achieved, everyone loses. We need to harness the energy of all in the group in as positive a way as possible. Sticking with the core values can help us work through the many conflicts, and achieve better collaboration among the group members.

When we discuss the stages of power, it becomes evident that true collaboration starts to occur when the leader is at a Stage Four or higher. A person at Stage Three is still concerned with selfish motives. Collaboration occurs when we realize that we need to be true to ourselves and to others equally. This is also a current societal dilemma:

> Very few people work by themselves and achieve results by themselves.... Most people work with others and are effective with other people.... Managing yourself requires taking responsibility for relationships. This has two parts. The first is to accept the fact that other people

are as much individuals as you yourself are. They perversely insist on behaving like human beings. This means that they too have their strengths; they too have their ways of getting things done; they too have their values. To be effective, therefore, you have to know the strengths, the performance modes, and the values of your coworkers.... Each [coworker] works his or her way, not your way. And each is entitled to work in his or her way. What matters is whether they perform and what their values are.... The first secret of effectiveness is to understand the people you work with and depend on so that you can make use of their strengths, their ways of working, and their values. *Working relationships are as much based on the people as they are on the work.* [my emphasis]

The second part of relationship responsibility is taking responsibility for communication.... Personality conflicts... arise from the fact that people do not know what other people are doing and how they do their work, or what contribution the other people are concentrating on and what results they expect. And the reason they do not know is that they have not been asked and therefore have not been told.... Even people who understand the importance of taking responsibility for relationships often do not communicate sufficiently with their associates. They are afraid of being thought presumptuous or inquisitive or stupid. They are wrong. Whenever someone goes to his or her associates and says, "This is what I am good at. This is how I work. These are my values. This is the contribution I plan to concentrate on and the results I should be expected to deliver," the response is always, "This is most helpful. But why didn't you tell me earlier?" [It is important for the leader to ask,] "What do I need to know about your strengths, how you perform, your values, and your proposed contribution?"... Trust... means that they understand one another (Drucker, 1999, pp. 71–72).

No one person is more important than another in a group. We all have our functions, or tasks, to accomplish and if we were without any member, the group would not function effectively. The problem here is that certain members of the group may perceive themselves as more important, i.e., the leader, or, in health care, the physician. In the pecking order of our society, the physician has importance. Yet if you talk with the most effective physicians, they are humble individuals who realize how much they count on the rest of the health care team to give care, and who realize that they do not have all the answers in treating patients. Even the physicians who are not yet as far along as this appreciate having a health care team they can count on to give patients the care that is needed.

The leader is only as effective as the team. After all, where would everyone be if no one cleaned the bathrooms for example? Part of leadership effectiveness is recognizing the individual differences in team members:

Some people work best as team members. Others work best alone. Some are exceptionally talented as coaches and mentors; others are simply

incompetent as mentors.... A great many people perform best as advis-
ers but cannot take the burden and pressure of making the decision. A
good many other people, by contrast, need an adviser to force themselves to think; then they can make decisions and act on them with
speed, self-confidence, and courage. This is the reason, by the way, that
the number two person in an organization often fails when promoted to
the number one position. The top spot requires a decision maker. Strong
decision makers often put somebody they trust into the number two spot
as their adviser—and in that position the person is outstanding. But in
the number one spot, the same person fails. He or she knows what the
decision should be but cannot accept the responsibility of actually making it (Drucker, pp. 68–69).

As East meets West in our generation, perhaps we will be able to meld the positives from
both cultures. In the West, we overemphasize individuality; while in the East, group collectivity—doing what is best for the group at personal sacrifice—is the mode. Each taken
too far to the extreme ignores the other. For instance, individuality can support competition, and conflicting people never enter into a dialogue with each other. Therefore, a better result is never achieved. Everyone is too busy trying to win, even if the opposition
loses. On the other hand, if all decisions are made based on what is best for the group as a
whole, someone's gifts may not be able to blossom. Bringing about a synergy between
these two opposites, individuality and group collectivity, may be part of our collective societal purpose presently. It may also help us to achieve better collaboration within conflicting viewpoints. Presently, our test seems to be remaining true to ourselves while doing
what is best for everyone concerned. Doesn't this sound like we are synergizing the East
and West philosophies?

Maintaining Objectivity

Collaboration is best achieved when we are able to maintain objectivity. Here it is important to understand people's different perspectives about an issue. This understanding
explains why they act as they do. With this knowledge, one is able to maintain this objectivity when dealing with difficult situations.

Staying in the Adult. Perhaps the best way to exemplify maintaining objectivity is to
use a transactional analysis model, or *staying in the adult*. Let's explain. Looking at
Exhibit 3–8, the P stands for the *parent* part of us. This side has many aspects. It can be
nurturing and helpful. It can be judgmental and be full of *should* statements. The C stands
for the *child* part of us. Children can be playful, or angry. They can be loving and responsive. Children often need direction and attention from parents to grow. Lastly, there is the
A, or *adult* part of us. This is the reasoning part. It is more like a computer in that emotion
is not attached to it, while emotion is attached to the parent and child part.

Now let's use this exhibit and look at interactions between two people. If Person A
comes from the parent when communicating with Person B, Person B will probably
respond from the child. If the parental communication is nurturing, the child response is
loving and uses the information to learn more about the world. When the parental approach

Exhibit 3–8 Parental Approach

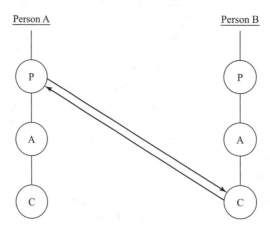

Person A   Person B

A parental approach will elicit a child response.

Key:

P = Parent
A = Adult
C = Child

is judgmental, the child may feel ashamed or angry and respond based on that response. Emotion is involved in the conversation. The same thing happens if the supervisor comes from the parent when interacting with staff.

Now let's move to **Exhibit 3–9**. Here Person A is coming from the child when communicating with Person B. The communication coming from Person A's child will hook into Person B's parent. So Person B will respond from their parent. If the child is angry, the parent may be angry. Or the parent may be calm and try to stop, or ignore, the angry outburst. Again, emotion is part of the interaction.

In **Exhibit 3–10**, Person A is in the adult when communicating with Person B. This is most likely to hook into Person B's adult. This is the reasoning, calm part of both individuals. Emotion is not involved. Person B still has a choice as to how to respond. If Person B chooses to stay in the parent or child mode, her/his response may switch to that approach. However, the greatest likelihood is that each person will communicate from the adult. Ideally, *the effective administrator uses the adult approach in communicating with others.* In fact, when we feel ourselves responding to someone using emotion, this is a clue that we are either in the parent or child part of ourselves. This is a time to rethink, "Do I really want to be in the parent or the child?" It may be time to exit to a place where one can become more calm and balanced before continuing with the communication!

When anyone is angry, the person is not as effective in responding to situations. Anger causes more anger and things escalate; this is not desirable. There is greater chance for success when one is able to stop and think before acting—or reacting—to a situation. If one is immediately emotional in a situation, it is generally better to wait, or step out of a situ-

Exhibit 3–9   Child Approach

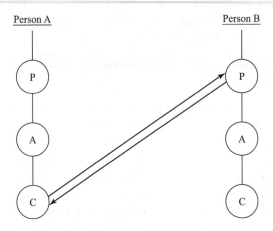

A child approach will elicit a parental response.

Key:

P = Parent
A = Adult
C = Child

Exhibit 3–10   Adult Approach

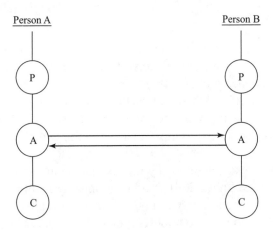

An adult approach will be more likely to elicit an adult response.

Key:

P = Parent
A = Adult
C = Child

ation, until one can get back into the adult before acting. Police know this—the best way to live to retirement is to remain calm in the midst of crises.

Even nurturing behaviors can get us in trouble. For instance, I often hear nurses say, "I will do this myself because I can do it better." This is their reason not to delegate tasks to others. This is dangerous because one person cannot possibly take care of everything alone! What the person often does not realize, is the child message this gives to others, "You cannot do this as well as I can." In fact, this attitude is dangerous because then others do not learn. For example, a new nurse is not appropriately mentored about the role; or a patient does not learn how to give his own insulin or appropriately care for himself. Or the parental nurse manager expects that all staff will check to see what the manager wants to do before taking action. This is also a trap—what are staff members to do when the manager is absent? Thus staying in the adult is very important in quantum leadership.

Objectivity, or staying in the adult, is very helpful when in conflict. It is easy for people to see each other as without a redeeming quality, even though the conflict is only caused by a person's behavior or by differences in opinion. It is helpful to identify the *real* source of the conflict. In this case, discussing the problem, and encouraging others to not attach the problem to the entire person can be helpful. It can be helpful to come back to the values when examining a conflict, asking, *"What is best for the patient?"*

Objectivity leads to better conflict management and decision making. To a certain extent, our own life experiences will always somewhat cloud our objectivity. But this is something that can be improved. Try to have a dynamic picture of the people involved, take into account all the different viewpoints, and stay in touch with what feels right intuitively. In this way we connect the past with the present, while working toward a better future. We can make the best of every challenge or opportunity. Doing so allows us to deal more effectively with chaos and complexity, and to bring clarity by cutting through the clutter.

Empathy

Collaboration is also enhanced by empathy for others. We are most effective when we can go beyond selfishness, and connect with something that is larger than ourselves. This empathy, or sensitivity, or connection with others and their predicaments, reflects an altruism that will better other's welfare. "Without feelings of deep sympathy and sorrow for others struck by misfortune and a genuine desire to alleviate suffering on the part of caregivers, patient care service would be no more than a robotic endeavor" (Porter-O'Grady and Malloch, 2003).

In emotional intelligence research, empathy means that we are able to learn from others' experiences and expertise (Snow, 2001), and that empathy is reflected in our actions. Empathy also reflects the connection between ourselves and a higher power, found in our integrity. It is the "caring" component so important in health care. It is what we give to others with no motivation other than what is best for them. Perhaps the best way to say this is, *we want what is best for everyone concerned.*

Empathy occurs when we understand another person's perspective. To achieve this understanding we will need to dialogue with others. In fact, as we get to know each other, we become able to anticipate a person's response to a situation, decision, or action. It is important to understand why someone chose to take a certain action, or to understand how a decision effects others. This understanding helps us more to effectively lead.

Conflict Management

Although good teamwork and collegiality decreases conflict, as groups work together to achieve collaboration, conflicts inevitably occur. Most often conflicts are caused by *expectations*. Think about this. If I have an expectation that you will (or should) respond a certain way, when you respond differently there is a conflict. This conflict could have been avoided if I had not had an expectation of how you should respond. The most effective leader lets go of expectations of others. After all, how a person responds is beyond our control.

Another issue is whether people feel free to express the conflict. This includes the leader having "a willingness to risk exposing thoughts and feelings and to acknowledge how these impact perception and behavior" (Perra, 2000). The more people are able to be honest about a situation in a calm manner, the better. The goal is to stay in the adult. To be "*in the storm of conflict and at the same time out of it and watching it in serenity*" (von Franz, p. 149).

For some reason in our society, we think conflict is a bad thing. In reality though, healthy disagreements and conflict provide different perspectives. By paying attention to different points of view we can make better decisions. Thus, conflict can be very helpful, and when handled appropriately, can help us determine better alternatives. Dialogue and disagreements allow us to consider other ramifications that could occur before choosing the action we will take. Thus instead of reacting, we can more thoughtfully consider the situation and prioritize matters. Dialogue coupled with good teamwork and collegiality can achieve better outcomes than any of us could accomplish alone.

Conflict management (**Exhibit 3–11**) is an important leadership competency. In the emotional intelligence research, this is further defined as developing consensus and mitigating conflicts (Snow, 2001). We would caution about mitigating conflicts. Trying to force everyone to "get along" and brushing the conflict "under the carpet," can be dangerous. Conflict is a natural occurrence—we cannot avoid it. It is a fallacy to think that everyone always totally agrees with each other. That is not the way life is. We are not a failure as a leader when conflicts occur in our work group. However, timing is important as sometimes we will need to mitigate conflict. In fact, conflict and healthy disagreement can help us to sense the best timing for a decision. Some decisions are best made right away, while others can wait. Some decisions are best made after input and dialogue has occurred between a number of people. Other times, when conflict is left unresolved, it interferes with the work getting completed. This is when immediate intervention is needed.

Developing consensus can be achieved when dialogue occurs between people who are experiencing a conflict. In fact, this can prevent war from occurring. Conflicts can be resolved in many ways. In an empowering environment, many issues can be resolved by

---

Exhibit 3–11   Conflict Management

- Encourage appropriate expression of conflict.
- Take into account different perceptions.
- Identify the real source of conflict.
- Stay in the adult.
- Always resolve the conflict using the value(s), such as, *What is best for the patient?*

other people, without any intervention needed from the administrator. Effective leaders know when to get involved, and when it is more appropriate to have others deal with the issue. So conflict can lead us to determine who is the most appropriate person(s) to deal with, and resolve, the conflict. Sometimes it is best for one person to make a decision, resolving the conflict, while, at other times, it is best for a group to come to agreement as to how to best handle a situation.

When we experience conflict, another emotional intelligence competency, *self-control*, is important. This is further defined as remaining poised even under pressure (Snow, 2001). Sometimes it helps to ask oneself, "Will I remember this five years from now?". If one is finding oneself having difficulty getting into the adult, and it is not an emergency, it may be time to just exit the situation, get oneself balanced again, and then come back and deal with the situation.

Conflicts can occur just as daily happenings occur. For example, administrators find that it often is not possible to start one project and finish it before starting another. In fact, one must be able to "multitask." A parent knows this as, for instance, when one interrupts doing dishes to rescue a child who has gotten into difficulties. An administrator might come to work expecting to accomplish certain things that day. Then an emergency happens, or someone is distressed about something, or someone takes an action that adversely affects the patient, etc. Sometimes the whole day passes with the planned activities not being accomplished. We can get upset about this, or we can think back—we really did what was best at each moment in the day. Perhaps it was not the right time to do the planned activities. After all, there is a right time for everything—it just may not be today! We can either experience a great deal of conflict—everything kept interfering with the goals we had set—or we can actually have a rewarding day. It did not go as planned but other more meaningful things were accomplished. Perhaps we were supposed to be of service to others on that day.

An administrator needs to know when it is important to get involved in a conflict, what the various viewpoints are in the conflict, and how to negotiate and resolve disagreements. Negotiating skills can be helpful in conflict resolution. Many times we cannot make decisions alone but must negotiate with others.[4]

In the administrative role, when we have two staff members in a conflict that is escalating, and it keeps them from effectively caring for patients, the nurse manager must get involved. Get both staff members together in a separate area, have each state their case with the other listening, ask both what is best for the patient(s) involved, and help both to reach some resolution to the problem. Honesty, staying in the adult, and dialogue to understand each other's perspectives are best in such situations. The resolution may happen as they understand each other's perspectives and reach an agreement; or they may agree to disagree but have a better understanding of the other person's perspective; or the administrator may have to make a decision as to how both should proceed. If a serious conflict is going unresolved and the nurse manager waits to intervene, patients may really suffer.

If the conflict is with a supervisor or someone at a higher level in an organization, one will need to decide what to do about it. (After all, it is best if we can prevent an unwanted trip to Abilene.)

---

[4] There is a wonderful book on successful negotiating, *Getting to Yes: Negotiating Agreement Without Giving In*, by Fisher, Ury, and Patton (1991).

Conflicts can occur simply because two people have different work styles. For instance, one person may pay close attention to detail while another only deals with the big picture. The detail person may think the big picture person is careless and needs to pay more attention to the details, while the big picture person does not understand why the detail person takes so long to do something and has more difficulty putting things into a larger perspective. In fact, each can learn a lot from the other.

Sometimes a patient is in a conflict with staff or physicians. It is best if we can be an advocate for the patient's position. This can be especially difficult when there are cultural differences, or when the patient is making a decision that we might not have made.

There are also conflicts between patients and families, or between family members. This is especially difficult if the patient is unable to tell us what s/he prefers. In fact, this can become so difficult that an effective ethics committee really has to grapple with how to proceed. We are not in these situations alone. In such cases it is important to try to determine what the patient would want and take that course, staying in the adult. This can be *very* difficult when we do not agree with the patient's perspective, or when family members do not want to do what is in the best interest of the patient.

Thank goodness there is diversity in this world! Wouldn't this world be a dull place if everyone was exactly alike??

Diversity means differences in our views of the world. Cultural differences, discussed in Chapter 2, can become a strong source of conflict, just because we do not understand someone's viewpoint. Such differences exist within work groups. Here is where empathy is put to the test. How well do we understand another person's perspective of the world? Are we comfortable to let them tell us about it, or are we so uncomfortable that we do not give them a chance to air their beliefs?

> The techniques for finding common ground, for sorting through the various landscapes representing the diversity inherent in each issue, are now required by every leader.... [Old leadership roles are] disappearing, and the new circumstances will demand new roles and challenge everyone to respond to a whole new set of questions. [This] will open up the door to uncertainty and a general lack of 'rightness.' The prevailing principles will be open to interpretation and will be applicable in a host of ways. No one response to a change or answer to a question will be clearly best. There might be many correct responses depending on the cultural and intellectual context. Leaders will have to respect the diversity embedded in every condition or issue (Porter-O'Grady and Malloch, p. 27).

Exhibit 3–12 shows some paradoxes we face. Many nurses who are presently very disillusioned with nursing are facing these paradoxes and not dealing with the paradoxes in an effective way. The first problem is that often nurses do not realize what the paradoxes are. Then, once recognized, nurses need to change their view of reality to include those factors. For instance, one paradox is chaos versus order. Remember the discussion on chaos theory in Chapter 2? We experience chaos at a point in time, and think that it should all be fixed. Yet, chaos research has shown that when the chaotic events are plotted together, a

---

Exhibit 3–12 Paradox

There are many paired elements of life that appear contradictory but at a deeper level are in fact complementary. These include the following:
- Chaos and order (there is order in all chaos and vice versa)
- Creativity and tension (tension leads to creativity and creativity causes tension)
- Conflict and peace (conflict is necessary to peacemaking, containing in it the elements upon which peace must be built)
- Difference and similarity (difference seen at a great distance appears as an integrated whole)
- Complexity and simplicity (complexity is simply the visible connection between aligned simplicities)

From: Porter-O'Grady, T., and Malloch, K. (2003). *Quantum Leadership: A Textbook of New Leadership*. Sudbury, MA: Jones and Bartlett, p. 27.

---

beautiful, orderly pattern emerges. ***So, are the differences actually differences?? Or does our perception need to be expanded??***

After further discussion and clarification, perhaps the differences are not really there, or perhaps we can agree to disagree. There is a wonderful book, Handy (1994) *The Age of Paradox*, that describes various paradoxes, and how to frame them. This helps us to deal more effectively with paradox.

Dialogue

We have already emphasized the importance of *dialogue*, or *honest communication*, between all involved. We take a risk when we expose our thoughts and feelings, but this sharing leads to achieving better decisions and more effective team work. Thus when conflicts occur, the leader needs to encourage appropriate expression of conflict as a way to achieve better decision making. No one is wrong or right; there just needs to be dialogue with each person sharing her/his perceptions and ideas about how to resolve issues. It is not a shouting match, but is a dialogue carried out using the adult.

In addition, when a problem occurs, there are usually many *different perceptions* about the problem. It can be very dangerous making a decision about an issue when only one perspective has been heard. Instead, one should find out different points of view about the matter before making a decision.

Part of the dialogue process includes listening to what others communicate both verbally and nonverbally. Then one can ask the right questions to further clarify the situation. For instance, sometimes a presenting problem is not the real issue. A leader may intuitively sense this; or find out by asking some questions—such as *why has this become such an important issue?*—to get to the bottom of the issue. Questions, both from the leader and from others in the environment, can help to identify additional factors that need to be considered before making a final decision. The best way to achieve this is through dialogue.

Once the decision is made, the person or people making the decision must effectively communicate this decision to others so that they can best understand it. This is also an important part of the dialogue process, or the decision can not be implemented, or implemented properly.

DECISION MAKING

Effective decision making is an art. (See **Exhibit 3–13**.) It involves: *finding and selecting the best alternative, and having the most appropriate person (people) make, and implement, the decision at the right time.* As one nurse executive said, "It is sifting out the new rules and building for an unknown tomorrow."

An effective leader possesses an ability to analyze difficult concepts; listen to, and understand, different perspectives; get appropriate facts needed to make a more appropriate decision; see the smaller picture and how it fits with the overall big picture; yet make a decision even when unknowns remain. Many times a leader does not know what to do. Some advocate that a leader bluff at such times, pretending to know the answer. The authors do not recommend this approach. Once people see through this (and they will), they lose trust for this leader. It is much more effective to admit one does not know what to do, to ask for other's ideas, and to say that one needs time to think on the situation. Or if something must be done right away, to listen to one's gut level after hearing other ideas, and take the action one intuitively chooses. We arrive at better decisions when we stay in touch with what feels right intuitively and encourage others to follow their intuition.

A number of factors can be helpful to determine the best way to handle a situation. Although many situations have similar themes, there are individual differences that occur that can change the way something should be handled. Using these processes can aid one to make the most appropriate decision.

First, go back to the core values. Decisions are best when the core values are supported. What is best for the patient? What is best for everyone concerned?

Second, decision making is tricky for another reason. *There are times when it is best to leave the decision making to others* who are fully capable of making better decisions on the matter than we would make. For instance, in the work setting each staff member has the best understanding of her/his work. We do not know the nuances of their work. They are the experts. Each person is a capable adult. They must make many decisions as they

---

Exhibit 3–13 Decision Making Factors

- Communicate, dialogue, listen.
- Understand the different perspectives.
- Have people make decisions at the appropriate level in an organization.
- Encourage healthy disagreement.
- Have empathy for others.
- Use our intuition.
- Always support the core value(s).
- Timing of the decision is very important.
- One must prioritize—What decisions are *really* important?
- Tenacity or persistence may be necessary.
- Accountability—Where does it lie?
- Take risks.
- Experience successes and failures. Celebrate successes. Correct mistakes.
- Use effective negotiation skills.

---

appropriately do the needed work. This is also true for patients—patients need to make the decisions that they determine are best.

Letting others make the decisions—actually *encouraging* staff to do this—can be difficult. Many nurses and nurse managers do not delegate enough. They say, "I can do it better." In this case, they have not expected others to make decisions. They have not treated others (this includes patients and families as well as other staff, physicians and administrators) as capable people deserving our respect. After all, if one person has to do it all because no one else can do it right, how does all the work get done? It is physically impossible for one person to do everything right. Meanwhile, patients suffer, staff members are unhappy and leave, physicians complain about staff, and so forth.

Instead, the workplace is most effective when all delegate effectively—this involves knowing, or learning about, others' capabilities, sharing information and teaching others if they do not know how to do something, and then letting the appropriate people do it at the most advantageous time. This means that others may go about accomplishing something very differently than we would. Unless this is harming someone, let them do it their way. They generally know more about themselves, or about doing their job, than we do.

When mistakes occur, help staff process what went wrong to prevent this from happening again. Perhaps the best question to ask when a mistake occurs is, "What did you learn from this?" We all make mistakes as we do our work. No one is perfect. Instead of punishing a person who has made a mistake (this is getting into the parent role), it is best to stay in the adult and factually find out what happened, listen to different perspectives, and try to help the person undo the damage that has been done. This is just as true for ourselves. Beating ourselves up for something does not help the situation. The situation does provide learning for us. It is important to go back and own up to the mistake, and then go on from there, undoing the damage as much as we can.

Third, another issue is *prioritizing*. One cannot do it all. In this information age, there is so much paper and information, one cannot know it all. Instead we need to listen to our gut level and concentrate our time and decisions on important issues. As previously discussed, this can be difficult for some as we will need to be delegating appropriately, and then prioritizing what we need to do. Certain things are VERY important, while other things can wait until tomorrow.

Fourth, *timing* is an issue. Knowing *when* to make the decision is another part of leadership effectiveness. Once again, it is important to stay in touch with one's intuition as well as to stay in touch with others in the environment. There are times when we must make the decision. But many times others need to make the decision. Knowing when to make the decision and when to leave the situation alone takes experience as well as being in touch with one's intuitive capabilities. Does it feel right to make the decision? If inexperienced, a good mentor can be very helpful in this area. At times it will be important to have the courage to make a difficult, or an unpopular, decision, even though others may disagree with it.

Another aspect of decision making is *tenacity*. Sometimes if one really wants something to happen one must be persistent, as discussed earlier in this chapter. For example, a nurse manager wants to start a new service. It gets turned down by the supervisor, the executive team, or the board. If this is really important, the nurse manager needs to bring it up again later.

Persistence is also needed in any change project. Just going through things once with everyone involved does not mean that the change will occur or that anyone will do it. Tenacity is important in its achievement. For example, a huge change occurs for the nursing staff when charts go from written to computerized. At first, most staff will find that it takes more time as they are unfamiliar with it, as unexpected problems occur, as the computer system goes down and nothing is available, etc. With persistence though (provided the computerized system was a good one) staff will love it and will find that it saves a lot of time.

With decision making comes *accountability* for the outcomes. As we lead, responsibilities follow. "The buck stops here." We are responsible for our decisions, as well as for the actions staff who report to us have taken. Were the outcomes what we expected? Was there an unexpected outcome? Should we have made the decision(s) or should others have been more involved? How could we have done it better? How can we fix/repair something that happened due to our decision(s)? Or due to our staff's decisions? An effective leader does not blame—oneself or others. A mistake was made. How can this mistake be rectified? What will we do differently next time? *Did we learn from our mistake?* is a better response.

> At times, an effective leader has to *take risks* on important issues.
>
> All decisions and actions are rife with risk. Risk cannot be eliminated and should not necessarily be decreased, for courses of action that possess great value tend to be associated with higher risk. What is important to determine is not whether the risk can be eliminated, but whether the level of risk is appropriate for the actions undertaken and, if so, what strategies can accommodate the risk (Porter-O'Grady and Malloch, p. 28).

Risk taking results in both successes and in failures. *Both success and mistakes are a natural result of change and of risk taking.* Celebrate successes with everyone involved. Give credit where credit is due. If a staff member did something wonderful, give her/him the credit for the success. Mistakes provide fodder for further learning. It can be easy to get bogged down when we know we have not been as effective in a situation, or when a situation really bombs. However, beating ourselves up about it can actually keep us from being effective in the next situation that presents itself. Instead, we can admit that we made a mistake, work to repair damage if needed, and move on, learning from our mistakes. If it is others who have made the mistake, dialogue with them. Why did they do what they did? What would they do differently next time?

Since this is an imperfect world, we will be experiencing successes as well as making mistakes as we move through life. Part of effective leadership is realizing that often we have had some role or influence in others' successes and failures. Plus we can learn a lot from our own mistakes. In his consulting, Tom Peters talks about the person who tried a new venture, lost a million dollars, and when the CEO asks to talk with the person, is afraid the CEO will fire him. Instead the CEO says, "Why would I want to fire you so you can go on and give another company the benefit of your experience?" The manager stayed but had learned a valuable lesson.

> Mistakes are the portals of discovery.
>
> —James Joyce

So What Is Effective Leadership Anyway?

Effective leadership will continue to evolve. It is a path of discovery. There is so much more to learn!

> In this chaotic world, we need leaders. But we don't need bosses.
> We need leaders to help us develop the clear identity that lights the
> dark moments of confusion. We need leaders to support us as we
> learn how to live by our values. We need leaders to understand that
> we are best controlled by concepts that invite our participation,
> not policies and procedures that curtail our contribution
> (Wheatley, p. 131).

Love one another.

> *The giving and receiving of love in whatever form it expresses itself can have a*
> *more lasting impact than any other single thing we do. All healing finds its roots*
> *in the expression of love.*
> *It can reach far deeper places than any pill can go.*
> *While it is imperative to give physical bodies the support they need,*
> *it is equally imperative to give spirits the love they need*
> *in order to access the tremendous healing power it carries (Joy, p. 26).*

References

Arbinger Institute. (2002). *Leadership and self-seception: Getting out of the box.* San Francisco: Berrett-Kohler.

Bass, B. (1998). *Transformational leadership: Industry, military, and rducational impact.* Mahwah, NJ: Lawrence Erlbaum.

Benner, P. (1984). *From novice to expert: Excellence and power in vlinical nursing practice.* Menlo Park, CA: Addison-Wesley.

Bennis, W., & Nanus, B. (1985). *Leaders: The strategies for taking charge.* New York: Harper & Row.

Bennis, W., & Thomas, R. (September 2002). Crucibles of leadership. *Harvard Business Review*, 39–45.

Bolman, L., & Deal, T. (2001). *Leading with soul: An uncommon journey of spirit.* San Francisco: Jossey-Bass.

Brooks, C. (1966). Report on work in sensory awareness and total functioning. In H. A., Otto (Ed.), *Explorations in human potentialities* (pp. 487–505). Springfield, IL: Charles C. Thomas Publisher.

Buhler, C. (1966). In H. A., Otto (Ed.), *Explorations in human potentialities* (pp. 19–26). Springfield, IL: Charles C. Thomas Publisher.

Burns, J. (1978). *Leadership.* New York: Harper.

Byham, W., with Cox, J., & Nelson, G. (1996). *Zapp! Empowerment in Health Care.* New York: Fawcett Columbine.

Campbell, D., Fleming, R., & Grote, R. (July–August 1985). Discipline without punishment–at last. *Harvard Business Review*, 162–178.

Chaffee, M., & Arthur, D. (September–October 2002). Failure: Lessons for health care leaders. *Nursing Economic$, 20*(5), 225–231.

Claxton, G. (2000). *Hare brain tortoise mind: How intelligence increases when you think less*. New York: Harper Collins.

Collins, J., & Porras, J. (Fall 1991). Organizational vision and visionary organizations. *California Management Review, 34*(1), 30–53.

Collins, J., & Porras, J. (1994). *Built to last*. New York: HarperBusiness.

DePree, M. (1989). *Leadership is an art*. New York: Dell.

Distefani, S., & Bledsoe, D. (September/October 2003). A balanced approach to leadership. *Nurse Leader, 5*(1), 32–35.

Dunham-Taylor, J. (July/August 1995). Identifying the best in nurse executive leadership: Part 2, interview results. *JONA, 25*(7/8), 24–31.

Drucker, P. (March–April 1999). Managing oneself. *Harvard Business Review*, 65–74.

Fisher, R., Ury, W., & Patton, B. (1991). *Getting to yes: Negotiating agreement without giving in*. New York: Penguin.

Frankl, V. (1984). *Man's search for neaning*. New York: Washington Square Press.

Gergen, D. (January 2003). How presidents persuade. *Harvard Business Review*, 20–21.

Gogoi, P. (November 20, 2000). As leaders, women rule. *Business Week*, 75–84.

Goleman, D. (1998). *Working with emotional intelligence*. New York: Bantam Books.

Hagberg, J. (1994). *Real power: Stages of personal power in organizations*. 2nd ed. Salem, WI: Sheffield.

Handy, C. (1994). *The age of paradox*. Boston: Harvard Business School Press.

Harvey, J. (1988). The Abilene paradox: The management of agreement. *Organizational Dynamics, 17*(1), 16–43.

Johnson, S. (1998). *Who moved my cheese?* New York: Putnam's Sons.

Joy, S. (March/April 2003). Is there enough room in my job for love? *Nurse Leader*, 24–27.

Khurana, R. (September 2002). The curse of the superstar ceo. *Harvard Business Review*, 60–66.

Kowalski, K., & Yoder-Wise, P. (September/October 2003). Five C's of leadership. *Nurse Leader, 5*(1), 26–31.

Krishnapada, S. (1996). *Leadership for an age of higher consciousness*. Columbia, MD: Hari-Nama Press.

Kuhnert, K., & Lewis, P. (1987). Transactional and transformational leadership: A constructive/developmental analysis. *Academy of Management Review, 12*(4), 648–657.

Lencioni, P. (1998). *The five temptations of a CEO: A leadership fable*. San Francisco: Jossey-Bass.

Lencioni, P. (July 2002). Make your values mean something. *Harvard Business Review*, 113–117.

Livingston, J. (January 2003). Pygmalion in management. *Harvard Business Review*, 121–130.

Luthans, F. (1988). Successful vs. effective real managers. *The Academy of Management EXECUTIVE, 11*(2), 127–132.

McClelland, D. (1973). Testing for competence rather than intelligence. *American Psychologist*, 46, 56–62.

Morris, T. (1994). *True success: A new philosophy of excellence*. New York: Berkley Books.

Murphy, G., & Murphy, L. (1966). Human nature and human potentialities: Imagination and the imaginary. In H. A., Otto (Ed.), *Explorations in human potentialities* (pp. 5–19). Springfield, IL: Charles C. Tomas Publisher.

Nauright, L. (January/February 2003). Educating the nurse leader for today and tomorrow. *Nurse Leader*, 25–27.

Nightingale, F. (1869). *Notes on nursing*. New York: Dover.

Perra, B. (Winter 2000). Leadership: The key to quality outcomes. *Nursing Administration Quarterly, 24*(2), 56.

Porter-O'Grady, T. (March–April 2003). Of hubris and hope: Transforming nursing for a new age. *Nursing Economic$,* 59–64.

Porter-O'Grady, T. (2001). Is shared government still relevant? *JONA, 31*(10), 468–473.

Porter-O'Grady, T., & Malloch, K. (2003). *Quantum leadership: A textbook of new leadership*. Sudbury, MA: Jones and Bartlett.

Porter-O'Grady, R. (February 2003). A different age for leadership, part 1: New context, new content. *JONA, 33*(2), 105–110.

Schultz, M. (1965). *Awakening intuition: Using your mind-body network for insight and healing*. New York: Harmony Books.

Senge, P. (1990). *The fifth discipline: The art & practice of the learning organization*. New York: Doubleday/Currency.

Senge, P., Roberts, C., Ross, R., Smith, B., & Kleiner, A. (1994). *The fifth discipline fieldbook: Strategies and tools for building a learning organization*. New York: Currency.

Sharpe, R. (November 20, 2000). As leaders, women rule. *Business Week*, 75–84.

Simons, T. (September 2002). The high cost of lost trust. *Harvard Business Review*, 18–19.

Snow, J. (September 2001). Looking beyond nursing for clues to effective leadership. *JONA, 31*(9), 440–443.

Stein, N. (October 2, 2000). The world's most admired companies. *Fortune*, 183–196.

Studer, Quint. (March 26, 2000). *Taking Your Organization to the Next Level. American Organization of Nurse Executives Annual Meeting*. National Nursing Network Inc., 4465 Washington St., Denver, CO 80216.

Sundeen, S., Stuart, G., Rankin, E., & Cohen, S. (1985). *Nurse-client interaction: Implementing the nursing process*. St. Louis: Mosby.

The Arbinger Institute. (2002). *Leadership and self-deception: Getting out of the box*. San Francisco: Berrett-Koehler.

Useem, M. (October 2001). The leadership lessons of mount everest. *Harvard Business Review*, 51–58.

Vitello-Ciccin, J. (April 2002). Exploring emotional intelligence: Implications for nursing leaders. *JONA, 32*(4), 203–210.

Von Franz, M. (1980). *Alchemy: An introduction to the symbolism and the psychology*. Toronto: Inner City Books.

Watzlawick, P., Weakland, J., & Fisch, R. (1974). *Change: Principles of problem formation and problem resolution*. New York: Norton.

Wheatley, M. (1999). *Leadership and the new science: Discovering order in a chaotic world*. San Francisco: Berrett-Koehler.

CHAPTER 4

Organizational Strategies

Janne Dunham-Taylor, PhD, RN

Tammy Samples, MSN, RN

Organizations are of, by, about and for people.

—James Autry

In today's environment, within organizations we must be able to change on a dime. To do this our administrative leadership needs to follow the quantum leadership model discussed in Chapter 3. We need to do regular rounds, dialogue as we come in contact with people, empower staff, and live the core ideology.

Staff need to have an awareness of what is going on in health care and beyond. Administrators, including nurse managers, need to discuss the current state of affairs with staff, as well as avail and encourage staff to be aware of current trends and developments that could impact patient care. Administrators should ensure that information is available as well as discussed. Staff (not just those at the top of the organization) need to attend conferences, network with others outside the organization, and access the internet. If staff are aware of the current information, they do better. What results is an organization that can rapidly change and survive.

> Our concept of organizations is moving away from the mechanistic creations that flourished in the age of bureaucracy. We now speak in earnest of more fluid, organic structures, of boundaryless and seamless organizations. We are beginning to recognize organizations as whole systems, construing them as 'learning organizations' or as 'organic' and noticing that people exhibit self-organizing capacity. These are our first journeys that signal a growing appreciation for the changes required in today's organizations. My own experience suggests that we can forego the despair created by such common organizational events as change, chaos, information overload, and entrenched behaviors if we recognize that organizations are living systems, possessing the same capacity to adapt and grow that is common to all life.
>
> What is it that streams can teach me about organizations?... This stream has an impressive ability to adapt, to change the configurations, to let the

power shift, to create new structures. But behind this adaptability, making it all happen, I think, is the water's need to flow. Water answers to gravity, to downhill, to the call of ocean. The forms change, but the mission remains clear. Structures emerge, but only as temporary solutions that facilitate rather than interfere. There is none of the rigid reliance that I have learned in organizations on single forms, on true answers, on past practices. Streams have more than one response to rocks; otherwise, there'd be no Grand Canyon. Or Grand Canyons everywhere. The Colorado river realized there were many ways to find ocean other than by staying broad and expansive....

Organizations lack this kind of faith, faith that they can accomplish their purposes in varied ways and that they do best when they focus on intent and vision, letting forms emerge and disappear. We seem hypnotized by structures, and we build them strong and complex because they must, we believe, hold back the dark forces that threaten to destroy us.... Streams have a different relationship with natural forces. With sparkling confidence, they know that their intense yearning for ocean will be fulfilled, that nature creates not only the call, but the answer (Wheatley, pp. 15, 17–18).

So what is a health care organization's ocean? Where are we headed? And, the greater question is, how do we get to that ocean? Our primary purpose, our ocean where we are headed, is *to provide appropriate, safe care that our clients will value.* This means that each person in the organization needs to provide the "radical loving care" described by Chapman (2004). What a powerful statement, steeped with meaning. Do you notice that money is not mentioned in this statement? The theme in Chapter 1 is that if we do what is right for the patient, the money will follow. We continue with that theme here.

We are mistaken if we think that our ocean, our primary purpose, is making money. Many health care organizations are run by administrators who believe that the bottom line runs the organization, antithesis to the mission statement above their entrance that spells out various values.

As the bottom line has gained importance, health care organizations have lost the soul of the organization (Bolman and Deal, 1997). Morale and job satisfaction of nurses has plunged. As budget cuts occur, workers feel depersonalized and suffer from battle fatigue. The problem is that staff do not feel valued. Problems spiral downward because clients coming there for care sense that they are not important, that staff do not care. Staff *know* this to be true. In bottom-line culture, the bottom line becomes the first priority rather than occuring behind the values. Any organization using this approach cannot survive in the long run.

It is amazing how *when we make the bottom line first, finances plummet;* while *when patients are first priority and bottom line second, finances are sustained or improved.* The research shows this to be true:

> **Profitability** is a necessary condition for existence and a means to more important ends, but it is not the end in itself.... Profit is like oxygen,

food, water, and blood for the body; they are not the *point* of life, but
without them, there is no life (Collins and Porras, p. 55).

If the CFO, and perhaps most of the executive team, really believes that the bottom line is the ocean, conflict and frustration occur for others in the organization who believe the patient comes first. The issue then becomes how much we decide to confront this, whether we leave, or whether we just work there and do nothing—or complain about it to the wrong people. The choice is ours.

This is not to say that revenue is unimportant. We still need money to operate. The money simply must remain secondary to the primary goal. Money is part of the meandering that the stream does while looking for the ocean. If revenues are unavailable from one source, there may be another source available. The first issue is, what services does the patient need or want? Then we go from there to determine our actions.

The ocean, or where we are headed, is *appropriate, safe care. Appropriate* means that it is what the *client* wants. If I am a chain smoker and I refuse to stop smoking, even though I have a terrible case of emphysema, I still have the right to make the decision about what is *appropriate* care for me. I can choose to continue to smoke, or I can choose to get some help to deal with this addiction.

It is easy to get into *shoulds* with our clients, (i.e., you should stop smoking and should lose weight). Sometimes we can get very frustrated when our clients choose to continue with the unhealthy practices. This "*should*" mentality is a waste of our energy; it is not our decision. We are not in the client's shoes. Consider yourself in the role of the patient, and ask: "Would I want some health care person to make my decisions for me?"

The word *safe* has acquired new meaning in this era, as many of the treatments we provide may cause further, more extensive problems. Examples of this include getting the wrong medication, experiencing complications including infections, and experiencing side effects to treatment that are very uncomfortable and perhaps are worse than the initial problem. As identified in Chapter 2, there are many ways that we could improve to achieve better safety.

"That our clients will value" can mean different things to different clients. This is where the "radical loving care" comes, as discussed in Chapter 2. This means that someone in the health care organization must listen to the client to glean what he/she actually values. For example, a stroke patient cannot button his shirt. What does he value? If he values getting help with buttoning his shirt, he will welcome a staff member who does it for him. If he values independence, he might not want help but instead will want to learn how to do it himself, even if the learning process is very frustrating with his first clumsy attempts at buttoning.

The *value* part is really what patient satisfaction is all about. In "Serving Up Uncommon Service" Doucette (2003) points out the difference between quality, the "measurement of outcomes," and service, "a measure of perception or what matters to the patient." "Quality outcomes are a baseline. The one feature that units demonstrating consistently high-ranking customer satisfaction scores share is satisfied employees. The conclusion seems clear: To improve patient satisfaction, improve staff satisfaction" (pp. 26–27). Remember discussing "love one another" in Chapter 3? This is a requirement for all administrators, as well as others in leadership positions throughout the organization. And all this love achieves healthier bottom lines.

How do we teach all this to staff? First we must agree on the ocean, the place that we are heading—*providing appropriate, safe care that our clients will value*. To arrive at this everyone needs to be involved in a dialogue about the words to be used, and the meaning of those words; they must understand that this applies to all patients, whether they can pay or not, whether they represent a different race or culture; whether or not it is a street person reeking of alcohol. After identifying words or scripts to be used, every-one needs to agree to support those words in their actions. This starts with us—the administrators. Do our actions support our words? Do we really mean it? When our actions do not support our words, staff believe the message contained in the *actions*, and do not believe the words. When our actions do not support the words, we need to catch ourselves, apologize, and change our actions accordingly. Once our actions are aligned with our words, we need to encourage and teach staff to align their actions with their words. All this takes time, but the time is worth it in the end. The expectation is that we are all heading to the same ocean.

The key to this chapter is that the goal and organizational strategies support going to the ocean—*providing appropriate, safe care that our clients will value, and that all adminis-trators and staff support this goal*. This is the "radical loving care" factor. The processes—which are the meandering rivers heading to the ocean—will vary from organization to organization. We provide some possible strategies, processes, or landmarks throughout this chapter, but in the case of each organization, there are differences in the strategies used as well as outcomes achieved. Just as no river is the same, no organization is the same. There are an infinite number of possibilities as to how to more effectively reach our ocean.

There are two additional energies necessary to successfully navigate the processes, or the meandering rivers heading to the ocean. They are soul and spirit. Understanding and believing in the ocean, that is the *soul*. It is the reason we are doing all this. It makes what we do meaningful. This is the most important part of our work. We feel it very deeply. Our relationships with each other reflect this soul. If relationships are not good, chances are we have lost touch with the soul part of our business. If the relationships are collaborative, chances are the soul part is present, alive, and well.

The *spirit* is the energy that fuels getting to the ocean. It is the synergy that exists between team members, physicians, suppliers, patients, and families. It is the energy that works to achieve getting to the ocean. It is the "radical loving care" that is given. "The fruits of spirit are enthusiasm, motivation, and performance" (Nobre, 2001, p. 288). Nobre (p. 287) suggests that:

Soul + Spirit + Resources + Leadership = Results

Core Ideology

Let's start with defining the ocean, the soul. This is where spirit gets its energy. Collins and Porras describe the ocean as the *core ideology* that actually has two components—*core val-ues* and *purpose*. Collins and Porras (1994) reported on an enormous research project with premier companies that have lasted 50–100 years, are known for excellence, yet have experienced multiple leaders and different product lines through the years. They report that:

> A visionary company almost religiously preserves its core ideology—changing it seldom, if ever. Core values in a visionary company form a rock-solid foundation and do not drift with the trends and fashions of the day; in some cases, the core values have remained intact for well over one hundred years. And the basic purpose of a visionary company—its reason for being—can serve as a guiding beacon for centuries, like an enduring star on the horizon. Yet, while keeping their core ideologies tightly fixed, visionary companies display a powerful drive for progress that enables them to change and adapt without compromising their cherished core ideals.

> There is no "right" set of core values.... Indeed, two companies can have radically different ideologies, yet both be visionary. Core values in a visionary company don't even have to be "enlightened" or "humanistic," although they often are. The crucial variable is not the content of a company's ideology, but how deeply it believes its ideology and how consistently it lives, breathes, and expresses it in all that it does. Visionary companies do not ask, "What should we value?" They ask, "What do we actually value deep down to our toes?" (pp. 8–9).

Core Values

Core ideology is better understood when core values and purpose are defined separately. Collins and Porras define core values:

> Core Values = The organization's essential and enduring tenets—a small set of general guiding principles; not to be confused with specific cultural or operating practices; not to be compromised for financial gain or short-term expediency (p. 73).

Core values can provide a common cause between people who work in an organization. The values actually represent *beliefs*. When sound, these beliefs provide the backbone of every policy or action people within the organization take. The core values come first, before goals, policies, or procedures. If a goal, policy, or procedure violates a core value, then it must be changed. Generally, there is one, or very few, core value(s) and they remain unchanged for many years.

Examples of core values include how we defined the ocean above: *to provide appropriate, safe care that our clients will value*. Examples of core values in other businesses are:

- To "treat the patient the way we would want a family member to be treated."

- Sam Walton's value for Wal-Mart: "[We put] the customer ahead of everything else.... If you're not serving the customer, or supporting the folks who do, then we don't need you."
- John Young identified the Hewlett-Packard (HP) core value: "The HP Way basically means respect and concern for the individual; it says 'Do unto others as you would have them do unto you.' That's really what it's all about" (quoted material from Collins and Porras, p. 74).

When determining the core value, it needs to be authentically identified by people in the organization, not copied from some other organization, even though it is possible that a core value for one company is the same as for another. The core value does not have to be unique, but it is imperative that all within an organization support it with words, actions, and goals.

Several authors discuss the importance of core values in rallying staff, but stress the difficulties of really living by the core values. For instance, Lencioni (2002) says that:

> Coming up with strong values—and sticking to them—requires real guts. Indeed, an organization considering a values initiative must first come to terms with the fact that, when properly practiced, values inflict pain. They make some employees feel like outcasts. They limit an organization's strategic and operational freedom and constrain the behavior of its people. They leave executives open to heavy criticism for even minor violations. And they demand constant vigilance (p. 114).

There is a good book, written as a story called *Walk the Talk... And Get The Results You Want* (Harvey and Lucia, date not given) that portrays the importance, and the difficulties encountered, when a company president begins to realize that it is important to match the company values with his actions.

The core values are extremely important and in the premier companies described in *Built to Last*, one *becomes an outcast* if one does not support the values (Collins and Porras, 1994).

> A visionary company creates a total environment that envelops employees, bombarding them with a set of signals so consistent and mutually reinforcing that it's virtually impossible to misunderstand the company's ideology and ambitions.... Because the visionary companies have such clarity about who they are, what they're all about, and what they're trying to achieve, they tend to not have much room for people unwilling or unsuited to their demanding standards, both in terms of performance and congruence (p. 121).

These companies promote from within, encouraging managers to immerse themselves in the company ideology for several years to make sure they understand what is expected from them, before being promoted.

Purpose

The other component of the core ideology is purpose.

> **Purpose** = The organization's fundamental reasons for existence beyond just making money—a perpetual guiding star on the horizon; not to be confused with specific goals or business strategies (Collins and Porras, p. 73).

Purpose, like the core values, remains unchanged for years. It may be a similar purpose to other companies. For instance, Merck's purpose, "fighting disease, relieving suffering, and helping people" may be similar to other companies who manufacture medications. Purpose is similar to quality where one is always working towards achieving it but never totally accomplishes it. Other examples of purpose are:

- Marriott's "making people away from home feel that they're among friends and really wanted;" or
- Disney's "bringing happiness to millions."

The purpose statements do not give a specific description of the products. Nor do they specifically define the customer. In fact the purpose:

> Get[s] at the deeper, more fundamental reasons for the organization's existence. An effective way to get at purpose is to pose the question, "Why not just shut this organization down, cash out, and sell off the assets?" and to push for an answer that would be equally valid both now and one hundred years into the future.
>
> … We did not find an explicit and formal statement of purpose in all of our visionary companies. We sometimes found purpose to be more implicitly or informally stated.… We've found that most companies benefit from articulating both core values and purpose in their core ideology (Collins and Porras, p. 78).

Purpose helps to give clarity and direction to all in an organization.

> When leaders make their strategic intent abundantly clear—as Wal-Mart's management has in proclaiming its strategy of "low prices, every day"—employees know what to do without requiring myriad further instructions. Achieving that clarity, however, is often far more difficult than managers appreciate (Useem, 2001, p. 57).

We are most successful in defining our purpose when it goes deeper than just surface direction. Have you noticed how people will accomplish the impossible for a cause?

> Ultimately the choice we make is between service and self-interest.…
> The antidote to self-interest is to commit and to find cause. To commit to something outside of ourselves. To be a part of creating something we

care about so we can endure the sacrifice, risk, and adventure that commitment entails. This is the deeper meaning of service (Block, 1993, pp. 9–10).

STEWARDSHIP

It is easy when determining the purpose to forget the company obligations to the community. An organization is part of a community. If the community flounders, the organization could be at risk. Just as all departments need to be integrated and working together within an organization, all organizations are better off if they are integrated and working with each other in the community, helping the community to better serve its citizens.

Walter Gast, a former professor at Saint Louis University's John Cook School of Business, rightly claimed that to be successful in the long term, "a business had to follow six laws: 1) provide a just return on capital; 2) produce a useful commodity or service; 3) increase the wealth or quality of society; 4) provide productive employment opportunities; 5) help employees find satisfying work; and 6) pay fair wages" (O'Hallaron , 2002, p. 125).

The Power of Meaningful Work

> *If there is light in the soul,*
> *There will be beauty in the person.*
> *If there is beauty in the person,*
> *There will be harmony in the house.*
> *If there is harmony in the house,*
> *There will be order in the nation.*
> *If there is order in the nation,*
> *There will be peace in the world.*
>
> —*Chinese Proverb*

The core ideology and purpose of the organization, or the soul, is the ocean towards which we are headed. Spirit comes from our belief that we are doing meaningful work. This intrinsic motivator is more important than pay. The research has, and continues, to show this. Still, we continue to get tripped up thinking that paying bonuses, or some other payment scheme, will achieve success with employees, forgetting that meaningful work comes first. The pay helps but is not the most important factor.

Motivation comes from within. There is not a magic wand we can wave to achieve a motivated workforce. Instead, in the right environment, under the right conditions, the opportunity is there for personnel to be motivated about their work; whether they are motivated is their choice. Herzberg (2003) has republished a classic that discusses motivation. In an early study he found that employee satisfaction was due to the following factors (in order of importance): achievement, recognition, the work itself, responsibility, advancement, and growth. Do you see the corollary this work has with Maslow's self-actualization need that we all have? For instance, if we love our work, chances are it is a match with our gifts, and, chances are, we think our work is meaningful because we are helping others. All this is related to the spirit part of the work we do. It is an intrinsic factor that comes from within.

Herzberg goes on with a list of dissatisfiers. These factors do not cause satisfaction but if there is something wrong in the workplace, these can cause employees to feel dissatisfied, and if not resolved, could result in people leaving for greener pastures. The dissatisfiers, in order of importance, are: company policy and administration, supervision, relationship with the supervisor, work conditions, salary, relationship with peers, personal life, relationship with staff colleagues, status, and security. Can you see how the dissatisfiers can erode spirit? It is a sad commentary on our present organizations that company policy and administration is at the top of the list.

For employee satisfaction, meaningful work gets back to the purpose and core ideology—and starts with how much we administrators live it. If our main concern is the bottom line, the soul is missing in the organization. But if our actions really support the purpose and core ideology, this is very powerful. Then we believe, and employees know that we believe because our actions show it. Our actions do not cause staff to be dissatisfied. Instead, staff spirit and motivation exists. Throughout history we have seen that when people believe in a cause, they will even die for it. The cause provides the backbone (the ocean) of meaningful work.

Trust is an important factor that relates to our spirit. When employees trust the administrators, any achievement is possible. Trust occurs when the administrator has integrity and always strives to achieve the core ideology and purpose. When dissatisfiers are present, chances are someone is not trusted and does not have integrity. When nurses complain of feeling depersonalized, something is seriously wrong with the administrative leadership, and the leadership must be fixed before the spirit can come back into the organization. Listen to the Studer (2000) tape. He was a CEO of a hospital in serious trouble both financially and in spirit. He discusses how he had to fix himself, go within, before he could work on fixing the rest of the organization.

Additionally, if the administrator has integrity, employee trust follows. Staff support decisions of an administrator who can truly empower them, by using group process in decision making, and encouraging all to support the core ideology and purpose. Trust is something to value very highly because it is not lightly given, and once lost, can probably never be regained.

This is the meaning that will permeate our feelings of belonging and engagement. It is the heart of teamwork and collaborative synthesis within an organization. The soul provides meaning so the spirit is alive and well. "Courage comes from the French word which means heart. Once our heart is engaged, we operate with passion and not power and we can find ways to transform our world together" (Kerfoot, 2002, p. 298). Meaningful work feeds our soul.

So when soul is there, and the spirit is missing, we need to start questioning within ourselves, are we doing something that is causing this problem? Curran (2000) reports that the Gallop organization, after doing 25 years of research on 400 companies with 80,000 managers,

Concluded that one could measure the strength of the workplace with 12 simple questions:

1. Do I know what is expected of me at work?

2. Do I have the materials and equipment I need to do my work right?

3. At work, do I have the opportunity to do what I do best everyday?

4. In the last 7 days, have I received recognition or praise for doing good work?

5. Does my supervisor, or someone at work, care about me as a person?

6. Is there someone at work who encourages my development?

7. At work, do my opinions seem to count?

8. Does the mission/purpose of my company make me feel my job is important?

9. Are my co-workers committed to doing quality work?

10. Do I have a best friend at work?

11. In the last 6 months, has someone talked to me about my progress?

12. This last year, have I had opportunities at work to learn and grow?

Buckingham and Coffman (1999) demonstrated that these 12 questions separate great organizations from average ones.... Individuals may join organizations, but it is their immediate manager who directly influences how long they stay and how productive they are. Employees do not leave organizations, they leave managers (p. 277).

Spirit is more likely to be present when these nine aspects are present at the workplace. Spirit comes from within each of us.

The condition of your employees' spirit is easily diagnosed. You can see spirit, or the lack of it, in their productivity. You can also see spirit in their eyes. You may see spirits overwhelmed and discouraged. And, in too many cases, you will see the depression of employees who have lost their spirit for healthcare work.... Employees want to be a part of an important work that is accomplished through collective effort.... Spirit and soul are not management techniques. They are available to us by personal commitment to their values. Soul and spirit are realities in us, as aspects of who we are. Soul and spirit are around us and available to energize our work relationships (Nobre, pp. 288–289).

Organizational Assessment

To best energize everyone's work with soul and spirit, let's look at administrative competencies that enable us to provide an energized climate for work. In administration, *organi-*

zational assessment is a critical thinking component necessary for role effectiveness. Organizational assessment is the ability to have a fairly accurate, dynamic picture of the total organization, such as how various people work together, which departments are more effective, how different departments have different cultures, how clients perceive the organization, and how the organization fits within the community that surrounds it. This picture is dynamic, and changes as various components, relationships, and people change within the organization. What was true yesterday will be different today, and what is true today will change tomorrow. This organizational assessment capability helps the administrator to know, with fair accuracy, how different individuals and departments respond to situations. No matter how well we know an organization, we still experience surprises, but this organizational assessment capability is a key factor for effectiveness.

This critical thinking capability can be developed and mentored. First, one needs to learn how to assess an organization. Assessment is dynamic, meaning that once one has assessed the current organization, the assessment must change as people and situations change. This is a lived experience that takes time and effort to learn. Actually, one's picture never is totally accurate because there are always hidden factors that we do not know, both about ourselves and about others; and because everyone in the organization is constantly changing. Thus at times we can surprise ourselves when we do not respond to something the way we had anticipated, or when someone else reacts in a way we had not anticipated.

ROUNDS

The best way to continually assess an organization is to do frequent rounds; do regularly scheduled, round-the-clock meetings, share information, and be open to questions and concerns of those attending; have roundtable gatherings around issues; and have an open-door policy. Our organizational assessment is dynamic and ever-changing.

It is critical that administrators at all levels of management do frequent rounds.

Rounds are where the administrator is regularly out visiting with patients and families, as well as staff, at the points of service. This also means that when there is full census, or a unit or department needs help, the administrators are empathetic to the situation and pitch in.

Tom Peters coined the phrase, Management By Walking Around (MBWA), but nurses have been doing rounds for years before MBWA became popular. One can find out all sorts of helpful information by visiting staff, physicians, patients and families, and other interdisciplinary staff while doing rounds. Rounds allow feedback from staff without having too many meetings. This is greatly facilitated when all administrators—from board members and the president on down to the nurse manager—are out doing rounds daily, being visible for the sake of more effective communication as well as giving support.

The research supports this concept in so many different ways. There are fewer lawsuits when the patient and family perceive that the caregivers—and administrators—care. A health care administrator is always more effective when doing rounds because the real patient issues are more likely to be identified and addressed.

While doing rounds, it is important to coach and mentor staff, rather than being too task oriented. One wants nursing staff to *think*, and not depend upon someone else, such as the physician or nurse manager, for all the answers. We also want to encourage staff to use systems thinking because one action will affect five other things. One can observe what processes can be improved, and what barriers exist that could be either eliminated or reduced.

There are some potential traps to avoid. First, the administrator—from the CEO and board member to the nurse manager—needs to exhibit certain behaviors. While walking down the hall of an inpatient unit, if the administrator does not pay attention to call lights or patients/families who are having obvious problems, the message the administrator gives is that patient issues are not important. If the administrator does not greet staff but just goes to find the manager, staff get the message that they are not important. They can view the administrator as not caring about them.

Second, it is best not to become Attila the Hun. If one reacts to a situation and heads roll, everyone becomes afraid of the administrator, literally hide, or hide information from the administrator, resent the administrator, and do not actually change their behavior—unless the administrator is around. It is more advantageous to converse with staff, and to help staff explore more effective options.

A third trap is to micro-manage. When an administrator micro-manages, the message to staff is that staff are not capable of doing the job right. However, the real problem is that the administrator has not learned to effectively delegate.

The most effective way to do rounds is to pay attention to everyone present, dialogue with people, demonstrate caring, and use rounds as a learning process. All actions support the core values and the purpose. As crises occur, remain calm and decisive, and, when necessary, pitch in and help resolve the situation. As problems become evident, dialogue with those involved to explore how best to handle a situation, or get into dialogue about what happened and determine what could have been done to more effectively deal with the problem.

Round-the-clock meetings enable everyone, regardless of shift or work schedule, to learn what is important from other perspectives. This way the midnight or weekend personnel do not feel as isolated. Administrators at all levels should hold these meetings regularly.

Roundtable gatherings can be a helpful way to deal with the many issues that staff experience as they do their work. It is best if all attend a gathering based on interest in the topic that will be discussed. It is especially helpful if those attending from administration represent various levels, and depending upon the topic to be discussed, special invitations should go out to departments that would be concerned with dealing with the issue being discussed.

An open-door policy means that when someone has an important issue we welcome the person coming to share it with us. An open door does not mean that a secretary intercedes for us, although, if the secretary is empowered, this person is invaluable to an administrator and actually deals with many issues directly, saving the administrator time.

ORGANIZING THE ASSESSMENT DATA

Collins and Porras (1994) suggest a way to organize the organizational assessment data one needs to know as an administrator. See **Exhibit 4–1**.

Exhibit 4–1 Organizational Assessment Categories

Category 1: Organizing Arrangements. 'Hard' items, such as organization structure, policies and procedures, systems, rewards and incentives, ownership structure, and general business strategies and activities of the company (e.g., acquisitions, significant changes in strategy, going public).

Category 2: Social Factors. 'Soft' items, such as the company's cultural practices, atmosphere, norms, rituals, mythology and stories, group dynamics, and management style.

Category 3: Physical Setting. Significant aspects of the way the company handled physical space, such as plant and office layout or new facilities. This included any significant decisions regarding the geographic location of key parts of the company.

Category 4: Technology.[1] How the company used technology: information technology, state-of-the-art processes and equipment, advanced job configurations, and related items.

Category 5: Leadership. Leadership of the firm since its inception: the transition between key early shapers of the organization and later generations, leadership tenure, the length of time the leaders were with the organization before becoming CEO (Were they brought in from the outside or grown from within? When did they join?), leadership selection processes and criteria.

Category 6: Products and Services.[2] Significant products and services in the company's history. How did the product or service ideas come about? What guided their selection and development? Did the company have any product failures, and how did it deal with them? Did the company lead with new products or follow in the marketplace?

Category 7: Vision: Core Values, Purpose, and Visionary Goals.[3] Were these variables present? If yes, how did they come into being: Did the organization have them at certain points in its history and not others? What role did they play? If it had strong values and purpose, did they remain intact or become diluted? Why?

Category 8: Financial Analysis.[4] Ratio and spreadsheet analysis of all income statements and balance sheets for every year going back to the date when the company became public: sales and profit growth, gross margins, return on assets, return on sales, return on equity, debt to equity ratio, cash flow and working capital, liquidity ratios, dividend payout ratio, increase in gross property plant and equipment as a percentage of sales, asset turnover. Also examine stock returns and overall stock performance relative to the market (if applicable).

Category 9: Markets/Environment.[5] Significant aspects of the company's external environment: major market shifts, dramatic national or international events, government regulations, industry structural issues, dramatic technology changes, and related items.

From: Collins, J., and Porras, J. (1994). *Built to Last: Successful Habits of Visionary Companies*. NY: Harper Business, pp. 259–260.

---

[1] Chapters 8 and 9 are concerned with technology.

[2] Products and services are discussed in detail in Chapter 2 on Quality factors and in Chapter 21 on Productivity. We are a service industry. This means that we rely on people to accomplish the output. This makes it difficult to achieve product consistency. It is further complicated because our patients have individual needs which will necessitate output variances if we are paying attention to what patients want.

[3] Core values and purpose have already been discussed in this chapter. Visionary goals are included with strategic planning in Chapter 15.

[4] Chapters 17 and 18 provide information on how to understand income statements and a number of financial ratios.

[5] Discussed in Chapter 14 on Budget Strategies.

Organizing Arrangements[6]

Following Collins and Porras example in **Exhibit 4–1**, we now turn to the various cate-gories within the organization. All the components, *when integrated together*, give us a more complete organizational assessment. If we use linear thinking, we can look at each aspect as separate entities. However, this does not represent reality, as the reality is that all aspects are interwoven. As we think of the organizational assessment, it is like describing a person. We cannot take a person apart and look at each component of the person or they will die. We can only describe how the whole person seems to operate. And each moment this whole person is changing as events happen and the person responds to the events. So although we describe the components to help get a better handle on this whole, please go beyond linear thinking and see the organization as a whole, ever-changing entity.

The first organizational assessment category describes *the organizing arrangements*. This includes structure and design elements. Structure and design is influenced by some new terms that come from chaos theory and the science of complex systems. This is fur-ther explained in **Exhibit 4–2**. These dynamics are present in organizations and will effect what happens in organizations.

Another term, *fractals*, is important when thinking about organizations. Have you heard the expression, *as above, so below*? This is what fractals are about.

> The notion of fractals is critical for understanding the order that exists in chaos and for appreciating the impact of complexity on organizations and human behavior. The smallest level of a single organization and the most complex array of a large aggregated system containing the organi-zation are connected inexorably through the power of fractals.
>
> If you have ever looked at a hologram, which is a three-dimensional pho-tograph of an image, you may have noticed that no matter what size sec-tion you focus in on, the entire image will still be present in the smaller piece. Holography thus can be used to explain the nature of fractals, for in a fractal the complete pattern is present in any component regardless of the level of detail or complexity. A tree is a good example from the so-called natural world, for its overall structure, including the trunk and branches, is similar to the branching pattern of each leaf.
>
> Fractals have tremendous implications for organizations. From the smallest structural elements to the very complex patterns of behavior existing throughout an organization, the same patterns appear and are played out in precise detail. This fact implies that at every level of the organization there exists a self-organizing capacity and that this capac-ity maintains a balance and harmony even in the midst of the most chaotic processes. To the extent that the balance and harmony are sus-tained, the organization's life is advanced. To the extent that they are upset or cannot be articulated, visualized, and acted upon at every level

---

[6] Ownership is discussed in Chapter 6. The chapter also defines for-profit, not-for-profit, and governmental structures, as well as various kinds of alliances and mergers that can occur. General business strategies are discussed in the second part of this chapter, as well as in several other chapters concerned with specific issues.

Exhibit 4–2 The Language of Complexity and Chaos

New words from the science of complex systems describe a different world than we have grown familiar with. They express a whole set of dynamics that operate just outside our field of vision, yet they have a defining impact on our experience of life and the human journey in which we each play an important but not always known role. Some of the more unusual words include these:

- **Autopoiesis.** The process by which living systems continually seek to renew and reinvent themselves yet maintain their core identity.

- **Autocatalysis.** A process in which information enters into a system in small fluctuations that continually grow in strength, interacting with the system and feedback upon itself.

- **Dissipative structures.** Structures in which disorder is the source of order and vice versa. In this "dance" between order and disorder, old form ends and new form begins.

- **Strange attractor.** The activity of a collective chaotic system composed of interactive feedback between and among its various "parts" and evidencing "attraction" to its pattern of behavior.

From: Porter-O'Grady and Malloch, (2003). *Quantum Leadership: A Textbook of New Leadership*. Boston: Jones and Bartlett, p. 13.

---

of leadership, the organization's actions will tend to impede its integrity and effectiveness. It is important, therefore, that the leaders of the organization be aware of the continuous and dynamic action of fractals in all organizational behavior and structure so that they can advance the consonance and value of the employee's activities and enhance the organization's ability to fulfill its mission.

Perhaps it is even more important for the leaders to recognize that, within the context of the fractal's dynamic action, their own actions have cascading and rippling implications in every other part of the organization. In fact, they should understand that no decision, action, or undertaking can occur any place in the organization without ultimately having an impact on every other action, decision, and undertaking. In addition, once they are cognizant of the web of interaction and interdependence that exists in the organization, the leaders will approach deliberation and decision making only with extreme care, caution, and thoroughness (Porter-O'Grady and Malloch, 2003, pp. 13–14).

STRUCTURE

Structure refers to the way an organization delineates jobs and reporting relationships, or the arrangement of roles within an organization (Gordon, 2002). "Advances are being made at an astounding rate in the medical, biological, and pharmaceutical fields, yet the structure of the health care delivery system in many places operates as it did decades ago" (McDonagh, p. 46). Although an organizational chart begins to define structure, it does not capture the various relationships between people on the chart or the resulting effectiveness of a group. We are all interconnected with each other to accomplish our work. The *design* of an organization describes the process of "setting up," or the "appearance" of the organization. Though the terms *structure* and *design* are closely related, there is a lack of consistency and clarity in the use of these words. Many times these terms are used interchangeably (Hodges, Anthony, and Gales, 1996). We use *design* as also having a broader definition that reflects the relationships and processes used within an organization.

Within the organizational structure and design, two forms are usually described: formal and informal. The *formal organization*, or "official" structure, is described within the organizational chart. The organizational chart displays the chain of command, or the relationship of authority. The solid lines that connect the boxes show the formal channels of communication and reporting relationships; the dotted lines show an informal reporting relationship.

Most often the organizational chart has the board and the CEO, or president, at the top of the chart. Some would suggest that this chart should be inverted with the *customer* at the top and the president at the bottom. The organizational chart provides clarity, and specifies areas of responsibility. However, it is a very imperfect picture because it does not capture the relationships that exist. The relationships are more important to getting the work accomplished than knowing areas of responsibility. Therefore the chart must be taken in context with the actual workings of the organization.

The formal structure also includes the regularly scheduled meetings that take place within the organization. Hopefully, these meetings aid those in the organization to function more effectively. However, there is a great divergence in actual meeting effectiveness—some being very helpful, some being ponderous, and some being a total waste of time. Some organizations have so many meetings the administrators cannot get their work done! Which comes first—the patient or the meeting?

Some questions to ponder with meetings follow:

- What is the outcome of this meeting?
- Is this meeting necessary?
- Could this meeting have been more efficient?
- Are we processing, or obsessing, too much on certain things?
- Are we concentrating so much on tasks that process is forgotten?
- Are we not spending enough time/or too much time in understanding each other's perspectives?
- Are meeting outcomes being effectively communicated with others who need to know the information?
- Are the right people attending the meeting?
- Most importantly, does the meeting support the organization's core values? What would patients think about how the meeting is conducted and about meeting outcomes? Were patients involved or represented in decisions?

The *informal*, or the "unofficial" structure of an organization includes all the relationships and people's personal characteristics. For example, if one department head is very difficult to work with, others in the organization know this and try to work around this person, or if the director's secretary is married to a board member, this needs to be taken into consideration.

The informal organization reflects all the interpersonal relationships between people that are not reflected on the organizational chart but that affect operations. For instance, a nurse manager may realize that the unit secretary's informal leadership can really enhance the nurse manager's effectiveness, and helps the unit to function much more efficiently. If the nurse manager chooses to ignore or suppress this person's leadership capabilities, unnecessary conflicts can result, patient care may suffer, and the dysfunctional situation would spiral downward from there.

When there are flaws or inefficiencies in the administrative leadership, such as being secretive and not sharing information, the informal information network becomes rampant. When most information is shared and there is trust in the leadership, the informal network becomes fairly inactive. Everything and everyone in an organization is interconnected. Some aspects of these links are given in **Exhibit 4–2**.

We are presently at an interesting juncture of time as an organization's structure is changing very significantly. As time is getting more compressed, discussed in Chapter 2, our present infastructure is changing dramatically.

This time compression, along with what we know about chaos theory and the science of complex systems (refer back to **Exhibit 4–2**) are working to change our organizational systems whether or not we actually want them changed. (Remember the Berlin Wall example?)

The compression of time is inexorably working to reconfigure the context for health care and restructure its framework without the consent of the participants. To be most effective health care leaders will focus on interpreting external demands and translating them into internal actions. They are being called into the chaos of creativity to produce a good fit between the new framework demanded and the infrastructure that needs to be constructed to support it.

Much of the current work of health care leaders involves deconstructing health services. The current infrastructure must be largely deconstructed so newer models of service and support can be implemented. Leaders need to perform a range of activities in reconfiguring health care to fit the coming age, when space and time will be further compressed, services will be more fluid and more highly mobilized, and the locus of control will shift from the provider to the user. The changes that will occur include:

- The hospital bed will cease to be the main point of service. During the next two decades, the number of hospital beds will decline by about 50 percent.

- The service structure will be decentralized. The health care system will deliver small, broadly dispersed units of service.

- Services will increasingly move out of the hospital. More than 70 percent of the medical services currently provided in hospitals will be provided in clinics and doctor's offices by the end of this decade.

- The core practices of the professions will be substantially altered. The institution-based, late-stage services that once predominated are being replaced by high-intensity interventions that do not require hospitalization, and these interventions will transform the roles of the various health professionals.

- Users of health services are becoming more accountable for their own health. Providers now have the major job of helping to transfer the locus of control for medical decision making and life management to individuals who have never had it and do not yet know what to do with it. [Providers'] work over the next two decades will include educating the users of health services and assisting [users] in acquiring the necessary skills (Porter-O'Grady and Malloch, p. 34).

SHARED GOVERNANCE

Shared governance is a structural framework that affords nursing—and all other organizational members—professional autonomy at the point of care.

> A system is always self-organizing and, given the appropriate support, will be self-sustaining and oriented toward thriving… Every member of a system has both a right to membership and the obligations that brings. Both must be clear to all who contribute to the system's work… Shared governance is simply a framework for whole-systems effectiveness providing a context for partnership, equity, accountability, and ownership… Shared governance is not a democracy. It is an accountability-based approach in which there is a clear expectation that all members of a system participate in its work. (Porter-O'Grady, Hawkins, and Parker, pp. 32–33, 40).

Shared governance operates in a true environment of empowerment. Remember in Chapter 3 on Leadership how empowerment does not even happen until a leader is at least at Stage 4 of Hagberg's power model? With shared governance, staff and leaders are empowered to contribute collectively to the decision making process related to clinical practice, standards, and procedures. Shared governance also provides the organization with a mechanism to make decisions that improve patient care and the workplace environment. For example, nurses know how processes can be improved, so the decisions can be made directly by the nurses that deliver the care.

O'Grady (2001) points out that in our current environment nurses can leave if they think they are being "controlled" and "devalued" in an authoritarian system. There are more jobs available than there are nurses to fill them. If there is an ideal time for shared governance and true empowerment, it is now. This is the only way to achieve retention.

The research supports this. Erickson's research shows the value of staff empowerment and collaborative governance (Erickson, et al., 2003). Kuokkanen and Katajisto (2003) found that nurses identified "factors that prevented empowerment included authoritarian leadership, poor access to information, and short working periods. Factors found to increase empowerment were job satisfaction, career consciousness, further training, and commitment" (p. 209). Laschinger et al. (2001) agrees:

> Decision latitude refers to the extent to which a worker has control over the nature of the job and how it is done. Nurses must be empowered with the authority to make autonomous decisions based on their expertise and professional judgment, and to have control over the implementation and outcome of these decisions. Organizational strategies designed to increase nurses' control over their practice and to promote accountabil-

ity include decentralized structures, participative management practices, and shared governance systems. Participatory management creates an atmosphere in which staff nurses are empowered to solve problems collectively, provide input into productivity measures, and improve clinical processes affecting patient care. Nurses have reported increased feelings of respect and value to the organization following the implementation of participatory management models. In shared governance systems, managers are accountable for ensuring that resources and support are available to assist nurses in providing high quality professional nursing care (p. 240).

Creating an empowering environment is hard work. It takes constant effort. It can be painful. It means staff should be making 90 percent of the decisions and may choose directions that never occurred to us. O'Grady suggests that staff needs to be involved in the decision making with "hiring, budgeting, allocating, discipline, and policy" (p. 469). He describes the leader's perspective of an empowering environment as "overwhelming, treacherous, noisy, slow, and time-consuming. It often is tedious, not glamorous, and painful to make the required changes in the system for real empowerment to become the modus operandi for an organization" (p. 471).

The main purpose of shared governance is to increase decision making at the point of service. In fact Porter-O'Grady, Hawkins, and Parker advocate that 90 percent of all decisions need to be made at this level. This is not just a nursing model as other health caregivers need to be making decisions at the point of service as well. Thus, even though in a health care organization, nurses may be making about 60 percent of the decisions, the medical staff, as well as other health care professionals, need to be involved in the point of service decision making.

The old model was either based on who had authority (physicians or executive group) or the location of the service (nursing, laboratory, radiology). "As discipline- and function-specific walls get broken down and partnerships increasingly form the foundation for functional clinical activity, integrating decision making and structures that support it becomes a critical task for the organization" (p. 35).

Porter-O'Grady et al. advocate a *whole-systems shared governance model* where each member has equal power and responsibilities in the decision making process, putting what the patient values and wants first. In this shared governance model there is an operations council (concerned with resources, linkage, planning, market strategy, implementation, and compliance), a patient care council (concerned with service delivery, system models, disciplines, service design, roles, quality and process), and a governance council (concerned with mission, strategy, priorities, policy, and integration).

The physicians have had a medical staff organization historically, but the authors advocate that "many of the current separate functions of the medical staff will disappear as they become more integrated within the system.... The real struggle for physicians is seeing themselves as a partner in the health system rather than the controllers of it" (pp. 219–220).

Using this model there is a *shared governance steering group* that shares information and integrates decisions between and amongst the three councils. It is important that "every key role in the system, staff or management, should be represented in the steering group. The majority of planners, however, should be from the staff, not from management" (p. 74). "Integration is evidence of the attempt to configure services around the point of care and to bring providers together in a service partnership.... compartmentalization is the death of integration" (pp. 36, 41).

To make all this work effectively, caregivers who are at the point of service need access to accurate information, need to tune in to what the patient values, need administrative support from the top down to make these decisions, and need to feel accountable for their decisions. Shared governance structure ensures "that the decisions made there are correct, 'implementable,' and do not require broad organizational approval or a long decision making process (which might reduce the efficiency and effectiveness of the clinical delivery system)" (Porter-O'Grady, et al., p. 72). It is a system based on accountability coming internally from staff who want to give their best effort to their work. The principles of shared governance can be found in **Exhibit 4–3**.

Policies and Procedures

One also needs to look at policies and procedures. Now that we are in the information age, policies and procedures can be available for staff via the internet (since the amount of information that we need to know is enormous, Chapter 7 outlines how to efficiently find necessary information using present technologies). One current flaw in health care is that often we have notebooks full of policies and procedures for RNs, the professionals, and few policies and procedures for nurse aides, the non-professionals. As a rule of thumb, more policies and procedures are needed for the non-professional group. For instance, doesn't *Love One Another* say it all? Look at what Nordstrom's set up for their policies:

> Nordstrom Rules:
>
> Rule #1: **Use your good judgment in all situations.**
>
> There will be no additional rules.
>
> Please feel free to ask your department manager, store manager or division manager any question at any time (Collins and Porras, 1994).

Don't we want nurses to be professionals? Isn't it better to have references for them to refer to when they do not know what to do? Does anyone really pay attention to all the policies and procedures anyway? Legally, don't we leave ourselves open for additional problems with all this volume if a nurse does not follow some procedure somewhere and something happens?

Creating policies and procedures for legal reasons brings up another example within this dilemma. We can have our hands tied by trying to have all the appropriate paperwork, and do all the actions that lawyers have told us to do to avoid legal issues. We are hamstrung. Our nurses do not spend nearly enough actual time with patients because of all the paperwork. We have turned into a society where we let the lawyers run us, rather than the other way around. How can we help those nurses have less paperwork so they have time to do what we, and they, really want them to do? Think of how this would help the retention issue.

Paige (2003) advocates taking a multidisciplinary approach to policies and procedures. This is because policies and procedures often apply to more than one department, so each department having a separate policy is redundant. Or worse yet, they may be different. It is possible that combining efforts can produce a better one. It can also help ensure that departments are consistent, and that legal problems do not result due to the inconsistencies.

Exhibit 4–3 Principles of Shared Governance

Partnership
- Role expectations are negotiated.
- Equality exists between the players.
- Relationships are founded upon shared risk.
- Expectations and contributions are clear.
- Solid measure of contribution to outcomes is established.
- Horizontal linkages are well defined.

Equity
- Each player's contribution is understood.
- Payment reflects value of contribution to outcomes.
- Role is based on relationship, not status.
- Team defines service roles, relationships, and outcomes.
- Methodology is defined for team conflict and service issues.
- Evaluation assesses team's outcomes and contributions.

Accountability
- Accountability is internally defined by person in the role.
- Accountability defines roles, not jobs.
- Accountability is based on outcomes, not process.
- Accountability is defined in advance of performance.
- Accountability leads to desired and defined results.
- Performance is validated by the results achieved.
- Processes are generally loud and noisy.

Ownership
- All workers are invested in the enterprise.
- Every role has a stake in the outcome.
- Rewards are directly related to outcomes.
- All members are associated with a team.
- Processes support relationships.
- Opportunity is based on competence.

From: Porter-O'Grady, T., Hawkins, M., and Parker, M. (1997). *Whole-Systems Shared Governance: Architecture for Integration*. Gaithersburg, MD: Aspen, p. 49.

Systems

Another aspect of this Organizing Arrangements category involves defining the systems used to accomplish the work. Senge (1990) coined the word, *systems thinking*, describing it as a framework for seeing wholes, or seeing interrelationships rather than things. Using systems thinking, we are able to picture the entire organization and how it functions, not just our own department. As we assess organizations as a whole, they differ—many have a high ethic of collaboration, while others are heavily authoritarian where administrators have difficulty with systems thinking. And, of course, there are combinations of both in the same organization.

What do we mean by systems thinking? This type of thinking takes into account the overall, dynamic organizational picture before making decisions. How will people across the organization, and even in the community, respond to a change? What outcomes might result if a decision is implemented? When decisions are made, they are carefully crafted to achieve the best result and avoid possible pitfalls that would actually worsen the issue. Without using systems thinking, it is easy to make quick-fix solutions that actually generate *more* problems and result in other unanticipated effects because solutions did not account for the entire system response to the change. This wholeness in systems thinking includes the way various departments work together within the organization. In today's complex organizations *systems thinking is a necessary administrative competency.*

In fact, systems thinking is so important that it is helpful if other team members, not just administrators, also use systems thinking. Work teams are more effective when the entire team can view the organization as a whole. Unfortunately, team members' confidence and responsibility can be undermined by the complexity of a situation. How often do we hear team members and front-line leaders comment, "You can't change the system". Systems thinking can drastically help to change this helpless feeling.

To accomplish systems thinking we must restructure the way we think. Senge states that systems thinking "lies in a shift of mind: seeing interrelationships rather than linear cause and effect and seeing processes of change rather than snapshots" (p. 73). As thinkers we often see things in straight lines, whereas reality is actually made up of circles.[7]

Understanding systems thinking begins with the concept *feedback*. The word feedback can be used in many different ways. When we ask for feedback we are often asking for someone's opinion, encouraging both positive and negative remarks. Systems thinkers use feedback for a broader concept. Senge (1990) describes feedback as any "reciprocal flow of influence," an "axiom that every influence is both cause and effect" and that "nothing is influenced in just one direction" (p.75).

The issue of responsibility often complicates the concept of feedback. As linear thinkers we are always searching for someone or something to blame. For instance, this blame-search occurs with patient safety. When we become accomplished systems thinkers, we renounce the idea that one individual is responsible. We begin to realize that responsibility is shared. However, this does not mean that everyone in the system has equal power.

---

[7] To explore thinking patterns, see two books by de Bono listed in the References.

Rewards and Incentives

In the organizational assessment, one must consider what is done within the organization to either reward various personnel, or is offered as an incentive for personnel. These incentives, if not carefully thought out, can produce very negative results. For example, one incentive for an executive team might be a bonus if they can keep costs below a certain amount for the quarter or for the year. This, however, has a downside as this is not linked with a quality dimension. So this encourages executives to save money even when it is at the cost of the patient, and patient outcomes may be worsened as a result of these decisions. In addition, these bonuses reward only executive level administrators for meeting standards, yet the people doing the everyday work with patients are not given bonuses.

Another disincentive for nurses is that they are professionals yet we make them use timecards to clock in and out. What if their patient(s) needed something beyond the shift time that the nurse wanted to provide? Some organizations have chosen to put nurses on annual salaries, rather than to use hourly pay. (Sometimes the salary issue has been abused by administrators as a way to avoid overtime. This is not the intent here. It should be a fair wage.) This is positive when nurses are given the freedom to come in as their patients need them. If this is an inpatient setting, some nurses could choose their hours while others cover actual shift times. The main thing is that nurses have meaningful work—satisfying experiences with patients and families that enhance nurse retention.

Another disincentive presently is the high salaries paid for traveler nurses, ignoring our best loyal workforce already present day after day working for us. Our message is that this loyal group is not as important as the traveler nurses.

It is important to give careful thought to the rewards and incentives provided because these should support desired behaviors. For instance, employee performance evaluations have no clout if they are not used to determine merit increases. Or, organizational performance evaluations are worthless if not everyone in the workplace is rewarded for meeting performance standards. For instance, in the preceeding example of the bonus-incentive, the organization has missed the boat for another reason. When rewards or incentives are used for certain behaviors, it is important to provide the staff with development activities that will teach them the specific behaviors. For instance, if all are rewarded for being *patient-centered*, it will be important to have staff development activities available to teach all staff what patient-centered actually means in daily behaviors including the thinking and decision-making process to be used. In addition, it is helpful if all, including top-level administrators, model and support the desired behaviors.

Another important incentive is to pay for staff to attend conferences. During budget cuts, staff development monies are often cut, a short-sighted decision. It is important that all staff, including aides and housekeeping staff, are up-to-date doing meaningful work. In fact, right now the research shows that these two groups spend the most time with patients in inpatient facilities. Budget cuts also often affect staff education monies, yet the executive group continues to attend national conferences with travel costs fully paid. This gets back to the fact that *our actions speak louder than our words.*

THE SOCIAL FACTORS

Social factors include the way people work together. It reflects the spirit aspect. It speaks to the "radical loving care," as well as our living "love one another" as administrators. Perhaps this is the most important factor within an organization because these social factors are what achieve the patient outcomes. Ideally, one hopes to achieve a culture of participation and teamwork around the core values.

Likert's Authoritarian versus Participative Model

To begin the organizational assessment, think about an overall picture of the organization. Likert (1973) identifies a classic organizational model that shows how various organizational variables interact with one another. See **Exhibit 4–4**. System 1 represents a very authoritarian model. Here there is little dialogue, communication only occurs in a downward direction (assuming the CEO is at the top–an authoritarian model), the informal rumor mill is rampant and needed because it is the best source of information for staff, decisions are made at the top, orders are given, no one dares to question the orders, often staff resist the orders covertly, and CONTROL is all important. Correspond this to a System 4, a very participative model. Here matrixes exist where there is communication between and within all levels, communication is open and shared, dialogue occurs, decisions are made at the appropriate level, the organization consists of well integrated staff, goals are determined by group action except in crisis, there is no need for an informal organization, because information is shared, and productivity is enhanced by each person, with everyone doing their own problem solving. System 2 and 3 fall between these two extremes with System 2 being slightly authoritarian while System 3 starts to become more participative.

Using Likert's model, we need to assess where our organization currently is, and base our actions on this assessment. For instance, if we are a transformational leader, believing in a System 4, yet we are in a System 2, we become very frustrated, and staff do not understand our leadership style, if we interact with staff as though it is a System 4. Instead we must start responding based on where the system currently is. So in a staff meeting, (which staff may not be used to having until we came!), we want to get feedback from staff on an issue or on a potential piece of equipment. When we ask for feedback, we might get none. It is easy to wonder what we have done wrong. (This is internalizing the problem.) Instead, realize that staff is sitting there being suspicious of us, thinking, "What does s/he want from me? I'm not going to stick my neck out." Repeated meetings where we ask for feedback are necessary, before staff begins to trust us enough to start offering suggestions. Even then, it only occurs on issues that are perceived to be safe, or not as emotionally laden. When this breakthrough happens, the group starts to move to a more participative model.

When we want to move an organization, department, or floor staff from a System 2 to a System 3, it may take repeated efforts for a *couple of years* before one begins to see movement in this direction. This cultural change is an enormous one, and is particularly hard when a number of administrators at the executive level are still into the authoritarian style. So it is important that we do not beat ourselves up for not being effective when we have not accomplished this sooner. The best place to begin is to look for small changes. Maybe

Exhibit 4-4 Likert's Organizational Systems

Organizational Variables	SYSTEM 1	SYSTEM 2	SYSTEM 3	SYSTEM 4
Leadership				
How much confidence and trust is shown in staff?	Virtually none	Some	Substantial amount	A great deal
How free do they feel to talk to supervisors about job?	Not very free	Somewhat free	Quite free	Very free
How often are staff's ideas sought and used constructively?	Seldom	Sometimes	Often	Very frequently
Motivation				
Is predominant use made of (1) fear, (2) threats, (3) punishment, (4) rewards, (5) involvement?	1, 2, 3, occasionally 4	4, some 3	4, some 3 and 5	5, 4, based on group
Where is responsibility felt for achieving the organization's goals?	Mostly at top	Top and middle	Fairly general	At all levels
How much cooperative teamwork exists?	Very little	Relatively little	Moderate amount	Great deal
Communications				
What is the usual direction of information flow?	Downward	Mostly downward	Down and up	Down, up and sideways
How is downward communication accepted?	With suspicion	Possibly with suspicion	With caution	With a receptive mind
How accurate is upward communications?	Usually inaccurate	Often inaccurate	Often accurate	Almost always accurate

continued

Organizational Variables	SYSTEM 1	SYSTEM 2	SYSTEM 3	SYSTEM 4
Communications (continued)				
How well do administrators know the problems faced by staff?	Not very well	Rather well	Quite well	Very well
Decisions				
At what level are decisions made?	Mostly at top	Policy at top, some delegation	Broad policy at top, more delegation	Throughout but well-integrated
Are staff involved in decisions related to their work?	Almost never	Occasionally consulted	Generally consulted	Fully involved
What does the decision-making process contribute to motivation?	Not very much	Relatively little	Some contribution	Substantial contribution
Goals				
How are organizational goals established?	Orders issued	Orders, some comments invited	After discussion, by orders	By group action (except in crisis)
How much covert resistance to goals is present?	Strong resistance	Moderate resistance	Some resistance at times	Little or none
Evaluation				
How concentrated are review and evaluation functions?	Very highly at top	Quite highly at top	Moderate delegation to lower levels	Widely shared
Is there an informal organization resisting the formal one?	Yes	Usually	Sometimes	No—same goals as formal
What are cost, productivity, and other evaluation data used for?	Policing, punishment	Reward and punishment	Reward, some self-guidance	Self-guidance, problem-solving

Modified from: *The Human Organization: Its Management and Value* by Rensis Likert. Copyright 1967 by McGraw-Hill, Inc.

a staff members starts to give honest feedback when alone with you, even though in meetings this person remains silent. This is an important start; it means that this staff member is starting to trust you.

System-level structure is important to use when looking for a job as well. One needs to ask what system level one is most comfortable with. For instance, if one is used to a System 2, and is comfortable there, moving to a System 4 department or organization may not be one's choice. In fact, the System 4 characteristics may seem like a foreign language that one does not know.

The author has seen nurse executives operating at a System 4 level move to a System 2 organization. This can work, but often it presents many problems. It is especially important to know what the nurse executive's boss is like. If the new boss functions as a System 2 administrator and likes this system, this new boss will not understand the nurse executive's leadership style and might even think that the nurse executive is not competent. After all, from the boss' perspective, when the new nurse executive asks staff what they think about issues, the boss might think, "Isn't the new nurse executive able to make his/her own decisions?" In other words, "Doesn't this nurse executive know what to do? Is this person incompetent?" The boss operates in a System 2 mode by giving edicts. Staff are to follow the edicts. No reasons for questions or dialogue. This approach could be very frustrating for the System 4 nurse executive unless the executive has appropriately assessed the situation.

In fact, in some previous research, the author found that when System 4 nurse executives had bosses who were in a System 1 or 2, often the nurse executive lost his/her job within the first year or two. In one case where this did *not* happen, the System 2 boss had hired the System 4 nurse executive to change the system because the boss knew it needed to be changed. In fact, the boss said that sometimes he did not understand the nurse executive but knew that she was leading her departments, and the hospital, in a needed direction. The System 4 nurse executive was effective, stayed, and helped to move the organization to a System 3. The end result was an increase in staff pride in the organization and in their work.

The Systems model can also help explain why a successful program in one facility will not work in another. Perhaps the successful strategy worked in a System 3 environment. Is it any wonder that it will not work in a System 2 setting?

Group Dynamics

In today's explosion of information technology, communication continues to be a complex process. Misunderstandings, misreadings, and unclear or selective hearing, all play into faulty communication exchanges within an organization.

Group dynamics can be very positive and helpful where team members support each other and do what is best for the patients. It can alternately become destructive if individuals are allowed to continue with more selfish behaviors such as never helping someone else, making their personal life and personal problems permeate their work, being negative about everything that happens, or complaining all the time. The nurse manager has an important role in this situation, because it may be necessary to counsel individuals exhibiting negative behavior to achieve positive group dynamics. It takes time to fix something that is broken, and there may be additional turnover as one is fixing the problem(s).

In the informal organizational structure, the free-flowing exchange of communication is known as the *grapevine*. This type of communication reaches every corner and level within the organization. When team members do not receive credible information, the grapevine takes over. Generally, information spread through the grapevine is about 75 percent correct. Leadership can use the "grapevine" to gauge employee responses by allowing new ideas and policies to be spread through the "grapevine". While it is critical for nurses to learn formal channels of communication, the informal communication networks can not be ignored by leadership.

In the past, there have been three common types of formal communication patterns defined in a formal organization: downward, upward, and lateral. *Downward communication* occurs from the top of the organization down (assuming the CEO is at the top—we advocate the patient belongs there). With the distance that is found from the sender to the receiver, there are often distortions in the content of information. (It is like the telephone game where one person whispers a sentence into one person's ear, and each person continues this process. By the end of the game the sentence is unrecognizable.) The various forms of downward communication are typically memos, policy and procedure manuals, and performance appraisal interviews. In authoritarian systems downward communication is predominant.

Upward communication occurs from the bottom to the top. It serves as a reporting system used by those in positions of authority to find out what is happening. This type of information is valuable to administrators, because the data received can be used to make critical decisions about such things as strategic planning, changes in procedures, orientation programs, and staffing patterns. Upward communication is invaluable because, without it, administrators may not have any idea what is "going on in the trenches," especially if administrators are not doing rounds. This information can facilitate improvements within an organization *as long as team members with this information feel that it is worth sharing with those in authority; and those in authority value the information.*

Lateral communication takes place among team members at the same organizational level. This type of communication serves as a basis for teamwork. It is generally used to discuss matters that concern the team, to formulate ideas, and to make suggestions to improve the work group or department. For lateral communication to be most effective there must be trust and respect between team members where each values input from others.

Presently we have realized that there is another communication pattern that is most effective. It is *circular and messy*. It is *people at all levels talking with one another*. It is talking with those within and those that touch our organization. For instance, as we do rounds we come in contact with people from across the organization, with patients and families, with physicians, with suppliers, and with anyone present. Rounds break the rigid barriers of the protected office with a secretary out front to prevent others reaching the administrator. This circular communication pattern is messy because it opens up the possibility that we have misperceptions about a situation. It changes our judgmental attitude to one of curiosity. At the same time it creates synergy and belonging.

> The most powerful way to make a significant change is to convene a
> conversation. But we know that often that is the most difficult thing to

do. It is easier to talk about the person than to the person, but no progress is made toward solving a particular problem or learning about new ways to interact to make a real change....

A sign of professional maturity is a person's capacity and appreciation for conversation. Our world and our organization's world would be in a much more peaceful state if the capacity for conversation between the parts were more mature.

The art and science of focused conversation [is]... a collaborative dialogue of discovery where you invite others to share differing views and you test your thinking and understanding in the context of this dialogue so you can hear in a different manner... trusting the wisdom of the person or group and believing that this is the right person or group to solve the problem... The leader will only succeed if he/she truly believes in the group's wisdom and does not come armed with solutions...

We must be open to seeing the issues in a much more messy context than our little world of making judgments has allowed us. When you open yourself to a conversation among equals, you open yourself to the necessity of questioning your positions and the "truths" from which you operate. The only way to enter a productive conversation is to give yourself permission and willingness to be disturbed... Real conversations change you and the people/groups you are talking to. That is the whole point: to make new relationships and synergies out of old dysfunctional patterns of parts interacting with each other. To have a conversation, you must allow for messiness and for being disturbed and confused as a way to make new growth.

The only way to improve the world is through relationships, and conversations are the prelude to creating that change (Kerfoot, pp. 298–299).

Communication is also messy because of gender differences, and the ways men and women do work. Rudan (2003) reports that nursing female nurse managers discuss "domestic, family, personal, and social issues before the meetings" and sometimes these issues are interwoven in meeting discussions while male leaders stick to business and work-related subjects. He describes the female leader:

[She] projected a warm demeanor and took a personal as well as professional interest in members of the group. The social dimensions of her behavior, when contrasted with those of the male... in the group who assumed leadership in her absence, did not clearly identify why she was an effective and respected leader. But a close analysis of the data revealed that her personal style facilitated a rotation of leadership and promoted the professional growth of individual team members (p. 181).

Another thing that occurred was that male leaders discussed meeting agenda items before the meeting in various locations, and once a meeting started,

> The male who began the discussion acted as a coach in charge of a team, with the other males helping him carry out the play. Female team members were never part of this 'meeting before the meeting.'... [During the meeting] the male participants communicated more actively, asking more questions, contributing information and data, and making frequent recommendations and suggestions. Males avoided both eye contact and exchanging personal thoughts and feelings. They were interested in getting to the point of issues by being assertive, dominant, competitive, independent, and aggressive (p. 184).

Females usually did not understand this dynamic and, instead, would bring ideas up in the meeting.

> Women see the leader's competence, respect, and fairness as significantly more important to team effectiveness than men do. Women see the team members' knowledge of their jobs as significantly more important to team effectiveness than men do. Women see the team members' liking, trusting, and helping each other as significantly more important to team effectiveness than men do (p. 184).

A nurse manager is more effective if s/he understands these differences. If female, it is important to not only be attentive to nurturing and socializing roles but to be task oriented with well-developed business and financial skills. Rudan suggests that the following learning needs to take place:

> Females must understand that males do not share personal experiences primarily because they do not want to appear vulnerable. Nurse leaders should... devote time prior to a formal meeting for idea generation, problem solving, and information sharing, just as the... male administrators... need to concentrate on being more open to new ideas as they are proposed or be prepared to present ideas and work out solutions while team meetings are in session (p. 185).

Staff development activities, identifying gender differences, but also encouraging everyone regardless of gender to understand and use the positive aspects of both perspectives will go a long way to achieve better team work. We recommend the Pat Heim tapes (1996) as a helpful tool to accomplish this goal.

Work Teams

A team is any group of two or more people who need to work together to accomplish something. When teams function using the core ideology as the reason for their actions, and are working to constantly improve their product, the outcomes can be phenomenal. With teams, the sum of their parts is greater than the whole. The converse is also true; if the team is not functioning properly the sum of its parts is lesser than the whole. For instance, the Washington Redskins paid tens of millions to lure top football players to their team, and then the team went nowhere. Teamwork was lacking. A lot of egos got in the way of success. The same can occur in organizations; some mergers have crumbled when egos have gotten involved and teamwork never happened. So group energy can increase, or decrease, what is accomplished. It is hard to measure effective teamwork quantitatively, but the outcomes usually are very clear. When outcomes are very positive, magic happens, and teamwork is excellent.

Teams can be led by an individual, an administrator, or can be self-managed. We advocate self-managed teams be used as much as possible because generally 90 percent of the decisions need to be made at the point of service. However, self-managed teams can go awry if the entire team never has to communicate with the rest of the organization. Communication is very important between various teams of people who are within an organization, including the executive team. Multidisciplinary teams tend to be very effective in health care organizations because the disciplines interface in so many ways with patients. Generally certain people within a team are better at certain team functions. Using sports as an example, a quarterback cannot win games alone; it takes a team working towards the same goal, with certain people more effective in certain positions within the team.

There are several reasons why using the team approach to decision making is more advantageous in organizations. First, synergy occurs with the knowledge and skills that each individual brings to the group. Second, we see an increase in creativity among the team members, often due to the diversity seen in multidisciplinary teams and the different worldviews that each brings to the group. Finally, because team decisions usually reflect a consensus, decisions are more readily accepted.

To achieve effective teamwork, trained group facilitators can work with a team to help the team members achieve better working relationships and more effective teamwork. Once the team functions effectively, the group facilitator may no longer be needed. In addition, other professional development activities can be helpful for all personnel. When one examines the costs of effective teamwork, further education and facilitation for the team can save countless hours of wasted time, and will enhance successful completion of the goal.

According to Wellins, Byham and Wilson (1991) there are six key factors in team development: commitment, trust, purpose, communication, involvement, and process orientation. These occur at every stage teams experience: getting started, going in circles, getting on course, and full speed ahead. Each one of these factors is critical to the success of any team, and if not resolved, can result in negative outcomes.

Commitment deals with team members seeing themselves as being part of a team. Team members need to be committed to the group goals, not just looking out for their own personal goals. Trust is involved both in having faith in each other, and providing support to each other. Purpose helps the team to understand its role within the organization, and how it fits into the business. Communication is crucial between members inside and outside the team. Just as in team sports, organizational teams must feel a sense of involvement or partnership. It is important that team members feel that their contributions to the team are respected. As in sports, everyone on the team has a special role. Finally, process orientation means understanding who you are, why you are here, and where you are going. It is the process of determining how to reach the final goal (Wellins, et al., 1991).

All six factors are found within each of the four stages of team development. In the first stage, *Getting Started*, a new group of individuals get together with no common goal. Members will be concerned with the purpose of the group and with what is expected. During this period it is crucial to reassure the team that support and training will be provided. There may be no basis for trust at this point because team members may not know one another. As the group clarifies the purpose, there may not be group motivation, unless the purpose is something that a person feels strongly about. The purpose, or goal, of the group needs to be clearly defined. If not, this can create a hurdle the group will never overcome. Communication is mainly in the form of questions and answers, and involvement is mixed with some members being more involved than others. As far as process orientation during the first stage, it is new and unfamiliar, and may even be confusing to certain individuals.

The second stage, *Going in Circles*, deals with the questions of, *now that we know who we are, and where are we going, how do we get there*? As we look at commitment, the team functions as subgroups, not as a whole. There is often an urge to pull out of the team and work alone. Members are sorting out those they trust, don't trust, and those they are not sure of at this point. There is a better understanding of purpose but the team still requires reassurance and guidance. Often much time is spent on how the meeting will be conducted, setting agendas, and setting up ground rules. Task completion is the goal.

In this stage we see conflict being to arise, especially if certain members attempt to dominate the team. This conflict is disturbing to members who want the team to succeed. Processes are just beginning to be unveiled, and are often difficult for the team to use or understand. Power moves will tend to decline as more effective group process develops, feedback occurs, and members begin to identify specific gifts each member brings to the table. However, if this does not occur, the team will be stuck and probably not accomplish the original purpose.

Getting on Course, the third stage, is exactly what it implies. The team is more comfortable with each other, more comfortable about their roles within the group, and they are committed to getting the job done. They are now developing trust, which comes from working together. Hopefully, dialogue develops as team members begin to develop relationships, and there is more sharing of ideas. The purpose is now focused on achieving the goal. The group process is more natural for the team as they now understand the purpose, are beginning to know and appreciate each other, and can begin to explore different solutions that may not be status quo. The major characteristic of this stage is cohesiveness and putting forward a united effort.

Wellins et al. identifies the final stage, *Full Speed Ahead*, as taking years to achieve. Teams are more comfortable with the benefits of being empowered. They are committed to both the team and the organization at this stage. Trust is a stable commodity and extended openly. There is a clear sense of mission and vision that is maintained and the team becomes more flexible. Changes in meeting frequency and communication occur at this level. There is constant involvement and the acceptance of new roles and responsibilities by members. The team focus is centered on quality and continuous improvement.

Porter-O'Grady and Malloch have divided this stage into three more levels, Competent, Proficient and Expert. At the Competent stage, team members want to hear each other's concerns and ideas, and may go around and ask each person about this. Then they integrate this information into a cohesive group collective. The members have established an effective set of ground rules. They may mentor and coach each other for increased effectiveness. They may find solutions that challenge the status quo.

> Teams at the competent stage can meet the requirements for standard success but find it impossible to become passionately optimistic while recreating the future or to maintain resilience in the face of negative events. They accomplish the assigned work but seldom move beyond the assigned boundaries (p. 214).

At the Proficient stage team members are more likely to have a total organizational assessment, be passionately optimistic, be aware of individual differences but able to arrive at consensus decisions, not just saying that the majority rules. They will honestly recognize team member failings, but give emotional support to help the person deal with personal failings. They will consider the emotional components of the conflicts, and work through these conflicts supporting both the emotions and the actual work that needs to be accomplished. Relationships stay intact and are based on honesty.

At the Expert stage, all the healthy internal group work is occurring, but the group is also recognizing the organizational issues and culture, and will make sure that the proposed solutions fit within the existing organizational components. "The members are aware of individual, team, and organizational emotions as an interactive whole. As a team, they have established norms that strengthen their ability to respond effectively to the kind of emotional challenges a group confronts on a regular basis" (p. 215). The group is proactive, affirmative with one another recognizing and dealing effectively with each member's emotional needs and undercurrents, yet arriving at effective solutions for the individuals, the group, and the organization. At times this could extend to the community as well.

Teams develop over time, and as each conflict occurs, if the team is able to resolve the conflict without decimating members, and use the situation as an opportunity for learning, the team is more likely to make good progress with group development. Teams progress at different rates depending on internal and external influences. In fact, if membership changes or goals are not well defined or change, the group may revert back to previous stages, or may never resolve the ensuing conflicts and never achieve the goal.

Unfortunately, it is easy to get tripped up with team development. *Five Dysfunctions of a Team* (Lencioni, 2002), written as a novel, presents some individual issues that can lead a team astray, and present how to fix these problems: invulnerability (absence of trust), artificial harmony (fear of conflict), ambiguity (lack of commitment), low standards (avoidance of accountability), and status and ego (inattention to results). These barriers create a tremendous cost to the organization. First, there is the cost of everyone's salaries that are wasted, but there are many larger costs—this lack of teamwork will occur in other work areas, conflicts not resolved will resurface, administration will be viewed as ineffective, patient care and patient outcomes will suffer, physicians will prefer to be somewhere else, legal issues will result. The higher the level of dysfunction, the more it will permeate the entire organization. If, for example, the board or the executive group cannot work effectively together, the rest of the organization will be in serious jeopardy, especially the patients.

Team development is not a linear process. Teams are often composed of very diverse members, with a variety of values and backgrounds. Some members may be into negative, selfish behaviors. The team will probably fail unless the team can reach such individuals and pull them into the team, or unless these individuals are effectively dealt with, or asked to leave the team, or even to leave the organization. Team development takes time, patience, and effort. If any one of the six factors go awry within a stage, the team may never progress to the next stage.

> Note that working together involves more than cooperation, participation, and commitment to goals. The team members must exhibit self-awareness, compassion, passionate optimism, and impulse regulation if they are to achieve their desired outcomes. According to Druskat and Wolff (2001), team success lies in the fundamental conditions that allow effective task processes to emerge and cause members to engage in these processes wholeheartedly. Three conditions—trust among members, a sense of group identity, and a sense of group efficacy—are essential to effectiveness. Without these, teams simply go through the motions of cooperating and participating, and members hold back rather than fully engage, reducing the level of effectiveness.... According to Orsburn and colleagues (1990), *most organizations experience a 20 to 40 percent increase in productivity when employees are deeply involved in their work* (Porter-O'Grady and Malloch, p. 207).

If the team is expected, and empowered, to make all their own decisions, the team can become self-actualized, and feel that they can make things happen.

> Self-actualized teams... use the whole potential of each team member to remain incredibly focused on 'their' work, and they use skepticism in a healthy and productive way. They are willing to live at the border and do not eliminate ideas, no matter how outrageous. All ideas are reviewed with the typical constraints of finance, practicality, time, and ethics. More importantly, self-actualized teams effectively deal with members who are congenital victims and continually tell us that this and that will not work now because it didn't work in 1947. Self-actualized teams regulate behavior and focus it toward innovation and away from the troubles of the day. They are able to be in the moment and image the future simultaneously, rearranging existing patterns into new and innovative strategies that will solve problem (Crow, p. 35).

Culture and Related Factors

A large portion of the social factor is culture. Culture has a lot of power. "Culture can kill the best strategic plan" (Curran, 2002, p. 257). Although there are many definitions of culture, according to Gordon (2002), an organization's *culture* "describes the part of it's internal environment that incorporates a set of assumptions, beliefs, and values that organizational members share and use to guide their functioning" (p. 374). A strong culture demonstrates internal consistency, and has great impact on team members, while a weak culture has more inconsistencies, having less positive, and more negative, impact on members. A strong, efficient culture results in goal fulfillment, innovations, and a strategic capacity (Gordon, 2002).

As organizations grow and diversify, changes in culture also occur. In every organization there is a particular culture of learned patterns, norms, values, beliefs, and customs. Culture is a pattern of assumptions or behaviors, often implied and not formally recognized, that are taught to new members as they enter an organization. For example, perhaps most nurses prefer to wear scrubs, or there is a taboo about wearing turtle-neck garments. This is not written anywhere, but everyone "knows" it and dresses accordingly. Perhaps there is a pattern that staff consistently take for lunch breaks, with certain people always going together. Maybe each staff member helps other staff complete the work when help is needed.

To assess the culture Curran suggests answering the question,

> Where does your organization [nursing department/you] spend its time and money?... When I see a physician's parking lot, a physician's lounge, and a physician's dining room, I conclude, 'this place values physicians.' I have never seen a nurse's parking lot or a nurse's dining room.... Things like meeting agendas and minutes tell a great deal about values. Most health care 'board packers' that I have seen are filled with financial information, and a long list of physician names for credentialing, but there is little about human resources and patient care (p. 257).

One common culture these days is described by Bohn (2000), who warns that if at least three of the following symptoms are present, the organization is in trouble, productivity will suffer, and everyone will be burned out rushing from crisis to crisis:

1. There isn't enough time to solve all the problems. [We do not have enough nurses present for the current number of patients.]
2. Solutions are incomplete. [As nurses try to deal with everything, they patch the present problem but do not fix it.]
3. Problems recur and cascade. [So the same problems come up again, or are even worse because they were not dealt with properly in the first place.]
4. Urgency supersedes importance. [There is never any time to examine processes or work on improvements because of all the crises the nurses are dealing with.]
5. Many problems become crises. [Smaller problems flare up to larger ones which may require heroic efforts on the part of the nurses.]
6. Performance drops (p. 84).

Think about this. We have people's lives at stake. This is where empowering nurses, such as giving the nurses options to close units to new patients with physicians and administrators not being able to override this decision, becomes a necessity. (This is discussed in more detail in Chapter 14 on Budget Strategies.)

Another culture is that nurses are very task oriented. We forget the importance of relationships with this culture. This can be fixed but will take a lot of time. Relationships are as important as getting the work done.

Authoritarian leadership can produce a culture of silence within the organization. Employees do not speak up about ideas, and do not disagree with anyone openly. This culture will quickly erode spirit. It creates a "we/they" mentality. In Chapter 3 we discussed the Road to Abilene situation where no one spoke out, and everyone did something no one wanted to do. In organizations if no one shares differences, decisions can be erroneous, products can fail, and processes can remain problematic with deleterious side effects. Along with silence, there often is a culture of secrecy, especially when the finances, revenues, or even vision are discussed at the executive level in an organization and are not shared with those at other levels in the organization.

> Our research shows that silence is not only ubiquitous and expected in organizations but extremely costly to both the firm and the individual. Our interviews with senior executives and employees in organizations ranging from small businesses to *Fortune 500* corporations to government bureaucracies reveal that silence can exact a high psychological price on individuals, generating feelings of humiliation, pernicious anger, resentment, and the like that, if unexpressed, contaminate every interaction, shut down creativity, and undermine productivity (Perlow and Williams, p. 53).

Psychologically, let's examine what happens. Perlow and Williams describe the downward spiral of silence. Often people are silent because they fear "a loss of status or even expulsion if we differ from the rest." Remaining silent

> Doesn't resolve anything; rather than erase differences, it merely pushes them beneath the surface. Every time we keep silent about our differences, we swell with negative emotions like anxiety, anger, and resentment. Of course, we can go on for a long time pretending to ourselves and others that nothing is wrong. But as long as the conflict is not resolved, our repressed feelings remain potent and color the way we relate to other people. We begin to feel a sense of disconnection in our relationships, which in turn causes us to become increasingly self-protective. When we feel defensive in this way, we become all the more fearful that if we speak up we will be embarrassed or rejected. Our sense of insecurity grows… a destructive "spiral of silence" is set in motion. We don't speak up for fear of destroying our relationships, but in the end our silence creates an emotional distance that becomes an unbridgeable rift (p. 54).

Breaking this cycle is possible but requires much work because the culture must change to one where people feel free, and are expected, to speak up. In administrative roles, this means that we never are directly or indirectly punitive to others when they do speak up. And if we really achieve this culture, they may be speaking up about not agreeing with us. The administrator must also encourage, and help, others when they disagree to learn how to express themselves in a way that explores differences, rather than blast each other with built-up anger. Conflict can actually lead us to better decisions, as long as the conflicts are honest, never put others down, and are resolved in a trusting environment. Haven't you known others who are just considered eccentric around certain issues? Everyone sees them as, "that is just the way they are."

Culture—The Hardest Organizational Component to Change

Culture is the hardest component of the organization to change, partly because much of it is unwritten or, at least, not recognized formally. It can reflect what has been emphasized through the years that have become patterns in work behaviors. Patterns can be very negative, such as one where staff members have been allowed to exhibit negative behaviors and never been counseled, or very positive, such as a work group that consistently thinks that no matter what happens they can successfully deal with it. So, depending upon the current culture, certain patterns may need to be directly dealt with or changed, while other patterns need to be continued, emphasized, or enhanced. As we pointed out earlier, it will take a couple years of consistent effort to change a culture.

> Two factors contribute to a deeply satisfying work culture. The quality of worker engagement at the point of service, the first factor, is similar to the caring concept of presence with the patient, which nurses find deeply satisfying. The second factor is the ability of front-line leaders to move out of supervision to focus on motivating and enabling workers to do their work effectively. These factors are challenged by emphases on efficiency and economics, such that employees often feel depersonalized as an expense item (Sherwood, p. 37).

Significant changes are occurring in both technologies and scientific discoveries that should be making the work more rewarding and exciting. This could affect the culture, and provides a way for us to better treat our patients.

We have spent the previous chapter describing the new paradigm of leadership needed to achieve a deeply satisfying work culture. The nurse administrator, using this kind of leadership, creates and manages a healthy work environment. However, if an unhealthy work culture exists, the nurse leader must deconstruct the work culture (Jones and Redman, 2000), while working to make it more healthy.

> Failure to purposely lead the workplace for growth and individual development allows contradictory paradigms of behavior and conflict. Shared values and group behavior norms are building blocks of corporate culture.... [For example,] does the group reward tardiness or positively reinforce timeliness?... The organization's culture is learned through the connection between behaviors and their consequences. Changing the culture means changing behaviors. Behaviors must match values. For instance, a hospital that values career progression, quality, and excellence will shift cultures from pay by seniority to pay according to performance and development (Sherwood, p. 37).

Both the administrator and staff must work to achieve the organizational mission, goals, and strategies as well as the core values. Everyone needs to know what the strategic plan specifies, and can realize how they can contribute to meeting this plan. It also means that they can adapt as problems occur, so that the goals can still be achieved, or that they have the power to change the goals when something else seems to be more appropriate for patients.

> A healthy work environment correlates to job satisfaction, primarily expressed as frequent and healthy communication with managers/leaders, recognition by direct managers and the organization, opportunities for professional growth and development, and support by peers. Organizational culture affects satisfaction, which affects retention and influences recruitment. Workplace culture is significant; yet few health care providers understand how to shape the environment for worker health and satisfaction.
>
> Job satisfaction is inversely related to centralized leadership, poor communication, powerlessness, alienation, reliance on policy and procedure, and stress. A positive work environment is essential for physical and mental well-being and for ensuring healthy outcomes for patients. Factors most favorably linked with job satisfaction are autonomy, communication with direct managers and peers, and recognition or feedback for good work (Sherwood, p. 37).

In building a credible culture, the most important thing to remember is to model the behavior that one wants to promote. *Actions speak louder than words.* Building trust and keeping it, is the key to the success of any organization. Bates (2003) gives us five tips for building a credible culture.

- Reward people who communicate openly and build trust in the workplace; [counsel] those who don't.

- Talk about the values of your organization from the top down and encourage conversation about issues.

- Build your own credibility bank by practicing open communication; if you make a mistake, you will get the benefit of the doubt.

- Encourage questions. Trust thrives on open lines of communication. The people who work for you know it's OK to question a decision or priority.

- Don't assume people know what is expected; be clear about the kind of behavior and communication you expect and find acceptable (p. 38).

Effective Counseling

Within the empowering culture that we want to achieve, there will be individuals who do not fit. Sometimes this can just be a style difference, or be an example of the Pygmalion effect discussed in Chapter 3. Moving to another work area with a different supervisor may better suit this individual.

If the individual is having a negative effect on the culture and needs to be counseled, the best way to counsel is to recognize that individual's personal responsibility for changing negative behavior(s). Campbell, Fleming, and Grote (1985) have published a classic on disciplinary action that involves the employee in solving the problem. This includes the use of *reminders* rather than *warnings*, and in the third step actually gives the employee a paid leave day to decide whether to change or to quit. This method of disciplinary action is preferable to action where the supervisor *tells* the employee.

A Culture of Giving It Our Best

What we are striving for is to establish a culture of teamwork and collegiality; a culture that is capable of making rapid changes; a culture where the expectation is that everyone gives their best. The problem with changing culture is that often we are trying to meld two opposing concepts or paradoxes. Consider some examples:

- We want to be able to change instantly, try things, improvise, experiment. Yet at the same time we want order, neatness, and consistency following procedures for patient safety.
- We want to be a risk taker and push beyond the limits of our comfort zone. We have trouble enough with ourselves on these issues, but we also need to encourage staff to be that way. Yet we continue to need status quo for comfort and stability.
- We need to balance data and intuition (Burns, 2001, p. 475).
- We need to balance planning and action (Burns, 2001, p. 475).
- We need to balance cooperation with competition (Burns, 2001, p. 475).

It is precisely these opposing concepts that provide us with the grist for the mill. Because these are seemingly opposing concepts if we think linearly, they will present sources of conflict for us. However, if we can realize that our responsibility is to rise above the seeming differences and find ways to combine the opposing forces, we can resolve these conflicts and create a better workplace. New tensions that need resolution always exist. It is like the piece of sand in the oyster causing friction that eventually results in a perfect pearl. Right now we cannot see the pearl, but it is there, and as we work through the tensions, the pearl manifests itself. We can choose to remain in our linear world with the pearl never manifesting, and feel the continuing frustrations.

Currently, we still grapple with these issues and are exploring avenues of resolution. This permeates our society. We all are working out these paradoxes. Exploration and tension come before resolution. That is to be expected. Our explorations eventually find the answers. Many times the answers come from unexpected sources. Some people, or work-groups, or organizations, are further along in this quest than others. Our mission may be to help fix our own organization, recognizing that there is a lot to do. Or we may need to move on to find an organization that is further along in this process than the one we work in presently.

Beglinger (2003) suggests the *importance of thinking* in working through these dilemmas. We need "to develop a culture that supports innovation and clearly communicates to its members that they are expected to think" (p. 40). Each person needs to be able to use his/her knowledge and judgment on issues because no issue is ever exactly the same. Take, for example, policies and procedures. We often have *books* of them for nurses in health care organizations. Nurses are professionals. Why is that amount of detail necessary? Isn't the main thing that people *do what is best for the patient*?

What conditions are present when we think best? Isn't it when we are taking a shower, driving the car, exercising, or even sleeping on it? Do we provide time for staff, or ourselves (!), to think? As an administrator, it is important to set aside two days a week with no meetings. This provides catch up time and time to think. Sometimes meetings can be more effective over lunch, or while taking a walk, or while riding to another location.

So thinking, and questioning everything, is where we want to go with cultural change. This begins with us. It is so easy to get in a rut and do the job the same way every day.

Other dilemmas that exist include what we have previously discussed; we are constantly working on improvement yet we know we will never totally reach that goal. There is always room for improvement, especially in leadership. Are we improving enough?? How can we have some job satisfaction yet continually work to make things better? Hope is a big factor, as is being in a job that matches with our gifts so that we will give more to the job, be happier with those around us, and actually achieve some satisfaction.

PHYSICAL SETTING

The physical setting can be a significant factor, and when a new building is needed, an expensive one. For instance, as we are having increasing numbers of elderly people navigating our health care systems, helping them to have easy access to services by not having to walk long distances is very important. The physical setting can also effect how well we can accomplish our work. If the environment is always too hot or too cold, or we only have double rooms available, or we have to go to different locations for equipment, supplies, a computer, a medication cart, etc., we are less effective. As we have added increased technology, many work settings, if older, are really not adequate to handle the newer technology necessary for care. One goal in many health care organizations is to have everything the health care worker needs present at the point of care. Fixing physical setting factors can create considerable expenses, but can be very important factors affecting work flow.

LEADERSHIP

In Chapter 3, we advocate using quantum leadership. Leadership has both internal and external components. In an organizational context, a person needs to have the ability to continually assess the organization, and use systems thinking to avoid quick-fix solutions.

Leadership can make or break organizational effectiveness. It is so important that when a work group is dysfunctional, the first place to look is the leadership. Most likely, the leader is ineffective. The person could be too authoritarian—not delegating, giving orders, and even showing favorites; wanting to be liked too much; being too laissez faire—not being involved with unit decisions and functions at all; having too much concern with personal achievement at the cost of others; emphasizing tasks and procedural efficiencies too much with little concern for human needs; or being too democratic and never stepping in to make decisions. All these dysfunctional styles, if used by an administrator at any level, create a downward spiral of negative outcomes.

To date, *quantum leadership*, as described in Chapter 3, is the most effective leadership style to use. Here one stays more in touch with oneself and one's vulnerabilities, and has effective relationships with those in one's environment, allowing staff to unburden themselves when they are unhappy. One's actions agree with one's words. One keeps promises. One shares information, is honest, and is vulnerable. One can make difficult decisions and take the heat for it. One recognizes and encourages staff leadership, and is even mentoring others to take one's place! Quantum leadership is needed throughout the organization.

Asselin (2001) has written an excellent article on the facilitator role that a leader must assume within an organization. The old authoritarian structure is obsolete. As a leader one no longer tells others what to do but must facilitate their thinking for themselves and their determining what is best to do. One is a group leader at staff meetings, but wants to achieve a lot of dialogue and sharing. Asselin suggests language to use that will fuel discussion, i.e., *What about . . .?* or *Are we on track?* as well as strategies for an administrator to use for better group effectiveness.

A leader in this new information age must go beyond being a facilitator. Porter O'Grady and Malloch (2003) describe it as mental fitness.

> Some providers appear tougher than others. In fact, their 'toughness' might be a kind of mental fitness resulting from their sense of commitment, perception of control, and ability to view change as a challenge. Mental fitness involves taking responsibility for one's reactions to adversity. Through this kind of fitness, individuals can prevent emotional exhaustion and turn stressful events into meaningful challenges (p. 318).

Mental fitness helps one to handle role modifications and reductions in the work force. Employees who lack mental fitness often develop an attitude of learned helplessness. For example, if they are laid off, they react with anger, believing getting laid off is beyond their control, blaming themselves, and generally feeling helpless. Their helplessness triggers a downward spiral of self-defeat in which they see themselves as increasingly unable to get ahead.

Goal setting, mental imagery, emotional mastery, and positive thinking are all part of the mental conditioning necessary to overcome this helplessness and to survive substantial changes. The mentally fit alter the perception of stress and mobilize effective coping techniques, lessening the trauma of stressful events. In fact, they transform these events into opportunities for increased meaning in life. Leaders who are mentally fit learn to manage the context of the work as well as the specific content of their discipline.

Mental fitness among leaders is associated with leadership resilience and leadership agility. As leaders become more mentally fit, they also become more resilient, decreasing the probability that they will experience burnout. Many leaders, particularly those at the vice-presidential level, work persistently to support and guide the chief executive in clinical matters as well as meeting their own responsibilities. The relationship between the head of the nursing department, for example, and the chief executive is not only intense but typically requires more from the nurse, who is likely to be continually providing feedback about the impact of decisions on patient outcomes and care provider satisfaction. Not surprising, the nurse leader, if lacking in mental fitness, will be prone to burnout.

Leaders who are downsized experience a much greater emotional and psychological impact than typically has been acknowledged, and their ability to deal with such trauma is minimal at best. For one thing, the skills needed to handle disappointment are seldom taught in educational programs. Therefore, downsized leaders spend considerable time second-guessing past decisions and become reluctant to make decisions for fear of further emotional insult. If they get follow-up counseling, it is directed toward helping them cope with their behaviors rather than preparing them for future disappointments. Becoming mentally fit, on the other hand, is a matter of learning to expect, anticipate, and plan for job-related disappointments and defeats and taking a proactive approach to managing one's personal destiny. Sometimes things are just meant to be!

Leadership agility is the ability to respond quickly and appropriately to input from employees and colleagues, the actions of competitors, and developing crises. Leaders with this ability are better able to manage the stress of situations and to calculate the odds of success or failure. Once they acquire agility, along with resilience and mental fitness, leaders are able to handle their responsibilities without becoming exhausted and incapable of experiencing the pleasures of their work. They also can appreciate the virtues of mental fitness and understand its importance for the organization as a whole. To ensure that the organization's entire work force is mentally fit, leaders should do the following:

- Create a culture that recognizes that good and not-so-good events occur, understand that employees need support when things do not go well, and provide the necessary support to those who require it.
- Develop a personal commitment to help others acquire mental fitness, resilience, and agility.
- Continually strive to increase their own mental fitness and create the culture that requires others to do the same.
- Extract hope and energy from the mission of health care.
- Establish a program of self-examination and self-renewal.
- Recognize that no individual is an island and that each person needs relationships, support, and feedback (Porter-O'Grady and Malloch, 2003, pp. 318–320).

Turning a Dysfunctional Group Around

When there is a dysfunctional work group, it is necessary to first assess the work group leader. Chances are that this leader is ineffective and either needs help to improve, or will need to step down. Consistent administrative support at higher levels in the organization must be given. For instance, as a leader tries to change dysfunctional behavior, staff may go to the leader's boss to complain about something. In this case it is very important that the boss support the manager and not undermine the efforts to turn the culture around. The best way to handle such complaints is to have all people involved in the same room engage in dialogue about the problem.

Whether the leader is replaced, or works on leadership improvement, it will be important for the leader to establish core values and standards of performance. Establishing core values, discussed above, and the resulting dialogue with all staff involved, is the first step to fix the dysfunctional situation/culture. The next step is to identify both existing problems *and* what could make the department more effective. The nurse manager will have some ideas about this as will staff and the nurse manager's supervisor. Dialogue with everyone about these issues. Ask for everyone's support on fixing the problems.

On the problem unit, dysfunctional behavior has been the norm. And no one likes to experience change. At first, as a manager establishes standards, staff will test these standards. Some staff will welcome this change. Some will fight it. All will be observing whether the administrative group is really serious and consistent about this change. It may seem that the situation gets worse before it gets better. Turnover will probably occur. Leaders should respond honestly to each incident making sure that decisions are always based on the core values, look for the small improvements, and take heart. The hardest thing to change in organizations is the culture. If one needs support—or just time to vent— go find your supervisor.

This kind of fix will require a cultural change. All in the group may not agree with the core values or standards because they have been living by other, more selfish motives that do not consider other's welfare. Or the group may agree, and then continue with their aberrant behaviors. If that is the case, the administrator may have to confront the behaviors, reiterating that this is an expectation for everyone. If necessary, disciplinary action may need to follow to improve aberrant behavior. And don't give up when the going gets rough. It will get better if you have been consistent. Weather the storms and you will turn the culture around. It will take time, but it will happen.

Designing the Organization

Once we have a fairly accurate organizational assessment, we can use this information to determine what organizational strategies are best suited to our organization. Status quo, although more comfortable because we are used to it, is actually the kiss of death. We cannot escape change. Change happens even when we cling tenaciously to the status quo, so our choice is whether we try to influence the changes in a certain direction. It's like they say in *Who Moved My Cheese,* we "need flexible people who are not possessive about 'the way things are done around here'" (Johnson, p. 17).

Thus in the administrative role we want to promote future-oriented system changes. After all, we are on a constant quest to improve clinical quality and safety, to enhance customer satisfaction, to stay viable with costs; we need to redesign systems so they are more efficient and effective, to improve each staff member's performance, to increase the team work between workers, and to stay updated on the latest outcomes research and technological advances. And if we are effective administrators, each person in the organization is working to improve these factors, regularly redefining our roles, improving processes, adding equipment, redesigning buildings, as new challenges present themselves. Sometimes we experience successes, and sometimes we fail and have to figure out some other way.

One fallacy that many of us hold is that as we develop strategies, the strategies are perfect from the get-go. The rule of thumb is that when the strategy is first implemented, it is full of problematic issues that will need to be resolved—even when we have used systems thinking, involved interdisciplinary groups to design it, and so forth. Expect that more changes are necessary after implementation. Try to pilot a new strategy with a small group first. At least some of the problems can be worked out before a large group is involved. But even when the pilot occurs, more changes will be necessary as the strategy is used by different groups or departments.

Using the quantum view of leadership, Senge (1990) tells us that leaders (leaders refers to both administrators and staff, in Chapter 3, the message is that our administrative aim is to have everyone be leaders in their areas of work) are designers, stewards, and teachers. Their responsibilities lie in building organizations where people can expand their capabilities, clarify visions, and improve shared mental models. Designing an organization starts with the purpose and core values, or mission statement, used to build a shared vision, but also includes all aspects involved in the organizational assessment. Design goes beyond assessment, not only looking at the parts (such as the assessment categories or department work units) but at how they are innerconnected both internally and externally. Senge (1990) stresses that trying to understand wholes by using systems thinking is the job of a true designer.

The main theme with designing the organization and selecting organizational strategies is our thinking, our perceptions, and what we do with this information. So often our picture of where we are going with the strategies is flawed in that we ourselves, as well as others in the organization, have too limited a picture of what we want to achieve.

Peter Senge has dealt with this issue in his book, *The Fifth Discipline: The Art and Practice of the Learning Organization*. This book has become a classic for administrators to understand. He suggests that what we want to achieve is a learning organization. This title is, in a way, a misnomer. An organization is not a person and therefore is incapable of learning. Yet people within an organization can change their picture of what they want the organization to be, and change the way they think by using systems thinking. Senge's description of a learning organization can occur.

The name of the book refers to the five disciplines that create the learning organization:
1. Building Shared Vision—the practice of unearthing shared 'pictures of the future' that foster genuine commitment;
2. Personal Mastery—the skill of continually clarifying and deepening our personal vision;
3. Mental Models—the ability to unearth our internal pictures of the world, to scrutinize them, and to make them open to the influence of others;
4. Team Learning—the capacity to 'think together' which is gained by mastering the practice of dialogue and discussion; and
5. Systems Thinking—the discipline that integrates the others, fusing them into a coherent body of theory and practice (Fulmer and Keys, p. 34).

FEEDBACK ISSUES

To be a more effective designer, and to get at our mental models, we must understand feedback issues. According to Senge (1990) there are two types of feedback: reinforcing and balancing. He describes *reinforcing feedback* as the "engine of growth," and *balancing* as a "goal-oriented behavior." We have seen *reinforcement feedback* in many places; examples may be in the workplace or in institutions of learning. Leaders often praise those who have done well and ignore or "label" low performers. Leaders fail to see how their own behavior influences others. This is called the Pygmalion effect or the "self-fulfilling prophecy" phenomenon first identified by psychologist Robert Merton.

Reinforcing processes may become vicious cycles. For example, one negative behavior results from another (i.e., one employee swears at another, that employee then gets angry at the person that swore, and so forth. Yet, there can be positive reinforcing processes such as healthy eating leads to weight loss and a healthier self image and body. It is important to remember that sometimes problems may go unnoticed until it is too late. For example, if a person is interfering with other team members' work and this behavior is allowed to continue, another more positive team member may leave for a healthier work environment.

The second principle in systems thinking is that of *balancing feedback*. This occurs as we encounter limits or boundaries. Senge (1990) gives us a classic example: managers under budgetary constraints will cut team members in order to help meet or decrease the budget. In turn the remaining team members are now overworked, and the budget does not improve due to an increase in turnover and required overtime. If the managers had used systems thinking, they would have anticipated this result and would have met the budget constraints in another way.

Everything that we do in our lives requires balancing. Our entire body contains balancing feedback processes such as eating when we need food and wearing clothes to maintain body temperature. Balancing feedback processes can be found within our societies and the organizations in which we work. Senge (1990) tells us that balancing feedback is often difficult to manage, because the goals are implicit.

Many times the goals go unrecognized and no one realizes that they even exist. One example that Senge gives us is the leader who tried relentlessly to decrease burnout among professionals by decreasing work hours and locking offices so that people stopped working late. This back fired with people taking work home, because the offices were locked.

Balancing processes are more difficult to handle than reinforcing processes, because we often do not see change occurring in them. Many times we think that things are status quo. Leaders may face resistance when attempting to make changes within the organization, and find themselves caught in a balancing act. Again this resistance is a result of unrecognizable goals. Hiring new employees is a balancing act with the goal of having an adequate work force to meet size and rate of growth (Senge, 1990).

Senge (1990) describes eleven laws of the fifth discipline in **Exhibit 4–5**. The first law, "Today's problems can come from yesterday's solutions," describes what it is like when one has to deal with a quick-fix solution that was made in the past but did not work in the long run. Quick-fix solutions, although they may seem best at the time, can actually create *more* problems, and may not even fix the original problem. For instance, a nursing shortage strategy has been to entice nurses with large "sign-on" bonuses and "crisis pay," only to find that once the time commitments are met for sign-on bonuses, staff move on to other positions. And crisis pay for one group can result in other staff groups feeling that they are disenfranchised and not valued. So yesterday's solution did not work in the long run. Instead, if administrators could look beyond these strategies by first examining the *real* problems, then these expensive quick fixes could have been avoided.

Exhibit 4–5 Senge's Eleven Laws of the Fifth Discipline Occurring in the Nursing Profession

Rules To Retain By

Law of systems thinking	Definition	Management Implication
"Today's problems come from yesterday's solutions."	Solutions that merely shift a problem from one part of a system to another aren't sufficient.	Because workforce issues cross all job categories, previous approaches such as substitution or shifting work to others are not longer viable. **Solution: Facilitate improvements in the way the work gets done by eliminating and/or automating. Voice-activated technology helps to streamline work processes.**
"The harder you push, the harder the system pushes back."	Well-intentioned interventions or solutions result in responses from the organization that off set the benefits of the intervention.	The "do more with less" mantra of the 1990s created harried work environments. **Solution: Redesign patient care in the context of fostering a meaningful work environment.**
"Behavior grows better before it grows worse."	In complex hospital organizations, you can always make things look better in the short run. But eventually, the feedback will haunt you.	The 1990s trend to broaden the scope of nursing leadership to manage more than one nursing unit may have short-lived benefits. Rising patient care complexity, outcome management, and a new emphasis on patient and staff satisfaction, and recruitment and retention challenges demand a new approach. **Solution: Implement the "one manager per one unit" model.**
"The easy way out usually leads back in."	We all find comfort in applying familiar solutions to problems. Pushing harder on familiar solutions while fundamental problems persist or worsen is a reliable indicator of non-system thinking.	The solution to hospital workforce issues doesn't lie in staffing and compensation alone. **Solution: Create environments that foster autonomy and decision-making.**

"The cure can be worse than the disease."	Sometimes the easy or familiar solution isn't only ineffective, it's addictive and dangerous. The long-term consequence of implementing non-system solutions is the need for more solutions.	Hospital workforce downsizing and flat wage rates of the 1990s seriously impeded new health care entries. Money saved in the last decade will be spent many times over as we finance the current workforce shortage. **Solution: In the future, initiate innovative recruitment and retention strategies *before* severe staffing shortages occur.**
"Faster is slower."	The tortoise many be slower, but he does win the race. When change in an organization becomes excessive, the system will compensate by slowing down.	Reengineering initiatives of the 1990s were often implemented too rapidly for the full acculturation of new values and practices. **Solution: Take your time implementing new initiatives and elicit staff feedback.**
"Cause and effect aren't closely related in time and space."	In complex organizations, there's a mismatch between reality and ways of thinking about a problem. The first step to correcting this is to recognize that a problem's causes aren't close to its effects.	Increasing nurse-physician collaboration is an age-old challenge for complex hospital organizations. **Solution: Challenge traditional paternalistic practices; reconceptualize male and female roles.**
"Small changes can produce big results, but the areas of highest leverage are often the least obvious."	The most obvious solutions don't always work—although matters may improve immediately, they most likely will worsen in the long run.	Reducing RN staff to save costs might save money, but its long-term impact on patient outcomes is troubling. **Solution: Think in terms of changing processes, not single actions.**
"You can have your cake and eat it too, but not all at once."	Either/or choices emerge as products of static thinking. Don't get preoccupied with what works at one fixed point in time.	Look for how choices can improve over time. Quality patient care doesn't necessarily have to come at higher costs over the long term. **Solution: Implement information technology initiatives to enhance patient care delivery. Although these involve high start-up costs, in the long run, you'll save money by reducing errors and streamlining documentation.**

continued

"Dividing the elephant in half doesn't produce two small elephants."	To understand the most challenging managerial issues, examine the entire system that's generating the issue.	The work of patient care can no longer be examined in silos. **Solution: Continue with a multidisciplinary care approach while designing new solutions to current issues.**
"There's no blame."	Although tempting, don't blame others or outside circumstances for problems. The solution lies in the relationships established with these outside forces.	Find solutions to today's workforce challenges by enlisting the help of colleagues. **Solution: Examine the relationships between problematic areas and their causes. Strive to improve relationships with these outside.**

From: Ritter-Teitel, J. (November 2002). "Sail Smoother With Systems Thinking." *Nursing Management, 33*(11), pp. 35–37.

"The harder you push the harder the system pushes back," discusses the phenomenon "compensating feedback." This occurs when the more effort you exert to improve or change matters, the more effort seems to be required. Instead it is better when a larger group has been involved and has decided to make the change.

Senge's third law, "behavior grows better before it grows worse," talks about systems that may make things look better in the short run, only to return in two or three years to haunt you. The sign-on bonuses worked at first.

"The easy way out usually leads back in," discusses how we often apply familiar solutions to problems. This idea of sticking to what we know best is comforting, but very often the real solution is not obvious and the answer is hiding somewhere in the darkness.

The fifth law, "the cure can be worse than the disease," is seen when familiar solutions are not only ineffective, but sometimes addictive and dangerous. For instance, many organizations become dependent on consultants, instead of training their own staff and solving problems themselves.

Senge's sixth law, "faster is slower," comes from the old story of the tortoise and the hare. Often when organizations grow excessively, the system compensates by slowing down. An example that Senge uses is the body's invasion of cancer and it's rapid growth, the body compensates by slowing down, placing its survival at risk.

"Cause and effect are not closely related in time and space," the seventh law that Senge explains, is about obvious symptoms (effects) that indicate a systems problem, for example, sagging profits and unemployment. The "cause" is the underlying interactions, such as companies moving beyond our borders for cheaper labor.

With the eighth law, "small changes can produce big results—but the areas of highest leverage are often the least obvious," Senge explains that large changes often have the least effect. This is related to Senge's seventh law describing time and space.

The ninth law that Senge explains is, "You can have your cake and eat it too—but not at once." For instance, high quality doesn't mean higher cost. Many times organizations can simply improve on processes and achieve better quality.

"Dividing an elephant in half does not produce two small elephants," is Senge's tenth law of discipline. Senge describes how many organizations can see problems within individual departments, but do not realize how they interconnect with the "whole" organization.

Many of the eleven laws that Senge (1990) describes can be applied to the "quick fixes" that we have experienced in many organizations. The real problem may include us. Senge's final law, "there is no blame," should send administrators a message. Many times organizations want to blame outside circumstances for their problems. They point the finger at competitors, economy, and the press, for doing the harm. Remember systems thinking tells us that there is no "outside" causing all the problems. "The cure lies in your relationship with your enemy" (Senge, p. 67). The enemy may be ourselves. A critical look at what we administrators are doing that chase people away can be a very difficult issue to be honest about. The book, *Leadership and Self-Deception*, previously mentioned in Chapter 3, can be a helpful resource for us, if we are willing to be honest about examining our part in all this.

So What Works?

Once we are aware of the eleven laws, we then need to more effectively change events using systems thinking. In the book, *The Dance of Change*, Peter Senge (1999) discusses organizational change. He tells us that for companies and organizations to survive they must be able to adapt attitudes and practices. Many companies have successfully initiated change, however, it can be hard to sustain the change over time. This happens because many organizations and companies have complex, "well-developed immune systems, aimed at preserving status quo" (Senge, 1999).

Time, energy and resources will need to be invested for change to occur. Senge (1999) lists several qualities that are seen in most successful change initiatives:

- They are connected with real work goals and processes;
- They are connected with improving performance;
- They involve people who have the power to take action regarding these goals;
- They seek to balance action and reflection, connecting inquiry and experimentation;
- They afford people an increased amount of "white space," opportunities for people to think and reflect without pressure to make decisions;
- They are intended to increase people's capacity, individually and collectively; and
- They focus on learning about learning, in settings that matter (p. 43).

Change initiatives can take on many different masks. They can be as simple as a series of meetings, or as large as an organizational transformation. Unfortunately, many leaders emulate Scarlett O'Hara: "I'll think about it tomorrow."

When you have disciplines that are less resistant, do you begin there? Senge (1990) reminds us not to push. Effective leaders do less crusading. The authoritarian model does not work. It is not as important to *tell* people what to do, as to *encourage* them to use their best judgment in situations, make their own decisions, with administrators providing ways that they can enhance their learning.

> The wise agent of change must know at the outset that there are people
> who have devoted their lives to preserving and assuring that change does

> not operate in their lives and, by reflection, in the lives of anyone around them.... These people are often addicted to negation. However, one blocking person can bring the entire change process to a grinding halt. The leader must name, identify, challenge, work with, and, if necessary, shift people who can't adapt. Staff must be empowered and inculcated in the process of their own transformation so they do not themselves become stuck in effectively forestalling what is necessary to assure the organization thrives in its new reality. Group barrier identification and strategic efforts to address them is a critical first stage in engaging staff in meaningful work (Porter-O'Grady, pp. 63–64).

Change is not just a one-time event; it is a journey. First, we must consider whether the present culture can even support the change. As a change occurs, it is better to think of it as a spiral that starts, touches many different people as it circles around, and that, hopefully, the spiral is leading upwards towards improved processes and relationships. The change may start with us, or may start with someone else, especially in an empowering environment. Even when we are masters at organizational assessment there are always surprises that we did not anticipate that may need our response. Some of the surprises may be about ourselves needing to change; change can expose our own vulnerabilities, as well as those of others. It also means that we are doing rounds and are available, and that our actions agree with, and support, the change.

> The clinical leader must look at change as a journey not an event.... It is premature to claim victory or arrival. Every arrival point is also a debarking point. There really is no permanent point of respite from change. Since everything in life is a journey, it is important for the nurse leader to keep an honest perspective. The arrival points are merely points of demarcation, of momentary rest. The wise clinical leader carefully balances the moments of rest and celebration with those of effort and action. Depending upon the demand, the timeframe, and the circumstances, leaders choose the moments of marking success carefully so that they can serve to reenergize when necessary, refresh when possible, and challenge when appropriate (Porter-O'Grady, p. 64).

REGULAR IDENTIFICATION AND IMPLEMENTATION OF MAJOR ISSUES THAT NEED TO BE FIXED

We have already discussed the importance of the administrator regularly doing rounds. Within the organization another important process for all administrators, as well as nurse managers, is to *regularly dialogue with the work group about major issues that need to be fixed; involve appropriate people to work on, and identify solutions to fix the problem issues; and then continue to involve appropriate people to implement the chosen solution, to tweak it when needed; and to evaluate the effectiveness of what occurred to make sure that the desired outcomes were achieved.*

This sounds fairly simple, but it is really very complex. Since 90 percent of decisions need to be made at the point of service, this process must be used by teams to improve their outcomes. If each team leader, or administrator, is using this process, it is easier to fix problems. However, if there are any cogs in the wheel, effectiveness may not be achieved because many of the problems need interdisciplinary involvement before they can be solved. Often when one department identifies a problem, another department identifies the same problem, and several departments must work together to solve it. After the work group decides upon a change, the implementation takes consistent follow-up before it can be successfully realized. This takes a lot of time and consistent effort.

> *It is important to regularly dialogue with the work group about major issues that need to be fixed; involve appropriate people to work on, and identify solutions to fix the problem issues; and then continue to involve appropriate people to implement the chosen solution, to tweak it when needed; and to evaluate the effectiveness of what occurred to make sure that the desired outcomes were achieved.*

Sims (2003), Abrams (2002), Drenkard (2001), Esler and Nipp (2001), and Boylan and Russell (1997) describe how to use this approach. (This same process is effective even when applied to strategic planning, discussed in more detail in Chapter 15 on Forecasting.)

Consider the following:

> Half the decisions in organizations fail. Studies of 356 decisions in medium to large organizations in the U.S., and Canada reveal that these failures can be traced to managers who impose solutions, limit the search for alternatives, and use power to implement their plans. Managers who make the need for action clear at the outset, set objectives, carry out an unrestricted search for solutions, and get key people to participate are more apt to be successful. Tactics prone to fail were used in two of every three decisions that were studied (Nutt, p. 75).

Or,

> Even the best concepts or strategies tend to develop incrementally. They rarely ever work the first time out or unfold just as they were planned (HBR, August, 2002, p. 122).

Or,

> The real voyage of discovery is not in seeking new landscapes but in having new eyes (M. Proust).

Or,

> In Honda plants,… even relatively routine… problems are solved by rapidly created, temporary teams assembled when needed from people who come from throughout the [facility]—not just from the specific area where the problem was first observed. The roots of even seemingly straightforward problems can be far-flung and thus require a surprisingly broad range of institutional knowledge to be resolved (Watts, p. 17).

Using the lessons from the disciplines, it becomes obvious that certain principles are important. For example, new projects or improvements have a better chance for success when the person assigned to the project believes in it. When the implementer burns with the issue, his/her belief in it helps the project to succeed.

Another principle is that an effective leader knows that when entering a new administrative role, it is best not to make a lot of changes in the beginning. Instead it is better to get to know people, build relationships, and get an accurate organizational assessment. Thus it is important to talk to staff both in groups and individually, make rounds, and come in at different times. This way the administrator has a chance to see how care is being delivered, to begin to understand processes, to identify systems problems, to ask questions, and find out what improvements staff suggest. After all this has occurred, then one can begin to plan and discuss changes with the work group.

A third principle is the importance of keeping one's boss informed about what is going on and what you plan to do. Or, if you are unsure what to do, to ask for help, thinking of ways you might deal with a particular situation before posing the problem with your boss. Having good chemistry with one's boss is important. The hardest issue with one's boss is when you do not agree with how he/she is handling something. Often in this case the boss has not realized a factor, but it can also be that the person has a blind spot about something.

> It requires tremendous diplomacy and tact to avoid a political blunder that can derail or end a promising career. At the same time, many great companies have floundered because of faulty decisions made at the top while middle managers sat on their hands.... In effect, we all need to be ready to lead even when we are not in charge (Useem, p. 58).

There are an infinite number of actions, improvements, and strategies that are possible. We need to use systems thinking and empower the appropriate people to make decisions. *Some of these strategies will enhance certain organizations, while they will not work, or not be as effective, in others.* Take self-scheduling, for example. If a unit is in a System 4, this can work very well. However, if this is introduced in a System 2 environment where there is ineffective leadership, it will inevitably fail. A nurse administrator must keep in mind the total organizational assessment, (i.e., such factors as staff personalities, the unit culture, the hierarchy, and the patients served). Then it is important the appropriate person chooses what seems to be best for the present moment under the present circumstances.

Conflict—Our Best Source for Change

Even when we are doing all this, conflicts occur. Why does this happen? Why do certain people really hit our hot button and bother us? Probably because they are a little too close to some problems that exist within ourselves that we have not yet resolved. Another issue is that culturally a lot of us are not encouraged to look at a person's *actions* that we do not like. Instead we just do not like the entire person. Historically, we were not encouraged to explore differences in opinion. Sometimes the difference is just a difference in style—for instance, one person is very detail oriented, never seeing the big picture, while another sees the big picture and does not pay attention to the details.

Therefore, an important administrative competency includes encouraging people to discuss issues when they do not agree—and it starts with ourselves. Who is pushing our hot button, and why? What do we need to face within ourselves? How is our problem affecting others? Are we willing to work on this issue, talk about it with others, and ask their help as well?

There are often conflicts between staff members. It is best when staff can discuss problems honestly with each other using assertive techniques, taking responsibility for their own actions. This is where the dialogue aspect (discussed in Chapter 3) is so important. In a disagreement, it is very possible that once we understand the other person's perspective, that we at least have a better understanding where they are coming from and why they are doing something a certain way. It is also possible that by listening to each other, the conflict may be easily resolved; or after all the dialogue, we may just decide to continue to disagree! Honest dialogue brings people closer together. There is also a possibility that we may both arrive at a better way of doing something that neither of us had thought about; that combining our approaches brought us to a better way of doing things than either of us had thought of in the first place.

This all relates back to the change process. We are more likely to consider making changes when we tune in to differences in opinion among people around us. Humility becomes important here. We want everyone in the organization to be a leader, and part of that role includes humility. All of us in the organization are flawed people, working together—or maybe not even working together—to provide *care* to and for others.

There will be more unresolved conflicts happening in an unhealthy workplace. This causes higher staff turnover; staff play more games, and may be passive-aggressive, talk behind other's backs, and complain. Often staff exhibiting poor performance are allowed to continue. All this is a sign that there is a problem. Most often, problems start with the administrative leader, assuming the present leader is not trying to clean up issues a poor past leader had caused. Here the first problem is to deal with the ineffective administrative leader, and then start cleaning up other issues that are causing conflict.

Conflicts can occur not only between people, but can also be caused by systems problems. These can create barriers to getting the work accomplished. They can create unnecessary hassles that, when they occur day after day, prompt one to finally leave.

For instance, if when admitting a patient the nurse has to fill out, or have the patient sign, 15 different forms, it is probable that this is something most of the nurses gripe about. However, it is also probable that none of the nurses have the tools to be able to cut back on the forms. Their nurse manager may routinely hear these grumbles, yet do nothing. In reality, the problem must be dealt with by an intra-organizational group representing different departments. In addition, there is probably a forms committee both contributing to the problem, and wanting to be involved in the change. Whoever chairs this group needs to facilitate discussion on the purpose of each form, on the identification of better ways to deal with/cut back on the forms, and on designing better forms for future use. It will be important that all departments and levels involved with the forms are represented in the group that is looking for a better solution. Then this is only the beginning, because the representatives from all the departments will have to get back to others in their department about the change. Others may not agree with the change, have additional issues that need to be considered, or have better solutions. Additionally, there is still the problem of getting the forms printed and introduced plus identifying and deleting old forms no longer to be used. All this from one systems problem that is causing conflicts for nurses!

Collaboration—The Best Way to Deal With Conflict

Because we are not taught to value conflict and see its many benefits in our society, most of us can do a better job with managing conflict, both within ourselves and within our work group. In fact, chances are, we have way more to learn. A very important goal is to achieve a *collaborative climate* where different views are encouraged, and where it is safe to express these views. This is part of "love one another." This is hardest to do when there are differences between us. We don't actually hate the whole person but, instead, do not like, or do not agree, with someone's actions or opinions. And if it is a patient, we have to be very careful not to superimpose our set of "shoulds" on the patient. Instead we need to help the patient explore what is needed, and find out what the patient needs from us. This is what "radical loving care" is about.

Regardless of with whom our conflict exists, we cannot superimpose our beliefs on someone else. It is up to the other person to decide what is best to do. If this action does not meet the standards set within the organization, this may need to result in counseling, but every person always is given respect for their differences.

Part of a collaborative climate within the workplace includes expecting proactive thinking from one another, i.e., that a person does not just list problems but thinks of a couple ways to solve the problem. Assertive behavior is a norm. Here if one person has a conflict with another, the expectation is that the two people discuss this conflict with one another, both knowing how to use "I" messages to describe what each sees as the problem, what each perceives to be the consequences of that problem, and how they each feel about the problem.

Past research has indicated that there are five ways that people deal with conflicts. *Collaboration* is most effective. Here individuals work together to come up with a mutually acceptable solution. Although this takes more time, no one loses. Other approaches that are not as effective can occur. For instance, some use *competition* where it is all important to win, regardless of the cost; one might *compromise*, where each person gives up something but agrees on the best alternative; one could *accommodate* where one concedes to others, letting them get their way; finally one could *avoid* situations and not take any action.

> Collaboration focuses on trying to reach agreement among divergent opinions to accomplish mutual goals. Weiss suggests that the conflicts between nurses and physicians are due to the overlapping nature of their domains and the lack of clarification between their roles. Adding to the difficulty of achieving agreement, doctors and nurses use different methods of conflict resolution. When resolving differences, physicians tend to bargain or negotiate while nurses avoid, accommodate, or compete.
>
> Collaboration... involves a high level of concern for others (cooperativeness), as well as a high concern for self (assertiveness)....

> Dechairo... found that self-confidence was a predictor of nurse case manager satisfaction with nurse/physician collaboration.
>
> The Thomas and Kilman model of conflict resolution is one of problem solving, and it is useful in complex situations where parties have common interests and the stakes are high. Inherent in this model is the assumption that conflict resolution [and mediation tools] can be taught and that effective collaboration will be the outcome. Using this model, willing participants can overcome the handicaps of a history of competition and style of avoidance or dominance (Dechairo-Marino, Jordan-Marsh, Traiger, and Saulo, p. 225).

Fisher, Ury, and Patton (1991) have published a classic that is very helpful on negotiation, *Getting to Yes: Negotiating Agreement Without Giving In*. This can be used in any setting, and is so successful that American Nurses Association (ANA) started using it to negotiate collective bargaining agreements. They advocate that it is best to "separate the people from the problem; focus on interests, not positions; generate a variety of possibilities before deciding what to do; and insist that the result be based on some objective standard" (p. 11). This is a must-read for administrators.

Collaboration is the glue that includes the relationships, teamwork between people, and the communication that occurs between everyone involved in the organization. The better the glue, the more effective the organization. This glue is not what we think of as permanently adhesive, nor is it removable. Instead this is a magic, dynamic glue. The bond is strong yet ever-changing. The bond is between people who know and trust each other. Magic happens when people work effectively together. Everyone, including the patients (residents, clients), staff, and physicians, fares better when this glue is present. This is where the spirit, or love, comes in.

Collegiality or collaboration between nurses and physicians, when effective, can affect patient outcomes. Kramer and Schmalenberg (2003) cite lower mortality rates in ICUs when this is achieved. In their research they came up with a five-category scale describing this relationship:

- Category 1: Collegial. Described as excellent, the essential ingredient in these relationships is equality based on "different but equal" power and knowledge.
- Category 2: Collaborative. In these "good" or "great" relationships, staff work together very well.... Nurses describe mutuality but not equality of power.
- Category 3: Student-Teacher. Physicians are willing to discuss, explain, and teach. Power is unequal, but outcomes are beneficial. Either nurse or physician act as the teacher.
- Category 4: Neutral. A near absence of feeling marks this relationship. Often there's only information exchange. But, physicians frequently fail to acknowledge receiving the information, which leaves the nurses feeling that they aren't contributing much.
- Category 5: Negative. Frustration, hostility, and resignation characterize this relationship. Power is unequal and outcomes are negative because of their reactions to power plays (pp. 36–37).

From this research, they suggest it is important to plant and nurture the "equal but different" seed; create a culture that values, expects, and rewards collegial nurse/physician relationships; and fosters, supports, and encourages education programs of all types (so all stay clinically competent). This collegiality improves with ongoing relationships over time.

Collaboration must happen in different ways now that we are in the information age. Richards (2001) suggests that "collaborative practice" involves a community of electronically connected practitioners providing a richer and more scientific foundation for practice" (p. 6).

STAFF DEVELOPMENT

Staff development is an important organizational strategy that enhances staff capabilities to better see what is coming in the future. It helps everyone to stretch and grow. By staff development, we mean that every member of the organization—from the board member to the housekeeping person cleaning the bathrooms—can benefit from additional learning opportunities. Opportunities can occur anywhere, and in many different environments. In fact, we probably could really help one another do better on the love aspect when differences occur. Generally, every staff member should experience learning opportunities both within and outside the organization. Since we learn differently—some by seeing, some by hearing, some by experiencing—we need to provide various opportunities that correspond to a person's learning style. And sometimes, we learn best when we have to teach someone else. The sky is the limit here, as there are an infinite number of possibilities.

Unfortunately, it is often the education budget that gets cut. This is unfortunate, and ignores the fact that we all need to do meaningful work and have opportunities to continue to grow. Scott (2002) makes the observation:

> When learning and professional development are viewed only in terms of an optional opportunity for improvement—rather than as a threat to your organization's survival if ignored—the commitment to sustain successful change will be missing. Thus, look at professional development from two angles: what you and your team will gain if everyone worked differently, and what you and your team will lose by simply maintaining the status quo. Bottom line, will you achieve your strategic goals if you and your staff continue to lead the way you are leading today (p. 17)?

We have discussed the shifts that all of us need to be living in this new information age. Scott names ten:

> From a provider orientation to customer obsession; from silo thinking to an organizational perspective; from directing to coaching; from status quo to courage, risk, and change; from busyness to results; from telling to facilitating dialogue; from protecting turf to building relationships; from a function manager to a business leader; from the employee as expendable to the employee as precious; and from pressure and overwork to perspective and balance (p. 18).

There are many more examples sprinkled throughout this book. The exciting thing is that there is so much more to learn, true for the nurse aide all the way through to the board.

Conclusion

This chapter is only the beginning. As we head towards the ocean, we take various paths. Some meander here and there. Some get there successfully despite many obstacles. Many experience temporary setbacks but know that sometimes it is these setbacks that lead us into a better direction. The charted course is different for each organization. Money can continue to be adequate, or, if bottom line thinking prevails, will be scarce. We always continue to evolve, either into better systems that run closer to the mission, or as antiquated relics of days gone by, floundering midstream. The choice is ours.

References

Abrams, R. (February 11, 2002). *A nurse's viewpoint*. Viewed online at HealthLeaders.com.

Arbinger Institute. (2002). *Leadership and self-deception: Getting out of the box*. San Francisco: Berrett-Kohler.

Asselin, M. (March 2001). Time to wear a third hat? *Nursing Management*, 25–28.

Bates, S. (January/February 2003). Creating a credible culture. *Nurse Leader*, 37–38.

Beglinger, J. (January/February 2003). The innovative organization for the 21st century. *Nurse Leader*, 39–41.

Block, P. (1993). *Stewardship*. San Francisco: Berrett Koehler.

Bolman, L., & Deal, T. (1997). *Reframing organizations: Artistry, choice, and leadership*. 2nd ed. San Francisco: Jossey-Bass.

Boylan, C., & Russell, G. (October 1997). Beyond restructuring: Futuristic rapid-cycle change to improve patient care. *JONA, 27*(10), 13–20.

Campbell, D., Fleming, R., & Grote, R. (July–August 1985). *Discipline without punishment—at last*. Harvard Business Review, 162–178.

Chaffee, M., & Arthur, D. (September–October 2002). Failure: Lessons for health care leaders. *Nursing Economic$, 20*(5), 225–231.

Chapman, E. (2004). *Radical loving care: Building the healing hospital in america*. Nashville, TN: Baptist Healing Hospital Trust.

Collins, J., & Porras, J. (1994). *Built to last: Successful habits of visionary companies*. New York: Harper Business.

Crow, G. (March/April 2003). Creativity and management in the 21st century. *Nurse Leader*, 32–35.

Curran, C. (November–December 2000). Musings on managerial excellence. *Nursing Economic$, 18*(6), 277, 322.

Curran, C. (November–December 2002). Culture eats strategy for lunch every time. *Nursing Economic$, 20*(6), 257.

DeBono, E. (1994). *De Bono's Thinking Course, Revised Edition*. Facts on File, Inc., 460 Park Avenue South, New York, NY 10016.

De Bono, E. (1976). *Teaching thinking*. New York: Penguin.

Dechairo-Marino, A., Jordan-Marsh, M., Traiger, G., & Saulo, M. (May 2001). Nurse/physician collaboration: Action research and the lessons learned. *JONA, 31*(5), 223–232.

Doucette, J. (November 2003). Serving up uncommon service. *Nursing Management*, 26–29.

Drenkard, K. (July/August 2001). Creating a future worth experiencing: Nursing strategic planning in an integrated healthcare delivery system. *JONA, 31*(7/8), 364–376.

Epstein, R. (2001). *Critical thinking*. Belmont, CA: Wadsworth.

Epstein, R. (2000). *The pocket guide to critical thinking*. Belmont, CA: Wadsworth.

Erickson, J., Hamilton, G., Jones, D., & Ditomassi, M. (February 2003). The value of collaborative governance/staff empowerment. *JONA, 33*(2), 96–104.

Esler, R., & Nipp, D. (July–August 2001). Worker designed culture change. *Nursing Economic$, 19*(4), 161–163, 175.

Fisher, R., Ury, W., & Patton, B. (1991). *Getting to yes: Negotiating agreement without giving in*. New York: Penguin.

Fulmer, R., & Keys, J. (Autumn 1998). A conversation with Peter Senge: New developments in organizational learning. *Organizational Dynamics*, 33–41.

Gordon, J. (2002). *Organizational behavior: A diagnostic approach*. 7th ed. Upper Saddle River, NJ: Prentice Hall.

Harvey, E., & Lucia, A. (Date not given). *Walk the Talk... And Get The Results You Want, 2nd ed. Copyright by Performance Systems Corporation*. Published by The WALK THE TALK Company, 2925 LBJ Freeway, Suite 201, Dallas, Texas 75234.

Heim, P. (1996). *Gender Differences in the Workplace Series*. Videotapes produced by Cynosure productions, LTD. And KTEH, Channel 54, San Jose, California.
The Power Dead Even Rule.
Invisible Rules: Men, Women and Teams.
Conflict: The Rules of Engagement.
Changing the Rules.

Herzberg, F. (January 2003). One more time: How do you motivate employees? *Harvard Business Review*, 87–96.

Johnson, S. (1998). *Who moved my cheese?* New York: Penguin Putman.

Jones, K., & Redman, R. (December 2000). Organizational culture and work redesign: Experiences in three organizations. *JONA, 30*(12), 604–610.

Kerfoot, K. (November–December 2002). Messy conversations and the willingness to be disturbed. *Nursing Economic$, 10*(6), 297–299.

Kramer, M., & Schmalenberg, C. (July 2003). Securing "good" nurse/physician relationships. *Nursing Management*, 34–38.

Kuokkanen, L., & Katajisto, J. (April 2003). Promoting or impeding empowerment? Nurses' assessments of their work environment. *JONA, 33*(4), 209–215.

Laschinger, H., Finegan, J., Shamian, J., & Almost, J. (May 2001). Testing karasek's demands—control model in restructured healthcare settings: Effects of job strain on staff nurses' quality of work life. *JONA, 31*(3), 233–243.

Lencioni, P. (July 2002). Make your values mean something. *Harvard Business Review*, 113–117.

Lencioni, P. (1965). *The five dysfunctions of a team*. San Francisco: Jossey-Bass.

McDonagh, K. (January/February 2003). Reaching for a dream: Challenges for the innovative nurse leader. *Nurse Leader*, 46–48.

Nobre, A. (June 2001). Soul + spirit + resources + leadership = results. *JONA, 31*(6), 287–289.

Nutt, P. (November 1999). Surprising but true: Half the decisions in organizations fail. *Academy of Management Review, 13*(4), 75–90.

O'Hallaron, R. (October 2002) Letter to the editor: Corporate values. *Harvard Business Review*, 125.

Paige, J. (March 2003). Solve the policy and procedure puzzle. *Nursing Management*, 45–48.

Porter-O'Grady, T. (October 2001). Is shared governance still relevant? *JONA, 31*(10), 468–473.

Porter-O'Grady, T., & Malloch, K. (2003). *Quantum leadership: A textbook of new leadership*. Sudbury, MA: Jones and Bartlett.

Porter-O'Grady, T. (March–April 2003). Of hubris and hope: Transforming nursing for a new age. *Nursing Economic$, 21*(2), 59–64.

Porter-O'Grady, T., Hawkins, M., & Parker, M. (1997). *Whole systems shared governance: Architecture for integration*. Sudbury, MA: Jones and Bartlett.

Porter-O'Grady, T., & Finnigan, S. (1984). *Shared governance for nursing: A creative approach to professional accountability*. Rockville, MD: Aspen.

Richards, J. (January–February 2001). Nursing in a digital age. *Nursing Economic$, 19*(1), 6–11, 34.

Ritter-Teitel, J. (November 2002). Sail smoother with systems thinking: Focus of big-picture strategies to devise clear retention initiatives that withstand time. *Nursing Management*, 35–37.

Rutan, V. (March 2003). The best of both worlds: A consideration of gender in team building. *JONA, 33*(3), 179–186.

Scott, G. (November/December 2002). Coach, challenge, lead: Developing an indispensable management team. *Healthcare Executive*, 16–20.

Senge, P. (1990). *The fifth discipline: The art and practice of the learning organization*. New York: Doubleday/Currency.

Senge, P., Roberts, C., Ross, R., Smith, B., & Kleiner, A. (1999). The dance of change: The challenges of sustaining momentum in learning organizations. New York: Currency.

Sims, C. (February 2003). Increasing clinical, satisfaction, and financial performance through nurse-driven process improvement. *JONA, 33*(2), 68–75.

Studer, Q. (March 26, 2000). *Taking Your Organization to the Next Level*. American Organization of Nurse Executives Annual Meeting. National Nursing Network Inc., 4465 Washington St., Denver, CO 80216.

Useem, M. (October 2001). The leadership lessons of mount everest. *Harvard Business Review*, 51–58.

Watts, D. (February 2003). The science behind six degrees. *Harvard Business Review*, 16–17.

Wellins, R., Byhams, W., & Wilson, J. (1991). *Empowered teams: Creating self-directed work groups that improve quality, productivity and participation*. San Francisco, CA: Jossey-Bass.

Wheatley, M. (1999). *Leadership and the new science: Discovering order in a chaotic world*. San Francisco: Berrett-Koehler.

CHAPTER 5

Ethics in Nursing Administration

Jo-Ann Summitt Marrs, Ed.D., RN

"The need today is not only to call attention to the value conflicts and ethical dilemmas facing us in health care and confronting us personally and professionally, but also to identify a process for examining these confusing areas and to offer a vision for change and a direction for growth."

—*Diann Uustal, 1993, p. 87*

Introduction

The list of corporations and individuals involved in corporate scandals seems to grow everyday. So much so, that the term "ethical leadership" has begun to sound like an oxymoron. While most of the court trials have involved business tycoon types, the health care industry has had its share of complex ethical dilemmas. These dilemmas have been complicated by technology, increased regulation, and the growing tensions between the business and the delivery side of health care (Heubel, 2000). Providers have used deceptive practices to secure insurance coverage; executives have engaged in health care billing fraud; hospitals have been forced to close beds due to unsafe staffing shortages; trustees have engaged in business with the institutions they advise; administrators have had conflicts with nurses over mandatory overtime; and employees have had to struggle with loyalties to organizations versus obligations to report unethical practices.

As ethical issues continue within our institutions and society, we must explore the issues further. We will begin with a discussion about ethics in general, and then move to a more specific focus on ethics in nursing administration.

Ethics

Ethics is the action of making a choice among competing values. The first definition of ethics in the American Heritage Dictionary (1983) defines the word as "a principle of right or good conduct, or a body of such principles" (p. 242). From the very beginning of the early human communities, ethics has been a strategy of how to get along in a specific community. As human populations migrated, organized religion and philosophy concerned themselves with what was right, wrong, fair, and just.

Since antiquity, which dates back to records in ancient Greece, philosophers have debated determinism vs. free will. Kantian philosophers have provided for reparations; utilitarian philosophers have given the notion of the greatest good for the greatest number; Marx has condemned the oppression seen in a class-based society; Rawls has examined justice in relation to the needs, duties, and resources of members of society. All of these philosophers have influenced our ideas about ethics and ethical decisions.

Because ethics is a specialized area of philosophy, like most specialized areas of study, it has its own language. The following are some key terms to help with the reading and comprehension of ethics. The following definitions have been taken from Aiken (2004):

Values	Ideals or concepts that give meaning to an individual's life.
Morals	Fundamental standards of right and wrong that an individual learns and internalizes, usually in the early stages of childhood development.
Laws	Rules of social conduct devised by people to protect society.
Code of Ethics	A written list of a profession's values and standards of conduct (see **Exhibit 5–1**).
Ethical Dilemma	A situation that requires an individual to make a choice between two equal unfavorable alternatives.

While definitions have allowed us to have a common language, laws and regulations have helped to code morality so that law and morality interlink extensively in our world. For example, the Ten Commandments, the Golden Rule, and the Old and New Testament are found throughout our legal systems. Our laws arise out of society's collective morality; therefore, one cannot separate ethical choice from legal principles. A capitalist ethic can be laid upon all human affairs in the United States, and it would be naïve to assume that generating profit has not been central to the provision of health care. As in all ethical issues, the context of the issue influences the outcome of the decision and the concept of right and wrong.

Organizational context also influences ethical decision making. Organizational policies and procedures dictate the actions that have an ethical content. In addition, the organizational culture creates the concept of trust and integrity (two concepts synonymous with ethics) in employees. The ethical/unethical conduct of the administrator has a profound effect upon the employee. The everyday actions of administrators, either omissions or commissions, help to create the ethical environment.

So in the end, our ethical action is the result of our experiences with religion, philosophy, society, culture, community, environment, family, codes, regulations, laws, and local context (Taft, 2000). While morality was not specifically mentioned in Taft's list it certainly plays a part in ethical decision making and certainly has a place in this chapter.

Exhibit 5–1 Code of Ethics for Nurses

American Nurses Association Code of Ethics for Nurses

1. The nurse, in all professional relationships, practices with compassion and respect for the inherent dignity, worth, and uniqueness of every individual, unrestricted by considerations of social or economic status, personal attributes, or the nature of health problems.

2. The nurse's primary commitment is to the patient, whether an individual, family, group or community.

3. The nurse promotes, advocates for, and strives to protect the health, safety, and rights of the patient.

4. The nurse is responsible and accountable for individual nursing practice and determines the appropriate delegation of tasks consistent with the nurse's obligation to provide optimum patient care.

5. The nurse owes the same duties to self as to others, including the responsibility to preserve integrity and safety, to maintain competence, and to continue personal and professional growth.

6. The nurse participates in establishing, maintaining, and improving health care environments and conditions of employment conducive to the provision of quality health care and consistent with the values of the profession through individual and collective action.

7. The nurse participates in the advancement of the profession through contributions to practice, education, administration, and knowledge development.

8. The nurse collaborates with the other health professionals and the public in promoting community, national, and international efforts to meet health needs.

9. The profession of nursing, as represented by associations and their members, is responsible for articulating nursing values, for maintaining the integrity of the profession and its practice, and for shaping social policy.

Reprinted with permission from American Nurses Association, Code of Ethics for Nurses with Interpretive Statements. (© 2001). nursebooks.org, American Nurses Association, Silver Springs, MD.

Morality

While the domain of morality has come to mean what is right and what is wrong, its theories must be included in a discussion of ethics, remembering that morality is but one aspect of ethics alongside laws, professional ethical codes, government regulations, culture, and context.

There are two notable moral development theories that were developed by Kohlberg and Gilligan. Both have different versions of how to measure moral development, and Gump, Baker and Roll (2000) has developed an instrument to measure dimensions of both theorists.

Kohlberg's theory finds its foundation in the cognitive and moral development theory of Piaget. Kohlberg has six stages found in three categories of progressive moral development: preconventional, conventional, and post conventional. In the preconventional level (Stages 1 and 2) people conceive of rules as external to oneself. Behaviors are based on expectations of reward or punishment. At the conventional level (Stages 3 and 4) people believe in a morality of shared norms, and at the center of this stage are individual needs/rules and expectations of others. Concern for others is crucial. The post conventional level (Stage 5) evolves around the maxim of "the greatest good for the greatest number." At Stage 6 people make decisions based on universal principles of justice, liberty, and equality, even if those decisions are in violation of laws and social norms. Kohlberg's cognitive moral-development theory employs the principles of justice in resolving moral conflicts. He believes that what was morally right was defined by justice, fairness, and the independent principle guidedness (Kohlberg, 1994).

Most of the early work of Kohlberg was conducted on men. The ideas for his theory were then transposed upon women's moral development. Gilligan was a later theorist who disagreed with Kohlberg's depiction of women being fixated at Stage 3, arguing that women's reasoning was contextual and deeply tied to relationships. Gilligan viewed women as moving from initial selfishness (Stage 1); to caring for others (Stage 2); and eventually to concern for both self and others (Stage 3). Gilligan formulated a moral theory in which moral rightness is interpreted to mean care, relatedness, and refraining from doing harm or violence. Later, lacking empirical support for her stage theory, she moved toward the concept of moral orientation or moral voice, for which she did have empirical evidence (Gilligan, 1982).

> **Defintion**
>
> *Moral Development*
> Kohlberg—The individual is the primary focus.
> Gilligan—Connections with others are the primary focus.

> **Definition**
>
> *Moral Maturity*—Permits difficult normative problems to be seen as tensions between conflicting goods.

Gilligan's morality considers *connections with others as primary*, while Kohlberg views *the individual as the primary focus*. The *Moral Justification Scale* developed by Gump, Baker, and Roll (2000) consists of six vignettes with two being justice oriented, two care oriented, and two incorporating both orientations. This scale could be used with groups to determine if educational sessions change moral orientations.

Scott (1998) has identified *moral maturity* as the maturity that permits difficult normative problems to be appreciated as tensions between conflicting goods, not between opposing good and evil. The movement toward resolution of polarization depends upon fostering a caring relationship and overcoming the barriers between the *us* and the *them*.

There have been other ethics studies done in specific areas of nursing. However, there has been a lack of tools to adequately measure the ethical issues in nursing practice. In 2001, Fry and Duffy developed the *Ethical Issues Scale*. This is a 32-item scale representing the three conceptual categories of ethical issues: end-of-life treatments, patient care, and human rights. This scale has been validated and found reliable, and could be used by nurse administrators to assess ethical dilemmas, or to develop continuing education programs.

Developing educational programs around ethical content is somewhat successful. For example, Bonawitz (2002) found in her research studies that students that took an ethics course appeared to have a higher level of moral development. Gomez (2001), advocated for an educational process whereby the individual is enabled to structure and to validate her or his own ethical development, with the institution serving as the common uniting factor and facilitator.

All of these theories provide a framework within which to view morality. There are also principles that can provide a framework for our thoughts and actions.

Ethical Principles

Principles give us direction and purpose to solve ethical dilemmas. They are neither rules (means) nor values (ends), but instead help guide us to organize our thoughts, to justify our actions, and to formulate resolutions to competing claims. While they are not absolute, they are universal in nature (Uustal, 1993).

> **Definition**
>
> *Autonomy*—The right to self-determination, independence, and freedom.

There are several key principles that form the underpinnings for ethical dilemmas. The first concept is *autonomy,* which is the right to self-determination, independence, and freedom. Under certain circumstances the right to autonomy may be taken away, especially if there is a potential harm for someone else's health, well-being, or rights (Aiken, 2004).

> **Definition**
>
> *Justice*—The obligation to be fair, and treated equally.
> *Distributive Justice*—to distribute services equally.

Justice is the obligation to be fair, and treated equally (distributive justice), regardless of sex, race, marital status, medical diagnosis, social standing, economic level, or religious belief (Aiken, 2004). This principle brings to the forefront the whole notion of health care access.

> **Definition**
>
> *Fidelity*—The obligation of the individual to be faithful to their commitments.

Fidelity is the obligation of the individual to be faithful to their commitments. Conflicts in fidelity can occur when nurse administrators are torn between obligations to the profession, the patients, and the organization (Aiken, 2004).

> **Definition**
>
> *Beneficence* occurs when the nurse administrator tries to determine, *what is good care?*

Beneficence occurs when the nurse administrator tries to determine, *what is good care?* Generally, good care includes making allowances for the patient's beliefs, feelings, and wishes, as well as those of the family and significant others (Aiken, 2004).

> ## Definition
> *Nonmaleficence* means that health care providers do no harm to their patients.

> ## Definition
> *Veracity* requires that the health care provider tell the truth and not mislead patients.

> ## Definition
> *Paternalism* implies that someone knows better than the patient.

> ## Definition
> *Rationalism* focuses on logical sequencing to form the basis for decision making.
> *Pragmatism* organizes thoughts by clarifying ideas objectively.
> *Standard of best interest* occurs when others decide what is best for the patient.

> ## Definition
> *Obligations* are demands that are made upon individuals, professions, society, or government to honor the rights of others.

Nonmaleficence means that health care providers do no harm to their patients. In real practice this principle is violated as the patient oftentimes suffers short-term pain for long-term treatment. This principle also extends to the health care provider protecting those who are vulnerable such as children, the mentally incompetent, the unconscious, and the elderly (Aiken, 2004).

Veracity requires that the health care provider tell the truth and not mislead patients. Of course, telling the truth can be difficult at times but feeling uncomfortable is not a good reason to avoid telling patients about their disease, treatment, or prognosis (Aiken, 2004).

Paternalism implies that someone knows better than the patient. This limits patients' liberty because without their consent, their wishes and desires are not realized (Aiken, 2004).

Rationalism focuses on logical sequencing to form the basis for decision making, while *pragmatism* organizes thoughts by clarifying ideas objectively. Sometimes decisions need to be made about an individual's health care when they are unable to make the decision for themselves. This is called *a standard of best interest* and is based upon what others decide is best for the patient. When the individual's desires are not considered, paternalism occurs (Aiken, 2004).

Obligations are demands that are made upon individuals, professions, society, or government to honor the rights of others. They are either legal obligations which are formal statements of law or they are moral obligations which are commitments based upon moral or ethical principles (Aiken, 2004). There are obligations to make up for a wrong (reparation) and obligations to make up for a good (gratitude) (Uustal, 1993).

Rights are something that is owed an individual as the result of just claims, guarantees, or moral/ethical principles. Rights can be classified as welfare rights (based on legal entitlements), ethical rights (moral rights), and option rights (freedom of choice and the right to live their lives autonomously) (Aiken, 2004). There is certain universality to rights as they are applicable to all people regardless of time, place, or persons involved (Uustal, 1993).

These principles form the basis for ethical dilemmas in general. But what ethical principles specifically speak to nurse administrators? Dr. Curtin is one of nursing's experts in the ethical arena and she has some thoughts regarding this topic.

> **Definition**
>
> *Rights* are something that is owed an individual as the result of just claims, guarantees, or moral/ethical principles.

Ethical Principles of Nurse Administrators

In 2000, Leah Curtin wrote an article addressing the ethical administration of nursing services. She felt that nurse administrators were responsible for assuring the safe care of patients, and for making the risks of practice tolerable, and the practice of nursing safe. Nurses should receive proper pay and benefits, and proper support and recognition. In her article she proposed eleven ethical principles to guide nurse administrator's dual responsibilities. They are as follows:

- Frugal and therapeutic elegance—promotes the right degree of economy of means with the right amount of resources necessary to assure competent care (respect for life, wisdom, stability, and fairness).
- Clinical credibility through organizational competence—requires disciplining professional practice through the application of current practice guidelines, regular self and peer evaluations, mutual teaching and counseling, and promoting.
- Organizational competence through consistent policies that advance the welfare of employees and provide discriminating and flexible staffing and scheduling patterns designed to safeguard patient care (tolerance, responsibility, freedom, women's place, and equity).
- Presence—promotes mutually trusting and beneficent relations with peers, collaborating professionals, patients, families, and members of the general public through communicating decisions in person and monitoring and altering decisions as necessary (love, responsibility, and unity).
- Responsible representation—ensures that the clinical and ethical concerns of nurses are heard at the highest level of organizational decision-making (courage, truthfulness, and justice).
- Loyal service—forbids exploiting the organization or the staff in order to advance one's own career (justice, responsibility, love, and stability).
- Deliberate delegation—demands that the delegation of tasks and duties includes enough authorization to accomplish them; requires an act of trust (fairness, unity, and courage).

- Responsible innovation—requires that organizational change be examined before it is implemented for its impact on patient care and employee morale (respect for life, love, and tolerance).
- Fiduciary accountability—provides value for the dollar in terms of the safety, quality, and relevance of services offered to the community (justice, truthfulness, freedom, responsibility, and hospitality).
- Self-discipline—ensures that decisions made and actions taken are based on careful deliberation, never made in anger or fear, and never for retribution or vengeance (love, tolerance, and responsibility).
- Conscious learning—recognizes that time and resources must be invested in self and staff in order to assure continued competence of care and excellence in organizational performance (love, truthfulness, and fairness)." (Borchert, 2001). (See **Exhibit 5–2**.)

Ethical Systems

Nurses constantly make ethical or normative decisions. *Normative decisions* are choices of action in which there is a conflict of rights or obligations between the nurse and patient, the nurse and patient's family, the nurse and physician, or any other combination. In order to resolve these issues nurses often use some type or types of ethical systems (Aiken, 2004).

Ethical systems do not provide a cookbook solution but instead offer a framework for decision making. By using a theoretical framework the nurse is able to curtail the use of emotions in the equation (Aiken, 2004). The following pages provide a summary of several ethical systems.

> **Definition**
>
> *Normative decisions* are choices of action, in which there is a conflict of rights or obligations. They are resolved by using some form of ethical system.

Exhibit 5–2 Curtin's Eleven Ethical Principles for Nurse Administrators

1. Frugal and therapeutic elegance.
2. Clinical credibility through organizational competence.
3. Organizational competence.
4. Presence.
5. Responsible representation.
6. Loyal service.
7. Deliberate delegation.
8. Responsible innovation.
9. Fiduciary accountability.
10. Self-discipline.
11. Conscious learning.

Data from: Borchert, W. (2001). Doing the right thing. *Nephrology Nursing Journal, 28*(3), 360.

One ethical system is that of *utilitarianism* (teleology, consequentialism, or situation ethics). This system is based upon the principles of "the greatest good for the greatest number" and "the end justifies the means." This system can be broken down into rule utilitarianism and act utilitarianism. In *rule utilitarianism* the individual formulates rules based upon some prior experience(s). With *act utilitarianism* the individual tries to determine the rightness or wrongness of a certain act and does not believe that any rule is permanently valid as all rules can change depending on circumstance. An act is determined to be good if it promotes happiness and bad if it promotes unhappiness. Utilitarianism is oriented toward the good of the population in general (Aiken, 2004).

Utilitarianism is easy to embrace; it is easy to apply because most people have a need to be happy and can justify almost any behavior in order to acquire happiness, even if it means breaking rules or telling lies. Unfortunately, by itself, utilitarianism does not work well in the health care system. When referring to the happiness concept, is it happiness for all or for a select few? Who determines what happiness or good is? If it is the greatest good for the greatest number, then what happens to minorities?

While utilitarianism is not a good fit with health care in general, it can be *combined with the principle of distributive justice*. Then questions can be asked such as, "How will resources be distributed?" and "Who will pay for these resources?" The tax system in the United States is an example of distributive justice as all people are treated equally based upon their income and situations. Distributive justice assumes that people are similar with regard to basic needs, freedoms, and goals. Combining utilitarianism with distributive justice ignores the idea that there are no fixed or unchanging rules, and more closely resembles deontology (Aiken, 2004).

Deontology (formalistic system) is a system of decision making based upon moral rules and unchanging principles. This system is based upon categorical imperatives where the results of an act are not judged based on right or wrong, but rather the decision of right or wrong is based upon the principles upon which the act was carried out. These principles come from the same universal principles that underlie most religions and are based upon the need for survival of the

> **Definition**
>
> *Utilitarianism* (teleology, consequentialism, or situation ethics). This system is based upon the principles of "the greatest good for the greatest number" and "the end justifies the means".
> *Rule Utilitarianism*—the individual formulates rules based upon prior experiences.
> *Act Utilitarianism*—the individual tries to determine the rightness and wrongness of a certain act.

> *While utilitarianism is not a good fit with health care in general, it can be combined with the principle of distributive justice. Then questions such as, "How will resources be distributed?" and "Who will pay for these resources?" can be asked.*

> **Definition**
>
> *Deontology* (formalistic system) is a system of decision making that is based upon moral rules and unchanging principles.

species. These principles are standard and do not change when the situation changes. A good example of some of these principles includes the American Hospital Association Patient's Bill of Rights (see **Exhibit 5–3**).

Exhibit 5–3 The Patient Care Partnership: Understanding Expectations, Rights and Responsibilities

When you need hospital care, your doctor and the nurses and other professionals at our hospital are committed to working with you and your family to meet your health care needs. Our dedicated doctors and staff serve the community in all its ethnic, religious and economic diversity. Our goal is for you and your family to have the same care and attention we would want for our families and ourselves.

The sections explain some of the basics about how you can expect to be treated during your hospital stay. They also cover what we will need from you to care for you better. If you have questions at any time, please ask them. Unasked or unanswered questions can add to the stress of being in the hospital. Your comfort and confidence in your care are very important to us.

What to Expect During Your Hospital Stay

- **High quality hospital care.** Our first priority is to provide you the care you need, when you need it, with skill, compassion, and respect. Tell your caregivers if you have concerns about your care or if you have pain. You have the right to know the identity of doctors, nurses and others involved in your care, and you have the right to know when they are students, residents or other trainees.

- **A clean and safe environment.** Our hospital works hard to keep you safe. We use special policies and procedures to avoid mistakes in your care and keep you free from abuse or neglect. If anything unexpected and significant happens during your hospital stay, you will be told what happened, and any resulting changes in your care will be discussed with you.

- **Involvement in your care.** You and your doctor often make decisions about your care before you go to the hospital. Other times, especially in emergencies, those decisions are made during your hospital stay. When decision-making takes place, it should include:

  – *Discussing your medical condition and information about medically appropriate treatment choices.* To make informed decisions with your doctor, you need to understand:

  - The benefits and risks of each treatment.
  - Whether your treatment is experimental or part of a research study.
  - What you can reasonably expect from your treatment and any long-term effects it might have on your quality of life.
  - What you and your family will need to do after you leave the hospital.
  - The financial consequences of using uncovered services or out-of-network providers.

    Please tell your caregivers if you need more information about treatment choices.

  – *Discussing your treatment plan.* When you enter the hospital, you sign a general consent to treatment. In some cases, such as surgery or experimental treatment, you may be asked to confirm in writing that you understand what is planned and agree to it. This process protects your right to consent to or refuse a treatment. Your doctor will explain the medical consequences of refusing recommended treatment. It also protects your right to decide if you want to participate in a research study.

– *Getting information from you.* Your caregivers need complete and correct information about your health and coverage so that they can make good decisions about your care. That includes:
- **Past illnesses, surgeries or hospital stays.**
- **Past allergic reactions.**
- **Any medicines or dietary supplements (such as vitamins and herbs) that you are taking.**
- **Any network or admission requirements under your health plan.**

– *Understanding your health care goals and values.* You may have health care goals and values or spiritual beliefs that are important to your well-being. They will be taken into account as much as possible throughout your hospital stay. Make sure your doctor, your family and your care team know your wishes.

– *Understanding who should make decisions when you cannot.* If you have signed a health care power of attorney stating who should speak for you if you become unable to make health care decisions for yourself, or a "living will" or "advance directive" that states your wishes about end-of-life care; give copies to your doctor, your family and your care team. If you or your family need help making difficult decisions, counselors, chaplains and others are available to help.

- **Protection of your privacy.** We respect the confidentiality of your relationship with your doctor and other caregivers, and the sensitive information about your health and health care that are part of that relationship. State and federal laws and hospital operating policies protect the privacy of your medical information. You will receive a Notice of Privacy Practices that describes the ways that we use, disclose and safeguard patient information and that explains how you can obtain a copy of information from our records about your care.

- **Preparing you and your family for when you leave the hospital.** Your doctor works with hospital staff and professionals in your community. You and your family also play an important role in your care. The success of your treatment often depends on your efforts to follow medication, diet and therapy plans. Your family may need to help care for you at home.

  You can expect us to help you identify sources of follow-up care and to let you know if our hospital has a financial interest in any referrals. As long as you agree that we can share information about your care with them, we will coordinate our activities with your caregivers outside the hospital. You can also expect to receive information and, where possible, training about the self-care you will need when you go home.

- **Help with your bill and filing insurance claims.** Our staff will file claims for you with health care insurers or other programs such as Medicare and Medicaid. They also will help your doctor with needed documentation. Hospital bills and insurance coverage are often confusing. If you have questions about your bill, contact our business office. If you need help understanding your insurance coverage or health plan, start with your insurance company or health benefits manager. If you do not have health coverage, we will try to help you and your family find financial help or make other arrangements. We need your help with collecting needed information and other requirements to obtain coverage or assistance.

While you are here, you will receive more detailed notices about some of the rights you have as a hospital patient and how to exercise them. We are always interested in improving. If you have questions, comments, or concerns, please contact _____.

The advantages of deontology are that the principles can be used in a variety of settings, and that this system takes into account a larger system of duties. The disadvantages of deontological thinking are that it does consider exemptions to the rules, circumstances where principles or duties and obligations conflict, or times when principles may actually harm a patient (Aiken, 2004).

The Theory of Obligation is based upon the two ethical principles of beneficence and justice as equal treatment. *Beneficence* is based upon four "oughts:" one ought not to harm, one ought to prevent harm, one ought to remove evil, and one ought to do or promote good. The principle of *justice* deals with equal or comparative treatment of individuals based upon individual need, individual effort, social contribution, and merit (Uustal, 1993).

The Theory of Justice as Fairness deals with the distribution of benefits/harms and good/evil in society. Rawls proposed that each person must have an equal right to the most extensive system of liberty for all and that social and economic inequalities should be arranged so that they are the greatest benefit to the least fortunate (Uustal, 1993).

The Ideal Observer Theory, which was formulated by Firth, describes the ideal characteristics of a person who is trying to resolve an ethical dilemma. They are as follows:

- Consistency: persons should be consistent in their decisions when reacting to a similar set of circumstances.
- Omniscience: persons should attempt to obtain all the information they need to know regarding a particular ethical matter.
- Normality: the mental and physical health of the person should be optimal for making a decision.
- Disinterestedness and Dispassionateness: the person should be impartial.
- Omniprecipience: the person should be able to see the implications and consequences of projected actions as if they are experiencing them (Uustal, 1993).

The Theory of Ethical Egoism proposes that the ethically correct thing to do is based upon whether something is good or comfortable for the ethical agent. Nurses may become ethical agents as they care for patients who are unable to make decisions. During the formulation of an ethical decision the ethical agent should consider his/her own standards (Uustal, 1993).

> **Definition**
>
> *The Theory of Obligation* is based upon the two ethical principles of beneficence and justice as equal treatment.

> **Definition**
>
> *The Theory of Justice as Fairness* deals with the distribution of benefits/harms and good/evil in society.

> **Definition**
>
> *The Ideal Observer Theory*, which was formulated by Firth, describes the ideal characteristics of a person who is trying to resolve an ethical dilemma.

> **Definition**
>
> *The Theory of Ethical Egoism* proposes that the ethically correct thing to do is based upon whether something is good or comfortable for the ethical agent.

The Theory of Social or Cultural Relativism presents the notion that what is ethical and unethical is determined by the customs, beliefs, and practices of a society or a culture (Angeles, 1992). While this may be true to some extent, ultimately the individual, and not society, determines what is ethical and unethical for him/herself.

The Theory of Emotivism holds the belief that feelings or emotions are forms of ethical knowledge. Supporters of this theory believe that every ethical decision is simply a disguised feeling. This theory in nursing might turn the nurse inward, away from the patient (Angeles, 1992).

While all of these theories have been used by various disciplines, they do not fit nursing well. Nurses function both as a professional and as a human being in a variety of contexts, and it is the context that influences how the nurse will function. There are two elements of context that guide ethical action: *context of situation* and *context of knowledge*. Knowledge of facts alone does not provide the information necessary to make a good ethical decision; one must also know the context of the case. However, knowledge of how to deal with facts is critical for good resolution of ethical dilemmas (Joel, 2004).

Nursing can always get assistance from other disciplines, such as business, when expanding knowledge related to ethics. The study of business ethics has evolved over the past 20 years, and many theories have been applied to business. The foundation for many of these research studies has been three basic theoretical frameworks: stockholder, stakeholder, and social contract theory. The *stockholder theory* supports the notion of the manager of a business being the agent for the stockholders of the company. The manager's job is to make as much money as possible while staying within the confines of the law. The *stakeholder theory*, on the other hand, includes not only the stockholders, but also customers, employees, suppliers, management, and the local

Definition

The Theory of Social or Cultural Relativism presents the notion that what is ethical and unethical is determined by the customs, beliefs, and practices of a society or a culture.

Definition

The Theory of Emotivism holds the belief that feelings or emotions are forms of ethical knowledge.

For nurses, there are two elements of context that guide ethical action: context of situation and context of knowledge.

Definition

Stockholder theory supports the notion of the manager of a business being the agent for the stockholders of the company. *Stakeholder theory* balances the needs of stockholders with that of customers, employees, suppliers, management, and the local community.
Social contract theory provides for the satisfaction of customer and employee interests, within the bounds of justice.

community (the stakeholders). In this theory the manager has to balance all constituencies' needs. The *social contract theory* provides for the satisfaction of customer and employee interests, within the bounds of justice. In this theory managers are bound by society's norms, values, and characteristics (Bell, 2003).

An instrument that was used by Bell (2003) in her study to measure ethical climate was the *Integrity Audit*, which is composed of 43 items. Six factors are identified in the scale: "(1) solving ethical problems directly and reflectively; (2) interacting responsibly; (3) modeling integrity; (4) sharing organizational purpose and direction; (5) valuing stakeholder perspectives; and (6) practicing personal integrity" (Bell, p. 135).

In the early 1980s, researchers in business theory began to investigate the variables within organizational climates that influence ethical decision making, or the organization's ethical climate. An interaction model of organizational climate postulated that both individual and organizational variables contribute to ethical behavior. Ethical climate is defined as the pervasive moral atmosphere of a social system, characterized by shared perceptions of right and wrong, as well as common assumptions about how moral concerns should be addressed. Ethical climate in organizations, as a product of the larger organizational culture, refers to the way in which an institution typically handles issues such as responsibility, accountability, communication, regulation, equity, trust, and the welfare of constituents (Bell, p. 134).

In the *Institutional Theory*, Agnew (1998) states that organizations de-couple along departmental lines with respect to ethical stances and are exemplary of closed systems. Therefore, non-boundary spanning departments are free to adopt ethical positions that are advantageous from an organizational efficiency and effectiveness perspective. On the other hand, departments that have significant interaction with the environment exhibit ethical climates characterized by concern for the greater good of society.

Another method of deliberating on ethical matters used in business to bring about resolution, is the synergistic combination of Casuistry and Virtue. *Casuistry* is an inductive method of ethical deliberation that uses case method, analo-

> ### Definition
>
> *Institutional theory* is where one adopts ethical positions that are advantageous from an organizational efficiency and effectiveness perspective.

> ### Definition
>
> *Casuistry* is an inductive method of ethical deliberation that uses case method, analogies, and maxims; it uses a taxonomy of cases that are arranged according to their moral certainty.
> *Virtue ethics* considers the character of the person or the "excellence of soul" that propels people to deliberate about moral matters to make the right decisions and to become better as people.
> *Casuistry and Virtue Ethics are best used in combination with each other.*

gies, and maxims. Casuistry uses a taxonomy of cases that are arranged according to their moral certainty. *Virtue* ethics considers the character of the person or the "excellence of soul" that propels people to deliberate about moral matters to make the right decisions and to become better as people. Casuistry and Virtue Ethics are best used in combination with each other (Calkins, 1998).

Role of Administrators in Ethical Decision Making

What role do nurse administrators play in ethical decision making? Those who lead in health care must do so by their own example, and through their actions. In her book on leadership, Wheatley (1999) writes:

> Organizations with integrity have truly learned that there is no choice but to walk their talk. Their values are truthful representations of how they want to conduct themselves, and everyone feels deeply accountable to them.... The organization's principles contain sufficient information about the intended 'shape' of the organization, what it hopes to accomplish, and how it hopes to. When each person is trusted to work freely with those principles, to interpret them, learn from them, talk about them, then through much iteration, a pattern of ethical behavior emerges. It is recognizable in everyone, no matter where they sit or what they do.... The leader's task is first to embody the principles of the organization and then to help the organization become the standard it has declared for itself. This work of leaders cannot be reversed or either step ignored. In organizations where leaders do not practice what they preach, there are terrible consequences (pp. 120–130).

Several studies support the fact that top management establishes the ethical tone of an organization (Forte, 2001; Kronzon, 1999). Kronzon's research found that if the company rewarded an employee for committing a transgression, then the participants viewed that action as legitimizing, and would be more likely to cheat in the future. A code of ethics did not prevent transgressions from occurring; in fact, if the code was weak it might encourage the commission of transgressions. In addition, Marta (1999) found that employees who worked in an organization with higher corporate ethical values were more perceptive of situations with problematic ethical content.

Torres' research (2001) reported that leaders can develop prudence and moral virtues, or character, by simply managing their own motivations through learning positively, by developing evaluative knowledge/capacity, by properly evaluating decisions on the basis of their consistency, and by deciding on the basis of rationally motivated transcendent motives. By developing integrity they acquire the dispositions of open-mindedness, sincerity, commitment, and courage, and they take the moral point of view (Carroll, 1996).

The factors involved in a decision to behave in an ethical or unethical manner can be organized under three basic determinants of ethical behavior: "incentives, behavioral control, and personal ethics. Incentives are those forces (such as financial, social or peer pressure) that cause the decision maker to choose one action over another. Behavioral control relates to attempts by a third party to control the behavior of the decision maker. Personal ethics are the internal beliefs of the decision maker regarding whether the action under consideration is ethical" (Bay, 1997, p. 1).

Steps in Ethical Leadership

What steps can administrators take to provide ethical leadership in their organizations? There are at least six that have been identified by Johnson (2002). They are:

- Reflect upon the values of the organization, commitments to others and the health care profession itself;
- Act in ways that are congruent with the values and principles of the organization;
- Behave like Socrates by asking the difficult questions and by creating forums for discussion;
- Create a culture of courage that encourages dialogue and not fear;
- Build processes and procedures that examine operations within a framework of ethical considerations; and
- Strive for simplicity in one's life and work environment by embracing one set of ethical standards for both realms of one's life.

While staff nurses often make judgments based upon personal justice, nurse administrators use the principles of distributive justice. Distributive justice can be approached in six different ways:

(1) That all people be treated the same way without regard to differences;
(2) That people are treated proportionately according to a person's social or institutional utility;
(3) That people are treated according to their level of excellence;
(4) That people are treated according to their rank;
(5) That people are treated according to their legal entitlement; and/or
(6) That people are treated according to need (Johnson, 2002).

Differences in perspective can lead to conflicts. For example, a conflict can occur when a staff nurse who believes #1 and an administrator who believes #2, if there is no understanding on the part of the two parties.

To reduce the conflicts between staff and administrators, *nurse administrators need to acquire as much information as possible about the situation; to decide who owns the decision (staff, physicians, administrators, staff nurse, group); to determine who will benefit most from the decision; and to designate who should implement the solution for the conflict* (Curtin, 2000).

> **Steps in Ethical Leadership**
> *(1) Acquire as much information as possible about the situation.*
> *(2) Decide who owns the decision.*
> *(3) Decide who will benefit most from the decision and decide how it will be implemented.*

Retention, Excellence, and Ethical Leadership

Registered nurses work in hierarchical organizations and face many constraints upon their autonomy and decision-making capabilities. This staff position can interfere with nurses' ability to act in accordance with their values and challenges—their ability to adhere to their own moral integrity.

In 2001, Pike conducted a qualitative study that identified what patterns nurses used to maintain their own moral integrity. These practices included: integrity-seeking practices, integrity-diminishing practices, integrity-repairing practices, and integrity-preserving practices. Data indicated that nurses fluctuate in and out of these categories. The findings challenge the notion of a conventional concept of moral integrity, and instead lend support to a sociological construct that considers moral integrity as a balancing of competing values. It suggests the maintenance of moral integrity might be a lifelong circular process rather than a linear process.

Administrators can do much to assist nurses in maintaining moral integrity by making a commitment to consistently live by the shared mission, vision, goals, and professional shared values of the organization. Then, a stable environment in which excellence exists can flourish. An ethical environment provides the framework necessary for resolution of moral conflict. Once conflict is decreased, then staff turnover will diminish, and retention, morale, and job satisfaction will increase (Hocker and Trofino, 2003).

Who would be the most successful with this notion of establishing an ethical environment? Surprisingly it would not necessarily be the most intelligent or most skilled; rather it might be the individual with the highest emotional intelligence. (Emotional intelligence is further explained in Chapter 3 on Leadership.) That is what Rehfeld (2002) found in her research study. She paired emotional intelligence with organizational trust.

Types of Ethical Issues Experienced by Nurse Administrators

Nurse administrators are often torn between the ethical responsibilities that they have for their organization, patients, nurses, and profession. They oftentimes find themselves at the crossroads of clinical ethics and organizational ethics. Riley (2001) found that they experienced three types of ethical conflict—professional role conflict, organizational conflict, and interpersonal conflict. Nurse administrators must now take into consideration the health needs of their clients and the financial ramification of the treatments.

Several nurse researchers have studied the ethical dilemmas that nurse administrators face and have found that most ethical decisions revolve around those related to the use or allocation of resources, and to the quality of care (Sietsema and Spradley, 1987; Borawski, 1995; Cumunas, 1994; Harrison and Roth, 1992; Silva, 1994). In a study by Redman and Fry (2003) they found that the six most frequently experienced issues by New England nurse administrators (in order of frequency) were, "protecting patient rights and human dignity (62.7 percent); respecting/not respecting informed consent to treatment (41.4 percent); use/nonuse of physical/chemical restraints (31.7 percent); providing care with possible risks to the RNs' health (TB, HIV, violence) (28.3 percent); following/not following advance directives (25.5 percent); and staffing patterns that limit patient access to nursing care (21.9 percent). The first five are human rights issues; the sixth issue is a patient care issue" (p. 152).

The six least frequently encountered ethics issues reported by New England nurse administrators were "participating/not participating in euthanasia/assisted suicide; reporting unethical/illegal practices of health professionals or agencies; caring for patients/families who are uninformed or misinformed about treatment, prognosis, or medical alternatives; ignoring patient/family autonomy; discriminatory treatment of patients; and breaches of patient confidentiality or privacy. The first issue is an end-of-life issue; the remaining issues are patient care issues (Redman and Fry, 2003, p. 152).

This issue arises again in a study done by Cooper, Frank, Hansen and Gouty (2004). They affirm that quality of service continues to be an issue, and that the perception of the concern extends beyond the nursing profession to include other providers as well. Despite its importance as a causative agent, economic constraints are not the key cause of the widespread disappointment in quality; it is instead the failure of health care executives to effectively manage the conflict that exists between the organizational and professional philosophy and standards in the health care agencies of today.

> *Most ethical issues a nurse administrator faces revolve around those related to the use or allocation of resources, and to the quality of care.*

In order to overcome the problem in quality, nurse administrators need to examine their own personal contributions to the problem by asking:

(1) Am I taking all appropriate steps necessary to help work through key ethical problems?

(2) Am I seeking more information regarding problems that have been identified by staff?

(3) Am I helping staff to see the need for the changes in nursing practice, and am I providing them with resources needed for the change?

(4) Am I encouraging staff to take risks?

(5) Am I motivating staff to focus on new opportunities created by change?

(6) Am I participating in and encouraging others to participate in ethics committees?

(7) Am I advocating changes to senior managers to improve productivity and job stability?

(8) Am I advocating changes to senior managers that I believe are essential in order to provide the best quality patient care?

Shared governance (shared governance is explained in Chapter 4 on Organizational Strategies) can serve as a starting point to change the work environment to one that more closely resembles both organizational ethics and professional ethics.

Nurses in administrative roles tended to report that 39 percent of the time they had experienced ethical issues; this was more frequent than that for the staff nurses. The most distressing issue for the nurse administrators was lack of patient access to nursing care, followed by that of prolonging the dying process with inappropriate measures.

Guidelines for Decision Making in Complex Ethical Situations

There is little doubt that addressing ethical issues consumes a large amount of the nurse administrator's time and energy, and that making these decisions is very difficult. Taft (2000) proposes the following guidelines for making decisions in ethical dilemmas:

- Consciously acknowledge the separate but related domains of philosophy, religion, economics, law and government regulation, culture, industry and disciplinary effects, and individual context as they contribute to ethical decision and action.
- Understand that conflicting obligations are the rule, not the exception. In any presenting situation, differentiate one's personal from societal values.
- Identify the ethical value hierarchy of authority that should prevail. Unless a compelling likelihood of immediate or future harm to others is present, the principles of law, government regulation, and explicit organizational policy should rule—in that order.
- When a compelling likelihood of harm to others does exist that is insufficiently addressed by law, regulation, or organizational policy, identify and discuss the ethical situation with trusted peers and managers. Consider both present and future scenarios, and acts both of commission and omission.
- Identify the process and people to engage in addressing the ethical challenge. Marshall peer support and initiate action.
- Understand the contingencies of the situation, including inherent risks for you, the nurse. Know what risks you can assume and what actions you personally are prepared to take as the situation moves toward a valid, or flawed, resolution (pp. 18–19).

Uustal (1993) also provides some questions to guide thinking in ethical issues. They are as follows:

- What ought to be done in this case?
- Who should be involved in the decision-making process? Who has the right to make the final decision? Why?
- For whom should the decision be made: for oneself, someone for whom you are acting as a proxy, for others?
- What guidelines should be used in a dilemma? How should they be prioritized? For example: physiological status, medical and nursing concerns, psychological condition, patient's values, economic concerns, legal factors, quality of life, allocation issues, social and family perspectives, spiritual considerations?
- What degree of consent should be obtained from the patient/client?
- What harm or benefits will come from the decision and resultant actions?
- What, if any, ethical principles and concepts are enhanced or negated by proposed choices for action?
- Just because it's possible to do something advanced or new, should we (p. 70)?

Another avenue of assistance to the nurse administrator is the formation of an ethics committee. This committee will set the stage for dialogue on difficult issues, and, hopefully, allow for open discussion of all ethical issues.

Ethics Committee

An ethics committee is a multidisciplinary committee established to consider and protect patient rights, to maximize benefits and minimize harm, and to establish moral ambiguous value issues relating to patient care, or organizational activities. These committees advocate standards and enhance quality. They could include physicians, nurses, social workers, chaplains, psychologists, and ethicists. Clinical ethics addresses patient concerns, such as end-of-life issues, while organizational ethics examines the overall health of the facility itself.

Establishing a formal ethics committee can provide all involved with the necessary support, guidance, and resolution of issues for staff members, patients, family members, and community members. In selecting members for the ethics committee, the American Society for Bioethics and Humanities identified some desirable traits. These traits include those of tolerance, patience, compassion, honesty, forthrightness, self-knowledge, courage, prudence, humility, and integrity (Angelucci, 2003).

It is helpful if committee members have skills in the following three areas:

- Ethical assessment skills in order to discern and gather relevant data, assess social and interpersonal dynamics of consultation cases, identify relevant values of involved parties, and clarify and critically evaluate the issue.
- Process skills in order to facilitate formal and informal meetings, identify key decision-makers, set ground rules, create an atmosphere of trust and respect, and negotiate between competing moral views.
- Interpersonal skills in order to listen well; communicate respect, support, and empathy to all involved parties and committee members; represent views of involved parties to others; and help all involved parties communicate effectively (p. 33).

Why establish an ethics committee? With all the things that are going on in our society and in nursing it appears that it is no longer a luxury but a necessity.

Ethical Inquiry in the Economic Evaluation of Nursing Practice

Nursing is experiencing a shortage and the numbers at the cash register are not reflective of the amount of excessive workloads, overtime hours, acuity levels of today's patients, complexity of nursing care provided, and so forth. It is time for economic inquiry to be married to ethical inquiry. Most of nurses' work has been, and continues to be, invisible because of the values inherent in economic measurement and health policy decisions. Without an ethical inquiry, nurses' work may continue to be invisible in the equation. What remains invisible is all too easy to dismiss. One important aspect of nurse's invisible labor is that of emotional support for the patient. Often times, due to the layout of the unit, location of resources, or allocation of the workload, nurses do not have time to talk with their patients. This results in emotional distancing from patients to preserve work time, or to rationing of care based on judgments of deservedness.

What are the results of being invisible? Because there was insufficient time to do the work that was expected many nurses freely gave of their own time; in fact, this is a frequent occurrence, making these donations for their own peace of mind. They simply did not want to go home being distressed over unfinished work. The impact of being unable to fulfill their work obligations left nurses with guilt, fatigue, illness, and stress. The ultimate destination is burnout.

"Ethical inquiry is an essential part of the philosophy of nursing insofar as it (1) describes moral phenomena encountered in the practice of nursing; (2) addresses the basic claims of rights and duties, and goods and values, as they arise within the practice of nursing; and (3) assesses the language of rights and duties, and of goods and values as a rational endeavor" (Fry, 1992, pp. 93–94). Ethical inquiry analyzes the value of what does and does not get measured, and also examines which values are socially constructed and reflective of broader social inequities. Certainly in our health care organizations there is conflict between the economic and service areas.

Ethical Conflict between Nurse Managers and their Organizations

An individual's personal values are a part of one's self-concept. They provide a framework for one's view of the world and for distinguishing right from wrong. When an individual's personal values clash with those of the employing organization, there is ethical conflict. In a qualitative descriptive study conducted by Gaudine and Beaton (2002) four themes of ethical conflict between nurse managers and their organizations are identified: voicelessness, where to spend the money, the rights of individuals versus the needs of the organization, and unjust practices on the part of the senior administration and/or organization:

Voicelessness:
- Nurse managers are hired because they are perceived to 'toe the party line.'
- Nurse managers are not present during decision-making on issues that affect nursing.
- Nurse manager positions are radically decreased, resulting in minimal nursing input.
- Nursing is not valued.
- Nursing is not understood.
- No effort is made to understand nursing.

Where to spend the money:
- Money is spent on acute care instead of long-term care; there is a failure to invest in staff development; the focus is on short-term issues instead of the quality of nurses' work life.
- Quality is sacrificed, e.g., there is substandard patient care; or patient/family rights are secondary to a balanced budget.
- Crisis management occurs rather than long-term budgetary planning.

Rights of individuals versus needs of the operation:
- Policies support the hospital's legal needs as opposed to patients' and nurses' needs as perceived by the nurse manager.
- The nurse manager is forced to make decisions that serve the needs of the organization but that will have negative implications for nurses.

Unjust practices on the part of senior administration and/or the organization:
- There are unfair policies used for the promotion and termination of nurse managers.
- Workloads for direct-care nurses and nurse managers are unfair.
- Senior administration fails to act even when aware of a problem.
- Decision making is centralized rather than decentralized.
- Non-nurses are given priority over nurses for first-line supervisory positions.
- There is a punitive absenteeism policy.
- There is a punitive medication-error policy.
- Underpaying of nurse managers.
- The hospital's stated values (e.g., integrity; consultation) are not upheld by the administration and the board.
- There seems to be a lack of interest and lack of information on the part of the board of directors (p. 22).

The study also examined factors that worsen nurse manager's ethical conflicts with hospitals. They were as follows:

Fallout from decisions the nurse manager did not agree with about:
- Poor or unsafe patient care,
- Poor treatment of friends/relatives,
- Increased number of patient complaints about poor nursing care, or
- Downsized nursing management that results in increased cost elsewhere.

Inability to resolve ethical conflict due to:
- Inability to speak out or to act,
- Unwillingness of staff nurses to speak out, often due to fear,
- Inability to make the needs of nursing understood,
- Knowing that senior management is aware of a problem but will do nothing, or
- Knowing that documenting required changes has been a waste of time.

Situational factors:
- Fear that the situation will escalate if the nurse manager speaks out,
- Poor communication with senior administration, either because of the organization's size or because the administration does not value nursing management,
- Some people refuse to negotiate,
- Opinions of physicians are more valued than those of nurses,
- The board of directors are uninformed,
- There are salary inequities among nurse managers,
- There are new nurses for whom nursing is just a job,
- There is difficulty in recruiting and retaining nurses,
- Nurses complain instead of taking constructive action,
- There are unfair comparisons to other hospitals regarding staffing levels,
- Staff know that other hospitals have better resources or have eliminated their deficits,
- Staff know that other hospitals go beyond the contract,
- Staff see money spent on physician retention,

- There is silence on the part of professional associations and other directors of nursing on an issue they are aware of,
- Staff know that the nurse manager's situation is not unique, and that nursing in Canada is in trouble, or
- There is a smear campaign against a nurse manager.

Factors relating to the nurse manager:
- The nurse manager is unable to identify what is right and what is wrong,
- Staff remember when nursing used to be valued,
- Staff need to have a mentor,
- Nurse managers feel trapped because of their number of years in nursing management,
- Nurse managers do not know if they are doing the right thing,
- Nurse managers feel responsibility to improve a situation, or
- Nurse managers fail to inform staff nurses of one's efforts to resolve issues of concern to nurses (p. 26).

Several factors were found that would mitigate the nurse managers' ethical conflicts with hospitals. They were as follows:

Support
- Support from other nurse managers, hospital administrators, physicians, hospital ethics committee, staff nurses, family, public;
- Internal strength gained from knowing that one is morally right; and
- Internal strength gained from knowing that one is following the Canadian Nurses Association's Code of Ethics.

Problem-solving and growth
- Problem-solving with other nurse managers, hospital administrators, physicians, hospital ethics committee, staff nurses;
- Learning to separate personal values from professional responsibilities; and
- Developing and presenting a proposal to senior administrators.

Refocusing
- Hoping that the next generation of [better-educated nurses] will improve nursing;
- Focusing on one's own goals and on what one can do;
- Focusing on the high quality of care that nurses do provide; or
- Dwelling on the positive when senior administration begins to address a problem (p. 27).

The negative outcomes of nurse managers' ethical conflicts with hospitals were as follows:

Negative feelings
- Frustration, anger, fear, stress, burnout, loneliness, demoralization, powerlessness and/or lack of fulfillment;
- Concern for well-being of nursing staff;
- Poor self-image as manager when over-budget;

- Unsupported and unvalued;
- Fear for patient safety;
- Torn between viewpoints of staff nurses and those of senior administration;
- Turnover, resulting in a changed profession; or
- Learning to remain silent (p. 7).

It is interesting to note that all four themes of ethical conflict were associated with distress and frustration. Jameton (1993) defined the stress he saw in ethical conflict as: moral dilemmas, moral distress, or moral uncertainty. A *moral dilemma* is present when an individual sees more than one right thing to do, whereas *moral distress* occurs when the individual knows the right thing to do but is prevented from doing so. *Moral uncertainty* is present when the individual is uncertain of which moral principle to apply. The ethical conflicts between the nurse managers and the hospitals were chiefly those of moral distress. The study results were disturbing and have widespread implications for nurse retention.

Despite the work that has been done on job satisfaction and retention, nurses continue to experience moral distress. Nurse administrators have shown some implicit acknowledgement of the problems, and have addressed the problems of staff nurses through better working hours, increased salaries, shared governance, and increased autonomy for professional nurses. Nurses who are empowered can take on the role of whistleblower and begin to address problems.

> ### Definition
>
> *A moral dilemma* is present when an individual sees more than one right thing to do.
> *Moral distress* occurs when the individual knows the right thing to do but is prevented from doing so.
> *Moral uncertainty* is present when the individual is uncertain of which moral principle to apply.
> *The ethical conflicts between the nurse manager and the hospital are chiefly those of moral distress.*

The majority of the nurse administrators did not feel in conflict with their professional organizations but instead felt supported by them. Professional organizations have established standards in an attempt to prevent or more effectively deal with ethical conflicts.

Another strategy to more effectively deal with ethical conflicts and to enhance nurse retention is the appointment of staff nurses to ethics committees. However, the benefit of having staff nurses participate is dependent upon the organizational environment and administrative support of ethical decisions with physicians. If the environment is not supportive of ethics committees and their decisions, then staff nurses may exhibit moral distress resulting in frustration, anger and guilt, and actually leading to nurses avoiding patients (Corley, 2002).

Much has been written in the literature about the lack of a voice among the nurse administrators and the effect that its absence has upon the organizational environment. For instance, in a study by Irby (2002) she found that:

(a) A transformational leader's voice cannot be greater than the sum of each employee's voice; leadership is a fluid consciousness that mentors, motivates, and summons the work community to produce, with excellence; (b) transformational leaders' spiritual or religious affiliations underscore their visions and ethics of care; apprehending their personal and collective voices, congealing collaborative consciousness, and exciting through insight; (c) leadership voices are the synchronized energetic vibrations of the work community, incorporating diverse personal core values orchestrated by proactive management principles; (d) proactive management goes beyond honesty and sincerity, requiring discipline, balance, dominion, and congruence between core values and actions; (e) transformational leaders must comprehend that they, and those to whom they delegate administrative authority, create their core values in the work environment (p. 1).

During this time an effective administrative leader, such as a quantum leader (explained in Chapter 3) has the ability to ensure that ethics is an essential part of every health care environment. It is the nurse, after all, that is ever-present and can make the difference. In addition, at the executive level, it is most often the CNO presenting the patient and family perspective.

Summary

There is little doubt that nurse administrators play a vital role in establishing and maintaining an ethical work environment. However, it is unlikely that this responsibility is found in their job description. Maybe if this expectation became a written requirement nurse administrators would take their charge more seriously. What do you think?

> *To be a nurse requires the willing assumption of ethical responsibility in every dimension of practice. The nurse enters a partnership of human experience where sharing moments in time—some trivial and some dramatic—leaves its mark forever on each participant. The willingness to enter with a patient that predicament which he cannot face alone is an expression of moral responsibility. The quality of the moral commitment is a measure of the nurse's excellence.*
>
> *Myra E. Levine*

References

Agnew, T. G. (1998). De-coupling organizational ethics: An institutional theory analysis of inter-departmental differences (Business Ethics). (Doctoral dissertation, Vanderbilt University, 1998). *Dissertation Abstracts International, 59*(03A), 881.

Aiken, T. D. (2004). *Legal, ethical and political issues in nursing.* 2nd ed. Philadelphia: F. A. Davis.

American Heritage Dictionary. (1983). New York: Houghton Mifflin Co.

American Nurses Association, Code of Ethics for Nurses with Interpretive Statements. (2001). American Nurses Foundation. Washington, DC: American Nurses Foundation/American Nurses Association.

Angeles, P. (1992). *Dictionary of philosophy.* New York: Harper Collins.

Angelucci, P. A. (2003). Ethics committees: Guidance through gray areas. *Nursing Management, 34*(6), 30–31.

Bay, D. D. (1997). Determinants of ethical behavior: An experiment (incentives, behavioral control, personal ethics). (Doctoral dissertation, Washington State University, 1997). *Dissertation Abstracts International, 59,* 3528.

Beauchamp, T. L., & Walters, L. (2002). *Contemporary issues in bioethics.* 6th ed. Belmont, CA: Wadsworth.

Bell, S. (2003). Ethical climate in managed care organizations. *Nursing Administration Quarterly, 27*(2), 133–139.

Bonawitz, M. (2002). Analysis and comparison of the moral development of students required to graduate with an ethics course. (Doctoral dissertation, Florida International University, 2002). *Dissertation Abstracts International, 63,* 1433.

Borawski, D. B. (1995). Ethical dilemmas for nurse administrators. *JONA, 25*(7/8), 60–62.

Borchert, W. (2001). Doing the right thing. *Nephrology Nursing Journal, 28*(3), 360.

Brannigan, M. C., & Boss, J. A. (2001). *Healthcare ethics in a diverse society.* Mountain View, CA: Mayfield.

Calkins, M. J. (1998). Casuistry, virtue, and business ethics. (Doctoral dissertation, University of Virginia, 1998). *Dissertation Abstracts International, 59,* 2544.

Carroll, R. (1996). Ethics education in the accounting curriculum. (Doctoral dissertation, Dalhousie University, 1996). *Dissertation Abstracts International, 63,* 259.

Cooper, R., Frank, G., Hansen, M., & Gouty, C. (2004). Key ethical issues encountered in healthcare organizations. *JONA, 34*(3), 149–156.

Corley, M. C. (2002). Nurse moral distress: A proposed theory and research agenda. *Nursing Ethics 2002, 9*(6), 636–650.

Cumunas, C. (1994). Ethical dilemmas of nurse executives, Part I. *JONA, 24*(7/8), 45–51.

Curtin, L. L. (2000). Ethics & nursing administration: Part I. *Curtin Calls, 3*(6), 4–5.

Curtin, L. L. (2000). The first ten principles for the ethical administration of nursing services. *Nursing Administration Quarterly, 25*(1), 7–13.

Forte, A. (2001). Business Ethics: A Study of the Moral Reasoning of Selected Business Managers. (Doctoral dissertation, New York University, 2001). *Dissertation Abstracts International, 62,* 2478.

Fry, S. T., & Duffy, M. E. (2001). The development and psychometric evaluation of the Ethical Issues Scale. *Journal of Nursing Scholarship, 33*(3), 272–277.

Gilligan, C. (1982). *In a different voice: Psychological theory and women's development.* Cambridge, MA: Harvard University Press.

Gomez, C. P. (2001). Nurturing an Ethics and Morality of Discovery: An Educator's Perspective. (Doctoral dissertation, University of Colorado at Denver, 2001). *Dissertation Abstracts International, 62*, 4008.

Gump, L., Baker, R., & Roll, S. (2000). The moral justification scale: Reliability and validity of a new measure of care and justice orientations. *Adolescence, 35*(137), 67–76.

Harrison, J. K., & Roth, P. A. (1992). Ethical dilemmas faced by directors of nursing. *Journal of Long Term Care Administration, 20*(2), 13–16.

Heubel, F. (2000). Patients or customers: Ethical limits of market economy in health care. *The Journal of Medicine and Philosophy, 25*(2), 240.

Hocker, S. M., & Trofino, J. (2003). Transformational leadership: The development of a model of nursing case management by the Army Nurse Corps. *Lippincott's Case Management, 8*(5), 208–213.

Irby, L. C. (2002). Leadership Voices (TM): Values, Proactive management, and Consciousness. (Doctoral dissertation, Seattle University, 2002). *Dissertation Abstracts International, 63*, 61.

Jameton, A. (1993). Dilemmas of moral distress: Moral responsibility and nursing practice. *Clinical Issues Perinatal Womens Health Nursing 4*, 542–551.

Joel, L. A. (2004). *Advanced practice nursing: Essentials for role development.* Philadelphia: F.A. Davis.

Johnson, J. E. (2002). Six steps to ethical leadership in health care. *Patient Care Management, 18*(2), 1, 5–9.

Kohlberg, I. (1994). *Essays on moral development: Vol. 2, The psychology of moral development.* New York: Harper and Row.

Kronzon, S. (1999). The Effect of Formal Policies and Informal Social Learning on Perceptions of Corporate Ethics: Actions Speak Louder Than Codes. (Doctoral dissertation, Princeton University, 1999). *Dissertation Abstracts International, 60*, 1897.

Marta, J. K. (1999). An Empirical Investigation Into Significant Factors of Moral Reasoning and Their Influences On Ethical Judgment and Intentions (Marketing Ethics, Hunt-Vitell Model, Religiousness). (Doctoral dissertation, Old Dominion University, 1999). *Dissertation Abstracts International, 60*, 1229.

Pike, A.W. (2001). "I don't know how ethical I am": An investigation into the practices nurses uses to maintain their moral integrity. (Doctoral dissertation, Boston University, 2001). *Dissertation Abstracts International*, UMI AA199991069, 234p.

Redman, B. A., & Fry, S. T. (2003). Ethics and human rights issues experienced by nurses in leadership roles. *Nursing Leadership Forum, 7*(4), 150–156.

Rehfeld, R. E. (2002). Organizational Trust and Emotional Intelligence: An Appreciative Inquiry into the language of the Twenty-first Century Leader. (Doctoral dissertation, Capella University, 2002). *Dissertation Abstracts International, 62*, 3669.

Riley, J. M. Nurse executives' response to ethical conflict and choice in the workplace. Nursing Ethics Network. Available at http://www.aone.org/practiceresearch/evolving nurse executive.htm. Accessed August 8, 2001.

Sietsema, M. R., & Spradley, B. W. (1987). Ethics and administrative decision-making. *JONA, 17*(4), 28–32.

Silva, M. C., & Lewis, C. K. (1991). Ethics, policy, and allocation of scarce resources in nursing service administration: A pilot study. *Nursing Connections, 4*(2), 44–52.

Taft, S. H. (2000). An inclusive look at the domain of ethics and its application to administrative behavior. *Online Journal of Issues in Nursing*, November 8, 25 pages.

Torres, M. B. (2001). Character and decision-making. (Doctoral dissertation, University of Illinois at Chicago, 2001). *Dissertation Abstracts International, 62,* 2485.

Uustal, D. (1993). *Clinical ethics and values: Issues and insights.* Jamestown, RI: Educational Resources in HealthCare, Inc.

Vaughn, R. H. (1935). *The actual incidence of moral problems in nursing: A preliminary study in empirical ethics.* Washington, DC: The Catholic University of America.

Veatch, R. M. (2002). The basics of bioethics. 2nd ed. Upper Saddle River, NJ: Prentice Hall.

Volbrecht, R. M. (2002). *Nursing ethics: Communities in dialogue.* Upper Saddle River, NJ: Prentice Hall.

Wheatley, M. J. (1999). *Leadership and the new science.* San Francisco: Berrett-Kohler.

PART TWO

Health Care and the Economy

Many times nurses do not understand how the health care economy affects their practice. They complain about all the administrative budget cuts or talk about the insurance companies as being the "bad guys," yet they do not realize why all this is happening to them. Thus here in Part II, we present an economic background that helps nurses to understand how we got here. Hopefully, we can now more effectively deal with all our current problems.

Chapter 6, Everything You Wanted to Know About Health Care and More!, shows how we became a tertiary care, illness-based system that often does not meet the needs of our population lucky enough to have health insurance.

Historically when most people were ill someone in the home cared for them. Amazingly, we are moving back toward that model again. Meanwhile, one can see how insurance companies surfaced, how Social Security, Medicare, and Medicaid coverage emerged as the most prominent player in health care; how Certificates of Need and legislation like the Hill-Burton Act drove the health care industry in a certain direction; and how prospective payment (managed care, HMOs, DRGs, RUGs, OASIS, and RBRVS) has affected the care given. This has led to an ineffective health care system, which probably cannot pay for itself in a few years. The health care industry fiber is further strained as the high cost of drugs, combined with health care personnel shortages and an aging population, are having a profound affect on all of us. Our current dilemma is that we have not figured out how to achieve all three health care components at once: universal coverage, paying for it, and containing costs.

Meanwhile, the system is driven by many legal entanglements and requirements that create more costs because our governmental players are mainly lawyers. All these laws create more legal business for lawyers. The latest example of a very costly, involved law is The Health Insurance Portability and Accountability Act of 1996 (HIPAA).

Many nurses do not understand the healthcare players: Consumers, Providers, Payers, Suppliers, and Regulators. A large portion of Chapter 6 describes all this so one can see how they all are interrelated, and can have a better understanding of each role.

Chapter 7, Is There Life After Capitation?, was adapted from a speech given to the 33rd Annual Meeting of the American Organization of Nurse Executives by J.D. Kleinke, a medical economist. During this presentation he spoke about health care, the future of hospitals, the future of managed care, and the future of the physician. This chapter covers Risk and Consumerism which define the supply and demand sides of health care. J.D. Kleinke goes back to the beginning of managed care through the DRG Payment system, and explains why we need managed care to control costs, and why managed care does not work because of the failure of the HMOs. He provides a look at surviving managed care through consolidation, branding, and niche marketing, and also shows how technology and data affect the healthcare industry.

CHAPTER 6

Everything You Wanted to Know about Health Care and More!

Janne Dunham-Taylor, PhD, RN

In ancient Asian cultures, citizens paid their doctors to keep them well.
If people got sick, it was the doctor's responsibility to take care of them
for free (Gottlieb, 2001, p. 23).

Economic Theory versus Quantum Physics

As we have moved from an agrarian society, where people were generally self-sufficient, into the industrial age that thrusts people into more interdependent relationships, *economic theory* has developed to describe the ebb and flow of resources. In economic theory, there is a need to find a balance between supply and demand. *Supply* is "the quantity of a service or product that providers are willing to sell at particular prices" (Chang, Price, and Pfoutz, p. 472); *demand* is "the amount of a service or a product that consumers are willing and able to buy at specified prices" (p. 469). The problem lies in correctly matching supply and demand to be most efficient.

Using economic theory, if the demand is suddenly great—need for RNs—while the supply is low—RN shortage—an economic problem occurs. The demand for nurses is greater than the supply of nurses. Thus RN employers may have to work around the shortage or take action—such as increasing RN salaries—so more RNs will choose to work for that organization. In the general community, as word gets out that RN salaries are good, more people will

> **Definition**
>
> *Economic Theory*—the ebb and flow of scarce resources.
> *Supply*—"the quantity of a service or product that providers are willing to sell at particular prices" (Chang, Price, and Pfoutz, 2001, p. 472).
> *Demand*—"the amount of a service or a product that consumers are willing and able to buy at specified prices" (p. 469).

choose to go into the nursing profession. When the demand for nurses is lessened and salaries level out, for example with managed care in this last decade, then the supply lessens. In fact, during this time some RNs lost their jobs and enrollments in nursing programs dropped.

Sometimes supply or demand can get out of balance because of our actions, and cause additional problems. Senge (1994) gives a wonderful example of a demand for beer going astray. As people began to buy a certain beer from stores and stores experienced a slow response from suppliers for this beer, store owners began to order extra beer and stockpile it. As many store owners stockpiled the beer, the company producing the beer could not keep up with all of the orders. Shortages occurred. If everyone could have talked together and worked out the problem together, by not stockpiling, a shortage would not have occurred. The company was producing enough beer for actual consumer needs. It was the stockpiling that caused the shortage of beer.

This happens in health care organizations. Let's use linen as an example in an inpatient setting. No one on the floors has enough washcloths. The laundry cannot figure out what has happened to all the washcloths and buys more. CNAs (certified nursing assistants) hide washcloths in places on the units because they know there will not be enough washcloths. The laundry buys more washcloths. Washcloths keep disappearing. The laundry spends over the budgeted amount for washcloths. The floors continue to complain about the problem. Actually, if the laundry personnel and floor personnel got together to discuss the problem, the shortage could have been averted, the laundry could stay within budget, and by putting a better system in place, washcloths would be consistently available on the floors when needed.

So in economic theory, it is important to keep supply and demand more even and constant. It becomes complicated because people from different parts of society all need to be involved to achieve this goal. If any groups overreact, an economic problem occurs, i.e., the run on banks during the Depression.

> Proponents of economic theory believe that resources are *scarce*.
>
> Accounting and finance are applied areas of microeconomics. The theory of economics forms the foundations upon which all financial management is ultimately built. The essence of economics is that society has a limited amount of resources, with competing demands for them. The economic system attempts to allocate those resources in an optimal fashion (Finkler and Kovner, 2000, p. 4).

According to the quantum physics theory (discussed in Chapter 2), what we believe and think is what we get. So believing in scarcity, rather than abundance, is problematic. It will cause many supply and demand problems.

We need to be careful about our thoughts as they can create our reality. I would rather choose abundance—not scarcity—in my thoughts as that is the reality I would rather live in. Applying this to nursing, if we believe—or enough of us think—that there is a nursing shortage, one will result. If we begin to believe that there are enough nurses, there will be enough.

Is the glass half full or half empty?? Using economic theory it is half empty; there is scarcity. Supply and demand occur in response to scarce resources. Using quantum physics theory, the glass is half full if we believe in abundance, or half empty, if we believe in scarcity.

How Did We Get into this Mess?

Presently health care is a wonderful, complicated economic quagmire and a lot needs fixing. The first problem is that it is "illness" based. The term "health" care is a misnomer; it is really "illness" care. We use the term, health care, in this book, but only because it is the common nomenclature for our illness system. Historically in this country, we have pursued treating illness, rather than researching what brings about good health. Research on promoting and achieving health is happening, but there are much larger amounts of money being spent on such things as treating cancer, heart problems, and strokes—the leading causes of death—rather than on how we can achieve health and avoid illness. Are we seeing the glass half empty, rather than half full? Perhaps if we could get beyond the causes of death (or rather concentrate on what happens as we live as we all will die anyway), we would be better off. Quality of *life* is what matters.

We know that our present "illness" care system has many serious problems. Throughout this last century, there have been a number of unsuccessful attempts to fix the health care system. However, this has often worsened the situation. Part of the problem is that all the players have not been involved as equal partners. So how did we get into this quagmire? Examining that will give us a better understanding of not only the present situation and unresolved dilemmas, but give us some idea of what may come next. Hopefully, we will use systems thinking (defined in Chapter 4) on a national level and learn from our past mistakes. Here's how we got to where we are.

Colonial Period to 1900

Historically, in this country, early medical care was provided by women in the family who took care of relatives in the home. There was no formal education or training for these women. Instead women relied on their knowledge and experience and, if they got any education or training, it was from other family members or neighbors, or, if they could read, from books. There is a definite correlation with the present and all the care givers in the home. The wealthy could pay for caregivers when sick. This was the forerunner of private duty nursing.

Physicians, if available, were consulted in more complicated or extreme medical situations. Formal education was not accessible until the 1800s. A person could become a physician by apprenticing with another physician. There was no mechanism for testing competence; anyone could hang out a shingle.

Hospitals and nursing homes existed but in those days were either voluntary hospitals existing on voluntary contributions, serving the indigent; or quarantine hospitals, opening and closing sporadically to deal with epidemic diseases such as smallpox, yellow fever, or later, tuberculosis; or were for the wealthy who could pay for the services, i.e., hiding a family member with a psychiatric illness in an insane asylum.

Florence Nightingale, well known for starting the *nursing profession*, started nurse training programs because she saw the need for training nurses to either work with the lay caregivers, to provide private duty nursing, to teach in nursing programs, or to be hospital administrators. Gradually these trained nurses expanded their roles and got involved with public health home visits, visiting several homes each day to teach and to provide better care to the sick. These nurses were often wealthy women of the community who provided charitable services. In addition to the nursing activities, they were also concerned with prevention of illness, sanitation, and better nutrition. In the 1800s, as hospitals were established, nurse training programs—early forms of the diploma schools—were started.

By the mid-1800s instruments such as the stethoscope, thermometer, sphygmomanometer, and microscope were introduced; air was viewed as a disinfectant so good ventilation became important; antiseptic procedures were introduced; better ways had been discovered to manage pain in surgery; and, later, the x-ray was invented. As all this developed, the wealthy started coming to hospitals for treatment because of the technology available there. This changed hospital design. Wards were replaced with semi-private rooms and, thus, the numbers of nurses needed to care for patients increased. Hospital financing was dramatically increased and resulted in more hospital construction. The matrons became nurse administrators. Nursing homes—supported by a community fraternal or church group—were also established for the poor, or for populations that were difficult to manage in the home including those experiencing mental illness, impaired children, and frail elders. Care tended to be better in the fraternal or church group sponsored nursing homes.

Public health activities first began in larger cities in the early 1800s. The main focus was sanitation and prevention of epidemics for such things as smallpox, typhoid fever, and diphtheria. They were concerned with waste removal, swamp drainage, and street drainage. If epidemics occurred, they would quarantine homes or ships. Later, as immunizations were developed, public health officials got involved with administering them. The first state board of health was formed in 1869 in Massachusetts. By the turn of the century, each state had a board of health that would work on the above issues with local boards of health.

1900s

In the early 1900s, early visiting nurse agencies were started, especially in the larger cities. If able, clients would pay a small fee for services provided. The visiting nurse agency board raised funds to support their work with the poor. Public health broadened to include maternal and child services in the slums of large cities to detect tuberculosis (which had become the leading cause of death), and to control venereal disease. This drew opposition from the physicians who thought that this was within their practice domain. In 1935 federal monies became available to local and state health departments for these purposes, thus strengthening the public health departments. By the 1970s, the communicable disease threat had been replaced by concerns with chronic and degenerative diseases. But, by the end of the century, public health departments were once again concerned with communicable diseases, the acquired immunodeficiency syndrome (AIDS) and the reemergence of tuberculosis.

Home care had its beginnings when in 1909 the Metropolitan Life Insurance Company began to provide home-based nursing services for its policyholders. The American Red Cross also provided home care services. This movement (life insurance companies providing home care services) lasted until about 1950.

BLUE CROSS/BLUE SHIELD

The emergence of health insurance was another significant change in health care. Initially, the coverage was either to provide health care for people involved in rail or steamboat accidents; or for mutual aid where small amounts of money were collected from worker groups—or occasionally employers—to provide a disability cash benefit for members experiencing an accident or illness including typhus, typhoid, scarlet fever, smallpox, diphtheria, and diabetes. In 1929 Justin Ford Kimball established a hospital insurance plan at Baylor University in Dallas, Texas. He had been a superintendent of schools, and noticed that teachers often had unpaid bills at the hospital. Examining hospital records he calculated that "the schoolteachers as a group 'incurred an average of 15 cents a month in hospital bills. To assure a safe margin, he established a rate of 50 cents a month.' In return, the school teachers were assured of 21 days of hospitalization in a semiprivate room" (Raffel and Raffel, p. 211). This was the beginning of the Blue Cross plans that developed across the country.

Then in 1939, the California Medical Association started the California Physicians Service to pay physician services. This became known as Blue Shield. In this plan doctors were obligated to provide treatment at the fee established by Blue Shield, even though the doctor might charge more to patients not covered by Blue Shield. Blue Shield was in effect for people who made less than $3000/year. In one of many unsuccessful attempts at national health care reform, physicians designed and agreed to this plan to prevent the establishment of a national health insurance plan.

Blue Cross offered service benefits rather than a lump-sum payment—*indemnity*—benefit that had been offered by previous insurance plans. If people having Blue Cross wanted a private room, the plan, which paid for a semiprivate room, would pay the semiprivate rate and the person would have to pay the rest themselves.

Blue Cross was quite successful. Blue Shield was not. As inflation occurred and patients made more money, the base rate was not changed, so fewer people were eligible for the Blue Shield rates. "Blue Shield made the same dollar payment for services rendered, but because the patient was above the service-benefit income level, the patient frequently had to pay an additional amount to the physician" (Raffel and Raffel, p. 213). Even when Blue Shield responded and changed the rates, the plan did not work well because inflation continued. There were also problems as radiology, pathology, and anesthesiology physicians moved out of the hospital and established their own billing. Blue Shield did not cover their expenses, yet Blue Cross could not pay the expense because it was no longer a hospital charge.

Both Blue Cross and Blue Shield faced similar situations in later years as new, often expensive, technology developed. If they paid for equipment,

> it would encourage hospitals to… [average] the new equipment with all
> other costs, [increasing hospital charges]. If Blue Cross covered such
> items, it would eventually force a rate increase, and if there was a rate
> increase, then competitors would gain an advantage. The pressures on
> both Blue Cross and Blue Shield became even more acute as they acted
> as fiscal intermediaries (the agency handling the payments) for
> Medicare. The federal government, bitten by rising costs, sought to pres-
> sure the Blues (a frequently used word for the Blue Cross/Blue Shield
> movement) and others to stem rising costs; pressure also came from state
> governments, which were bitten by the rising costs of Medicaid (Raffel
> and Raffel, pp. 214–215).

SOCIAL SECURITY ACT

As insurance plans were emerging, another major societal shift occurred that dramatically affected health care. In 1935, in the midst of the Depression, the Social Security Act
was passed. Until this event, local and state individuals and governments had been responsible for services for the poor. The Social Security Act shifted that responsibility to the
federal government. This also started the era of *entitlement*. Perhaps Peter Drucker summarizes this best.

> During the last fifty years, society in every developed country has
> become a society of institutions. Every major social task, whether eco-
> nomic performance *or health care* [italics added], education or the pro-
> tection of the environment, the pursuit of new knowledge or defense, is
> today being entrusted to big organizations, designed for perpetuity and
> managed by their own managements (1974, p. 3).

The Social Security Act of 1935 dramatically affected the nursing home industry. This
Act specified that money be given to private nursing homes and excluded—later
repealed—from public institutions. Thus for-profit and proprietary nursing homes (privately
owned) proliferated to serve the welfare patient. These homes would give first priority to paying patients because the government reimbursement was substantially lower. Sound familiar?
A 1948 Amendment made construction grants available to private and non-profit nursing
homes. Later the proprietary homes did succeed in getting Congress to make Federal
Housing Authority (FHA) construction grants available for investor-owned facilities.

HEALTH CARE CHANGES FOLLOWING WORLD WAR II

Our health care system, as we know it today, emerged post-World War II. Hospitals were
built as anesthesias, medicines, and technologies became available—along with government money to build hospitals (Hill-Burton Act). National legislation now emphasized
secondary/tertiary care—highly technical hospital-based care—rather than primary care,
defined as preventive, restorative, or medical treatment given while the patient lives at
home. By this time communicable diseases were no longer a concern. With this change in
care, many of the life insurance companies, and the American Red Cross, stopped sup-

porting nursing services. Economic survival became an issue in home health as home health agencies merged with public health departments. As Hill-Burton money became available for hospital construction, hospital-based home health emerged.

In many states after World War II, private insurance companies offered health insurance policies both to individuals and to employers. Suddenly large employers were expected to offer employees health care benefits. Unionization played a major role. Health insurance became an entitlement. Soon private insurance companies (third party payers) enrolled more than half the US population. The McCarren-Ferguson Act of 1945 "gave states the exclusive right to regulate health insurance plans. . . . As a result the federal government has no agency that is *solely* responsible for monitoring insurance" (Finkelman, p. 188).

Psychiatric treatment also changed dramatically. With the advent of psychotropic medications, more psychiatric patients were able to be treated in outpatient settings. In 1963, the federal government established community mental health centers for this purpose. Thus, many psychiatric patients who had been hospitalized for years were able to leave the hospitals and function in the community setting. Unfortunately, those who were more severely mentally ill suffered, as less money was available for their care. Funding for community mental health centers has continued to decline.

MEDICARE AND MEDICAID BEGIN

Until 1965, the federal government financed little in the way of health care, concentrating only on some public health issues and providing services for military personnel and Native Americans. State and local governments established and supported special facilities for mental illness, mental retardation, and communicable diseases such as tuberculosis. Less than half of the elderly, and disabled Americans, had health insurance. Then in a wave of entitlement programming, the federal government *really* became involved in health care by establishing Medicare and Medicaid. Naturally, this Social Security Amendment benefitted the elderly and the poor, and gave them more access to health care; but providers— hospitals, other health care organizations, physicians; and even suppliers and the building industry—really benefitted as well. Medicare often became the largest source of revenue for health care providers, resulting in more hospital and long-term care building programs. As more personnel were needed for all the expansion and new building, additional federal programs were funded to supply more physicians, nurses, and technicians. Providers quickly learned how to use methods to maximize reimbursements. Where possible, documentation to support certain diagnoses that provided higher reimbursement was used.

This focus of long-term care services changed.

> With the advent of Medicare and Medicaid and the accompanying large sums of money that would become available for nursing home care, the federal government had to establish definitions for the types of institutions that would fall within the framework of those eligible for reimbursement, as well as standards to govern and ensure quality of care in those homes eligible to participate. No longer could a "home for the aged" be synonymous with a "nursing home." If a home for the aged wanted to be paid under Medicare or Medicaid for care to eligible patients, the home had to meet certain standards. The federal government now recognizes two types of homes as being eligible. The first is a

skilled nursing facility (*SNF*), and the second is an intermediate care facility (ICF). The U.S. Department of Health and Human Services provided these definitions:

> A *skilled nursing facility* (SNF) is a nursing home that has been certified as meeting Federal standards within the meaning of the Social Security Act. It provides the level of care that comes closest to hospital care with 24-hour nursing services. Regular medical supervision and rehabilitation therapy are also provided. Generally, a skilled nursing facility cares for convalescent patients and those with long-term illnesses.
>
> An *intermediate care facility* (ICF) is also certified and meets Federal standards and provides less extensive health-related care and services. It has regular nursing service, but not around the clock. Most intermediate care facilities carry on rehabilitation programs, but the emphasis is on personal care and social services. Mainly, these homes serve people who are not fully capable of living by themselves, yet are not necessarily ill enough to need 24-hour nursing care (Raffel and Raffel, p. 183).

Medicare and Medicaid also infused the home health industry with the money to expand both agencies and services. Where there had been about 250 home health agencies in 1960, by 1968 there were 1,328 official agencies providing home health services. Federal funding over the next 20 years gradually refocused home health on post-acute services. Unfortunately, money became unavailable for the chronically ill client needing longer term services. Services also changed in the home health industry as home health funding began to include rehabilitative services—physical therapy, occupational therapy, speech therapy, and social work services. This continues today.

To administer these programs, the federal government started the Health Care Financing Administration (HCFA), now Centers for Medicare and Medicaid Services (CMS), within the Department of Health and Human Services. Payment was based on the *retrospective cost* of the care—figured by health care organizations and by physicians seeing patients. (This subsequently changed to prospective payment, explained later in this chapter.)

Suddenly the federal government was spending a tremendous amount of money on health care. In fact, the gross domestic product (GDP) for health care grew from 6 percent when Medicare and Medicaid were introduced to 13 percent presently. To find money to support these programs, the government was faced with increasing taxes, shifting money from other services such as defense or education, or curbing hospital and physician costs. The federal government chose to continue to support tertiary and secondary care rather than less expensive primary care and prevention. Another huge problem resulted. Tertiary care became an entitlement. However, more money was needed for long-term care, public health, and home care services. Where would this money come from?

Federal legislation mandated the states to share costs for Medicaid. The states now had to find money for this purpose. The problem has worsened each year as Medicaid costs continue to rise. For instance, by 1995, 17 percent of the Medicaid beneficiaries were disabled, but accounted for 37 percent of the health care costs ($8,422/person). States, because they pay a sizable portion of Medicaid, adopted various laws to regulate hospital costs and charges. The most common strategy has been to establish HMOs for this population, and mandate Medicaid recipients to receive care in the HMOs.

This Social Security Amendment also established *utilization review* (UR) for Medicare patients to try to counteract the rising costs, and two years later utilization review was started for Medicaid patients. Hospitals receiving Medicare "were required to certify the necessity of admission, continued stay, and professional services rendered to Medicare beneficiaries" (CMS—Centers for Medicare and Medicaid Services).

In 1965, the Older Americans Act of 1965 mandated and funded Area Agencies on Aging (AAA). The AAAs fund a wide array of services for the elderly: senior centers with nutrition and recreation programs; health promotion and screening programs; mental health evaluation and treatment; respite care; case managers to plan care for elders so they can stay in their homes rather than be institutionalized; and services to the homebound such as meals, homemaker services, chore service, and transportation.

As Medicare standards required hospitals to renovate and rebuild, the 1970s and 1980s brought about a rapid growth of for-profit or investor-owned hospitals. For-profit hospitals, like many other businesses, had publicly traded stocks. Stockholders expected the for-profit hospitals to make a profit so stocks would both increase in value and provide good dividends. In this arrangement, hospitals had to pay attention to stockholder interests. These interests might not always be what ethically was best for the patient. Actually not-for-profit hospitals made profits too—using the profits for pay increases, new equipment or building projects, and investments—but never wanted to call it "profit," calling it "excess of revenue over expenses." Investor-owned nursing homes and home care facilities also increased.

With this movement, cost remained an issue and serious concerns about quality arose. Professional review organizations (PROs) were implemented to do preadmission reviews, and to review cases when length of stay went beyond what was expected. Yet this action did not bring down the cost of health care. PROs began to deny payment for medically unnecessary care, care given in an inappropriate setting, or substandard care.

CERTIFICATE OF NEED

Along with starting Medicare and Medicaid, the federal government mandated that states adopt laws requiring health care facilities to establish a certificate of need for a major expansion, or for major capital expenditures because an overbedding problem began to occur in hospitals. Home care was exempt and continued to increase at an exponential level. Congress repealed the certificate of need requirement in 1987, saying it was up to the states. Today some states still require this for new construction, although many do not.

HEALTH MAINTENANCE ORGANIZATIONS

In another attempt to hold down health care costs, the Health Maintenance Organization (HMO) Act of 1973 provided grants to develop HMOs. This Act required employers with more than 25 employees to offer an HMO health insurance option to employees. HMOs had a good track record of bringing down health care costs because they had traditionally been serving younger, healthier populations. (Traditional insurance plans serving a wider range of people were more expensive.) Thus starting more HMOs sounded like a way to cut health care costs. This Act provided a specific definition of what an HMO was, and gave the states oversight (or licensing) responsibility for HMOs. At first, although more HMOs were started, not many people chose this option. However, as health care costs increased, HMOs gained in popularity. HMOs became a popular option for employees in lower wage categories because no out-of-pocket money was needed to see the health care provider for care. As HMOs' began to serve older people with chronic illnesses, their costs began to rise dramatically.

MARKETING

As health care organizations realized that if they did not pay attention to the volatile shifts in payer structures and employer needs, they might find that they had no patients, they began to implement more strategic planning. "Overt promotion was considered unethical by physicians and inappropriate by not-for-profit hospitals until 1978 when a ruling of the U.S. Supreme Court held the proscription to be in violation of antitrust laws" (Griffith, 1999, p. 496). Thus health care organizations began to *market* their services to consumers. Hospitals and health care systems often added marketing departments, or combined this function with the public relations responsibilities. Although marketing efforts were aimed at the patient consumer, some were asking whether the decision makers also should include the employers who were purchasing the plans. Actually, to effectively market services, every employee who comes into contact with patients or their families should market services. If hospital employees are perceived as non-caring, patients might prefer to go somewhere else. In addition, physicians and physician services are now being marketed, especially in areas where there is a lot of competition.

OCCUPATIONAL SAFETY AND HEALTH ADMINISTRATION (OSHA)

Other changes were occurring in the 1970s. As more public attention was being given to workplace injuries or death, the Occupational Safety and Health Act of 1970 was implemented to ensure a safe, healthy workplace. This act established the National Institute of Occupational Safety and Health (NIOSH) to do research and set standards to be enforced by another establishment, the Occupational Safety and Health Administration (OSHA). The law states that if an employee reports a facility to OSHA, the employee cannot be punished or fired.

EMPLOYEE RETIREMENT INCOME SECURITY ACT (ERISA)

As plants closed or merged in the 1970s, many individuals lost their pensions. Thus the Employee Retirement Income Security Act of 1974 (ERISA) took away some of the state responsibility for insurance plans, and "established federal jurisdiction over self-insured, employer-sponsored health benefit plans" (Finkelman, p. 189). This Act also mandated "reporting and disclosure requirements for employer-sponsored benefits such as pensions, group life and 'self insured' health plans" (p. 482).

1980s

EMPLOYER COST CUTTING

Employers, like the federal government, were experiencing increased health care costs as their employees used more health care services. Employers followed the government's lead by using utilization review (where a payer reviews the appropriateness of care), a gate-keeping strategy, before a patient could receive treatment. Thus the payer would have to approve all specialist referrals and potential hospitalizations before the patient could receive treatment.

Employers began to pass the cost of health insurance plans on to employees. Employees would pay a set monthly fee for the health insurance benefit. Now, if spouses each had an insurance plan, it became important to delineate what plan would first cover family health care needs, with the other plan picking up uncovered expenses only. This was followed by offering *cafeteria plans* for employees. In this arrangement an employee would choose the amount and type of health care coverage (and other benefits) needed, within certain limits set by the employer. If the employee's spouse had a good insurance plan it was possible the employee would not require health insurance at all. This saved employers money. Another strategy used by employers turned to a capitated method of payment, i.e., PPO (preferred provider organization) or HMO (health maintenance organization). (Managed care and capitation is further explained in the payers section of this chapter.)

In 1985 CMS joined employers, developing HMOs to serve the Medicare population. This allowed Medicare beneficiaries to choose which plan they preferred to use. Not many beneficiaries chose the HMO option because by this time, there was negative press being given to managed care plans. When they did choose HMOs, HMO costs escalated because Medicare serves the elderly, many of whom have chronic illnesses requiring a lot of medical care. It was not until 1999 that the large HMOs began to be profitable by boosting rates and dropping unprofitable lines—often the elderly Medicare population. Many HMOs went out of business entirely.

In managed care, payers were paying providers a per member per month fee to be used to provide health care for all members of the plan. This *capitation* payment model caused a dramatic incentive for providers (physicians, hospitals) to change their practices because suddenly revenues were not related to the volume of services provided. Instead, according to the plan, if members used too many services in a month, the provider would lose money. However, if plan members did not use as many services in a month, it was possible for the provider to make a profit. Now the incentive for providers was to only provide needed services and to provide services in the least costly way. For example, in a hospital an acutely ill patient would be transferred from an ICU bed to a stepdown unit to a subacute unit and then to outpatient and home care as quickly as possible.

Managed care resulted in additional problems. For example, there are many hospital readmissions because some patients are discharged too soon. Hospital "re-admissions account for 22% to 37% of all hospital admissions for older people" (Merrill, p. 127). As patients began to realize that care was suffering, managed care began to receive a lot of negative publicity.

Employers were hit with additional expense when the COBRA legislation mandated employers to continue benefits for terminated employees for a certain length of time. This was mandated federally to ensure health care coverage for people who were unemployed or between jobs.

PHYSICIAN CHANGES

With the advent of managed care plans, the traditional single physician having a separate office began to erode. Groups of physicians began to band together for cost and coverage reasons, but also because it became important for them to be part of different insurance plans. As employers changed to managed care, patients suddenly had to go to certain specified physicians. If a physician was not a part of various insurance plans, patient numbers (and thus revenues) dwindled. Physicians had to pay attention to the various plans being offered by employers to make sure that they would still have a large enough patient group. This process created more unbillable time. By being in a physician group, more attention could be paid to the insurance plans, they would continue to have patients, and thus continue to have revenue. As physician group practices became larger, the major insurers in that area would be more likely to want to include the group in the plan. Then insurers, expected to guarantee a certain amount of business to providers, began to expect discounts from providers in return. Group practices became more of a necessity.

By the 1970s, the specialty physicians, especially surgeons, received more reimbursement than primary care physicians. Many new physician graduates began to choose a specialty. It was not uncommon in rural and inner city areas to have a shortage of primary physicians.

Malpractice costs began to spiral, especially in surgery, anesthesiology, and obstetrics. High awards were being given as malpractice rates climbed. It was not uncommon by 1989 for a physician to pay $15,000 a year for malpractice insurance. Currently malpractice awards have declined as some states passed laws limiting the amount or type of damage awarded, as specialty groups established standards, and as physicians began to realize that if they treated the patient well, fewer lawsuits would result. However, malpractice insurance costs are still too high.

Managed care brought about a another change for physicians. Physicians actually started to be employed by the HMO instead of being an independent practitioner. This had happened to a small extent earlier, as various employers might pay a physician to do employee physicals or provide medical coverage for accidents that occurred in the workplace. With the advent of managed care and the issues that arose with the need to be included in insurance plans, many physicians chose to become employed by the HMO. The downside was that the HMO might expect that they see a certain number of patients, or that they refer very few patients for more expensive treatment.

NURSE-MANAGED CARE

Both home care and public health services, drastically underfunded in our illness payment system, can only partially provide needed community health services. Thus, numerous consumer health care needs are left untended. This leaves many underserved rural and inner city populations at the poverty level with no resources for health care. To partially meet this need, parish nursing, Community Nursing Centers (CNCs), Community Nursing Organizations (CNOs), and Nursing HMOs have been sponsored by local communities, community groups, churches, and by university schools/colleges of nursing who donate not only money, but nurses and supplies (Lundeen, 1997; Spitzer, 1997; Storfjell, Mitchell, and Daly, 1997; Ethridge, 1997; Harris, 1997). Many of these centers are also partially supported on the federal level by the Division of Nursing located within the Center for Nursing Research in the Department of Health and Human Services.

HOSPITAL PROSPECTIVE PAYMENT BEGINS

Congress passed two bills: the Tax Equity and Fiscal Responsibility Act of 1982 (TEFRA) and the Social Security Amendments of 1983 mandating a prospective payment system for inpatient hospital services for Medicare patients. Under *prospective payment*, fixed rates are set for various diagnoses; for Medicare these are called *diagnosis-related groups* (DRGs). HCFA, now CMS, would determine the DRG fixed rates. Fixed rates were established for medical/surgical and obstetric diagnoses, not for pediatric and psychiatric diagnoses. However, utilization review was started for psychiatry and substance abuse patients. Managed behavioral health care companies were formed. If hospitals could provide the service at a rate lower than the DRG, the hospital could keep the difference. If more was spent, the hospitals would have to come up with the extra money. The DRGs started with Medicare patients but other insurance companies, including Medicaid state plans and Blue Cross, adopted this concept for their insurance payments. TEFRA gave bonus incentives when home care, or less expensive alternatives, could be used to replace inpatient care.

Financially, this meant driving the point of service to the least expensive option, because doing extra tests or having a long length of stay would incur more costs. It was more advantageous to cut out unnecessary costs and drive down costs as much as possible. Primary care is cheaper than tertiary care, thus it was less expensive to set up subacute or rehabilitation units and transfer hospital patients as quickly as possible to these units. Providing home care services was less expensive than continued stay on any inpatient unit. Nurse practitioners, nurse anesthetists, and nurse midwives could provide certain services more cheaply than physicians (Catlin and McAuliffe, 1999). It became important to make sure that services were provided on a timely basis so the length of stay would be shorter. Prevention of complications became critical as complications would increase length of stay, which increased cost.

When some for-profit hospital emergency rooms refused to treat patients that could not pay, the Consolidated Omnibus Budget Reconciliation Act of 1985 (COBRA) mandated that if hospitals participated in Medicare they must provide emergency care to indigent and uninsured patients. This means that the emergency personnel must screen patients to determine if they have a true medical, psychiatric, alcohol-related or substance abuse emergency. If so, treatment must be provided or, if a transfer is necessary to a specialized facility, that facility must accept the patient.

Emergency rooms have a common dilemma. The primary purpose of an emergency room is to provide care to people in emergency situations. However, the emergency room has become a place to go to when a person does not have a primary physician, or when one cannot get in to see their physician. In light of this new use of the emergency department, JCAHO developed standards of care related to continuity addressing repeated visits, immunizational status, and nutritional screening. To maintain accreditation, emergency departments are obligated to address these standards and respond appropriately. These issues cost insurers a lot of money because it costs significantly more to provide care in an emergency room than in a physician's office. Hospitals face real dilemmas with this issue as part of the patients need acute critical care facilities while part of the population is better served by a primary care physician or nurse practitioner. Patient wait times can be extensive. A common practice today is to have a separate nearby area—or free-standing clinics around the community—set up for the primary care group with the actual ER set up for more acute emergencies.

This cost-cutting movement was having a domino effect on health care. As hospitals dramatically cut patient length of stay, the acute care hospitals began to seem more like critical care units. Numbers of hospital beds decreased, and hospitals closed or merged. Same-day surgery became the new buzz word and the observation patient (or 23-hour patient)—the patient who would come in for surgery but be discharged before 24 hours had elapsed—emerged.

LONG-TERM CARE BECOMES MORE ACUTE

As prospective care was implemented for hospitals, skilled nursing units grew. When ill patients were not ready to go home but were discharged by the hospital, the patient was transferred to a skilled nursing unit.

Then another piece of federal legislation had additional impact for long-term care. The Omnibus Budget Reconciliation Act of 1987 (OBRA '87) specified minimum requirements for long-term care staffing:

- one LPN on each shift,
- at least one RN for at least eight hours per day,
- seven days a week (states may have additional staffing requirements),
- creation of a long-term care national data base (MDS),
- state licensing of nursing assistants, and
- a defined knowledge base and competencies required for nurse assistant certification.

State requirements can vary but have to include those federally mandated. "In addition to personal care and communication skills, CNAs must be trained in the psychosocial and restorative needs of residents, including resident rights. . . . A CNA must have at least 12 hours of in-service education annually to satisfy the federally required curriculum" (Mitty, p. 120). CNAs are required to submit proof of the additional education to the state board in order to be recertified. By 1987, long-term care facilities were subject to many federal mandates for licensure and certification, (further defined in the Regulator section of this chapter). (The CNA requirements are also mandated for home care and hospice, but have never been mandated for hospitals.)

Long-term care insurance policies, for both in-home care and for institutional care, have gained popularity. Meanwhile, some nice models for community-based long-term care were developed, including the PACE program (Program for All-Inclusive Care for the

Elderly.) Then in 1996, the Health Insurance Reform Act was passed, making long-term care expenses, including home care, tax deductible.

HOME CARE EXPANDS

In 1980 the Omnibus Budget Reconciliation Act aided home care by expanding the Medicare benefits to 100 visits per year with a $100 deductible. Previously a three-day hospitalization had been required before giving home care. This requirement was lifted. For the first time, for-profit home care agencies could become Medicare-certified providers. In addition the advanced technology, such as ventilators, renal hemodialysis, and infusion therapy, originally found only in hospitals, all moved into the home, expanding the need for a home care nurse. This need was coupled with prospective payment for hospitals, and resulted in earlier discharges and greater use of home care. The number of home care agencies increased exponentially.

In response, in 1984 the federal government restricted home care significantly by limiting home care services to consumers who were home bound, and only required "part-time" and "intermittent" home care. (The "and" changed to "or" in 1989). The need for home care had to be documented in the patient record. This resulted in a *Duggan v. Bowen* court ruling requiring CMS to clarify its eligibility criteria for home care. So in 1989, CMS redefined and eased home care eligibility.

AMBULATORY CARE INCREASES

Ambulatory care changed dramatically with the advent of Medicare and Medicaid, and more importantly, later with DRGs. This change was coupled with advanced technology making available new, less invasive procedures for treating certain health problems. For example, laser surgery dramatically changed gall bladder, eye, and knee surgeries. Surgeries could occur, and patients could go home the same day. Ambulatory care grew exponentially. In addition, freestanding surgery centers were started by groups of surgeons and renal dialysis moved to ambulatory facilities, often owned by physicians or for-profit companies.

1990s

THE HEALTH INSURANCE PORTABILITY AND ACCOUNTABILITY ACT OF 1996 (HIPAA)

HIPAA addresses several significant issues.

- This act "establishes that insurers cannot set limits on coverage for preexisting conditions, . . . guaranteed access and renewability [of health insurance], . . . [and] addresses issues of excluding small employers from insurance contracts on the basis of employee health status… In addition the law provided for greater tax deductibility of health insurance for the self-employed" (Finkelman, p. 192).
- HIPAA started the *medical savings accounts*, a tax-free account provided by employers. Here the employee can annually set up an account, and pay in the amount of money the employee expects to have to pay for health coverage for the year. The money paid into the account takes place before taxes are taken out by the employer.

At the end of the year, if the money is not spent it goes back to the employer.

- A major portion of HIPAA mandated patient privacy procedures. This can vary from state to state as long as the minimum federal requirement is met.[1] HIPAA ensures confidentiality and privacy of paper, oral (telephone inquiries and oral conversations), and electronic (computer or fax) patient health information to or from any source. The following three standards must be met:
    - **Standard One:** This set governs the proper use and disclosure of personal health information (PHI) by the facility, its workforce, and certain business associates such as lawyers, auditors, consultants, and other third parties who handle PHI.
    - **Standard Two:** This set allows patients to request access to their PHI, request reasonable amendments to it, and receive an annual written report of all of the facility's uses and disclosures of their PHI that they didn't authorize in writing… the patient may request certain restrictions regarding disclosure of PHI to certain third parties such as family members.
    - **Standard Three:** This set requires facilities to complete several administrative tasks, including appointing a privacy officer, making the various written changes to its operating procedures, educating its workforce about these changes, and establishing an effective method for patients and others to communicate complaints, questions, and concerns about its privacy practices (Ziel, pp. 28–29).

THE BALANCED BUDGET ACT OF 1997 (BBA)

The BBA significantly lowered payments for psychiatric care, rehabilitation services, and long-term care. Since ambulatory services, skilled nursing facilities (SNFs), and home care services were rapidly expanding and costing more health care dollars, the idea was to curb spending by placing these services under prospective payment. Prospective payment means that the payer determines the cost of care before the care is given; the provider is told how much will be paid to give the care. Thus the government could limit provider reimbursement. For instance, an *Ambulatory Payment Classification* system was established giving a fixed dollar amount for outpatient services diagnoses; skilled nursing facilities experienced prospective payment through the RUGs system; and home care was regulated via the OASIS system. Even physician services changed to payments based on a *resource based relative value scale (RBRVS)*. Hospitals, already experiencing prospective payment, had major, mandated payment reductions limiting DRG and resource based relative value scale (RBRVS) payment rates. BBA reduced capital expenditures, graduate medical education, established open enrollment periods and medical savings accounts for Medicare recipients, increased benefits for children's health care, and created new penalties for fraud.

One positive aspect of BBA was the creation of the Children's Health Insurance Program (CHIP) which "expands block grants to states increasing Medicaid eligibility for low-income and uninsured children, establishing a new program that subsidizes private insurance for children or combining Medicaid with the private insurance" (Finkelman, p. 398).

---

[1] See www.hhs.gov/ocr/hipaa.

BBA had a major impact on health care, causing a number of hospitals, long-term care facilities, and home care companies to fold. A direct result of BBA has been to erode profit margins of hospitals and make cost shifting very difficult. For example, in 1997 it recommended no pay increases. Whereas hospitals averaged a 6 percent profit margin in 1997, in 1999 the profit margin was 2.7 percent. Rural hospitals were most drastically affected, and hospital bond ratings have been downgraded due to this Act. This means that it is harder to get credit and interest rates are higher. BBA had such profound cost-cutting effects that in December 2000, Congress passed relief legislation providing additional money for hospitals and managed care plans.

If hospitals hadn't already been outsourcing services like housekeeping, food service, and grounds keeping, this Act encouraged more of this to occur (Contract Management Survey, 2001). "The basic premise of outsourcing is that a specialist organization can perform a particular service more efficiently than can internal operations because a specialist organization has an inherent advantage in producing and delivering a service" (Roberts, p. 241). Outsourcing has been around for a long time. Instances include contracting with physicians to staff a hospital emergency room, contracting with anesthesiologists to staff an operating room, contracting with pharmacies to provide pharmaceuticals for long-term care patients, and contracting with companies to provide patient satisfaction measurement. Now outsourcing is happening with many health care functions/services.

BBA had a major impact on the nursing profession. Under BBA, nurse practitioners (NPs) and clinical nurse specialists (CNSs) practicing in any setting could now be directly reimbursed for services provided to Medicare patients at 85 percent of physician fees. This occurred to both better serve populations not receiving medical care and to save costs as studies had determined that NPs could deliver as much as 80 percent of the medical care at less cost than primary care physicians. This federal legislation overrode state legislation that, in some cases, required NPs to work under direct physician supervision with reimbursement being made only to physicians.

Another problem confronted by hospitals was that Medicare and managed care companies have slowed payments to health care organizations resulting in poor cash flow due to lengthening days of accounts receivable. Slow payment is caused in part by slow or erroneous provider billing and claims denials by insurers. The problem is that a provider is often dealing with different payers that all have different forms and policy provisions. Receiving money for services has become very complicated. The cash flow problem is compounded by antiquated computer systems that cannot handle the current requirements and complexities. In general, electronic medical records and electronic billing now ensures more prompt payment.

2000s

ILLNESS CARE CONTINUES TO BECOME LESS INVASIVE AND MORE PERSONALIZED

As our medications, genomics, and technologies improve, health care is becoming less invasive. Gene Roddenbury's picture of health care in *Star Trek* is very likely where we are going.

e-Health Opportunities

As our telehealth capabilities increase, health care is expanding so that a clinican does not need to actually be present to treat a patient (Greenberg and Cartwright, 2001). (See Chapter 14 on Budget Strategies for more details.)

In addition the internet has vastly improved clinician information on evidence-based practice. (See Chapter 8, written by two dedicated librarians, showing how easy it is to access information at the point of care, to determine the best way to treat a specific patient.) Consumers continue to access the internet, both about their specific illnesses, but also to determine which providers are most effective. They use this information to evaluate how effectively their provider is determining their care (Meadows, 2001).

Genomics

"While genetics is the study of inherited traits, genomics is the study of the complete set of human genes, the way genes are assembled (sequence), how they are expressed (what they do), and the relationships between different sequences" (Larson, p. 77). Presently scientists have joined forces with private companies who supply enormous funds to map genes. With commercial enterprises involved, it has created *great* ethical implications, as business leaders think this information can produce future profits. Enriquez and Goldberg (2000), state:

> Optimism reigns that we are on the cusp of a wholly new style of medicine. Ever since Hippocrates, curative regimens have been one-size-fits-all. Until recently it simply wasn't possible to truly dispense custom cures that had been designed for this person, right now. However, suddenly medicine is becoming "personalized medicine" where cures are concocted in line with an individual's genetic makeup. Computer simulation will let medical scientists see exactly what will happen when this person is administered that dose of a medicine. The upshot will be pinpoint cures. When will this genetics-based medicine be widely available? Scientists are not making hard predictions, but the whispered word is that we will benefit from personalized medicine probably before this decade ends. And that just may rank as the biggest revolution in medicine in the last couple millennia (McGarvey, p. S1).

Who knows? Health care may be adding a genetics department into the caregiver mix.

> As researchers investigate the human gennome, they've discovered that most health conditions result from a combination of genetic and environmental influences and interactions. These discoveries already allow clinicians to diagnose some conditions prenatally and to identify genetic susceptibility prior to symptom onset. Increasingly, genetic discoveries are used to tailor particular medications and dosages to an individual's genetic makeup, pointing the way toward future therapies and even cures for many devastating diseases.
>
> Nurses should firmly understand the role genetics plays in health and disease and incorporate genetic questions into patient assessment. In the

near future, individual risk profiling based on a person's genetic makeup will be used to customize prevention, treatment, and ongoing management of health conditions.

Researchers believe that every human carries at least six recessive genes that could create genetic conditions in his descendants if his partner carries the same gene. In addition, many people carry genes predisposing them to conditions such as arthritis, diabetes, or cancer. The term 'genetic disease' no longer refers only to rare syndromes and illnesses because research continues to demonstrate how many common conditions have a genetic component (Lea, p. 19).

Lea goes on to explain how important it is for the nurse to get genetic and family information, going back at least three generations if possible, in the initial assessment of a patient. Suggestions for a genetic history are listed in **Exhibit 6–1**.[2]

PERSONNEL SHORTAGES

Health care has been experiencing many personnel shortages—nurses (average age of the staff nurse is mid-forties), nursing faculty (average age is mid-fifties), pharmacists, technicians/aides, and medical coders, to name a few. Newer generations have more choices for professions and proportionately are not choosing these professions. This is exacerbated by the large number of baby boomers who will be retiring.

Exhibit 6–1 What to Ask Patients

For each family member in the genetic history, ask:
- age at onset of any serious illness and chronic conditions.
- cause of death and age at death.
- if any family members have birth defects, mental disabilities, or such familial traits as shortened limbs or extra fingers.
- whether the patient or his relatives are related by blood to people who entered the family by marriage. People who share common ancestors have more genes in common than those who are unrelated; for example, first cousins share one in eight genes. The more genes parents have in common, the higher the risk of having children with birth defects and genetic conditions.
- about reproductive history, including if a woman has or had a history of miscarriages, stillbirths, or conditions such as gestational diabetes, seizure disorder, or phenylketonuria, which increase the risk of birth defects. Also ask a woman whether she used alcohol or took medications during pregnancy.
- age of a pregnant woman. Those age 35 or older should be offered prenatal diagnostics such as amniocentesis because of the association between advancing maternal age and chromosomal abnormalities.

Adapted from: Lea, D. (November 2003). Look back to move forward: how genetics changes daily practice. *Nursing Management, 43*(11), p. 22.

---

[2] Two good references on genetics for nurses are: Cummings (2003) *Human Heredity: Principles and Issues*, 6th ed.; and Lashley (1998) *Clinical Genetics in Nursing Practice*, 2nd ed.

Presently the faculty shortage is most critical because someone must educate the new generations. In fact, the American Association of Colleges of Nursing (AACN) estimates that:

> 5,800 qualified applicants were turned away from baccalaureate and master's programs in 2001 because of an insufficient number of nursing faculty as well as clinical sites, clinical preceptors and classroom space. Furthermore, many states now face huge budget constraints, which will decrease their ability to fund additional capacity. The greatest need is for doctorally prepared faculty, with schools reporting that over 64 percent of their faculty vacancies were for faculty holding doctorates. . . .Studies have shown that on average, nursing faculty are not only older than their clinical and administrative colleagues, but are paid less than other tenured faculty within the same institutional setting. Compounding this problem is that the average salary for a master's prepared nurse practitioner can be $20,000 more than the average master's prepared nursing faculty member (Webb, p. 3).

ALTERNATIVE THERAPIES

In the midst of all the cost-cutting in our illness care system, by 1999 "alternative medicine visits (629 million), including those to chiropractors and massage therapists, now outstrip visits to primary care physicians (427 million)" (Hospital and Health Networks, April 1999). Studies indicate that two out of every five Americans use some form of alternative medicine. Alternative therapies have been enjoying increased popularity with the American public even though consumers most often pay "out of pocket" for the services. This is a reflection of the problems inherent in our current illness system—treating "disease," not promoting health. As patients visit physicians and receive medications for diseases, they discover often that does not cure the problem. In many cases, the medications cause further medical problems. In addition, many of the tests and treatments are very painful. The alternative therapies provide a way to stay healthy as well as to treat disease, bring comfort, and they do it in a way that does not produce as many side effects and pain.

As part of the alternative therapy movement, people are purchasing vitamins and herbs; beginning vegetarian; they find other therapies, such as massage, meditation, wellness centers, biofeedback, acupuncture, and chiropractic. The public is getting health information from many sources: books, i.e., Balch and Balch, 2000, *Prescription for Nutritional Healing*, in its third edition, presents the current research results on vitamins and herbs; the internet; the alternative care giver; some physicians and nurses; and even personnel in health food stores. The alternative therapy business continues to grow.

This increase has brought about changes in the traditional illness care industries. For instance, the pharmaceutical industry has realized that it has missed a great deal of income with the vitamin and herb movement so is working to increase market share, as well as asking the Food and Drug Administration (FDA) to control this industry. The FDA has developed a number of regulations for the vitamin/herb industry.

Although most medical schools predominantly teach illness care, medical and nursing education programs have often added more about health in their curriculums. Because many of these health activities are new to Americans, more research is needed to determine their efficacy. The National Institute of Health (NIH) has funded some initial research examining various alternative therapies, and the Food and Drug Administration has been involved with developing regulations for this industry. Achieving health has been pursued in various countries, such as use of herbs in China and homeopathy in Europe. Presently, this movement is bringing together the best information and practices from many cultures worldwide.

It is important to note here that remaining healthy and promoting health has become a national concern with consumers—even though our payment system does not reflect this interest. A single hospitalization can wipe out a person's life savings. Thus, staying healthy is advantageous even from a financial perspective. Now, even though demographically the elderly population is increasing, they are healthier than they were a generation ago. This has resulted in new habits, such as people walking the malls each morning and a new awareness of personal control at home, for example, by using glucometers, and checking cholesterol levels.

HIGH COST OF PHARMACEUTICALS

Pharmaceutical costs to both the consumer and to the health care organizations have been increasing with double digit inflation. "Prices are two to five times higher here than abroad. Industry profits soar as senior citizens on fixed incomes are forced to forgo needed medications. . . . Drugs now account for 15% of health care expenditures" (Carpenter, p. 49). One reason for the increased costs can be attributed to the Food and Drug Administration which requires costly studies of new drugs, conducted by the pharmaceutical companies, before the FDA will even consider the drug. Then it takes FDA a long time to review the drug and authorize it to be sold in the United States. At this point the pharmaceutical company can charge monopoly prices until the patent expires in seven years. All this additional cost gets passed on to the consumer.

The prospective payment has never been used to curtail drug costs. Canada has chosen to subsidize drug studies and the review process using tax dollars. The actual costs of the drugs are reduced for consumers. Congress and state legislators are analyzing models to control high drug costs, including prescription plans.

One reimbursement strategy used by payers to counteract this cost problem has been to specify less expensive generic drugs in formularies and mandate providers to prescribe these. Although this system works effectively in many case, it can be problematic if the generic drug efficacy is not as effective.

Another issue, resulting in more profits for the pharmaceutical industry, has resulted when pharmaceutical companies could start doing consumer ads. This boosted pharmaceutical sales by 16 percent.

Despite all this additional money going to pharmaceutical companies, at times we are experiencing critical drug shortages. Part of this has been caused by the just-in-time strategy used in business and industry to keep supply stockpiles down to bare minimum. The problem with this strategy is that if there are suddenly more patients than usual using a certain drug, or if shipments are delayed, or if drug companies do not produce enough of a certain drug, there may not be enough for all the patients who need the drug.

INCREASED ELDERLY POPULATION

Our elderly population is increasing as the baby boomers reach retirement age. "The number of elderly will double in 20 states between 1995 and 2025" (Lanser, p.7). At the same time we are living longer. This means that even though the elderly are becoming healthier, there are more elderly needing health care services, especially for chronic illnesses. Women especially feel the impact as they live longer, and as they face possibly living at the poverty level when old. Today, women in the workforce—and 92.5 percent of nurses are women—continue to be paid 75 cents to every dollar a man makes. Retirement incomes will continue to reflect this problem. In addition, women at retirement are usually paid lower monthly annuity benefits because they live longer then men. Thus incomes for older women actually average 55 percent of what older men make. This problem could be further compounded if there is not enough money to pay Social Security benefits. "It is estimated that by 2032, payroll taxes will cover only 70% to 75% of promised benefits" (Meier, p. 168). To make matters worse, Medicare continues to raise premiums, Medicare eligibility may be raised to 67 years, and Medicare does not cover the costs of most prescription drugs.

WHERE IS THE MONEY FOR CONSUMER HEALTHCARE?

> In a new survey of some of the largest U.S. employers—conducted by the Kaiser Family Foundation and Hewitt Associates prior to passage of the new Medicare prescription drug legislation—10% say they eliminated subsidized health benefits for future retirees in the past year, while 20% say they are likely to terminate retiree health coverage for future retirees in the next three years. These changes primarily affect new hires, rather than current retirees. The study also finds that 71% of surveyed firms increased retiree contributions, 'Based on current trends, we can expect that fewer retirees will have health coverage in the future and those who do will be paying more for their health care' (http://www.kff.org/medicare/011404package.cfm).

We have already discussed the large number of uninsured in the United States, and that many elderly are concerned because one illness episode can wipe out their life savings. As baby boomers approach retirement, it is possible that many will have no source of health care benefits other than Medicare, and Medicare may be bankrupt!

OUTCOMES RESEARCH

One exciting research development presently is the emerging interest in examining patient outcomes resulting from various treatments. Outcomes research is at the infancy stage. It will be exciting to see where this leads us as the research results will provide us with more effective answers for care. Now that more outcomes data is available, especially due to availability of Medicare and Medicaid data, quality *report cards* are now available, and provide performance data about health care organizations, for example, linking staffing with patient outcomes. Performance data (discussed in Chapter 2) is becoming available to the general public. In fact, sometimes the patient is better informed about this than the provider.

PATIENT SAFETY

Patient safety is a huge issue in health care. This is discussed in detail in Chapter 2.

BIOTERRORISM

Bioterrorism has come to the fore as a significant force to be reckoned with in this decade. This is discussed in more detail in Chapter 2.

MANAGED CARE—A THING OF THE PAST?

Today, a decade of managed care restrictions—gatekeepers, prior authorizations before receiving care—is starting to be a thing of the past. Many of the large insurers have changed their policies, and have eliminated prior authorizations and gatekeepers, letting the physician determine the needed care. Some of these plans are not charging capitated amounts but are reverting back to fee for service for physician payment. This way the consumer can go directly to a specialist for care. Marketing is becoming an important strategy for providers as insurers are beginning to contract with many providers again. This offers market choice to consumers.

The problem is that health care costs are still high with many individuals and employers finding health care unaffordable. Present health care dilemmas are captured in this editorial quote from the provider perspective.

- The new reality is that we have to give as little care as we can possibly get away with.
- The new reality is that we have to spend as little money as possible.
- We need to figure out how to give as much care as we possibly can in this new era.
- Our challenge is to promote as much health as possible.
- Our task is to determine how to promote the maximum amount of health care for the minimum expenditure of money. The real question is how to accomplish this task rather than how much care to give (Finkelman, pp. 81–82).

Health Care Expenditures Predominantly Spent for Illness Care

National health expenditures were $1,424.5 billion in 2001, 14.1 percent of the gross domestic product. This total includes expenses from the following, in order of greatest amount received: hospitals, physicians and clinical services, nursing home care, prescription drugs, dental services, other durable or nondurable medical products, other professional services, other personal healthcare, and home health care. *Notice here that home health care is last in expenditure amount and no where is prevention, health promotion, or public health service even mentioned.* In addition the gross domestic product for health care includes construction and research. How does this compare with other national expenditures?

> Approximately 81 percent of total federal government expenditures in 1997 were spent on four major items: Social Security, defense, interest on the national debt, and health care services. Social Security is the largest component, but health care programs are a close second and

exceed expenditures on national defense. In fact, federal government
expenditures for Medicare and Medicaid (over $300 billion) exceeded
all other federal expenditures (such as education, transportation, space
exploration, etc.) combined (Whetsell, p. 1).

In 2002, total CMS program outlays were $377.2 billion, 18.6 percent of the Federal
Budget. Medicare skilled nursing facility benefit payments declined from $14.2 billion in
2002 to $13.6 billion in 2003. Medicare home health agency benefit payments increased
between 2002 and 2003 from $12.2 billion to $13.6 billion. The national health expenditures per person were $205 in 1965 and grew steadily to reach $5,035 by 2001.

Providers

The number of inpatient hospital facilities decreased from 6,770 in December 1975 to
6,002 in December 2002. Total inpatient hospital beds have dropped from 46.5 beds per
1,000 enrolled in 1974 to 24.5 in 2002, a decrease of 47 percent. The total number of
Medicare certified beds in short-stay hospitals showed a steady increase from less than
800,000 at the beginning of the program and peaked at 1,025,000 in 1984–1986. Since that
time, the number has dropped to 844,000. Note: A portion of this decline is due to the
reclassification of some short-stay hospitals as critical access hospitals.

Between 1990 and 2001, the number of short-stay hospital discharges increased from
10.5 million to 12.2 million, an increase of 16 percent. The short-stay hospital average
length of stay decreased significantly from 9.0 days in 1990 to 6.0 days in 2001, a decrease
of 33 percent. Likewise, the average length of stay for excluded units decreased significantly from 19.5 days in 1990 to 12.0 days in 2001, a decrease of 3 percent.

The number of psychiatric hospitals grew to about 400 by 1976, where it remained until
the start of the prospective payment system (PPS) in 1983. After PPS, the number
increased to over 700 in the early 1990s and has since dropped to 494.

The number of skilled nursing facilities (SNFs) increased rapidly during the 1960s,
decreased during the first half of the 1970s, generally increased thereafter to over 15,000
in the late 1990s and again decreased, reaching 14,755 in 2001.

The number of participating home health agencies has fluctuated considerably over the
years, most recently almost doubling in number from 1990 to almost 11,000 in 1997, when
the Balanced Budget Act was passed, and then decreasing by a third to just over 6,800.

Consumers and Third-Party Payers

Who paid for this health care? A low percentage are out-of-pocket expenditures (18 percent in 1999). You and I paid this. This amount is increasing. The rest was paid by third
party private health insurance, state and federal funding, and other private funds.
Uninsured (4 percent) consumed part of the private funds.

The ratio of Medicare aged users of any type of covered service has grown from 367 per
1,000 enrolled in 1967 to 916 per 1,000 enrolled in 2002. About 30 million persons

received a reimbursed service under Medicare fee-for-service during 2000, and almost 43 million persons used Medicaid services or had a premium paid on their behalf in 2000. 28.8 million persons received reimbursable fee-for-service physician services under Medicare during 2000, and 19.1 under Medicaid during 2000. 20.5 million persons received prescribed drugs under Medicaid during 2000.

Persons enrolled for Medicare coverage increased from 19.1 million in 1966 to a projected 40.6 million in 2002, a 113 percent increase. On average, the number of Medicaid enrollees in 2002 is estimated to be about 39.9 million, the largest group being children (18.4 million or 46 percent). In 2000, 12.3 percent of the population was enrolled in the Medicaid program. Medicare enrollees with end-stage renal disease increased from just under 67 thousand in 1980 to 356 thousand in 2001, an increase of 431 percent. Medicare state buy-ins have grown from about 2.8 million beneficiaries in 1975 to over 5.7 million beneficiaries in 2001, an increase of about 104 percent. The average number of dually enrolled persons (that is, persons covered by both Medicare and Medicaid) during 2000 amounted to about 6.4 million persons.

Looking at these statistics, some problems with our health care system are immediately evident. First, we do not stress prevention in our health care system. Contrast this with Japan, which spends about half of what we do per person for health care spending by heavily stressing prevention. Knowing this, some US employers have health screening programs to promote healthy lifestyles with employees. The idea behind such health promotion programs is to reward those who do not smoke, who are at their ideal weight, and who regularly exercise. By sponsoring these programs, employees are less likely to need expensive illness care. Second, with the many chronic health care needs of an aging US population, having very little spent on home care, coupled with insufficient public health services, seems very inadequate. Contrast this with the Australians who have kept health care costs down by using an extensive public health system (which includes home care). Third, look at the overbedding problem (63 percent occupancy rate) in hospitals. This represents whole floors or wings—or facilities—not being used. Hospitals have closed. Another downsizing strategy has been to merge health care systems. Fourth, uncompensated care is another issue. We have 43 million uninsured people here in the United States. If they need any health care, they need to either pay for it themselves, or the health care provider takes the loss to provide care to them. In addition to the poor, this group includes many people working for small businesses, who cannot afford to offer health insurance benefits for employees.

Health Care Dilemma

Can you see how interrelated all the issues in **Exhibit 6–2** are? Many of our societal illness care dilemmas are caused by a series of events that all contribute—or add—to the problem. For instance, Hill-Burton funding for hospitals emphasized tertiary care, created overbedding, influenced more expenditures for tertiary care than primary care, and changed responsibility for hospital funding from a local or state level to a federal level.

Exhibit 6–2 Health Care Issues

- Quality.
- Cost.
- Access.
- Entitlements.
- Health care personnel shortages.
- Focus on illness rather than health.
- Fraud and abuse.
- Overbedded hospitals.
- Health maintenance and prevention are not a priority.
- Health care has become a business transaction.
- We have lost the "family doctor for life" concept.
- Caring is often absent.
- Health care is administered by lay caregivers in the home who are not always aware of patient care needs.

Advancements such as antibiotics, anesthetics, and new technology that had made previously untreatable illnesses treatable compounds this. More people then required hospitalization, and expected health care entitlements for cadillac care. People were either unaware of health promotion and prevention, or not taking responsibility to do it. Each of these issues, and the measures taken to deal with them, can easily result in more societal dilemmas that make things worse, while improving something else.

Peter Kongstvedt, a proponent of economic theory, observed that there are three major dilemmas in health care: universal coverage, paying for it, and containing costs. According to economic theory, it is possible to achieve any two but not the third. For example, if you achieve universal coverage and pay for it, costs will be very high. If you contain costs and pay for it, you will not be able to achieve coverage for everyone. See **Exhibit 6–3**.

On the other hand, if one subscribes to the quantum physics theory, then it becomes important that all of us think we will be successful in solving our health care dilemmas. Here we must believe that we can conquer all three economic dilemmas. We just have not figured out how to do it yet! Perhaps if we could change to a health perspective we could avoid many of the present illness costs. As a side note, it would be interesting to see whether we could all fix our societal health care problems if we made a massive effort to truly believe that it could be fixed!!

Finkelman (2001) sums it up very nicely:

> The United States has struggled for some time to determine the best way to 'achieve reasonably equitable distribution of health care, without losing control of total spending on health care, and without suffocating the delivery system with controls and regulations that inhibit technical progress.' This struggle continues today. Most industrialized countries have chosen to focus on equitable distribution of health care by providing universal coverage; however, the United States continues to vacillate

Exhibit 6–3 Pick Any Two

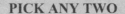

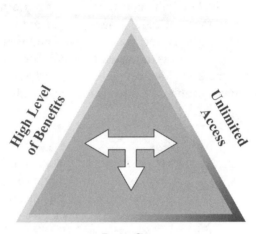

Low Cost

From: Kongstvedt, P., MD, FACP. Capgemini, US, LLC.

between equity and innovative dynamism. The result has been one of limited success on both sides. [Author note: Neither have been successful.]

A definite result of this struggle has been the development of the medical-industrial complex. Health care has changed from a social good to a product. Health care delivery has become commercialized, and health care professionals, such as hospitals and physicians, have turned more toward business techniques, such as advertising, to survive. The rapid growth in hospitals and other types of health care facilities puts pressure on all providers to find patients. This pressure has led to economic problems, increasing costs, and new health care delivery approaches. Not all of these factors have been negative as some changes have resulted in improvement with better management and increased focus on community care (p. 3).

Five Players: Consumers, Providers, Payers, Suppliers, and Regulators

To better understand this complicated health care system and where it is presently, it is necessary to examine the five key players in the health care arena: consumers, providers, payers, suppliers, and regulators. Simplistically, *consumers* receive the health care, *providers* give the care, *payers* finance the care, *suppliers* provide supplies to the providers, and *regulators* set laws, rules and regulations that must be followed while giving and paying for the care. Yet realistically, these terms are more complicated. First, these players are all integrated together in a health care system where actions taken by one player affect the other players. So as the federal government passes a law establishing a set of regulations, the providers must make sure they effectively meet the regulations; the payers may be involved in meeting or policing the regulations; the consumers can be affected; and the suppliers may have to change supplies to meet the regulations. Second, at times players intermingle functions. For instance, the consumer receives the care but is a payer when paying deductibles; the federal government owns the Veterans Administration hospitals (provider) yet is a regulator with the Centers for Medicare and Medicaid Services (CMS) office; or Kaiser Permanente (payer) owns health care organizations (provider).

Consumers

Definition

Consumers receive health care. Consumers directly pay for health care in the following ways:
- Share premium costs with employers;
- Pay *deductibles*—the amount of money a consumer must pay before the insurance company will pay for health care services
- Make *copayments*—the amount of money a consumer must pay out of pocket for every health care service received;
- Pay for services not covered by the insurance plan;
- Pay amounts above what the payer considers "reasonable and customary";
- Can choose to pay cash for services

Consumers are patients in hospitals, residents in long-term care, clients in home care, or enrollees in managed care organizations who receive health care. Another insurance term for the consumer is "covered life." (Don't we have a wonderful way of dehumanizing people?) This concept seems simple enough, but in the US system it is complicated by several factors. First, who pays for the health care? Some consumers pay cash for care. Examples include the wealthy or the Amish. More often, consumers use health insurance. However, even with health insurance, consumers pay up front in several ways—by sharing insurance premium costs; by paying deductibles, the amount of money a consumer must pay before the insurance company will pay for health care services; by paying copayments, the amount of money a consumer must pay out of pocket for every health care service received; by paying for any services not covered by the insurance plan such as alternative therapies or plastic surgery; by paying the amount above what the payer has established as a reasonable and customary charge,[3] such as for outpatient services; or by choosing to pay cash for a health care service so

---

[3] As mentioned previously, this is true for coinsurance deductibles, and what is above the reasonable and customary costs with regular insurance. However, with Medicare Part A and Medicaid, other than billing the deductible and coinsurance, it is illegal to bill the patient for the amount of reimbursement not paid by the government. In Medicare Part B providers can bill up to 15 percent more for services than the cost covered by Medicare.

it will not be necessary to go through the insurance company. One advantage for employed consumers are the medical savings accounts, using pre-tax dollars.

As the price of health care rises, consumers are paying more and employers are paying less. **Exhibits 6–4** and **6–5** illustrate how deductibles and copayments can add up for the consumer. All employer-based plans now have a limit the employee has to pay annually— often $1,000 for an individual or $2,000 for a family. Once an employee has reached the limit, the employer pays 100 percent of the medical expenses. However, there are no limits for the Medicare consumer. Thus for the non-working elderly, health care costs can quickly deplete life savings. Let's look at two typical scenarios. An elderly couple, Mr. and Mrs. Oldfield, have a nice savings and own a home. Mr. Oldfield experiences an expensive illness resulting in the savings being entirely depleted—even with insurance and Medicare. What are Mr. or Mrs. Oldfield to do in case either experiences another costly expense or illness? In a second scenario, Mrs. Ancient has lost her husband, is below the poverty level, has no savings, and has no insurance other than Medicare. Mrs. Ancient develops a heart problem that results in her needing to take expensive medications. How can she pay for the medications when her entire monthly income is already spent on food and lodging expenses? Medicare does not cover the medication expense.

> **Definition**
>
> *Medical savings accounts*—a tax-free account provided by employers. Here the employee can annually set up an account for an amount of money the employee expects to spend on health care for the year. At the end of the year, money not spent goes back to the employer.

Exhibit 6–4 Deductibles and Co-Payments: A Patient Example

Hospital bill	$20,000	
Patient deductible	-$ 200	
	$19,800	Medical charges after deductible paid
Medical charges after deductible paid	$19,800	
	x .20	
	$ 3,960	Amount of medical expenses to be paid by patient/copayment

Deductible must be paid before the insurer will pay its portion.
Patient must pay deductible and copayment.

Deductible	$ 200	
	+$3,960	
	$4,160	Total amount to be paid by patient

Despite insurance coverage, the patient must still pay $4,160, which is not a small amount.

Source: Finkelman, A. (2001). *Managed Care: A Nursing Perspective.* Upper Saddle River, NJ: Prentice Hall.

Exhibit 6–5 Out-Of-Pocket Expenses: More Than You Think—An Example

Physician's bill for office visit: Bronchitis	$120
Insurer's reasonable and customary charge for this visit	$100
Patient's co-payment of 30 percent ($100 x .30) =	$ 30
Uncovered part of bill to be paid by patient ($120 - $100) =	$ 20
Patient's total out-of-pocket expenses	
Co-payment ($30) + uncovered portion ($20) =	$ 50

The $50 represents 41.6 percent of the total charge of $120.

Source: Finkelman, A. (2001). *Managed Care: A Nursing Perspective*. Upper Saddle River, NJ: Prentice Hall.

Then there are *uninsured* consumers, over 43 million in the United States. This includes 15 percent (11 million) of our children. The uninsured includes several groups that one would expect such as the unemployed, rural, or migrant workers. However, this group also includes people who are self-employed, are employed in small businesses, are college students, or are early retirees not old enough for Medicare but not poor enough for Medicaid. Even when employers offer health insurance, 6 million employees turn it down. Why? Because the employers are sharing the cost of health insurance with workers. And workers making less than $7/hour generally need all their money for living expenses. The health insurance premium costs are too expensive.

Thus *access* to health care remains a problem for many in the United States. This reduced access actually can create more expenses in the long run societally because it is less expensive to provide care based on prevention or early interventions than to let illness progress and become very serious before giving the care. As the numbers of uninsured rise, do they have a right to health care? If so, who will pay?

Presently there are some trends eroding health insurance coverage:

- Rising premium costs, both for persons who have access to insurance through their employers and for those who buy insurance individually.
- An increasing number of temporary and part-time workers, who seldom receive health care coverage.
- A reduction in explicit coverage, most notably pharmaceutical benefits.
- Greater de facto limitations on covered care, especially by health maintenance organizations.
- A broad shift from traditional HMOs requiring very low out-of-pocket payments to point-of-service plans and preferred provider organizations requiring high payments by patients.
- Loss of Medicaid coverage due to welfare reform.
- The rising cost of "Medigap" coverage for the elderly, which leads to substantial underinsurance.
- The crackdown on illegal immigrants and the reduction in services to legal immigrants.

- The trend away from community ratings of individual insurance premiums, which results in rising costs and, hence, reduced rates of coverage for middle-aged persons (Finkelman, p. 43).

Another problem with the uninsured—although others with insurance do the same thing—is that they often use the emergency room as their primary care provider. This clogs the emergency room with patients who have primary care needs and increases patient wait times.

Managed care (more completely defined in the Payers section of this chapter) has had a tremendous impact on consumers. For example, the consumer may have to change providers based on the insurance plan their employer chooses. Or, if consumers experience an acute illness, they are transferred to various units or facilities, yet still are not well enough to care for themselves when discharged. If no one at home can care for them, what can the consumer do? (This often becomes a major problem for the provider as well as the consumer. The provider faces the financial and ethical dilemma of discharging the patient, versus providing additional care at a financial loss.)

This problem has resulted in more uncompensated, untrained caregivers—most often relatives with no nursing training—having to care for the consumer in the home. They need more basic care information on how to appropriately care for their loved ones. They need basics like turning frequently to prevent bedsores, and encouraging hydration and better nutrition, which a public health nurse could spearhead in the community if public health programs were more adequately funded.

> Psychiatric care has been coping with managed care for a long time.... Decreased [length of stay] has led to the need for rapid inpatient assessment, which is not always effective. Most of the medications that are used require time for results, and thus most patients are discharged with limited improvement and... with few choices for follow-up care. The InterQual Intensity, Severity, and Discharge psychiatric criteria (InterQual ISD) has been used as the managed care standard for decision making about patient admissions and discharges from inpatient treatment. Some research has indicated that these criteria may not be appropriate and may decrease lengths of stay when they should not be decreased.
>
> Psychiatrists, psychiatric nurses, psychologists, and social workers who provide psychotherapy have been confronting decreasing reimbursement rates, fewer number of authorized visits, a growing pile of forms to complete, and increasing time required to negotiate with insurers over reimbursement (Finkelman, p. 402).

Along with this problem, as the US population is aging, more people are experiencing chronic illness. If on Medicare or Medicaid, there is inadequate health care coverage for chronic illness. This is where both home health and public health, both drastically underfunded, could make a significant contribution. Often a consumer must deal with lack of medical care, and this has only worsened with managed care, not to mention expensive drugs, and, if necessary, no one to care for them in the home. More serious ill-nesses, and/or acute admissions to other health care facilities, that might have been pre-vented with better home care, have also resulted.

Another consistent problem for consumers is *patient education* and *prevention* meas-ures. Physicians are illness oriented, and with managed care, have to see many patients to make money, so, most often, patient education does not occur. When patients are acutely ill, have just delivered a baby, or are admitted for immediate surgery, they are so ill or exhausted that it is not possible to provide patient education. The good news is that most same-day surgery pre-operative programs will provide educational information to patients. Other sources are the physician's office, the internet, the alternative therapist, or the health food store. One obvious answer, used by other countries, is to have the public health department do more population-based education and prevention programs. However, pub-lic health continues to be drastically underfunded in the United States.

Aside from the problems with paying for health care, *consumer protection* has resulted in various public policy mandates being adopted at the local, state, and national levels. For example, the Health Insurance Portability and Accountability Act of 1996 (HIPAA) is con-cerned with confidentiality of the medical record; Joint Commission on Accreditation of Health Care Organizations (JCAHO), and many states, now requires organizations to report sentinel events[4]; and The Institute of Medicine's Committee on the Quality of Health Care in America is regularly releasing quality and safety consumer issues and the need for better mechanisms to prevent the reoccurrence of these issues.

Providers

> **Definition**
>
> *Providers*—The individuals (nurses, physicians, dentists, and other health care personnel) and organizations (hospitals, outpatient facilities, long-term care facilities, home care agencies, or other health care organizations) providing the health care services.

Providers are the individuals (nurses, physicians, dietitians, social workers, pharmacists, physical or respiratory therapists, dentists, and other health care personnel), and organizations (hospitals, outpatient facilities, long-term care facilities, home care agencies, or other health care organizations) providing the health care services. Some common provider organizational terms are: MCO, *managed care organization* ("an HMO, PPO, provider-sponsored network, or other health plan models that integrates the financing and delivery of health care") (Finkelman, p. 485); or *health services organization* (HSO). Health care organizations are groups of people working within an organizational structure to provide health care services to consumers. Health care services can be provided across the continuum of care, from how to achieve health, such as alternative or preventive care, to treating disease, such as acute, chronic, restorative, or palliative care.

---

[4] A sentinel event is an unexpected occurrence involving death or serious physical or phsycosocial injury, or the risk thereof. Serious injury specifically includes the loss of limb or function. The phrase, "or risk thereof" includes any process variation for which a recurrence would carry a significant chance of a seri-ous adverse outcome (www.jcaho.org/sentinel). Examples of such events include: patient suicide, infant abduction or discharge to the wrong family, rape, surgery on the wrong body part or on the wrong patient, and unanticipated death.

Health care organizations are classified in several ways based on profit status:

- *not-for-profit* (where profit is used by the health care organization for additional capital needs, working capital needs, capital replacement needs, or improving services or quality);
- *for-profit* (where the profit is paid to owners or investors);
- *sectarian* (affiliated with a particular religious group such as Catholic, Methodist, or Seventh Day Adventist) as opposed to non-sectarian;
- *governmental or publicly-owned* (where cities, counties, states, or the federal governments own, partially finance, or control the health care organizations). For example, a city governs a city hospital, the county runs a health department, the state gives partial funding to a university hospital, and the federal government owns the Veterans Administration facilities.

The federal government also provides other public health services as previously mentioned. In fact, the Office of Disease Prevention and Health Promotion in the Department of Health and Human Services has published a national set of health objectives called *Healthy People 2010* (*www.health.gov/healthypeople*). It will be interesting to see how much of this gets accomplished in our tertiary-based health care system.

A health care organization can be a single, small free-standing clinic or long-term care facility, or a much larger thousand-bed hospital. It can be multiorganizational where two or more organizations have grouped together in various ways to better achieve delivery of care. The combinations are limitless with multiorganizational arrangements—alliances, cooperative linkages, networks, and joint ventures. They can result from management contracts, umbrella corporations, mergers, and other consolidations. The arrangements may be with other similar organizations,[5] or may include a wide range of health care services. A single organization may actually be linked in several different arrangements, such as a hospital that has merged with another hospital, which also belongs to Voluntary Hospitals of America, a nationwide purchasing alliance. Generally there are three types of multiorganizational arrangements. The first, and most common, is for market transactions. Examples are: joining Premier Alliance (to purchase supplies or equipment at lower costs) and having contracts with insurance companies or employers who supply patients. The second multiorganizational arrangement is where the health care organization must participate with another entity. This arrangement might include collective bargaining agreements, federal or state regulatory bodies, bond rating services, and utilization management companies. The third arrangement is a voluntary one. Here a mutual benefit or gain is realized by the organizations in the arrangement. For instance, a rural hospital is linked with a medical center. The rural hospital can then refer patients who need more specific tertiary care to the medical center; the medical center needs "feeder" hospitals for patients.

Health care organizations, regardless of category, have an owner or a governing body or board. The body's role is trifold: 1) to establish/approve the mission, vision, and strategic objectives of the organization (formulated by the organization's executive senior management group) and the broad responsibility to make sure these objectives are fulfilled (this includes having an appropriate budget to accomplish the objectives); 2) to hire and

---

[5] For more information on multiorganizational arrangements see: Longest, B., Rakieh, J., & Darr, K. (2000). *Managing Health Services Organizations and Systems*, 4th ed. Baltimore: Health Professions Press.

evaluate the chief executive officer (CEO) of the organization; and 3) to ensure the quality of the medical care.

Choosing board members often becomes a political process. A board member should be familiar with the community, have a good reputation, be familiar with good business practices, have served well in the past or had experience on other boards, and have an understanding of the patient care process. In health care, often boards are self-perpetuating, meaning that present board members select new board members. At times the CEO has voting privileges on the board, as do physicians. In a way it is a conflict of interest for the CEO or physicians practicing in the organization to be on the board; however, at times they best understand the issues involved with delivering care. In fact, JCAHO recommends physician board members (remember that JCAHO was started by physicians). Compensation of board members is rare, about 20 percent in all non-governmental hospitals (Griffith, 1999).

Unless the medical staff is directly hired by the organization, the health care organization will have a *medical staff organization* in hospitals, sometimes called a *professional staff organization* in other settings. The medical staff organization is a separate association with its own bylaws and governing structure. It has a dotted line responsibility (meaning that the CEO does not have supervisory responsibility for them) to the CEO. Thus the group members are not employees of the organization, and are paid independently for their services. Although the medical staff group is mainly physicians, it can also include other professionals such as dentists, clinical psychologists, podiatrists, nurse midwives, nurse practitioners, and chiropractors. In order to receive *practice privileges* in the facility, the physician has to be recommended by the medical staff organization who examine credentials and competency, the recommendation has to be approved by the governing board, the medical staff organization extends the privilege of membership, and the physician then accepts the bylaws of the medical staff organization. Another title for this group of physicians is *attending physicians*.

Typical functions of the medical staff organization are illustrated by the committee structure often used for hospitals.

- The *credentials committee* reviews qualifications of the membership and recommends practice privileges to the executive committee (and ultimately to the governing board).
- The *pharmacy and therapeutics committee* develops the drug formulary, monitors drug use, and sets drug usage policies.
- The *surgical case review committee* reviews need for surgery and evaluates the pre- and post-operative diagnoses.
- The *medical records review committee* checks on the timely completion and quality of the medical record.
- The *utilization review committee* examines length of stay and use of ancillary services.
- The *quality assessment committee* examines the appropriateness of patient treatment. (This committee can replace the surgical case review and medical records review committees in smaller hospitals.)

Additional committees can include infection control, risk management, safety, blood use, disaster planning, bylaws, and nominating committees. If there are problems with medical staff performance, the medical staff organization will deal with the problems. One common problem is that the physician has not completed the medical record in a timely fashion. In this case, the physician will not be able to admit patients until getting caught up with documentation. If a serious problem occurs, this becomes an issue, not only for the medical staff organization, but for the CEO, the health care organization executive group, and the governing board as well.

The executive group in a health care organization includes the following members: the chief executive officer (CEO), the chief operating officer (COO), the chief financial officer (CFO), the chief nursing—or patient services—officer (CNO), general counsel, and other vice presidents from human resources, plant services, medical officer, and/or information services. Membership depends upon the size of the organization as well as upon the CEO's and governing board's orientation.

In multiorganizational arrangements, such as strategic alliances, there are a couple governance models used. In the *centralized model*, there is one governing board responsible for all health care facilities in the alliance. The advantage is that there are not as many stakeholders to deal with, but the disadvantage is that they may not be aware of local issues and differences. The individual health care organizations may have an advisory board that has no legal or fiduciary authority. In a *decentralized model*, there is a system governing board that shares governance responsibilities with other smaller individual boards within the system. The smaller boards can be set up for specific organizations such as for each individual health care facility; for specific functions such as insurance companies, hospitals, or physicians; or for regions. With this model there can be more local autonomy. The disadvantage is that with the many boards, confusion and conflict can result within the system as a whole. In multiorganizational arrangements, there is usually a corporate executive, along with a corporate executive team, for the entire system as well as having a CEO, and executive group, for each facility.

Providers generally have several payer contracts, each can pay differently and use different formats for payment. It is generally necessary to electronically send information to payers.

As managed care has been implemented, health care organizations have responded by using a number of strategies. Providers, such as health care organizations and physicians, have merged to serve more patients; they have expanded services—such as hospitals expanding ambulatory and long-term care services, or physicians opening free-standing surgical centers—or organizations have closed and physicians have retired. The hospital often serves regional needs, or links with other hospitals to serve regional needs, and has survived.

One survival strategy has been to develop an *integrated delivery system* (IDS) to provide a broad range of services, rather than just to have one free-standing health care organization. An integrated system is economically and clinically linked through ownership or by contract. In *horizontal integration*, a facility combines with like facilities. A prime example of horizontal integration has been occurring since the mid-1980s with a number of hospitals in a community merging into multi-hospital systems, or, at least, affiliating with other hospitals in some fashion. Examples of the largest multi-system health care groups include Kaiser Permanente, Columbia/HCA Healthcare, and Tenet Healthcare. In long-term care, the largest multi-system is Beverly Enterprises while in home care, it is Gentiva Health Care. In 1985, 35 percent of community hospitals were affiliated with a health care system while, by 1998, 42 percent (2,142 hospitals) were affiliated with a health care system. Presently this movement has stagnated, perhaps because it now exists in most communities. Other problems with these affiliations are the loss of autonomy, as well as less sensitivity to local community health care needs.

Horizontal integration achieves cost-savings in several ways. First, services can be consolidated to save money. For instance, only one human resource department or business office is necessary, and policies can be developed, or technology can be purchased for the whole system. Second, economies of scale can be achieved when purchasing supplies, saving considerable money. Third, larger organizations have better bargaining positions when negotiating with managed care plans allowing one person or department to negotiate for all the facilities. Fourth, marketing can occur for all the facilities. Fifth, each facility can benefit the other by broadening available services, i.e., "the small rural hospital would provide basic general care; the moderate-sized hospital, more specialized care and equipment; and the regional hospital, the most sophisticated and expensive special types of care" (Raffel and Raffel, p. 137). Services can be broadened in the specialty areas as well. Let's use cardiovascular services, one of the few remaining profit centers for hospitals, as an example. Between 1985 and 1999, open-heart surgery programs increased by 47 percent, and cardiac catheterization services grew by 70 percent.

In *vertical integration*, an organization integrates as many different health care services as possible, services offered are "womb to tomb," or, to put it another way, they offer a continuum of care—primary to tertiary. The idea behind this strategy is that patients rarely or never have to leave the system for health care services, and, while there, have convenient accessibility to the care. In addition, it is advantageous to have various care delivery sites in close proximity based on patient needs. For example, it is helpful to have the lab and X-ray departments near the primary care physician, or nurse practitioner, offices. Or, for same day surgery, to have all the needed pre- and post-operative services near the operating room. The idea is to provide quick, efficient services so patients do not need to spend a whole day just getting needed health care services.

Services in an integrated system might include:

- Acute care,
- Primary care,
- Specialty ambulatory care,
- Acute rehabilitation,
- Subacute care,
- Home care,
- Long-term care,
- Traditional skilled nursing care,
- Assisted living, and
- Durable equipment services (Finkelman, p. 64).

Although vertical integration is a popular concept, in reality some of it has been difficult to achieve. "Health care organizations poured $5 billion into integration strategies over the last decade, but now those organizations acknowledge that their investments didn't always pay off and say that future integration activities will be sharply reduced" (Haugh, pp. 33–34). Two examples of unsuccessful vertical integretion have been: 1) hospitals buying physician practices; "hospital-owned practices turn out to be 50 times less profitable than those owned by medical groups or practice management companies . . . the median loss of $47,000 is typical" (Hudson, p. 26). Now many hospitals are selling off the physician practices and restructuring loans. Presently, the best options with physicians seem to be contracting with physician groups for services. 2) Some of the large multi-hospital systems expanded their services by developing managed care insurance lines that could compete with existing insurance plans. Most of these hospital-based plans are losing money and many have closed. What most health care organizations choose to do is to take the middle ground in vertical integration, doing part of the services themselves and outsourcing other services.

In making the decision to outsource (for such things as billing or housekeeping), it is helpful to evaluate how effective this collaborative arrangement will be. Chyna (2000) presents a weighted evaluative tool that can be used to determine whether to outsource. Hospitals and Health Networks (2001) published a helpful insert on what has been outsourced, how it is evaluated, what is included in contracts, and levels of satisfaction with outsourced services.

Within health care organizations, a consistent, nagging communication problem keeps occurring. Ideally, during an episode of illness, all providers need to communicate well with each other, as well as with the patient and the patient's family, and work as a team to provide the patient care. Unfortunately, this often does not happen. If anything, care has become more fragmented with managed care. Providers often do not communicate and the quality of care suffers. It is common for a patient to be transferred to several divisions or facilities to receive care. Important information about the patient may not be communicated from one location to another. Most often, the patient experiences new staff members who provide the care. Relationships with care workers, already established, do not continue in the new division or facility. Patients', not to mention health care workers', emotional needs, or support connections, are often disregarded. The result is fragmentation of care— even when one has a good insurance policy.

Another problem providers experience is *uncompensated care*. If a patient is uninsured and is unable to pay for care, what should the provider do? Care for the patient anyway and take a loss? Or refuse to care for the patient? What about the ethics of all this? Historically, the Hill Burton Act, and later COBRA legislation, specified that hospitals receiving money from the federal government for building projects or for Medicare reimbursement, must agree to provide care for the uninsured. So hospitals would "cost shift" this expense, charge more to the wealthy or insured patients, and use the resulting profit to pay for the uninsured. Now, as profit margins have been curtailed, most health care providers do not have enough "cost-shift" money to offset uncompensated care. Too often providing care for the uninsured represents a true loss of money to the provider. Because of this, some providers will refuse to provide care unless a patient can pay. This translates into the patient having insurance or paying cash before services are rendered.

Along similar lines, providers are concerned with *payer mix*. The issue is that different payers actually pay different amounts for services. For example, if most of the patient population have Medicaid or Medicare payers, it is probable that the provider will lose money as neither will pay the full amount needed to care for the patients. (In fact, it is possible that they pay less than 50 cents for every dollar spent.) Providers prefer having a majority of private-pay patients who will provide better reimbursement. Even with private-pay patients, if discounts are given to payers, (discounts may be just a flat discount on all services rendered, or the discount may be a sliding scale based on volume), the provider must know whether the true reimbursement amount can still provide a profit, or at least cover costs. If the discount is "too deep," losses will be incurred.

Presently providers face another issue. Consumers via the internet, regulators, and payers are examining *provider performance*. Here data is collected on patient outcomes—length of stay, readmission rates, adverse reactions, complications, infections, deaths, number of medications per patient, and consumer satisfaction/complaints. (This is discussed further in Chapter 2.)

Payers use the performance data to compare providers' performance and determine who gives the best care and who is less expensive. This is called *performance-based reimbursement evaluation*. Payers will use this evaluation before contracting with providers for health care services. The contract will be for a specified time and for specified services. In addition, the provider will be expected to provide evaluation data. Before the contract is renewed, the payer will again evaluate provider data.

With managed care, another provider issue emerged—*provider protection*. In HMOs, there are often rules that physicians are expected to meet to continue working for that HMO. For example, they will not order expensive or frequent diagnostic tests, nor authorize many patient hospitalizations. The idea behind the rules is to keep down expenses. Often there are monetary incentives—withholds or bonuses—paid to physicians to ensure costs do not skyrocket. *Withholds* happen when the HMO holds part of the physician or hospital income until the end of the year and pays it back to the physician or hospital based on the physician's or hospital's performance. Withholds may never be paid back to the provider, being used to cover other expenses the HMO is experiencing. *Bonuses* are another method used by payers. Here the provider receives a bonus at the end of the year based on the provider's performance, or based on the total plan performance. Such practices have recently resulted in legislation aimed at either limiting the incentives, or revealing the incentives, to consumers. Providers need protection for due process in their relationship with payers in these matters, because payers may expect that providers remain quiet about the incentives (*gag rules*). Because of all this, physicians are experiencing "frustration in their attempts to deliver ideal care, restrictions on their personal time, financial incentives that strain their professional principles, and loss of control over their clinical decisions" (Finkelman, p. 103).

Nurses are also providers; though at times we are not treated as such. One problem has been that historically, with the exception of private duty nursing, nursing costs have been bundled into room charges. Only a few organizations have broken away from this model. It is such a problem in long-term care that the therapies receive higher reimbursement, and a higher acuity level, than nursing care gets. It is another example of what is wrong with health care reimbursement as it presently exists.

Payers

Payers directly pay for health care services, i.e., individuals, employers, insurance companies, or the government. *Individuals* who directly pay for health care services are payers as well as consumers.

Employers are payers when they choose to provide health care benefits for employees. They can do this in one of two ways: 1) purchase (or make available) health insurance for employees. In this scenario, the employer is not a direct payer of health care services. Or 2) the employer can be self insured (usually only larger employers are self insured), directly paying employee health care costs. In this case, the employer is the payer, and pays the insurance company to administer

> **Definition**
>
> *Payers*—directly pay for health care services, i.e., individuals, employers, insurance companies, or the government.

the insurance plan. The employer sets up the limitations of the plan including annual limits per employee, provides claim forms for employees, verifies employee claims, and pays providers from the employer budget. Employees can be confused and think that they have insurance, such as Blue Cross, when in actuality their employer is self-insured and Blue Cross is only the intermediary administering the insurance plan. When self-insured, health care costs are listed as a line item on the employer budget. This can create the need for huge mid-year budget readjustments for unexpected large costs such as an employee experiencing a catastrophic illness costing the employer $500,000. In this situation the employer must find the additional money to cover the health care line item in the budget.

Insurance companies provide individual or group insurance coverage for *covered lives*—the individuals included in the plan—for a contracted amount of time, often a year. The purchaser(s) pay a premium to the insurance company. In group plans, the premium payment often is shared with employees. Generally individuals, or even small business employers, pay more for insurance premiums than large employers. To counteract this problem, Hawaii established several health maintenance organizations (HMOs) for small businesses, and aggregated the entire small business population together to get lower rates for small businesses.

Governments are the biggest force in the health care payer arena. The *federal government* is a major payer, covering about 45 percent to 55 percent of the total health care revenue. Federal government insurance programs include Medicare, part of Medicaid, the Federal Employees Health Benefit Program (FEHBP), TriCare, and the Civilian Health and Medical Program of the Uniform Services (CHAMPUS). Thus, as the federal government starts some payment strategy, the other insurers will follow suit. The *state governments*, often the state's largest employer, have been responsible for health insurance for state employees, in addition to sharing responsibilities for Medicaid programs with the federal government.

The term, *third party payers*, or *insurers*, refers to insurance companies, employers, or government agencies who provide health care insurance. The insurance company acts as an administrator of the pool of money collected from all its members, paying, or

> ### Definition
>
> *Third party payers*, or *insurers*, are the insurance companies, employers, or government agencies who provide health care insurance.

> ### Definition
>
> *Retrospective payment*—payment for care occurred after the care was given. This occurred with *indemnity insurance*. Here the consumer chose the provider, the provider determined what was charged, and the insurance company paid it (*fee-for-service*). The insurance contract was with the individual or employer.

> ### Definition
>
> The current insurance reimbursement model generally used is *prospective payment*. Here the payer determines the cost of care *before* the care is given. The provider is then told how much will be paid to give the care. This is an example of *managed care*—any method of health care delivery that is designed to cut costs yet provide needed health care services. In managed care, payers determine the amount they will reimburse for medical services.

underwriting, the defined illness care coverage to a provider when the consumer has received health care services. With insurance there is a risk to the insurance company. What if more people need coverage than anticipated? Obviously, it will benefit the insurance company to serve a larger population. This reduces the risk, and has the additional benefit of costing less to administer the plan. It is also better to have healthier people in the plan. The federal government, with Medicare, has a problem with this issue because it serves an older population who are more likely to need illness care. To determine the risk, the insurance company uses *actuarial data*—a statistical method that takes into account such factors as the age and sex of enrollees, past use, and cost of medical services—to determine both premium costs and definition of coverage. The purchaser's perception of risk is also an issue. Insurance is only worth purchasing if people perceive that they may experience a risk, such as expensive surgery or other care.

RETROSPECTIVE PAYMENT

Historically, the typical health insurance was *indemnity insurance*, where payment occurred after the care was given. This was called *retrospective payment*. Here the consumer chose the provider, the provider determined what was charged, and the insurance company paid it (*fee-for-service*). The insurance contract was with the individual or employer. Except for those who pay cash, true indemnity insurance is largely nonexistent today because health insurance plans use some form of managed care, or financial incentives, to be cost effective.

PROSPECTIVE PAYMENT

Like the name implies, *managed care* refers to any method of health care delivery that is designed to cut costs yet provide needed services (i.e., use the least expensive option for delivery of care, only pay for necessary services, control costs by contracting and telling providers what will be paid for services *before* the services are delivered, and involve consumers in paying for part of their care). In managed care, *payers* determine the amount they will reimburse for a medical service.

Generally the reimbursement strategy is *prospective payment*, where the payer determines the cost of care before the care is given. The provider is then told how much will be paid to give the care. This is called the *prospective payment system (PPS)*.

Service Benefit Plans

Service benefit plans, an example of both prospective payment and managed care, directly pay providers after negotiating and specifying the prices paid for each health care service. In service benefit plans, the patient pays part of the costs with deductibles and coinsurance. Medicare, and preferred provider organizations (PPOs), such as Blue Cross, have service benefit plans. (This can be confusing because Blue Cross and Medicare also offer HMOs, a direct service delivery plan, discussed in the next section.)

Medicare, supported from payroll cash contributions put into the Medicare Trust Fund, pays for health care services for Americans age 65 and older, for some people with disabilities under age 65, and for people with End-Stage Renal Disease. Medicare covers about 75 percent of the health care cost. Presently, there are approximately 34 million older adults and 5 million disabled people with Medicare benefits. In fact, "Medicare beneficiaries comprise one in seven Americans, and this proportion is expected to grow to one in five by 2030, when the number of beneficiaries will exceed 76 million people" (Longest, Rakich, and Darr, p. 97). There has been some debate whether there will be enough Medicare payroll cash contributions once the baby boomers are all eligible.

Medicare is administered by the Centers for Medicare and Medicaid Services (CMS), formerly called the Health Care Finance Administration (HCFA). Medicare usage is monitored by the Medicare Payment Advisory Commission (MedPAC), that independently advises Congress about more effective, or less costly, ways to manage Medicare. CMS pays an administrative fee to *fiscal intermediaries* to carry out the actual payment system for Medicare. Fiscal intermediaries are other insurance companies who already have experience with processing insurance claims—companies such as Blue Cross. Fiscal intermediaries pay Part A and some Part B bills, which are discussed in a following section. See **Exhibit 6–6**.

Medicare divides defined services and payments into Part A, covering hospital inpatient

> **Definition**
>
> A *service benefit plan* directly specifies and pays providers after establishing and negotiating prices. In this plan, the patient pays part of the costs with deductibles and coinsurance. Medicare, and preferred provider organizations (PPOs), such as Blue Cross, use service benefit plans.

> **Definition**
>
> *Fiscal intermediaries* are other insurance companies who already have experience with processing insurance claims—companies such as Blue Cross. Fiscal intermediaries pay Part A and some Part B bills.

Exhibit 6–6 Medicare Part A

Medicare Part A (Hospital Insurance) Helps Pay for	What YOU pay in 2004* in the Original Medicare Plan
Hospital Stays: Semiprivate room, meals, general nursing, and other hospital services and supplies (this includes care in critical access hospitals and inpatient mental health care). This does not include private duty nursing, a private room unless medically necessary, or a television or telephone in your room.	**For each benefit period YOU pay:** • A total of $876 for a hospital stay of 1–60 days. • $219 per day for days 61–90 of a hospital stay. • $438 per day for days 91–150 of a hospital stay. • All costs for each day beyond 150 days.
Skilled Nursing Facility (SNF) Care: Semiprivate room, meals, skilled nursing and rehabilitative services, and other services and supplies (after a 3-day hospital stay).	**For each benefit period YOU pay:** • Nothing for the first 20 days. • Up to $109.50 per day for days 21–100. • All costs beyond the 100th day in the benefit period. If you have questions about SNF care and conditions of coverage, call your Fiscal Intermediary.
Home Health Care: Part-time skilled nursing care, physical therapy, occupational therapy, speech-language therapy, home health aide services, durable medical equipment (such as wheelchairs, hospital beds, oxygen, and walkers) and medical supplies, and other services.	**YOU pay:** • Nothing for home health care services. • 20% of the Medicare-approved amount for durable medical equipment. If you have questions about home health care and conditions of coverage, call your Regional Home Health Intermediary.
Hospice Care: Medical and support services, from a Medicare-approved hospice, for people with a terminal illness, drugs for symptom control and pain relief, and other services not otherwise covered by Medicare. Hospice care is given in your home. However, short-term hospital and inpatient respite care is covered when needed.	**YOU pay:** • A co-payment of up to $5 for outpatient prescription drugs and 5% of the Medicare-approved payment amount for inpatient respite care (short-term care given to a hospice patient by another care giver, so that the usual care giver can rest). The amount you pay for respite care can change each year. If you have questions about hospice care and conditions of coverage, call your Regional Home Health Intermediary.
Blood: Pints of blood you get at a hospital or skilled nursing facility during a covered stay.	**YOU pay:** • For the first 3 pints of blood, unless you or someone else donates blood to replace what you use.

Source: Health Care Financing Administration, 2004. (See www.questions.medicare.gov/Publications/ Pub/pdk/yourmb.pdf for updated information.)

services, skilled nursing, and some home care; and Part B, including physician services, outpatient services, diagnostic tests, laboratory services, cancer screening, home health services not covered under Part A, and medical equipment costs. Most people receive Part A automatically on their 65th birthday. They do not have to pay a premium because they, or their spouse, paid Medicare taxes while they were working. There are deductibles ($876 in 2004, which covers the first 60 days of care) and coinsurance costs for consumers in Part A. Coinsurance starts by charging $219/day for days 61 through 90, and $438/day for hospital stays beyond 90 days (2004 rates). However, under Part A providers cannot further bill consumers for services. **Exhibit 6–7** further describes Part A services and payments.

Exhibit 6–7 Medicare Part

Medicare Part B (Medical Insurance) Helps Pay for	What YOU pay in 2004* in the Original Medicare Plan
Medical and Other Services: Doctors' services (not routine physical exams), outpatient medical and surgical services and supplies, diagnostic tests, ambulatory surgery center facility fees for approved procedures, and durable medical equipment (such as wheelchairs, hospital beds, oxygen, and walkers). Also covers second surgical opinions, outpatient physical and occupational therapy including speech-language therapy, and outpatient mental health care.	**YOU pay:** • $100 deductible (pay once per calendar year). • 20% of Medicare-approved amount after the deductible, except in the outpatient setting. • 20% for all outpatient physical, occupational, and speech-language therapy services. • 50% for outpatient mental health care.
Clinical Laboratory Service: Blood tests, urinalysis, and more.	**YOU pay:** • Nothing for Medicare-approved services.
Home Health Care: Part-time skilled nursing care, home health aide services, durable medical equipment when supplied by a Medicare-approved home health agency while you are getting Medicare-covered home health care, and other medical supplies and services.	**YOU pay:** • Nothing for Medicare-approved services. • 20% of Medicare-approved amount for durable medical equipment.
Outpatient Hospital Services: Hospital services and supplies received as an outpatient as part of a doctor's care.	**YOU pay:** • A coinsurance or co-payment amount which may vary according to the service.
Blood: Pints of blood you get as an outpatient, or as part of a Part B covered services.	**YOU pay:** • For the first 3 pints of blood, then 20% of the Medicare-approved amount for additional pints of blood (after the deductible), unless you or someone else donates blood to replace what you use.

Note: Actual amounts you must pay may be higher if the doctor or supplier does not accept assignment, and you may have to pay the entire charge.

Source: Health Care Financing Administration, 2004. (See www.questions.medicare.gov/Publications/ Pub/pdk/yourmb.pdf for updated information.)

If one has paid Medicare taxes before age 65, one is eligible to sign up for Part B; signing up for Part B is a choice that is up to the individual. If people choose to sign up, they will pay monthly for Part B ($66.60/month in 2004) as well as paying deductibles and copayments. Rates change each year based on set formulas—25 percent of estimated program costs have to be covered by the enrollee monthly charge. The rest (75 percent) is from federal tax dollars. When the Medicare beneficiary needs skilled care the coinsurance is $109.50 for days 21 through 100 (2004 rates). To get the cheapest rates, one needs to sign up three months before one's 65th birthday. If one does not sign up for Part B when they first became eligible (age 65), the Part B premium goes up 10 percent for each year one was eligible but did not sign up! About 95 percent of Medicare beneficiaries have enrolled in Part B. In Part B, providers can bill patients up to 15 percent more for services than the cost covered by Medicare. **Exhibit 6–7** further describes Part B services and payments.

Medicare covers very little prescription drug costs, has high deductibles, and has no cap on out-of-pocket spending. (Note that the federal government mandated employers to cap out-of-pocket spending but does not do this for our elderly!) This means that additional insurance is needed. As of 1995, about 33 percent of our elderly had private health insurance. Approximately 25 percent purchased *Medigap plans*, sponsored by private insurance companies, not the government. Medigap plans provide supplemental insurance for Medicare consumers. Plans vary. Consumers can choose coverage for "medical care, SNF coinsurance, coverage of Medicare deductibles for Part A or Part B, coverage for health care needs during foreign travel, home care, preventive care, and[/or] prescription coverage... Medigap HMOs cannot require higher premiums based on age; however, Medigap non-HMO plans can require higher premiums" (Finkelman, p. 302) based on age. Some Medigap premiums are quite expensive and many elderly cannot afford them. Another 14 percent of the elderly are below the poverty level so are eligible for Medicaid benefits; the 9 percent enrolled in HMOs receive more benefits automatically from the HMO as well as paying lower costs for deductibles and coinsurance.

> Despite the prevalence of public and private supplemental coverage, beneficiaries face substantial out-of-pocket expenses. Medicare covers less than half of older adults' total health spending and is less generous than health plans that are typically offered by large employers. On average, older adults spend 20% of their household income for health services and premiums. The most vulnerable, . . . those with incomes below the poverty level, spend more than 33% of their income; those in fair/poor health spend more than 25% (Longest, Rakich, and Darr, p. 98).

Medicare's service benefit plan uses prospective payment mechanisms for care. In hospitals *diagnosis-related groups* (DRGs) are used for reimbursement, while *resource utilization groups* (RUGs) were adopted for long-term care reimbursement, *ambulatory payment categories* (APCs) were started for ambulatory settings, *resource-based relative value scale* (RBRVS) were developed for physicians, and home care is regulated using the *Outcome and Assessment Information Set* (OASIS). In DRGs,

> "discharged Medicare patients are assigned to one of almost 500 DRGs based on diagnosis, surgery, patient age, discharge destination, and gender. Each DRG's weight is based primarily on Medicare billing and cost data, and reflects the relative cost—across all hospitals—of treating cases that are classified in that DRG. Hospitals that can provide services at lower costs keep the difference. Those exceeding the DRG rate must recoup the difference elsewhere" (Longest, Rakich, and Darr, p. 71).

The physician is responsible for identifying the principle diagnosis, which has to be the reason for admission, using the *International Classification of Diseases*, 9th Revision, Clinical Modification (ICD-9). (For more information, see *www.hcfa-1500-forms.com/coding-books/icd-9-cm.html#Volumes 1 and 2*.) Up to four secondary diagnoses can be documented. If the physician does not adequately document all this, payment will not be forthcoming. Outliers occur when either costs or length of stay are longer than expected. Hospitals need to do as much as possible to prevent outliers. (See the Staffing Chapter for research linking fewer patient complications with higher RN staffing.) The biggest concern with Medicare presently is that it does not adequately reflect severity of illness.

> Ambulatory payment categories (APCs) are being developed for the whole range of ambulatory services. APCs group thousands of procedure and diagnosis costs into more than 300 categories, with separate classifications for surgical, medical, and ancillary services. Each group includes clinically similar services that require comparable levels of resources. A relative weight based on median resource use is assigned to each classification. Payment for each APC is determined by multiplying the relative weight by a conversion factor, which is the average rate for all APC services. The system is expected to apply to all Medicare Part B outpatient facility costs, except those covered by a separate schedule, such as ambulance, durable medical equipment, laboratory, and implantable-device costs (Longest, Rakich, and Darr, p. 72).

In addition to APCs being developed for Medicare Part B, a physician fee schedule, resource-based relative value scale (RBRVS), was started in an attempt to even out payments to specialty physicians (who were paid more) compared with family and general practice physicians (receiving less). Presently, physicians are paid for each treatment so there is an incentive to overuse services.

In long-term care, Medicare reimbursement has been based on the resource utilization groups (RUGs), now into RUG-III. "It set 44 reimbursement levels (26 for Medicare, 18 for Medicaid) based on resident condition and use of services. RUG-III uses 300 elements of care to measure a resident's acuity based on differences in ADLs [activities of daily living]; need for specialized therapies, nursing, and ancillary services; and presence of depression" (Longest, Rakich, and Darr, p. 72). RUGs:

> measure resident characteristics and staff care time for various categories of patients. RUGs have seven categories of patient severity.

> Caregivers derive the classifications from assessments recorded in the res-
> ident Minimum Data Set (MDS) assessment instrument required for days
> 5, 14, 30, 60, and 90 during a Part A stay. Facilities must also complete a
> comprehensive assessment if a patient's condition changes significantly. .
> . . To establish payment . . . caregivers need to record and code MDS data
> and use it to assign patients to case mix groups (Knapp, p. 14).

So in long-term care, reimbursement is determined by how effectively staff complete the MDS data.

Home health care, driven by having to use OASIS, is presently serving patients follow-ing acute care episodes. There is no money allotted for chronic illness needs. Yet the great-est percentage of Medicare dollars is spent on acute tertiary care—a major problem with our current health care system.

The problem with all these payment changes, aside from those for the physicians, is that there is a tendency to discharge patients too soon. For example, a patient might still be medically unstable when leaving the hospital or the patient may not be able to care for themselves and need medical care but have used up their home care allotment.

Medicaid predominantly pays for custodial long-term care of more than 100 days, rep-resenting 48 percent of Medicaid expenses. If people need custodial long-term care, they must be at the poverty level, as established by each state, before Medicaid will pay. If peo-ple are not at the poverty level, a person can pay cash, or if the person has long-term care insurance (including Medigap insurance) that covers custodial care, the insurance plan can pay. If a person does not have one of these two options and is above the poverty level, it is possible to receive Medicaid benefits for custodial long-term care by "spending down" all assets (income, property, and other assets) until the patient is below the poverty level. Then Medicaid benefits will begin. The other option, used by a significant number of elderly needing custodial care, is to be cared for by a relative in the home. This avoids spending down life savings.

Definition

Medicaid, a cost-sharing program involving both state and federal funds, provides services for med-ically indigent people including children, and for people with severe and permanent disabilities that are under age 65–although elderly over 65 receiving welfare are also included in Medicaid.

Medicaid, a cost-sharing program involving both state and federal funds, provides services for medically indigent people including children, and for people with severe and permanent dis-abilities that are under age 65–although elderly over 65 receiving welfare are also included in Medicaid. The federal government mandates certain basic coverage—inpatient and outpatient hospital services, physician, midwife, and certi-fied nurse practitioner services, laboratory and x-ray services, nursing facility and home health care, early and periodic screening, diagnosis, and treatment (EPSDT) for children under age 21, family planning, and rural health clinics/fed-erally qualified health centers. States can add such things as prescription drugs, clinic services, prosthetic devices, hearing aids, dental care, and intermediate care facilities for people with mental retardation to this coverage. Services and reimbursements vary widely from state to state.

Medicaid is quickly becoming a federal-versus-state rights issue. The federal government has mandated the states to support Medicaid, yet in 2003 forty-nine states cut Medicaid spending. This is nearing crisis proportions because the state governments do not have the money to pay. The situation is exacerbated because of the increased population needing Medicaid services.

Medicaid programs face special challenges. Often consumers do not have a primary care physician, unless they are in an HMO program where one is assigned. When they need care, a usual practice has been to go to the local hospital emergency room for care. Also, this consumer group may not keep appointments because of lack of transportation or lack of childcare options. Sometimes nurse case managers are assigned to these patients to better, and less expensively, serve them.

PPOs, another example of a service benefit plan, consist of a group of providers–such as physicians and hospitals–who have agreed to provide services at lower than usual rates to enrollees. The PPO acts as the intermediary between providers and consumers. The PPO pays prearranged fees for services provided. The enrollee incentive is to use the providers in the plan and not have to pay for many of the services provided. If an enrollee chooses to go to a physician not included in the PPO, the PPO only pays part–or none–of the fee, with the enrollee having to pay the remainder. Capitation, or prepayment by enrollees, generally does not occur with a PPO.

Direct Service Delivery Plans

A *direct service delivery plan*, is another type of plan used by *health maintenance organizations (HMOs)*. This plan is different because it pays the provider in advance. Generally, there are five types of HMOs:

- Staff HMOs that employ physicians individually.
- Group model HMOs that contract with one multispecialty group of physicians. A per capita rate is paid to the physician, as specified in the contract.
- Network model HMOs operate just like group models, except that they contract with more than one group of physicians.
- Individual practice association (IPA) members include both individual and group practice physicians. The HMO contracts with the

---

Definition

Preferred Provider Organizations (PPOs) consist of a group of providers–such as physicians and hospitals–who have agreed to provide services at lower than usual rates to enrollees.

Definition

In a *direct service delivery plan*, *health maintenance organizations (HMOs)* use a capitation model for reimbursement. Here the payer prepays the provider on a monthly or annual basis. Under this arrangement, providers agree to provide all specified services enrollees would need for that month or year, receiving no additional monies. This is another example of *managed care*.

IPA for physician services. IPA physician members provide services for the HMO, but also treat other patients.
* Point-of-service HMOs came about more recently. Here an HMO patient can go to a physician or hospital outside the HMO but pays more out-of-pocket expense.

HMOs use *capitation* as the reimbursement mechanism. The word, capitation, comes from the "per capita" (per person) fee the purchaser pays. To purchase HMO services, the employer (or individual purchaser) pays a monthly (*capitated*) fee to the HMO. The HMO agrees to provide health care services specified in the contract for no additional costs to the employer or the individual. The HMO either contracts with, or hires, providers who agree to be paid in advance a monthly, or yearly, fee in return for providing all services enrollees will need for that period. Under capitation, a provider could lose money if too many services were provided in the covered period; alternately, the provider could make money if fewer services were given to enrollees and the cost was less than the prepaid amount. For example, a physician would not want to order too many tests; or a hospital would want to quickly transfer an acutely ill patient from ICU, to a stepdown unit, to a sub-acute unit, and then to outpatient treatment and/or home care. Capitation established a *provider* incentive to cut costs.

In addition to capitation, HMOs use another managed care strategy. When consumers need care, they must first see a *gatekeeper* provider, such as a primary care physician or nurse practitioner. The gatekeeper determines if care is necessary, and if so, makes the decision whether the patient should be referred to a specialist. The advantage to the patient is that there is no charge to see the gatekeeper, and no insurance paperwork is necessary for reimbursement. In addition there is no charge for specialty care, as long as the gatekeeper makes the specialty referral. The consumer disadvantage with an HMO is when the gatekeeper does not think specialty care is needed. In this case, if the patient still wants specialty care, the patient would have to pay for the specialty service or go without.

In the HMO system, gatekeepers are constantly under scrutiny for *practice patterns*. This includes collecting data on such things as *bed days per thousand*, the number of hospital inpatient bed days used by 1,000 health plan members in a year. Capitated payments have forced down patient length of stay, resulting in all health care services treating more acutely ill patients. This has created many conflicts and ethical dilemmas, as well as bad publicity, between the various health care players.

HMOs use another managed care strategy, *disease management*, with chronic, long-term illnesses. Here the physician, or provider, is given a mandated systematic, population-based approach that defines the patient diagnosis or problem, and the specific intervention(s) to take with all patients that meet this definition. The HMO then collects data on the physician practice patterns and the patient clinical outcomes to determine how effectively the physician followed these mandates. "Examples of illnesses that are often targeted for disease management are asthma, arthritis, cancer, diabetes, hypertension, osteoporosis, high-risk pregnancy, congestive heart failure, depression, high cholesterol, and human immunodeficiency virus/acquired immune deficiency syndrome (HIV/AIDS)" (Finkelman, p. 96). Disease management identifies the best practices to achieve fewer poor outcomes, or at least to slow down the degenerative aspects of these chronic diseases.

Pricing Strategies

As managed care has developed, various pricing strategies have been used. The terms at the beginning of the following list reflect more payer risk, while the terms toward the end have shared more risk with the provider. This dispersed risk has been a goal of managed care as it has developed (Harris, pp. 535–536).

Fee for service or *reasonable and customary charges* reimburse the provider a specific amount of money for each service and/or product that is provided. A *discounted fee-for-service* reimburses the provider for the service and/or product but here a discount, either a fixed amount or a percentage, is subtracted from the fee. The discount is specified in the payer-provider contract. *Per diem rates*, or fixed rates on a per day basis, cover all the services or products used in that day. *Per case rates* are paid per visit or procedure.

> Today, a shift has been made to a fixed per-member/per-month fee for primary care practices and the Medicare fee schedule for specialists. The hospitals negotiate their rates separately and probably are paid on a per diem rate something that is usually much less than their costs. No connection is made between payment and patient need in the per diem methodology. In fact, the incentive for the hospital could be to keep the patient longer since the first few days of providing care are very expensive and keeping the patient an "extra day or two" might pay for the total cost of care (Anderson, p. 12).

Per episode rates reimburse the provider for an episode of illness. Examples of this include the DRGs used for hospital reimbursement, the RUGs used for long-term care reimbursement, the Ambulatory Payment Classification system, the OASIS system in home care, and the resource based relative value scale (RBRVS) for physicians. In these systems, a *relative value unit* is developed where payment is based on the complexity of a procedure. For example, a more complex procedure might be paid the equivalent of two relative value units converted to dollars, as compared with a less complicated procedure where reimbursement is only one relative value unit.

Capitation, already discussed, is used when the provider is paid a per member per month fee. The provider can make money if fewer services are provided but loses money if too many services are given.

Risk sharing is where the provider shares the cost of care given to a specified risk population.

Outcomes-based pricing pays the provider a specified amount per case based on expected outcomes.

In the United States, four stages of managed care development have been identified. (We are in different stages because managed care penetration has reached certain states more than others.) The stages are outlined in **Exhibit 6–8**.

Who Is the Bad Guy?

A common fallacy is to view the third party payers as the "bad guys"—the cause of our societal dilemmas (such as the inadequacy of health care coverage, creating limitations on health care coverage, paying predominantly for tertiary illness care, and being responsible

---

Exhibit 6–8 Stages of Managed Care Development

Stage I: Unstructured Markets
An unstructured market is essentially a non-managed care market and includes the following:
- independent hospitals
- independent physicians
- unsophisticated purchasers
- fee-for-service pricing
- 0% to 20% managed care market penetration, such as rural United States, Iowa, Alaska, and Wyoming

Stage II: Loose-Framework Markets
Managed care organizations (MCOs) enter the market, and providers receive contact from case managers, utilization reviewers, and other personnel who are interested in reducing costs. This is characterized by the following:
- proliferation of HMOs and PPOs
- formation of provider networks
- declining hospital bed capacity
- discount and per diem pricing
- 20% to 50% managed care market penetration

Stage III: Consolidation Markets
MCOs compete heavily for patients, and this causes some MCOs to lose business or to go out of business. It is difficult for providers to distinguish the appropriate targets in this market. Stage III is characterized by the following:
- the shakeout of marginal MCO players
- the emergence of dominant MCOs
- the formation of provider/payer alliances
- per diem, per case, per episode, and capitation pricing
- 50% to 75% managed care market penetration

Stage IV: Managed Competition
The majority of alternate-site referrals are controlled by MCOs. Providers without MCO contracts have difficulty generating nongovernmental business. This is characterized by the following:
- fewer MCOs
- fully integrated systems
- direct employer/provider contracts
- high MCO penetration
- pricing strategies that are capitation, risk sharing, and outcomes based
- 75% to 100% managed care market penetration, such as Los Angeles and Minneapolis (Harris, 1997, 535).

From: Harris, M. (1997). *Handbook of Home Health Care Administration*. 2nd. Ed. Gaithersburg, MD: Aspen. p. 535.

for the high cost of health care.) However, who is really the "bad guy"? Reviewing the history of health care in this country, one sees a much larger societal problem. Employers are spending large amounts of money on illness needs of employees who expect the best tertiary care possible and want someone else to cure all their illnesses. This cost is shared with employees in the form of deductibles and copayments; the majority of the cost then gets passed on to whatever widget or service the employer sells. As consumers purchase the widgets or services, consumers complain about the high costs. Who is really to blame? It turns out that finding the bad guy is really a much larger, societal dilemma that holds many implications. This societal dilemma includes us—the general public or consumers, employers, payers, providers, suppliers, and regulators. We *all* contribute to the problem and *all* will have to be involved if we ever fix it.

Workers' Compensation

Another group of payers cover *workers' compensation costs*, providing health care benefits to persons injured on the job. This is a $26 billion health care business. State laws vary but generally require employers to purchase insurance to cover workers' compensation. Employers are required to give cash benefits, medical care, and rehabilitation services for work-related injuries. In addition, diseases associated with specific occupations are automatically covered. Employees do not need to supply proof that the employer was at fault. However, in this arrangement employees give up the right of legal action and awards. Employers therefore benefit by having limited liability for occupational illnesses and injury. A current trend with workers' compensation is to have managed care companies take over the insurance. Since state laws differ in this area, it is best to consult the human resource department if an employee is injured on the job. Along with worker's compensation, most employers offer disability insurance to employees. Currently 55 percent of all workers' compensation expenditures are for disability costs.

SUPPLIERS

Suppliers—individuals or companies—provide supplies, equipment, and services used by the health care providers.

Nursing interacts with suppliers in a number of ways. For instance, the product evaluation committee is used to determine the best deal on major equipment or supplies. The infection control nurse can become very involved with equipment and supplies that adversely affect either the patient or the health care worker. In the late 1970s, in response to the importance of cutting costs, nationwide purchasing alliances—Premier Alliance, Voluntary Hospitals of America (VHA), SunHealth, and American Healthcare Systems—were formed. The idea was that materials and supplies could be purchased at less cost (many touted a 10 percent savings) because of the higher volume that could be purchased at once by the alliance. Presently Premier Alliance and VHA contract volume includes approximately two thirds of the nation's hospitals. This has caused other issues:

> **Definition**
>
> *Suppliers*—individuals or companies—provide supplies, equipment, and services used by the health care providers.

size brings big discounts, however, not everyone wants to use the products. From a nursing perspective, it can be an issue when everyone is trained to use one supply, but the purchasing alliance gets a better deal on another similar supply that staff have not been trained to use properly. The purchase itself may save money, however, staff education may cause the organization to actually spend more on this purchase.

When health care organizations join a purchasing alliance, they still must rely on local companies for certain supplies and services such as waste removal, physician contractual services to staff the emergency room, and laundry facilities (if contracted outside the health care organization).

Warren Bennis has called the physician group "suppliers" for health care organizations. This seems to be the most appropriate term. However, you often hear physicians being referred to as customers. Many hospitals market to physicians to be sure that there are enough primary care physicians to refer patients to specialty physicians, and to make sure there are enough specialists to meet community needs and keep hospital beds filled. At times the recruitment process also involves providing assistance such as loans for office practices or homes, along with a certain amount of reimbursement for relocation expenses, to physicians.

REGULATORS

> **Definition**
>
> *Regulators* are the organizations/agencies that set the rules, regulations, and/or standards that providers must meet to stay in business. This includes many groups, such as the federal, state, and local governments and judicial systems, accrediting bodies, regulators of professions such as medicine and nursing, and professional organizations.

Regulators are the organizations/agencies that set the rules, regulations, and/or standards that providers must meet to stay in business. This includes many groups, such as the federal, state, and local governments and judicial systems, accrediting bodies, regulators of professions such as medicine and nursing, and professional organizations. The standards used by regulators come from many sources including consumers, providers, payers, professional organizations, and even state or federal laws or executive orders.

Federal Regulation

In health care, the federal government, as a regulator, has the overall responsibility for both achieving quality and holding down costs. The Constitution specifies that the federal government has the authority to regulate interstate commerce and provide for the general welfare of its citizens. Through the years this has resulted in so much federal regulation that the Centers for Medicare and Medicaid Services (CMS) has created an advisory committee to recommend changes that will streamline the regulatory process.

The main federal health care regulators are the Centers for Medicare and Medicaid Services (CMS), established to administer Medicare and Medicaid and enforce national health care regulations. For example, federal legislation, in a 1972 cost reduction strategy, mandated *utilization review*, "a formal assessment of the medical necessity, efficiency, and/or appropriateness of health care services and treatment plans on a prospective, concurrent, or retrospective basis" (Finkelman, p. 490). (Most other payers have adopted this strategy as well.) Utilization review is accomplished using several mechanisms:

- *Preadmission Certification*—The insurer approves care in advance. If this is required, and certification is not obtained, the insurer can refuse to pay for the care.
- *Concurrent Review*—Some insurers will monitor patients' lengths of stay to ensure the patients are discharged quickly. If an insurer determines that the patient has received all the appropriate tests and treatments, [the insurer] will not authorize additional care and will refuse to pay for additional days.
- *Discharge Planning*—Discharge planning has always been important. However, now it is critical. It is important to keep lengths of stay as short as possible. The discharge plan may include additional care needed by transferring the patient quickly to long-term care, home care, and/or ambulatory care, which will be less expensive than the hospital stay.
- *Case Management*—More information about case management is in Chapter 16. In this case, care plans are developed for complicated patients to provide the needed care in the least expensive way. For example, perhaps a hospitalization can be prevented by providing home care seven days a week.
- *Second Surgical Opinions*—For elective surgeries, insurers may require that the patient go to a second physician to determine whether the surgery is necessary. Additionally, the insurer wants to do the surgery in the least expensive way—outpatient is preferred but if hospitalization is needed, this needs to be specified.

Another example of CMS regulation is the special handicap access standards developed by the American National Standards Institute (ANSI) and the federal government. For instance, corridor width needs to be at least eight feet wide and a bathroom needs to accommodate two CNAs assisting a resident in a wheelchair. In long-term care, "design principles for the elderly focus on safety, privacy, lighting, texture, color, signage, independence, orienting features, access, and social contact. . . . For example, it is difficult for an older person to distinguish colors of similar intensity such as pastels and combinations of blues and greens; smooth textures make colors appear lighter; rough textures make colors appear darker" (Mitty, p. 312).

Another important federal regulator for health care is the Occupational Safety and Health Administration (OSHA), implemented to ensure a safe, healthy workplace. OSHA uses Center for Disease Control (CDC) standards in health care organizations. The CDC's mission is to prevent and control disease, injury, and disability. OSHA regulations are very complicated and change each year. To find more information about either OSHA or CDC current requirements, go to their websites (www.osha.gov or www.cdc.gov). Employers are required to be aware of unsafe conditions (vague wording), are responsible to inform employees about OSHA standards, and are expected to provide safe conditions and appropriate safety equipment for employees. In addition, an employer is expected to accommodate employees who are disabled unless it causes an unrealistic disadvantage on the employer (more vague wording). It is advisable to consult with the human resource department for more details on the disability issue. (Federal OSHA standards can be expanded, but not reduced, by a state.)

Employers violating OSHA regulations can be cited, fined, and, if serious enough, a workplace can be closed. OSHA is not well staffed, having fewer than a thousand inspectors for the country. However, they make unannounced comprehensive safety and health inspections, and if an OSHA inspector arrives at the workplace, they have a right to enter and inspect. (Most OSHA cases do not involve an inspector.) Generally, a safety committee at the workplace takes responsibility for meeting OSHA standards. If an employee is injured in the workplace, the safety committee investigates workplace conditions at the site where the employee was injured and evaluates the situation, and, if necessary, makes recommendations for changes. The safety committee then has the responsibility to make sure the recommendations have been followed. Safety committee records are to be regularly audited. Most often, accreditation standards include meeting OSHA regulations.

To accomplish quality monitoring, the federal government delegates specific responsibilities to each state's licensure and certification agency. For a facility to participate in Medicare and Medicaid programs, they must undergo this licensure and certification process. States vary as to actual requirements. In addition, health care organizations must be accredited to be eligible for Medicare reimbursement. Joint Commission of Accreditation of Healthcare Organizations (JCAHO) has become the main organization for health care accreditation although there are a number of other accreditation bodies (i.e., The American Osteopathic Association Healthcare Facilities Accreditation Program (HFAP), listed in the Regulator section of this chapter) that meet the Medicare accreditation standard.

There are other federal regulators that affect health care.

- The Department of Justice and Federal Trade Commission enforces antitrust issues, which prohibits anticompetitive practices.
- The National Labor Relations Board regulates union organizing and collective bargaining.
- The Food and Drug Administration regulates drugs and medical devices as well as dietary regulations and inspections.
- The Securities and Exchange Commission regulates how investor-owned health care organizations can market, sell, and trade stock.
- The Nuclear Regulatory Commission regulates hazards arising from storage, handling, and transportation of nuclear materials.
- The Equal Employment Opportunity Commission enforces Equal Employment Opportunities (EEO) in hiring, equal pay, civil rights, and age discrimination issues (Longest, Rakich, and Darr, p. 74).

Judicial Regulation

> Additional laws can be enacted when case decisions are made in the state and federal judicial systems. Two central doctrines make courts a source of formal law. *Stare decisis* is a Latin phrase meaning that courts will stand by precedent and not disturb a settled point. The doctrine of

> *stare decisis* is based on the principle that the law should be fixed, definite, and known. Courts and litigants are guided by previous cases with similar facts. Predictability and consistency are important attributes of the law. Whimsical changes and uncertainty are to be avoided with judge-made law and legislative enactments. Nevertheless, precedents are sometimes overturned.
>
> The second doctrine is reflected in the Latin phrase *res judicata*, which means a matter has been judged or a thing has been judicially acted on or decided. Thus rehearing will occur only if there is a substantial problem in the original judgment because of factual error, misrepresentation, or fraud, or if significant new information becomes available. *Res judicata* adds stability and predictability to the law because, after appeals are exhausted, the case is settled and usually will not be reopened (Longest, Rakich, and Darr, pp. 693–694).

State Regulation

> When the states delegated certain powers to a federal government and ratified the U.S. Constitution, they retained a wide range of authority... known as the police powers, defined as the powers to protect the health, safety, public order, and welfare of the public. Consistent with the police powers, states have enacted legislation to regulate and license a wide variety of [health care organizations]. . . that are required to obtain and retain a license [and] must submit to inspections and other regulation (Longest, Rakich, and Darr, p. 69).

Health and safety issues include radiation safety, sanitation of food and water, and disposal of wastes. States may delegate some of the safety, sanitation, and waste disposal responsibilities to city and county governments. Therefore, the states regulate, inspect, and license health care organizations on physical plant safety issues, as well as license and regulate various health care professionals and nursing education programs. In addition, "each state has an insurance commission. This commission is responsible for regulating both the solvency of insurers and the marketing of insurance.... A particularly important responsibility is the regulation of the level of reserves [savings to cover future claims] that the insurance companies must maintain" (Finkelman, p. 43).

Because states were already conducting annual inspections of health care inpatient facilities when Medicare was established, the federal government mandated an annual state inspection of hospitals and long-term care facilities receiving Medicare funding. Home care was added to the list for state licensing if treating Medicare and Medicaid patients. State licensure and certification agencies have a number of responsibilities. First, to be eligible for Medicare and Medicaid funding the health care organization must be licensed by the state. For example, in long-term care, the state will "authorize a nursing home to provide certain services when particular criteria are met: minimum staffing levels, personnel qualifications, educational requirements for the administrator, quality assurance systems, compliance with fire and safety codes, service delivery capability, bylaws and administrative organization" (Mitty, p. 248). After the inspection, the states make recommendations to CMS for Medicare certification.

Second, annual inspections then must occur with organizations treating Medicare and Medicaid patients. Certification is needed each year to receive Medicare reimbursement. Medicaid regulation is shared between the federal government and the states.

> Licensure and certification standards may exceed federal requirements...
> but states may not eliminate a standard or requirement or create one in
> conflict with federal regulations. The federal government has the
> authority to conduct independent inspections... of certified nursing
> homes in order to audit the state's certification activities in both the
> Medicare and Medicaid programs (as a rule, 10 percent of homes annu-
> ally) (Mitty, p. 248).

Because of this, each state has designed a different version of Medicaid. This is why Medicaid has different titles in many states, such as TennCare in Tennessee and MedCal in California.

Since 48 percent of Medicaid funds are for long-term care, the federal government has mandated each state to do a more involved annual inspection of long-term care given to each Medicaid-funded resident. As part of the inspection:

> A multidisciplinary survey team must ensure that the care reimbursed
> with Medicaid funds is necessary, available, adequate, appropriate—and
> of acceptable quality to maximize the physical and mental potential and
> well-being of the resident. The review also includes an assessment of
> [each] resident's continued placement in the home and the feasibility of
> meeting his needs through alternative institutional or non-institutional
> services. The survey team looks for evidence that the resident's dis-
> charge potential was evaluated (Mitty, p. 248).

If the facility meets all the federal requirements, the state, representing CMS, then certifies or recertifies the long-term care facility on the day of the survey.

Another important state responsibility concerns individual licensing and certification for various health occupations. Perhaps, as nurses, we are most aware of the *board of nursing*. (In addition, there are other professional boards, such as the board of medicine or the board licensing long-term care administrators). Each state has a Nurse Practice Act(s) that defines nursing practice and establishes the board of nursing. The professional boards define professional practice, license caregivers (to become licensed a person must show that they have achieved minimum competencies with the board keeping an official roster of all who are licensed), and set standards. Boards of nursing also license LPNs and nurse assistants. Generally, the practice acts specify that RNs can treat patients independently, while licensing for LPNs or nurse assistants specify that licensees are dependent on the orders of an RN or physician. In addition, the board holds regular hearings, regulates practice, determines what is improper professional conduct and takes disciplinary actions when this occurs, introduces legislation to better define professional practice, licenses new nursing education programs, and oversees the quality of current nursing education programs. Most states have mandated that nursing education programs achieve an 85 percent student pass rate on the National Council Licensing Exam (NCLEX). Having representation on the board of nursing can be an important role in policy making.

Although it is not a state regulatory body, it is important to note here that there is a National Council of State Boards of Nursing (NCSBN) whose purpose is to provide a national organization where boards of nursing can "act and counsel together on matters of common interest and concern affecting the public health, safety and welfare, including the development of licensing examinations in nursing" (www.ncsbn.org). NCSBN has been involved with several important issues: 1) They have developed computerized licensure examinations, the NCLEX-RN and the NCLEX-PN, which are administered by a national test service to all individuals who want to be newly licensed as an RN or LPN. 2) NCSBN has established a multistate Nurse Licensure Compact. Presently, nurse practice acts are not uniform in all states. A state legislature can pass a law to become a part of this Compact. Once passed, nurses can practice across state lines, without getting licensed in another state, as long as the nurse follows the practice provisions in place in the state in which the nurse is practicing. One can find the list of states that currently belong to the Nurse Licensure Compact at the NCSBN website.

Credentialing

Credentialing of health care occupations takes place in several ways: licensure, registration, certification, and competency. With *licensure* a person must show that they have achieved minimum competencies to the state licensing board such as the board of nursing. *Registration* is the official roster, kept by the board of nursing, listing all who are licensed. *Certification* is awarded to individual providers by a non-governmental organization/registry when the individual has met certain educational requirements, and passed an examination. For example, family nurse practitioners or CNAs are certified. **Exhibit 6–9** lists various nursing specialty organizations that certify nurses. In turn these professional certifying organizations are certified by The American Board of Nursing Specialties (ABNS), a certifier of certifiers (Bernreuter, 2001). Boards of nursing, as well as employers, require that people in certain health occupations are certified, i.e., the nurse practitioner. Voluntary certification for nurse administrators can be obtained from the American Nurses Credentialing Center (ANCC) at two levels: the nurse manager level and the nurse executive level. Nurse executive certification can also be obtained by admission to the American College of Health Care Executives, and for home/hospice care nurse executives, through the National Association for Home Care's (NAHC) Executive Certification Program. (Certification can also be given to organizations that have met specified qualifications, such as providers needing Medicare and Medicaid certification to receive payments.) See **Exhibit 6–9**.

A component of organizational accreditation includes the standard that employees are properly *credentialed* to do their assigned work. The evaluation process for this standard examines licenses, certification, educational background, and *competency* (evidence of current, safe practice or performance quality) of personnel, as well as that of the physicians.

Exhibit 6–9 Nurse Specialty Certification Organizations

American Academy of Nurse Practitioners Certification Program NP-C	www.aanp.org
American Association of Critical Care Nurses Certification Corporation ACNP; CCRN®; CCNS®	www.certcorp.org
American Board of Neuroscience Nursing CNRN	www.aann.org
American Board for Occupational HealthNurses COHN®; COHN-S®; COHN/CM; COHN-S/CM	www.abohn.org
American Board of Neuroscience Nursing	www.aann.org (click on ABNN)
American Board of Perianesthesia Nursing Certification, Inc. CAPA; CPAN	www.cpancapa.org
American Holistic Nurses' Certification Corp.	ahna.org/certification.html
American Legal Nurse Consultant Certification Board® LNCC ®	www.aalnc.org
American Nurses Credentialing Center RN,C; RN,BC; APRN,BC; CNA,BC; CNAA,BC	www.nursecredentialing.org
Board of Certification for Emergency Nursing CEN; CFRN	www.ena.org/bcen
Canadian Nurses Association Certification Program CCN(C); CNCC(C); ENC(C); GNC(C); CNeph(C); CNN(C); COHN(C)®; COHN-S(C)®; CON(C); CPN(C); PNC(C); CPMHN(C)	www.cna-nurses.ca
Certification Board Perioperative Nursing CNOR®; CRNFA®	www.certboard.org
Certifying Board of Gastroenterology Nurses and Associates, Inc. CGN; CGRN	www.cbgna.org
Council on Certification of Nurse Anesthetists CRNA®	www.aana.com
Infusion Nurses Certification Corporation CRNI	www.ins1.org
Intravenous Nurses Certification Corp. CLNI; CRNI	www.ins1.org/certify2.htm
National Board for Certification of Hospice and Palliative Nurses CHPN	www.hpna.org
National Board for Certification of School Nurses, Inc. NCSN	www.nbcsn.com
National Certification Board for Diabetes Educators	www.ncbde.org
National Certification Board of Pediatric Nurse Practitioners and Nurses CPNP®; CPN®	www.pnpcert.org
National Certification Corporation for the Obstetric, Gynecologic and Neonatal Specialties WHNP; INPT; NIC; NNP: LRN; MN	www.nccnet.org
National Certifying Board for Ophthalmic Registered Nurses CRNO	webeye.ophth.uiowa.edu/ asorn/certif.htm

Nephrology Nursing Certification Commission CNN; CDN	www.nncc-exam.org
Oncology Nursing Certification Corporation OCN®; CPON; AOCN®	www.oncc.org
Orthopedic Nurses Certification Board ONC	naon.inurse.com/certification
Plastic Surgical Nursing Certification Board	asprsn.inurse.com/psncb/default.htm
Rehabilitation Nursing Certification Board CPSN	rehabnurse.org/index5.htm
Vascular Nursing Certification Board CVN	www.svnnet.org
Wound Ostomy Continence Nursing Certification Board CCCN; CETN; COCN; CWCN; CWOCN	www.wocncb.org
Rehabilitation Nursing Certific ation Board CRRN®; CRRN-A	www.rehabnurse.org

Source: Smith, N. (1997). "Chapter 44: Managed Care" from Harris, M., p. 535.

Economic credentialing of physician patient volume and practice patterns, including patient outcomes, is now a common practice for hospitals. These factors are considered when renewing physician privileges.

Accreditation

> *Accreditation* is the process by which organizations are evaluated on their quality, based on established minimum standards. There are two major reasons for accrediting [health care] organizations. Health care purchasers want objective data to make informed decisions about health plans to support a good return on their investment. Data from accreditation, as well as accreditation status, can supply some of this objective data. In addition, consumers have become more interested in data about health plans as they make their own decisions about which plan to select from the choices available to them. Purchasers and consumers are interested in two critical elements: cost and quality. They want greater accountability for the quality of services (Finkelman, pp. 230–231).

Accreditation of health care organizations has gained popularity in the last 30 years. This is partially because, when Medicare was established in 1965, accredited organizations were given "deemed status" for Medicare reimbursement eligibility. There are many accrediting bodies, as shown in **Exhibit 6–10**. Generally, *accreditation* involves two steps: reviewing written materials (self study) and making an on-site visit, to determine whether the minimum standards have been met. Personnel in health care organizations must have ongoing education about current/new standards to maintain accreditation.

Health care organizational accreditation began when in 1918 the American College of Surgeons (ACS) began surveying hospitals to improve medical practice. In 1951 ACS, the American Medical Association (AMA), the American Hospital Association (AHA), the American College of Physicians (ACP), and the Canadian Medical Association formed the *Joint Commission of Accreditation of Healthcare Organizations* (JCAHO). JCAHO began by emphasizing minimal standards; this has changed to an emphasis on optimum

Exhibit 6–10 Accreditation Organizations

Name of Accrediting Body	Website Address	Accredits
The Accreditation for Ambulatory Health Care (AAAHC)	www.aaahc.org	Ambulatory Health Services Organizations, Medical and Dental Group Practices, Surgery Centers, Managed Care Organizations, Urgent and Immediate Care Centers, Community and College Health Centers, Occupational Health Services, and Hospital-sponsored Ambulatory Care Clinics
The American Assembly of Collegiate Schools of Business (AACSB)	www.aacsb.edu	Health Services Management Programs in Colleges of Business
American Association of Colleges of Nursing (AACN)	www.aacn.edu	
The American Osteopathic Association Healthcare Facilities Accreditation Program (HFAP)	www.aoa-net.org/Accreditation/ HFAP/HFAP.htm	Hospitals, Laboratories, Ambulatory Care/surgery, Mental Health, Substance Abuse, and Physical Rehabilitation Medicine Facilities
Commission for the Accreditation of Freestanding Birth Centers	www.BirthCenters.org/ naccinaction/commission.shtml	Birth Centers
Commission of Collegiate Nursing Education (CCNE)	www.aacn.nche.edu/ Accreditatopm	Bachelor's and Graduate-Degree Nursing Education Programs
Community Health Accreditation Program, Inc. (CHAP)	www.chapinc.org	Home Health
Commission on Laboratory Accreditation (COLA)	www.cola.org	Laboratories
Council on Education for Public Health (CEPH)	www.ceph.org	Schools of Public Health

Exhibit 6–10 continued

Name of Accrediting Body	Website Address	Accredits
Joint Commission of Accreditation of Healthcare Organizations (JCAHO)	www.jcaho.org	Hospitals, Long-term Care Organizations, Home Care Agencies, Clinical Laboratories, Ambulatory Care Organizations, Behavioral Health Organizations, and Health Care Networks or Managed Care Organizations
The National Committee for Quality Assurance (NCQA)	www.ncqa.com	HMOs
National League for Nursing Accreditation Commission (NLNAC)	www.nlnac.org	Practical Nurse, Diploma, Associate Degree, Baccalaureate Degree, and Master's Degree Nursing Education Programs
The Rehabilitation Accreditation Commission, CARF	www.carf.org	Medical Rehabilitation, Assisted Living, Behavioral Health, Adult Day Services, and Employment and Community Services
Utilization Review Accreditation Commission (URAC)	www.urac.org	PPOs and Workers' Compensation Programs

achievable patient outcomes, and developing ORYX, an outcomes and performance measurement system. Only recently has JCAHO had a nurse commissioner in their governing body. Presently JCAHO accredits 15,000 health care organizations including hospitals, long-term care, home care, clinical laboratories, ambulatory care/surgery, mental health, substance abuse, and physical rehabilitation facilities.

One of the earliest accreditation bodies, *The American Osteopathic Association Healthcare Facilities Accreditation Program (HFAP)* was started in 1945 to survey hospitals each year and assure that osteopathic students were training in facilities that provided a high quality of patient care. Since 1966 they have been surveying a broad spectrum of health care facilities. HFAP accreditation is a recognized alternative to JCAHO.

The National Committee for Quality Assurance (NCQA), accredits approximately half of the HMOs. NCQA developed the Health Plan Employer Data and Information Set (HEDIS), to "standardize how health plans calculate and report performance information. . . . About 90% of accredited health plans currently submit HEDIS data" (Finkelman, p. 234). This provides a wonderful, national data source so that both employers and employees can see whether their plans are effective. However, this potentially invaluable data is not used very much by employers, and even less by employees. HEDIS measures include examination of: effectiveness of care, accessibility or availability of care, satisfaction with experience of care, health plan stability, use of services, cost of care, and other descriptive information. CMS reviews this data for Medicare contracts. Eventually CMS could require other health care organizations to report this data.

Accreditation of ambulatory care varies. JCAHO accredits ambulatory surgery centers, emergency and urgent care centers, family practice centers, and multispecialty group practices. A second accrediting body, *The Accreditation for Ambulatory Health Care (AAAHC)*, begun in 1979, also accredits ambulatory health services organizations. This accredits medical and dental group practices, surgery centers, managed care organizations, urgent and immediate care centers, community and college health centers, occupational health services, and hospital-sponsored ambulatory care clinics. Birth centers are accredited by the Commission for the Accreditation of Freestanding Birth Centers.

In addition to JCAHO, the National League for Nursing (NLN) subsidiary, *Community Health Accreditation Program, Inc. (CHAP)*, started to accredit home health agencies in 1965. Now its focus has broadened to community health organizations such as home health agencies, hospice, public health, home care aide services, private duty services, supplemental staffing services, home infusion therapy, home dialysis services, home medication equipment, pharmacy services, day care, community nursing centers, and community rehabilitation centers.

The Foundation for Hospice and Homecare's National HomeCaring Council accredits home care aide and private duty nursing services. This now has reciprocity with JCAHO.

The American Accreditation Health-Care Commission Utilization Review Accreditation Commission (Commission/URAC) accredits managed health care organization services, such as utilization management, health networks, health care practitioner credentialing, workers' compensation utilization management or networks, and PPOs. In addition they have established standards for case management, credentials verification organizations, and telephone programs for health information and triage.

Other patient-oriented accrediting bodies include the *Commission on Laboratory Accreditation (COLA)* that accredits laboratories. Educational accreditation for nursing education programs can be from one of two accrediting bodies: the *National League for Nursing Accrediting Commission (NLNAC)* that accredits diploma, associate degree, baccalaureate degree, and master's degree nursing programs for registered nurses as well as practical nursing programs; and the *Commission on Collegiate Nursing Education (CCNE)*, affiliated with the *American Association of Colleges of Nursing (AACN)*, that accredits baccalaureate and master's nursing programs. Aside from the overall university or college accreditation, educational accreditation bodies exist for other professions: the Council on Education for Public Health (CEPH) for schools of public health, the American Assembly of Collegiate Schools of Business (AACSB) for colleges of business, and graduate education programs in health services management are accredited by the Accrediting Commission on Education for Health Services Administration (ACHEHSA).

International Organization for Standardization (ISO)

Although not technically a regulatory body for US health care organizations, the International Organization for Standardization (ISO), a non-governmental quality management organization, was started in Geneva, Switzerland, in 1947. Health care organizations are beginning to use ISO standards. "The ISO 9000 family is concerned primarily with quality management, which means that the features of a product or of services conform to customer requirements. The ISO 14000 family is primarily concerned with environmental management, which means what the organization does to minimize harmful effects on the environment caused by its activities" (Longest, Rakich, and Darr, p. 76).

Professional Organizations

Professional organizations, such as the American Nurses Association (ANA) and the American Organization of Nurse Executives (AONE), continually examine professional scope of practice and professional standards. AONE, ANA, American Association of Colleges of Nursing (AACN), and the National League for Nursing (NLN) has formed a national Tri-Council on nursing. Together, they represent nursing on certain national issues. In long-term care, directors of nursing can belong to the American Association of Directors of Nursing Administration in Long-Term Care, or to the National Conference of Gerontological Nurse Practitioners (NCGPN). The American Academy of Ambulatory Care Nursing (AAACN) focuses on ambulatory nursing practice. The National Association for Home Care (NAHC) represents home care professionals. Nursing Professional Organizations are listed in **Exhibit 6–11**. *Nursing Management* (2001 Guide to Nursing Organizations, pp. 57–59) publishes a list of nursing professional organizations anually. The authors suggest that the nurse manager belong to both clinical and administrative professional organizations that are appropriate for the area of practice in which one is working.

In addition to nursing organizations, there are other professional organizations nurse administrators might want to consider.

- the American College of Healthcare Executives (ACHE) serves hospital administrators,
- the American Hospital Association (AHA),
- the American Osteopathic Hospital Association (AOHA),
- the Federation of American Health Systems (Federation) for investor-owned hospital administrators,
- Catholic Health Association of the United States,
- the American Health Care Association (AHCA) for assisted living, nursing facility, and subacute care for-profit and not-for-profit providers,
- the American Association of Homes and Services for the Aging (AAHSA) for not-for-profit nursing facilities, continuing-care retirement communities, senior housing facilities, and assisted living and community services,
- Medical Group Management Association (MGMA) focuses on group practice management with members who are administrators, practice managers, and some physicians,
- the Institute of Health Improvement (IHI) concerned with improvement processes with members who are administrators, physician managers, and practice managers,
- the American Association of Health Plans (AAHP) for HMOs, PPOs, utilization review organizations, and other network-based plans.

Exhibit 6–11 Nursing Organizations

Academy of Medical-Surgical Nurses	www.medsurgnurse.org
Air & Surface Transport Nurses Association	www.astna.org
American Academy of Ambulatory Care Nursing	aaacn.inurse.com
American Academy of Nurse Practitioners	www.aanp.org
American Academy of Nursing	www.nursing-world.org/ann
American Assembly for Men in Nursing	www.aamn.org
American Association of Colleges of Nursing	www.aacn.nche.edu
American Association of Critical-Care Nurses	www.aacn.org
American Association of Diabetes Educators	www.aadenet.org
American Association of Legal Nurse Consultants	www.aalnc.org
The American Association of Managed Care Nurses, Inc.	www.aamcn.org
American Association of Neuroscience Nurses	www.aann.org
American Association of Nurse Anesthetists	www.aana.com
The American Association of Nurse Attorneys	www.taana.org
American Association of Occupational Health Nurses, Inc.	www.aaohn.org
American Association of Office Nurses	www.aaon.org
American Association of Spinal Cord Injury Nurses	www.aascin.org
American Board of Nursing Specialties	www.nursingcertification.org
American College of Nurse Practitioners	www.nurse.org/acnp
American Holistic Nurses Association	www.ahna.org
American Long Term & Sub Acute Nurses Association	www.alsna.com
American Nephrology Nurses' Association	annanurse.org
American Nurses Association	www.ana.org
American Nursing Informatics Association	www.ania.org
American Organization of Nurse Executives	www.aone.org
American Psychiatric Nurses Association	www.apna.org
American Radiological Nurses Association	www.arna.net
American Society for Long-Term Care Nurses	
American Society of Pain Management Nurses	www.aspmn.org
American Society of PeriAnesthesia Nurses	www.aspan.org
American Society of Plastic Surgical Nurses	www.asprsn.org
Association for Professionals in Infection Control and Epidemiology, Inc.	www.apic.org
Association of Nurses in AIDS Care	www.anacnet.org
Association of Pediatric Oncology Nurses	www.apon.org
Association of PeriOperative Registered Nurses	www.aorn.org
Association of Rehabilitation Nurses	www.rehabnurse.org
Association of Women's Health, Obstetric and Neonatal Nurses	www.awhonn.org
Case Management Society of America	www.cmsa.org

Council on Graduate Education for Administration in Nursing	www.unc.edu/ ~sengleba/CGEAN/
Dermatology Nurses' Association	www.dna.insure.com
Emergency Nurses Association	www.ena.org
Endocrine Nurses Society	www.endo-nurses.org
Home Healthcare Nurses Association	www.nahc.org/hhna
Hospice and Palliative Nurses Association	www.hpna.org
Infusion Nurses Society	www.ins1.org
International Council of Nurses	www.icn.ch
International Nurses Society on Addictions	www.nnsa.org
International Transplant Nurses Society	www.itns.org
League of Intravenous Therapy Education	www.lite.org
National Association of Clinical Nurse Specialists	www.nacns.org
National Association of Hispanic Nurses	www.nahnhq.org
National Association of Home Care	www.nahc.org
National Association of Neonatal Nurses	www.nann.org
National Association of Nurse Massage Therapists	members.aol.com/nanmt1
National Association of Orthopaedic Nurses	naon.inurse.com
National Association of Pediatric Nurse Associates & Practitioners, Inc.	www.napnap.org
National Association of School Nurses	www.nasn.org
National Association of Vascular Access Networks	www.navannet.org
National Black Nurses Association, Inc.	www.nbna.org
National Council of State Boards of Nursing, Inc.	www.ncsbn.org
The National Federation of Specialty Nursing Organizations	www.nfsno.org
National Federation of Licensed Practical Nurses, Inc.	www.nflpn.org
National Gerontological Nursing Association	www.ngna.org
National League for Nursing	www.nln.org
National Nursing Staff Development Organization	www.nnsdo.org
National Organization for Associate Degree Nursing	www.noadn.org
National Student Nurses' Association	www.nsna.org
Oncology Nursing Society	www.ons.org
Respiratory Nursing Society	www.respiratorynursingsociety.org
Sigma Theta Tau International Honor Society of Nursing	www.nursingsociety.org
Society for Vascular Nursing	www.svnnet.org
Society of Gastroenterology Nurses and Associates, Inc.	www.sgna.org
Society of Pediatric Nurses	www.pedsnurses.org
Society of Urologic Nurses and Associates	www.suna.org
Transcultural Nursing Society	www.tcns.org
Wound, Ostomy and Continence Nurses Society	www.wocn.org

Source: *Nursing Management*, September 2001.

Public Policy

Steele, Rocchiccioli and Porche (2003) suggest a framework that can help us to more effectively deal with health policy.[6]

> Health policy comprises the entire set of public policies that are related
> to or influence health and illness. . . . Health policies usually emerge in
> the form of laws, rules and regulations, judicial decisions, resource allo-
> cations, and broad global health care budgets. As nursing has matured as
> a discipline, nurses are becoming more cognizant of the need for
> activism in health policy and politics at all levels. Nurse manager par-
> ticipation in the policy process as mentor and facilitator to staff nurses
> ensures inclusion of nursing's unique perspective in private and govern-
> mental health policy decisions (p. 80).

Public health care policy at the local, state, and national levels will continue to impact health care and nursing. Nurses and nursing organizations have become involved with these issues. For instance, the American Nurses Association (ANA) and the American Organization of Nurse Executives (AONE) have been involved regarding managed care reform, patient safety, nurse safety, funding for nursing education and research, and resolving the nurse shortage. The nurse shortage issue has resulted in many legislative actions at both federal and state levels.

Professional organizations have been involved with public policy in several ways. First, they establish professional standards and ethics. These standards may be adopted by regulatory groups, as well as setting guidelines for professional practice. Second, some professional organizations have *lobbyists* working at state and federal levels who keep abreast of current legislation, notifying members of significant developments; follow legislation important to the professional membership; and provide input to legislators on the professional organization's position on current legislation. Third, some professional organizations support *political action committees (PACs)*, who get involved with both health care policy and election processes. Political action committees are comprised of professional members, such as nurses, who work closely with the lobbyists to stay current on legislative issues. They collect monies that will be used for political campaigns. The nurses also talk directly with legislators and other government officials about the issues, provide expert testimony to congressional committees, take back issues to the professional organization to get more feedback or member involvement, and keep track of voting records of legislators. Once legislation passes into law, nurse's work is not done. As regulations are developed to implement the legislation, nurses continue to provide input on regulation development. Fourth, when public hearings are held, the professional organizations alert members so they can also be present for the hearings. The hearings give various constituents a chance to be heard. Fifth, occasionally professional group(s) will introduce legislation that will benefit the professional membership.

---

[6] A good reference for nurses on both policy and communication with the media is Buresh and Gordon's *From Silence to Voice: What Nurses Know and Must Communicate to the Public* (2000).

Many involved in health care are already involved in public policy issues. Consider the following:

- During the 2000 election cycle, the health industry gave over $94 million in campaign contributions, vastly exceeding the $8.5 million given by tobacco interests.
- According to *Public Citizen*, in 1999, drug companies hired 297 lobbyists—the equivalent of one lobbyist for every two members of Congress—on the Medicare drug benefit alone.
- Since the early 1990s, manufacturers of medical devices have successfully petitioned the Food and Drug Administration (FDA) to provide firms with advance notice of inspections—including the products to be inspected—and to keep any violations uncovered during the inspection process out of the public's eye.
- The health insurance and HMO indiustry spent over $35 million on lobbying in 1999 and contributed nearly $10 million to campaigns during the 2000 election cycle. Meanwhile, the industry strives to keep managed care liability out of the federal patients' rights legislation (Their money or your health: who owns health care, pp. 64–65).

Policy development is critical to solving our health care dilemmas. So far, our piecemeal fixing in policy development has not been effective. Now we have the opportunity to fix the problems. All the health care players, including nursing, must be involved as equal partners in planning efforts to reach more effective health care delivery, reimbursement strategies, and the education of our health care professionals/workers. We will have the best chance of success if we all picture that we *have effectively fixed* the problems.

Personal Changes

Besides policy development and all of us working together to find the answers, we have personal responsibilities for change. One such responsibility, is to decide what we are willing to do for our own health; this responsibility includes facing the consequences if we choose not to be healthy in our day-to-day living. The consequences are not only quality of life issues but monetary. Someone else may not want to pay for the problems that we have caused.

Another personal change advocated in this book (see Chapter 1), is that if we do what is right for the patient we will make money. The money *follows*, rather than precedes, the value.

In nursing, we face a future dramatically changed from present practice. We are already experiencing compressed time, or less time available, for our work. Many of us cling to past rituals and stay in our nursing box, however we have defined it. Nursing practice is changing. Nursing administration is changing. There is comfort in chaos theory (discussed in Chapter 2) that shows that even though everything around us seems to be in chaos, overall it makes an orderly picture. In this context, consider the following:

> Out of the chaos are signs of a pattern of changes that give us a glimpse
> of the direction of change in healthcare. Some of these factors are as
> follows:

1. Healthcare is moving from residency-based delivery models of health service to mobility-based approaches as medical therapeutics become more portable, less invasive, and require less treatment and recovery time.

2. Much of the emerging medical care models do not require that patients stay for a long time to get service; however, much of nursing education is still based on learning and practices that require patients to stay around long enough for nurses to do the work they learned.

3. There is an accelerating movement from inpatient care structures to a fast growing outpatient care marketplace where service is speedy and patients do not stay long.

4. Much of the aftercare following procedures is now rendered in the patient's own environment instead of in the healthcare facility, shifting accountability for subsequent procedure and activity from professional caregivers to patients and their significant others.

5. Payment models are changing their form and application. Those processes once paid for without question are now subject to review driven by the shift in technology, location, and procedure affecting both the substance and amounts of remuneration.

6. Staff shortages of all kinds are contributing to the stress of providing services and scheduling and assigning sufficient staff to meet the demands of a changing population and shifting therapeutic environment.

7. The behavior of the worker is now changing from an 'institutional' model to a 'mobility' model of work. The conflict emerging between the mature worker, inculcated in loyalty to the workplace, and the new worker, loyal only to the work, increases the stress in the work relationship.

8. The pace of technology creates a demand in process and procedure that changes faster than providers can cope. When a new technique is learned, even newer technology arrives that makes the recently engaged learning obsolete, often before the provider has had time to entrench previous new learning.

9. Managers are leading temporary workers employed by others, yet are accountable for the care these workers render in the institution. Issues of managing people you do not employ raise the stress level of leadership and affect the ability to assure quality and positive outcomes.

10. The demands of management work appear to be increasing, taking the manager away from the unit and service much more frequently

to address systems issues. The staff is on its own more often, problems remain unresolved, and crises emerge more frequently because the manager is not able to anticipate them, accelerating the degree of stress in the manager's role (Porter-O'Grady, pp. 105–106).

So the question is: Are we able to see the patterns, help to translate these patterns to others as we go about our work, and constantly revise our picture of what our work entails? It is up to us, keeping in mind that:

> *That which is, already has been; that which is to be, already is.*
>
> *—Ecclesiastes 3:15*

References

American Association of Managed Care Nurses. (2000). *A Nurse's Introduction to Managed Care*. Glen Allen, VA: American Association of Managed Care Nurses.

Anderson, R. (Summer 2000). Are our systems really integrated? *Nursing Administration Quarterly, 24*(4), 11.

Anonymous. (September 2001). 2001 guide to nursing organizations. *Nursing Management*, 57–59.

Anonymous. (2001). *2001 contract management survey*. Hospitals & Health Networks, centerfold.

Balch, P., & Balch, J. (2000). *Prescription for Nutritional Healing*. 3rd ed. New York: Avery.

Bernreuter, M. (March 2001). Spotlight on… the american board of nursing specialties: Nursing's gold standard. *JONA's Healthcare Law, Ethics, and Regulation, 3*(1), 5–7.

Buresh, B., & Gordon, S. (2000). *From silence to voice: What nurses know and must communicate to the public*. Ottawa: Canadian Nurses Association.

Carpenter, D. (August 2000). Bitter pills. *Hospitals and Health Networks*, 49–52.

Catlin, A., & McAuliffe, M. (Second Quarter 1999). Proliferation of non-physician providers as reported in the Journal of the American Medical Association (JAMA), 1998. *Image: Journal of Nursing Scholarship, 31*(2), 175–177.

Chang, C., Price, S., & Pfoutz, S. (2001). *Economics and nursing: Critical professional issues*. Philadelphia: F.A. Davis.

Chyna, J. (May/June 2000). From alliances to outsourcing: Making good connections. *Healthcare Executive*, 12–16.

Cumings, M. (2003). *Human heredity: Principles and issues*. 6th ed. Pacific Grove, CA: Thomson.

Curran, C. (January–February 1996). An interview with John Kitzhaber. *Nursing Economic$, 14*(1), 5–8.

Drucker, P. (1974). *Management tasks, responsibilities, practices*. New York: Harper & Row.

Enriquez, J., & Goldberg, R. (March–April 2000). Transforming life, transforming business: The life-science revolution. *Harvard Business Review*, 96–104.

Finkelman, A. (2001). *Managed care: A nursing perspective*. Upper Saddle River, NJ: Prentice Hall.

Finkler, S., & Kovner, C. (2000). *Financial management for nurse managers and executives*. 2nd ed. Philadelphia: W.B. Saunders.

Gottlieb, S. (March 2001). One doctor: One patient. *Cost & Quality*, 23–24.

Grenberg, M., & Cartwright, J. (November–December 2001). Identifying best practices in telehealth nursing: The telehealth survey. *Nursing Economic$, 19*(6), 283–285.

Griffith, J. (1999). *The well-managed healthcare organization*. 4th ed. Chicago: Health Administration Press.

Guo, L., Schmidt, S., & Scheer, S. (May–June 2001). Use of acute and subacute services by hospitalized stroke patients: A comparison across payers. *Nursing Economic$, 19*(3), 107–114.

Harris, M. (1997). *Handbook of home health care administration*. 2nd ed. Gaithersburg, MD: Aspen.

Haugh, R. (January 1999). Medicare fraud busters. *Hospitals & Health Networks*, 16.

Haugh, R. (January 2001). Hospitals rethink their integration strategies basics. *Hospitals & Health Networks*, 33–35.

Hudson, T. (December 1977). Necessary loses? *Hospitals & Health Networks*, 26.

Knapp, M. (May 1999). Nurses' basic guide to understanding the medicare pps. *Nursing Management*, 14–15.

Kongstvedt, P., MD, FACP. Capgemini, US, LLC.

Lanser, E. (January/February 2003). Our aging population. *Healthcare Executive*, 7–11.

Larson, L. (March 2000). Genomics: Medicine's future in our molecules. *Hospital & Health Services Networks*, 75–82.

Lashley, F. (1998). *Clinical genetics in nursing practice*. 2nd ed. New York: Springer.

Lea, D. (November 2003). Look back to move forward: How genetics changes daily practice. *Nursing Management, 34*(11), 21–24.

Longest, B., Rakich, J., & Darr, K. (2000). *Managing health services organizations and systems*. 4th ed. Baltimore: Health Professions Press.

Lovitky, J. (November 1997). Health care fraud: A growing problem. *Nursing Management, 28*(11), 42, 44–45.

McGarvey, R. (May 2003). Biotech advances: Transforming out lives with new drugs, better crops, even personalized medicine. *Harvard Business Review*, S1.

Meadows, G. (November–December 2001). The internet promise: A new look at e-health opportunities. *Nursing Economic$, 19*(6), 294–295.

Meier, E. (May–June 2000). Medicare, social security, and competitive benefits are neglected nursing issues. *Nursing Economic$, 18*(3), 168–170.

Merrill, P. (May–June 2001). Wake-up call for us health care system and apns. *Nursing Economic$, 19*(3), 127.

Mitty, E. (1998). *Handbook for directors of nursing in long-term care*. Albany: Delmar.

Mohr, W., & Mahon, M. (September 1996). Dirty hands: The underside of marketplace health care. *Advances in Nursing Science, 19*(1), 28–37.

Porter-O'Grady, T. (February 2003). A different age for leadership, part 1: New context, new content. *JONA, 33*(2), 105–110.

Raffel, M., & Raffel, N. (1994). *The U.S. health system: Origins and functions.* 4th ed. New York: Delmar.

Retiree Health Benefits Now and in the Future. Found at http://www.kff.org/medicare/011404package.cfm.

Roberts, V. (July/August 2001). Managing strategic outsourcing in the healthcare industry. *Journal of Healthcare Management, 46*(4), 239–249.

Rognehaugh, R. (1996). *The managed health care dictionary.* Gaithersburg, MD: Aspen.

Senge, P. (1994). *The fifth discipline: The art & practice of the learning organization.* New York: Doubleday Currency.

Smith, N. (1997). "Chapter 44: Managed Care" from Harris, M. *Handbook of Home Health Care Administrators.* 2nd ed. Gaithersburg, MD: Aspen, p. 535.

Steele, S., Rocchiccioli, J., & Porche, D. (March–April 2003). Analyzing and promoting issues in health policy: Nurse manager's perspective. *Nursing Economic$, 21*(2), 80–83.

Succi, M., Alexander, J., Jelinek R., & Lee, S. (November/December 2001). Change in the population of health systems: From 1985 to 1998. *Journal of Healthcare Management, 46*(6), 381–396.

Tahan, H. (March–April 1999). Home healthcare under fire: Fraud and abuse. *JONA's Healthcare Law, Ethics, and Regulation, 1*(1), 16–24.

Teisberg, E., Porter, M., & Brown, G. (July–August 1994). Making competition in health care work. *Harvard Business Review*, 131–141.

Their money or your health: Who owns health care? (February 2002). *JONA, 32*(2), 64–65.

Webb, J. (April 2003). The washington report. *Voice of Nursing Leadership*, 3.

Wheatley, M. (1992). *Leadership and the new science.* San Francisco: Berrett-Koehler.

Whetsell, G. (Summer 1999). The history and evolution of hospital payment systems: How did we get here? *Nursing Administration Quarterly, 23*(4), 1–13.

Woodward, S. (May 1995). Oregon: Philosophy collides with finance. *Business & Health*, 51–61.

Ziel, S. (2002). Get on board with hipaa privacy regulations. *Nursing Management, 33*(10), 28–29.

CHAPTER 7

Is there Life after Capitation?
The Economics of the U.S. Health Care
System after the Managed Care Revolution

Adapted from a speech given to the 33rd Annual Meeting and Exposition of the American Association of Nurse Executives (AONE), Tuesday, March 28, 2000, Nashville, Tennessee[1]

J.D. Kleinke[2]

Recently, I finished *Bleeding Edge*, a book about health care in the United States (Aspen).[3] One of the great frustrations in trying to write the book was that everything I wrote was out of date before I could hit the print button. The first draft of the book was driven by headlines:

The Future of Hospitals—*Columbia HCA*

The Future of Managed Care—*Oxford Health Plans*

The Future of the Physician—*PhyCor*[4]

Generally, the headlines were obsolete before the ink was dry. One of the hardest things I had to say was, "Okay, I'm going to ignore the headlines. I'm going to stand back and focus on the big picture—the 100-year problem."

---

[1] Thank you to Dr. Penny Marquette for this transcription.

[2] A medical economist with an MSB in finance (Johns Hopkins) and a BS in economics (University of Maryland), J.D. Kleinke is a frequent contributor to the *Wall Street Journal*, *JAMA*, *Barron's*, *Modern Healthcare*, *Business and Health*, *Managed Healthcare*, *Health Affairs*, and *Compensation and Benefits Management*. He also serves on the editorial board of *Health Affairs*. During the 1990s, Kleinke was a driving force growing HCIA from a small firm engaged in data analysis for the health care industry, into a publicly traded corporation providing analysis and software products to a broad spectrum of health care providers. Kleinke's background also includes experience with Sheppard Pratt Health Systems, where he was instrumental in developing and managing a provider-based, managed health care system. Sheppard Pratt, the largest psychiatric hospital in the United States, was the first to develop such a system.

[3] J.D. Kleinke, *Bleeding Edge* (Gaithersburg, Maryland: Aspen Publishing, Inc., 1998).

[4] PhyCor is a physician management company that grew rapidly by buying large group practices and smaller physician management companies. PhyCor quickly ran into financial and operating difficulties.

The truth is that we have 100 years of history in our health care system and much of it was built by accident. The fact that employers are involved in providing health care (or at least paying for it) is a complete accident, dating to World War II. The fact that we have hospital-centric capacity goes back to the turn of the century and is not part of a well thought-out master plan. The cultural conflict between physicians and hospitals as business entities is equally old—a conflict that can be dated to the start of the 20th century. And finally, the fact that we have fee-for-service, versus a pure risk-based payment system, goes back to the rejection of that payment model by physicians at the turn of the last century as well. *Managed care* is trying to fix a 100-year-old problem, and that fix cannot occur overnight as many expected.

Competing Tensions

Whether you're reading headlines about Columbia, or Oxford, or the impact of the internet, or about hospitals merging together and later unbundling, it all fits into the tension between two things: (1) risk, and (2) consumerism. Risk and consumerism define the supply (risk) and the demand (consumerism) sides of health care. Further, supplying health care is expensive, and *managed care* is part of the continuing attempt to rationalize producer behavior and remind providers that there are financial consequences to what they do. Everything else occurs downstream from that; everything else is a consequence.

The other goal of managed care (in addition to managing the money) is to manage consumer's expectations. We all grew up believing that medicine was free, the budget was unlimited, access was immediate, and we expected that it would always be that way. We never questioned the value of irrational, recreational medicine. An article in the *Wall Street Journal* reports that people are having full-body CAT scans as part of their executive physicals. Recreational CAT scans. (Sounds like a great time.)[5] In truth, for most of us, it will never be that way again. And I won't lie to you. Re-educating patients is a tough process and it's a miserable one.

What I'd like to do in this chapter is provide you with some history to explain why we have the type of managed care system we do today, give you my opinion on why it isn't working the way it was intended, and provide some advice on how to survive (and even prosper) in a managed care environment.

DRGs—The Beginning of Managed Care

Look back over the past twenty years. What is the most significant thing that has happened to health care legislatively? What one stroke of the legislative pen, what one act of Congress, changed *everything* about the health care delivery system? Clearly, it was the DRG—the Diagnosis Related Group. The DRG said that we could no longer manage our hospital care costs on a lab-by-lab, radiology-study-by-radiology-study, drug-by-drug basis.

---

[5] I guess this was a next logical step after the oxygen bar.

Speaking (theoretically) for Medicare only, Congress said, "Let's give providers a fixed amount of money, a lump sum payment, based on the DRG and let them figure it out." At that time it was the conventional wisdom that hospitals would all close because they were overstaffed, utilizing too many resources, and making tons of money doing things that really weren't necessary (the public alarm about the outcome of DRGs suggests that Congress had a point). But the alarm was premature. Within three years the average length of stay for Medicare patients went from nine days down to six.

In the process, DRGs had other positive side effects. One was the collection of detailed data, previously unavailable from providers. Those data, as we will see later, are an important element in surviving managed care. Another positive side effect was the creation of the home health care business, and the sub-acute business, both of which can often provide adequate care at a far lower cost than in-hospital service.

All of this was the result of one simple idea: Based on the diagnosis, reimburse a fixed lump-sum payment, for a hospital *episode*, and let the provider figure out how to provide care cost-effectively. It is a very inspiring story, and because it's so inspiring, and because the numbers are so powerful, the managed care industry got a little too excited and took one more step, a step into global capitation—turning doctors and hospitals into insurance companies.

Global Capitation

With the success of DRGs fresh in their minds, the policy makers said, "Oh well, if we take one more step and change to a lump sum payment *per person* (rather than *per hospital episode*) we won't have to worry about micro-managing doctors and hospitals and everyone working for them. We'll get to avoid sick people entirely." Unfortunately, global capitation was a total over-correction (common in health care) because it mixed two kinds of risk: (1) case risk and (2) insurance or actuarial risk. With case risk, like the DRG, you have to figure out how to do the best job you can for a fixed payment. That is something that you, as the provider, can (within limits) control, particularly because the size of that fixed payment will vary depending on the severity of the diagnosis.

Insurance or actuarial risk, on the other hand, holds providers responsible[6] "for the health of their insured population. They are "responsible" for the occurrence of breast cancer or HIV in the population. Clearly, these are things over which providers have *minimal control*. In essence, you're punishing providers for serving the wrong clientele.

This over-correction had some pretty significant consequences. For one thing, global capitation turned everyone *against* managed care, both because it was an over-correction, and because the rates it paid were usually unreasonable. The popular solution has been to destroy managed care entirely, and I think that if I could, I would (at least managed care as it is currently practiced).[7] But unfortunately, the messages of managed care are important and they are historically salient. They've just been delivered in a very unpleasant way. And one of the valid messages of managed care is that we need to shift the form of payment in

---

[6] Providers make more money when fewer services are provided and when patients remain healthier.

[7] Unfortunately, unlike computer systems, there is no [CONTROL-ALT-DELETE] button on the managed care system.

managed care away from fee-for-service—the blank-check wielding patient and the blank-check signing employer. That system simply doesn't work. That's the strongest message of managed care.

Why We Need (Ugh) Managed Care

Managed care is trying to make a set of statements about provider behavior. In essence, managed care says that "provider behavior is dysfunctional." The problem—how do we fix it? And the answer is that we fix it with nothing less than a cultural revolution. And, for better or worse, nurse administrators are as much in charge of trying to lead people through this revolution as physicians and hospitals. Let me give you an example of dysfunctional behavior (not from health care); a parable that we can refer to later.

Recently, when I moved to Denver, I discovered all these culinary delicacies. I found that I really like blue corn chips and blue corn pancakes. One day, when I was shopping in one of our health food stores, I discovered blue corn flakes. So I threw the box in the cart and it wasn't until I got to the check-out counter that I realized that this stuff is $5.00/box (and not a very big box at that). The Kellogg's Corn Flakes are $3.50/box and the generic stuff is even less (was that a clue?). What, I asked myself, am I paying an extra $1.50/box for?

Well, on the box, the manufacturers have written the slogan "made from the blue corn that the Hopi ate for strength." Sounds good enough to me; I bought the blue corn flakes.

The next morning I'm eating this cereal (it tasted awful by the way, but since I paid $5.00 for it, I'm wolfing it down) and I'm feeling pretty noble because this is the stuff that gave the Hopi strength. But then I begin thinking about it, and remembering some of the things I've read since moving to Denver, some of which includes ancient history about the Hopi, I double check my facts.

It turns out that the average life expectancy of the Hopi was 19.4 years and that they reached an average height of 4 feet 10 inches tall. In defense of the Hopi, it wasn't their fault that they had a life expectancy of 19.4 years. Typically in the Hopi tribe if you were febrile for some reason (and remember that they had no understanding of germs and didn't know about pneumonia or otitis media and those things), they threw you off a cliff. Of course you died and then the tribe moved away.[8] So much for the powers of $5.00/box blue corn flakes.

Let me give you an example of "made from the blue corn that the Hopi ate for strength" in the real US health care system—not experimental procedures, not even alternative medicines, just *extra money for a claim that may not have the most rigorously tested clinical evidence to support it.*

A good example is the storage of umbilical blood. Right now there is a business that did not exist two years ago. It's a commercial business, about $40 million in sales, and there are three companies in the industry. These companies will store umbilical cord blood for a pregnant woman for $2,000. Then, if the woman's child develops leukemia later, say five years down the road, the umbilical cord blood will provide an excellent source of stem cells.

---

[8] Actually this is very similar to the clinical protocol that Aetna thought they were buying when they acquired U.S. Health Care.

Consider the emotions of the parent. "I'm pregnant and I'm terrified of anything happening to my child." In this situation, the "rational" health care *consumer* (who is irrational by most economic standards), says, "Okay, I'll pay the $2,000." And remember, it probably isn't the parent's $2,000, it's the health insurance company's $2,000, or the employer's $2,000. In other words, it's free.[9] So the mom says, "Two grand? I'll sign." But the HMO's job is to say, "No, you can't have it." The HMO has medical economists whose job it is to say, "There's no family history of leukemia here; the likelihood of this woman's child ever getting leukemia is so remote that there is *no cost-benefit model* that would justify paying this for a population. We're not paying $2,000."

So the mom has two choices (aside from suing the HMO). She can go without, because the HMO controlled and rationalized the resource, or she can pay for it from her own pocket. *And that's the purpose of managed care. Ultimately, managed care is in the business of sorting people into consumer segments based on how much of their own money they are willing to spend on stupid things—for recreational medicine, for things that aren't necessary.* That's the ultimate theory—that if we rationalize enough of the dumb stuff, we'll have more money left over for the stuff we now go without—stuff that we really need like prenatal care, well-baby visits, and immunizations.

I'm not trying to defend managed care—only to explain it, and that is still the message of managed care—to keep people away from the box of blue corn flakes or make them pay for it out of their own pockets. The rationalization of managed care is not going to go away, because our current reality needs to be changed. I've given you an example from the patient's side, let's look at one from the provider's side. An example from North Carolina may help explain both the complexity of the issues and the reason that the current health care situation needs to be fixed.

In 1994, North Carolina had a terrible hysterectomy rate, totally out of whack with the rest of the country. It was also out of whack from place to place *within the state of North Carolina*. When researchers analyzed their data, they found that it wasn't the payer mix, or the urban-rural breakdown (in fact, rural populations had *higher* hysterectomy rates, which is totally counterintuitive), or anything they could define about the patient's condition. They simply couldn't find anything in the *patient population* to explain the rate. Finally, they controlled enough of the variables to identify the driving factor, and it had nothing to do with the patients. It was *something about the physicians*. Once they found what they were looking for, they could adjust for the age of the patients, the co-morbidity and everything else, and still separate the physicians into two groups. One group was doing 70 percent more hysterectomies than the other. If you haven't already guessed, the two groups were *based on gender*. Male physicians did 70 percent more hysterectomies than female physicians.

Another of the legitimate things that managed care has had to say is that when it comes to medical and surgical and treatment issues, the gender of the physician should not matter. This is supposed to be science.

---

[9] And don't forget, in the world of self-insured employers, and pre-tax insurance benefits, spending your employer's money is like getting a $2,000 raise.

Why Managed Care Doesn't Work

Micro-Managing Payments

Having defended the need for managed care, I don't want to go so far as to defend its primary provider—the HMO. HMOs have not done the job that managed care thought they would, and there are a number of reasons why. The first is the fact that physicians are what economists call *rational economic actors*.

> *Rational Economic Actors—Put obstacles in the way and physicians will figure out how much money they "need" to make, and hospitals will figure out how much money they "need" to make, and then they will firgure out how to back around the system and make that amount of money.*

Every now and then when you're talking about the future of the US health care system, it is occasionally useful to talk about medicine, and since most of you have clinical backgrounds, I hope you'll humor me while I tell you an apocryphal story. This story will make a point about where managed care has taken us as an industry over the past ten years and where it may take us in the future. I will do this by referring to a particular clinical case.

In front of me I have an x-ray of the pelvic region of a patient. On the film you would see a tiny fixed object just right of center. It looks kind of gnarly, but no less twisted than the story behind it. I learned of this case from a physician friend in Denver—a gastroenterologist. Every Saturday he and I get together for a bike ride, and we indulge in a little contest to see whose workweek was worse. Since my friend is a practicing physician, he usually wins this contest (which is, of course to say, he really loses). One week he tells me that I'm not going to believe the case he had: The patient whose film I am looking at came in with abdominal pain and then, on the film, there's this gnarly fixed object. It was a *dental bridge*.

The patient had swallowed the dental bridge and it ended up in his colorectal tract and perforated the intestine. Of course, my physician friend went in and took it out. The procedure took four hours, and because of the perforated intestine, the patient wound up spending three days in the hospital.

After he tells me this story, my friend says that as difficult as it was to surgically wrestle this object out of this guy's colon, that was *nothing* compared to what he had to do to get paid. Just when he thought his problems were over, he received a letter from HCFA[10] (this is a Medicare patient). This letter and my friend's reaction to this letter, embody everything that's wrong with trying to line-item-by-line-item manage fee-for-service medicine:

> Dear Provider:
>
> Pursuant to our review of reference claim for reimbursement for CPT 4, procedure code 74632, Extraction of Other Foreign Objects from

---

[10] HCFA—Health Care Finance Administration is now called CMS—Centers for Medicare and Medicaid Services

> Colorectal tract, we have reviewed provider's contention that said object consists of one type 77 B dental bridge in conjunction with said beneficiary's enrollment record. As a result of such review we're referring this matter to the Inspector General's Office for the investigation of possible fraud. Fiscal intermediaries' records show that the beneficiary is not enrolled in a managed care risk contract, and therefore we find no clinical basis for provider's contention that a third party is taking a bite out of said beneficiary's ass.

Of course my friend does what every rational caregiver does. He calls his lawyer. Then he calls his wife. Then he calls his lawyer again. But, he also talks with one of his Ernst and Young consultants and together they figure out that, while this is a problem, the web also makes it an opportunity. What he can do is use the web to attract more patients like this one. So he starts a web site called *dental-bridge-swallowers.com*. And it works. He's getting a lot of these cases coming in and he's gotten very good at doing them surgically. But equally important he's gotten really good at avoiding this letter.

For these procedures, my friend knows that he needs a three-day length of stay. So he goes to the Milliman and Robertson Guidelines,[11] looks for a three-day length of stay in the column, and then he looks across to the left to find an appropriate diagnosis. No problem. Now he takes these bridges out of his (mostly male, mostly elderly) patients' colorectal systems using a C-Section.

All kidding aside, the reaction I've just described, and the reaction we have come to expect from all physicians (self-trained), is to figure out *how to work the system*, how to cope.

Under the old fee-for-service system, people would arrive at the clinic bearing a blank check of their bosses' money and the provider would say, "Ooh! A blank check," and fill it out. The first wave of risk-based payments (DRGs) was an attempt to deal with that kind of dysfunctional system. It did work to a degree, but patients learned to cope and providers learned to cope. For providers there is the simple coping technique of dealing with the system *as they find it* and figuring out a way to get through the gates, and over the humps, and through the hoops, and take care of patients and *make a target income*. HCFA figured this out a long time ago (but they never bothered to tell any of the rest of us).

Initially, when HCFA wanted to reduce the cost of a surgery, they would reduce the price by a certain amount. If they wanted to reduce the cost of a procedure by 5 percent, they would reduce the price by 5 percent, expecting the total cost to go down by 5 percent. What they found, however, was that the *frequency* of that procedure would go up just enough to offset the reduction in price so that the total outlay was the same the following year. It's called the "Target Income Effect."

The fact of the matter is that everyone in the health care system, just like everyone else in our economy, is a rational economic agent, and it took managed care about ten years to figure this out. Put the obstacles in the way and physicians will figure out how much

---

[11] The Milliman and Robertson Guidelines are developed by physicians and nurses who identify target lengths of stay for various types of hospital patients. Although they have been used widely by managed care organizations to monitor hospital stays, they are highly controversial.

money they "need" to make, and hospitals will figure out how much money they "need" to make, and then they will figure out how to back around the system and make that amount of money. This is something that managed care did finally figure out—*reimbursement* reform is health care reform. If you really want to change something clinically, change the way you pay for it. If you want to improve quality, or rationalize resources, rationalize the economic motives for using those resources.

A good example can be found in C-Section rates in Pennsylvania. At the crest of the C-Section wave, the C-Section rate reached a national high of 24.5 percent. Twenty-four point five percent of all deliveries were done by C-Section in that year, *except in Pennsylvania* where the rate was 29 percent. Twenty-four point five was the national norm, but it was 29 percent in Pennsylvania. Why?

Easy. Pennsylvania had two commercial insurers, Blues in the West and Blues in the East. They were paying $2,500 for a normal delivery, and $4,000 for a C-Section. When the Blues saw the data they said "We have a real problem here, let's do something about it." What they did was go to a "global payment" system. They decided to pay physicians and hospitals the same number of dollars for a delivery regardless of the manner of delivery and let them figure out when to do a C-Section. Surprise. They put this payment plan in place and the next year the C-Section rate in Pennsylvania was 24.5 percent. Back to the national norm, based on one fine-tuning of the payment system. The message is clear. Unregulated fee-for-service medicine doesn't work. Trying to regulate health care costs with line-item-by-line-item managed care doesn't work either. If you really want to change something, change the way you pay for it.

HMOs in Conflict with their Mission

There are a million examples of how HMOs find themselves in conflict with their own mission statements. Why? Because better health care costs more money, not less. For example, do you want to know, according to *Readers' Digest*, the "top ten things that women doctors want you to know?" Seven out of ten of them involve having a lab test, another type of diagnostic workup, or seeing a physician or physician extender for some kind of exam. Essentially they are ten top reasons to encounter the health care system. Imagine. You're standing in the grocery line and you're feeling fine and suddenly you're told that you need a medical encounter—something that's going to consume the time of a nurse or the time of a doctor. And if five of those seven things tested return less than a normal outcome, you're supposed to get on a drug. Is that good news for HMOs? No, it's terrible news for HMOs, because most of those people are perfectly healthy.

HMOs are hurting because of a contradiction in their own mission. The fundamental flaw in the HMO theory is that better informed patients, people who will take care of themselves, will result in decreased health care costs. In the long term that may make sense, but in the short run it does not. Doing the right thing for your members costs money.

Another example. Recently, there was a study of a pneumococcal pneumonia vaccine from Kaiser. Kaiser immunized 19,000 infants against pneumococcal pneumonia. It was a four shot regimen and expensive. They also put 19,000 infants on placebo. The vaccine was very successful—it was able to prevent 38 cases of pneumococcal pneumonia that occurred in the placebo group. Assuming that each one of these kids who actually gets sick goes into the hospital (a worst case scenario), the vaccine saves about $5,200 per infected infant. Multiply that times 38 cases and you have a $200,000 savings. Unfortunately, immunizing 19,000 infants costs a million bucks. That's a reverse ROI (Return on Investment) of 5:1. For every dollar they save, it costs them five. This is terrible accounting because it chafes against everything we believe. We believe that the right thing is to immunize people against disease. But it doesn't work from the managed care perspective. It's exactly backwards. The HMO that invests a dollar in this vaccine, loses five. So who has a vested interest in this? It's not Kaiser.

The vested interests lie with the parents of the children who don't have to watch a child get sick, don't have to suffer with a child in the hospital, don't have to miss work or encounter all the other hardships that go with it. The HMO really doesn't have a vested interest in this, the parents do, the consumers do. And this is the real shot heard round the managed care world; this is the sad truth they're facing. At least in the short run, an HMO loses money doing the right thing. This is the central contradiction facing the HMOs and it is why they are falling apart in the court of public opinion.

Not Everyone Can Afford It!

One final example. I have a friend whose wife is a dermatologist with a high-end practice in Denver. She has a lot of society patients and powerful business people. One of them came to her recently with a "thing" on her arm. Now this patient is a high-powered investment banker, perfectly healthy other than the "thing," and she came to her dermatologist and said, "I'd like you to remove this thing on my arm." The doctor replies, "Yep, that's a thing on your arm, and I'd love to take it off, but you have Health Net.[12] You have to go to your primary physician who will look at it and say, 'Yeah, that's a thing on your arm,' and then he'll send you to me (the dermatologist-specialist), and then I can say, 'Yes that's a thing on your arm' and I can take it off." In other words, you have to go through the gate keeper. Essentially your primary care physician has to tell you what you already know.

As one might expect, the woman said something like, "That's outrageous, I make $350,000 a year and I don't have time for this," and her dermatologist said to her, "Then you should have bought real insurance." If your time is that valuable, then the cost of cheap insurance is turning out to be pretty expensive. That is also part of the process of cultural re-education that managed care is affecting. It's not a fun task but it is forcing all of us, as patients, to consider the value of access, the value of choices, the real value of the blue cornflakes.

---

[12] Health Net is a commercial HMO with a large presence in the Western United States.

Surviving Managed Care—Consolidation, Branding, and Niche Marketing

The Overall Strategy

I'm going to start this section with another story—a true story about firefighters. When I relocated to Denver a few years ago, one of the things I learned about my adopted state is the way they put out forest fires. It's fascinating, and there's a true story from the late 1940s about a particular fire which provides a lot of parallels to what is happening in health care now. Through the rest of this talk I'm going to refer to it again and again.

Obviously, there aren't any fire hydrants in the wilderness, and so you put out forest fires by parachuting fire fighters into the wilderness. There's a whole science to how you fight a fire. Typically the fire fighters, called smoke jumpers, drop into an adjacent canyon and work a fire line down the other canyon. This happened in 1949 in the Mann Gulch. Eighteen smoke jumpers parachuted into a canyon adjacent to a roaring fire and due to an unfortunate confluence of factors—topography, weather, humidity, and heat—these 18 guys parachuted in just as the fire jumped the ridge next to them. Fanned by cold rushing wind from a stream at the bottom of the canyon, the fire raged, forcing a fireball up the canyon into which they had landed. It's a terrifying story. They stood there, trying to get their parachutes off, and looking at a wall of fire coming at them at 200 miles an hour. They knew they were doomed and they did the only "rational" thing—they ran. Fifteen smoke jumpers died as a result, but three of them survived. How they survived is very illustrative.

Two of the men had been lucky. They had parachuted in close to a cave and they hid in the cave until the fire blew by them. The remaining guy, the foreman of the crew, saw the fire coming, saw people trying to outrun a 200 mile an hour fire, and knew they were doomed. He looked around and spotted an area of waist high, tinder dry grass nearby. He pulled matches out of his pocket and lit the grass on fire. When it had burned down into smoldering ash, he jumped into the middle of it, crouching down in the ash, and the fire blew over him. He survived. *But to survive, he had to burn his own grass. He had to have the courage to burn his own grass, and he had to have the knowledge and tools to do it.*

What does this story have to do with managed care? Well, everyone I encounter in this industry tells me that managed care is evil and we should destroy it. That, I would contend, is the equivalent of hiding in the cave. Some would compare the cave to the academic medical center, or to joining a consulting firm. But I would argue that a better, more generally applicable way to survive the 200 mile per hour fire that managed care is sending toward patients *and* providers is to burn your own grass—not an easy thing to do.

Burn your own grass—what does that really mean? How do you translate that into health care? I'll tell you what I say to physicians, and it's particularly good news for nurses, especially advanced practice nurses. I tell physicians that *everything they were trained and taught represents dry grass.* For physicians that means stop the bickering among specialties, stop the bickering between academic doctors and community doctors, stop the bickering between doctors and hospitals, *stop bickering with advanced practice nurses.*

Burn your own grass means adapting to economic pressures. If managed care is going to pay you a lump sum to deliver a baby, Dr. OB-Gyn, then maybe a nurse midwife—whom you've been trained to criticize for substandard clinical skills—isn't such a bad thing. Maybe a nurse midwife is an excellent way to leverage your clinical talent, embracing the message of managed care, which is that we need to manage cost, and that everything you've been taught to revile about nurse midwives (like the fact that they have half the C-Section rates of physicians) is good for you when you're getting paid a lump sum. There's an old saying: the enemy of my enemy is my friend, and managed care is the enemy. And it's *not* going away.

Beyond physicians embracing alternatives to deal with managed care, I don't believe in the philosophy that, *"We're all in this together."* I think that surviving managed care is a bare knuckles, zero-sum game. At HCIA, I worked and negotiated with managed care companies, acted as a data intermediary in dealings between HMOs and doctors, and between HMOs and hospitals, and the fire that is managed care has always been a zero-sum game. There is a fixed dollar amount out there and that dollar isn't getting any bigger very fast. Whatever does get bigger seems to go to the drug industry. And everyone else is left to fight over whatever's left. In the next section we're going to look at some strategies to survive managed care. Primarily we will look at consolidation, branding, and niche marketing. Each of these is related to defining the local market for health care.

There's an old cliche that says if you've seen one health care market, you've seen one health care market. And, to a large extent, that's true. But just as everything else in health care is changing, the definition of a local health care market is changing as well. In my six years at HCIA we compiled databases for 27 state hospital associations and I was involved in a lot of our HMO and drug company work. As a result, I saw a lot of commonalities between health care markets across the United States. While the descriptions in the sections that follow may not exactly describe any *specific* health care market, they generally describe them all. For example, even the smallest single system town will have problems of competition and consolidation because somewhere, about twenty miles away, is another single system town and it is providing effective competition. That's why the Federal Trade Commission can't seem to win health care anti-trust suits. These single system towns do have competition; it's just 20 miles down the road. As long as everyone has access to emergency room services, you can reasonably expect people to go 20 miles for a CAT scan.

Consolidation

Consolidation and branding occur at many levels. Historically, the process began (and it is a slow, miserable process) when Columbia/HCA or Tenet went into a medium sized town and found nine hospitals, each with a 50 percent occupancy rate, with MRIs and cardiac cath labs at two or three of them. So the for-profit buys up three hospitals, shuts down one of the cath labs, moves the patient traffic over to the other hospital, shuts down one of the MRIs entirely, and moves that traffic to another hospital. They get the occupancy rate up from 50 percent to 65 percent and they lay off nurses. In the process, they take three hospitals which were underutilized with too much fixed cost and overhead and create a much more rational system.

Then the plot thickens. The Nuns at the Catholic hospitals are appalled that three not-for-profit hospitals have been replaced by for-profit hospitals. Clearly the other not-for-profit hospitals are at risk of a similar fate. Blasphemy! So one of the Catholic systems swoops in and sees three Catholic hospitals sitting side by side in the same market, and each hospital has a 50 percent occupancy rate, and two of the three have MRIs and cath labs. So the Catholic system buys the three hospitals, shuts down one of the cath labs, shuts down one of the MRIs entirely and moves the patient traffic to the other hospital. And they get occupancy up from 50 percent to 65 percent and they lay off nurses. But it's not-for-profit. And then the two systems position themselves, one against the other: You're for-profit, you're evil—you're not-for-profit, you're inefficient. (But we'll get into the marketing messages later.)

This type of consolidation and integration is a natural outcome of the shift from fee-for-service to managed care, and the economic pressures that it represents. At the same time, there are pressures working *against* successful consolidation. The reality is that no CEO or CIO or CFO wants to find himself or herself out of a job. As a result, mergers of facilities and vertical integrations often don't work very well because everyone still wants to defend his or her piece of turf.

A second type of consolidation and integration is going on at the same time. The motivation is different. It is *consolidation in response to managed care*. I would venture to say that the real function of this type of consolidation and integration isn't efficiency, or running a better system of care, or coordinating care across the continuum (although, by accident, these things may happen). Consolidation and integration in response to managed care are really about *negotiating leverage*. If managed care consolidates in a market and Aetna or PacificCare winds up owning two-thirds of the covered lives, the hospitals, the doctors, and all the other providers in that market have no option but to consolidate *in reaction*.

It's like a game of chicken, with all the providers running to cry that, "You can't exclude me from your network." Patients, the final health care consumers, will ultimately pick a system. And when they do that, *they'll start by picking a doctor*, and then another doctor, and eventually, a hospital. If "we" can put those providers in "one bucket," then whether it's Aetna or PacificCare doesn't matter. They can't exclude us from their network—they can't pick us off.

The reality is that *87 percent of people pick their physician first*. I have seen three separate studies, using three different methodologies, over the past three years with virtually identical results. People pick their physicians first. Then they find a way to wrap the insurance coverage around their choices. When someone signs up with Aetna, the first thing they do is go to the back of the provider book and find their doctor and their hospital. Then they figure out how to deal with the inconvenience of insurance. If their doctor isn't in the HMO, but he or she is in the PPO/POS, then the *consumer* has to decide whether it's worth paying another $8 in premiums to get that doctor into the network and have immediate access to one's own personal physician. For some people it is worth it, and for some it isn't.

The HMOs have reacted to this consumer behavior by attempting to "brand" the HMO. That's what the idea of Columbia/HCA, or the Catholic Systems, or the Teaching Hospital Systems, is all about. It's about creating a brand that's big enough and robust enough that the HMO is neutralized in terms of patient loyalty. And clearly it is also an attempt to neutralize Aetna's and PacificCare's leverage. Ultimately, however, the one who wins in this fight is the provider. I think the provider always wins because the attempt to brand is not generally successful. Kaiser has been the most successful, only because it has been around for so long. In health care, the provider is the market.

Another aspect of consolidation flows from the zero-sum, Darwinian game created by managed care. We are in a period of price compression. There are very few new dollars and, as I mentioned earlier, any that show up will probably go to the drug companies. Information technology, advertising and branding, are expensive and increasingly necessary in order to attract consumers. Combining resources to undertake these activities is another important aspect of consolidation.

Don't confuse rational consolidation with the huge over-correction of massive consolidation. The idea of Columbia/HCA or PhyCor rolling up hundreds of hospitals or thousands of physicians nation-wide, and negotiating *en masse* is ridiculous. Equally irrational is the old-fashioned extreme of nine stand-alone hospitals and multiple groups of three to five doctors. Nevertheless, I am talking about *local* consolidation, and *local* branding. Between the two extremes of (1) everyone being a part of PhyCor, and (2) "we're out here by ourselves and Aetna's picking us off like sniper fire," there is a properly sized group that can meet the needs of the local market and still be large enough to ensure inclusion in the network. Right now, I think the optimization point between the two extremes is about 400 physicians in an Independent Practice Association (IPA). That allows the group to include every specialty patients need, get plenty of flow, variability, and traffic, and allows for the option of adding nurse midwives, advanced practice nurses, and physician assistants (PAs). It's big enough to answer the call of consolidation, but it's still small enough to be manageable.

Branding and Niche Marketing

We started the discussion of branding and niche marketing when we discussed the for-profit and the Catholic system coming into a market, consolidating three hospitals each, and then labeling themselves and their mission. The Catholic System brands the for-profit hospital's motives as evil, and the for-profit system brands the Catholic system as inefficient. Said another way, one caters to the employers and the other caters to the community. And, depending on the market, one generally goes mid-market with traditional third party payers, and one goes down-market. So, the first type of branding and niche marketing we'll examine is vertical—who gets the private patients and who gets Medicaid?

It doesn't always come out the way you might think. I can name markets where the Catholic, not-for-profit system is mid-market and the for-profit system is down-market dealing with charity care and Medicaid. But regardless of who is positioned where, they will basically fight to stay out of last place. And they keep each other honest and offer market segmented service to the community.

The plot really thickens when someone fills the final niche and goes up-market. Where I came from, it was the Johns Hopkins Health Plan (read that in bold, sonorous tones). The very name of the plan and the way it is spoken says, "We don't do managed care, we're Johns Hopkins. We don't need to be in your network, you need us in your network. We're Johns Hopkins."

And Hopkins does a terrific job of managing that brand. They do every kind of transplant, they're big in pediatric oncology, they separate siamese quadruplets, and they get this stuff on the news all the time. And, because they are doing these incredible things, you're supposed to believe that Hopkins is the best place for an angioplasty (because that's what branding is all about).[13]

Branding works at the low end too. We have a great public hospital in Denver called Denver General Hospital, which serves a largely Hispanic, indigent population. This is definitely a down-market hospital which has also done some amazingly consumer savvy things. For example, they had a large cafeteria next to a very small smoking area. They took out the cafeteria and put in a McDonalds and increased the size of the smoking area. Then they renamed the hospital "Denver Health."

Denver Health knows who their market is. They're making money on Medicaid. They advertise in Spanish on the Spanish language TV station in Denver. They have done a terrific job of finding out who their market is and branding it. And that branding creates a sense of consumer appeal that transcends all efforts by the HMOs in telling patients where to go.

When you move into a new community you can tell which health care system is up-market, mid-market, or down-market by reading the billboards:

Quality Health Care You Can Afford

That's the billboard you see for the down-market.

Quality Health Care for Your Whole Family

That's the billboard for the mid-market. And then there's the up-market position:

Medical Miracles Every Day

People will, irrationally, assume that if it costs more it's better. People will still pay twice as much for Bayer Aspirin even when they know, intellectually, that it's no different from the generic. The real task of managed care is to sort people into buckets of price tolerance and perceived quality differences.

An analogy may help. People really like Fed Ex. Fed Ex is not really that much more reliable than the Post Office. Although Fed Ex is truly reliable when it matters, on average, the Post Office will get it there, and not much later. So what's the real issue? When the mail

---

[13] So, is Hopkins the best place for angioplasty? Well, maybe, if you want it done by a resident who hasn't been to bed since 1998.

shows up on someone's desk, what happens? Is it important to you that your package is opened *first*? People open the Fed Ex package first because it is *perceived to be* a more valuable package. Actually, Fed Ex is the best thing that ever happened to the Post Office. Fed Ex keeps the Post Office innovative, honest, and pushing hard.[14]

Let me give you a very quick MBA in marketing: *Match your product to your market.* Your product is your practice, and your market is your payer mix. Figure out who your patients are because they are very different depending on the market you're working in.

If you have an upscale practice with wealthy patients, spend more time with each person. They have money, they have traditional insurance, and if the insurance doesn't cover something, they can pay for it out-of-pocket. Often, physicians with well-insured patients believe that because of managed care, they have to have high volume. That's wrong, because you can't do a good job for your particular market. Well-heeled patients don't expect to wait and they don't expect to be rushed through. They'll pay for red carpet service.

Then there are physicians with high-risk, heavily managed care populations who are still trying to do medicine the old way, calling back all the normal labs, not burning their own grass by using physician extenders or nurse midwives or having the PAs do the lab call backs. They have high volume, low price patients, and they need to use clinical leverage. And that leverage involves using nurse midwives for normal births and using PAs for things like first line otitis media. That is the right thing for these hospitals and physicians to do. If they don't change and learn to serve their market, there will be less health care for poorer patients.

This discussion of market niche is an arrow pointing toward everyone in this room. *Your greatest opportunities exist where the market is demanding the most clinical leverage.* In the down-market to a large degree, in the mid-market to a lesser extent, and big time in certain ancillary services in the up-market. And if you are the boss and you are hiring people, match your product (your employees) to your market (your clients). Understanding that is not radical. It's just Business School 101, but it really *sounds* radical in health care.

A final note of hope about learning to find your market. Fed Ex didn't start putting drop boxes in yuppie residential neighborhoods until it had been in business for 13 years. At first you (and they) would think that Fed Ex sells to *businesses*, but the reality is that the *businesses' employees* are their customers, and by putting boxes in residential neighborhoods, they are matching their product to their market. But as great a company as Fed Ex is, it took them 13 years to do that. So take heart.

Consumerism and Patient Power

If nothing else had changed in the world, the job of the HMO would have been simple: keep people away from the blue corn flakes, and make them spend their own money for things that made no sense. The problem is, that while there are lots of blue corn flakes out there, there's also a lot of good information in various media, and there's the internet.

---

[14] Not *everyone* loves Fed Ex. We once spent weeks developing a proposal for UPS. It was a great proposal, but we didn't get the job. It was weeks later when we realized that we had Fed Ex'd the final paperwork.

When I say that there's lots of good stuff going on in the media, I'm not talking about *Scientific American*. I'm talking about *Readers' Digest*, available near every cash register, in every grocery store checkout counter in America. And it isn't just the print media. Fifteen years ago, you could watch NBC News every night and *maybe* you'd see one medical story a week. And that story was usually about a multi-organ transplant or something major that wasn't really relevant to the lives of most people. But turn on NBC News now—Monday through Friday you will probably see a story from *JAMA*, or the *New England Journal of Medicine*, or *Lancet*—a medical story every night of the week, and every one of those stories is there because the treatment group had a positive outcome. NBC doesn't talk about how the placebo group did really well. So it's always good news and it's an inducement for viewers to go out, demand more medicine, and rack up more costs. And, as we said before, that's something that the HMOs didn't count on. They never expected their own rhetoric about people taking care of themselves, rhetoric about wellness and prevention, to catch up with them.

This is one reason that managed care in the United States is going the opposite way of the rest of the world. With *Readers' Digest*, and NBC News, and everyone else out there, telling patients how to manage their own care, do we really need an HMO "adding" that value? Especially when the HMO is conflicted because that "value" isn't providing any value to them???

Tom Emerick, who is responsible for health care benefit's purchasing for Wal Mart, is one of the most articulate spokesmen for why HMOs not only don't work, but actually aggravate things. Emerick likes to color these debates by holding up this old, yellowed copy of a bill from 1951 for a normal delivery of a newborn, six-day length of stay. The bill is $191. You know what the deductible for health insurance was in 1951? It was $200. You couldn't deliver a baby in 1951 and exhaust your deductible. That's because in 1951, health insurance was really *health* insurance. It wasn't about the ten things women's doctors want them to know. It was about cancer and heart attacks. It was about catastrophe. Most significantly, it was not about putting an administrative layer on every inch of the health care system and complicating it. And it's easy to underestimate the cost of that extra layer. Let me give you an example.

A typical otitis media encounter with the medical establishment involves a PA or an advanced practice nurse (maybe a doctor), and a generic antibiotic, about $28 worth of medicine. *Maybe* it's a total of $35 in a high cost market. Do you know what it costs, across the whole system, to administer all the claims related to that generic drug and that nurses' or doctors' time? It's about $35. *In primary care we spend as much money administrating and hassling and dickering with the system as we do delivering care.* And the medical side isn't free either. The doctor or the PA or the nurse has to deal with the system too, and probably spends another $10 on input into the system that supports the reimbursement of the $35.

Ultimately it simply does not make sense for people to have everything managed down to the first dollar. If you need proof of that concept, think about what happens to your automobile insurance when you go from a $100 deductible to $500 to $1,000. Your premium gets cut in half at each stage. The HMO is an anachronism, a system of paternalism in a society where people want to manage their own health care and their our own pension funds.

This is why the idea of a Medical Spending Account (MSA) can work so well. By having insurance coverage to take care of catastrophic illness, along with a pot of money that can be spent out of one's own pocket, you can increase independence and decrease cost at the same time. It is similar to any insurance plan where the deductible is high.[15]

TECHNOLOGY AND DATA

When I gave this talk at AONE, I was grateful to be using slides. Normally I love technology and usually I use PowerPoint slides with my laptop. But a few weeks before AONE, I was talking to about 1,200 physicians and physician assistants about (of all things) the process by which information technology was going to revolutionize healthcare. We're talking about point-of-care clinical decision making, software right at the point of prescribing, and how this was going to change everything we know about health care today, and in the middle of this presentation, my lap top crashed. I had what we refer to as a *Microsoft Moment*.[16] Despite these moments, I remain a relatively unscathed true believer.

In the early 1990s, we all believed that computers would change everything. That given enough data, we could figure out which was the right drug, and what was the best timing for preoperative antibiotics, and what was the right mix of nursing skills, and who was a good doctor, and which hospital was a bad hospital. And we still believe that, although it's gotten to be a lot more complicated than I would have ever guessed ten years ago.

If the task of managed care is to re-engineer health care, we might reflect on when health care was engineered in the first place. We have $1.3 trillion dollars being churned through a system based on a bunch of peoples' habits, and feelings, and expectations, and needs, and it has not been penetrated by a lot of analysis or a lot of data. Earlier, I told you how reimbursement rates were driving the frequency of C-Sections in Pennsylvania, and how physician gender was determining the rates of hysterectomies in North Carolina. This should be a no-brainer. This is medicine, it's science, it shouldn't be practiced based on personal biases or economic motives.

This is the most useful thing the HMOs ever really had to offer. *"In God We Trust...all others must submit data"*—it's a slogan from a medical director at a large HMO. Along with all the dumb things managed care has done, and all the dumb ways that they have tried to do smart things, like rationalize the hysterectomy rate, they have run up against resistence. So the HMO positions and justifies itself by saying that the providers just can't figure it out. Providers have hysterectomy rates based on their own gender. Providers scream a lot of rhetoric about how they need to use an RN instead of an LPN, but they have no data to support their position. So, the HMO says, it falls to us to be the information broker. We will decide who's a good doctor, a bad hospital, the best drug to be on.

---

[15] I know that the whole MSA idea is very political and not well agreed upon and there are many things about the MSA with which I don't agree. For example, with an MSA you get to keep unspent money at the end of the year; a bad idea because it doesn't encourage you to take care of yourself. (I would prefer a plan like an FSA (Flexible Spending Account) where you either use it or lose it. That gives you an incentive to both take care of yourself and plan your medical spending.)

[16] It's also interesting that as I addressed AONE, Microsoft was about to be broken up by the Federal Government. About a week after the Justice Department was scheduled to announce how it would break up Microsoft, HCFA was going to issue a $20,000,000 RFP to figure out how we could develop market-driven standardization of health care software.

I understand the problems that people have with data. But I also believe that a good deal of this resistance is being driven by an attitude of "don't measure me, don't profile me; my patients are sicker."[17] So the physicians have said, "No, you can't measure it, everything's too different, the data stink, the patient mix is too different." This represents a complete unwillingness to burn their own grass, to accept the messages of managed care and embrace them.

I believe that all physicians and all the people in this room can ultimately make their case using data. If you really believe that a certain skill set improves an outcome, document and prove your position. Sometimes in health care, as in the rest of the world, the best outcome does cost more. If you are higher cost, but you believe that you have better outcomes, prove it. Correlate the outcomes and tell patients about it. If you do have the best outcome, that's where patients will want to go, and if you can prove it, and the HMO won't let patients use your services, their lawyers are going to sue and they are going to win. But this isn't what's happening. The physicians have abdicated. They have run away from the information and by default the HMOs have picked up the ball and have used the worst kind of data to set the rules.

I keep reminding my friends that it was a physician who started all this stuff, not an HMO. It was back in 1985 when John Wennberg, an MD/PhD working out of Dartmouth, was one of the first people to get his hands on data regarding hospital-based surgeries. And these data were available because the existence of DRGs had created a data base. (Data gathering and availability is another unintended outcome of DRGs that has made the system work better). Looking at hospital-based surgeries in Vermont, he found six to nine-fold differences in prostatectomy, tonsillectomy, hysterectomy—ridiculous variations in care that made no sense at all. And when he was done, Wennberg wrote an article, published in 1986, that should be required reading in every business of medicine course.[18]

The article, which appeared in the *New England Journal of Medicine* was called "Which [surgical utilization] Rate is Right?" And in the last paragraph of this article, published in 1986, Wennberg says, "In this coming era of cost containment, if we as physicians do not determine which rate is right, someone will [do it] for us." That is one of the most prophetic things I have ever read. And as I said before, the physicians abdicated. So I'll tell you who is determining which rate is right—it's the HMO.

And the problem continues to exist today. If providers don't figure out the "right" number of nurses, the right amount of surgeries, which drugs to use, and all of that, if they don't seize the opportunity and seize the information, if they don't burn their own grass, guess who will be figuring out that stuff out for you? The insurer. And if your data are weak, and you have big variability and weak arguments, guess where the insurer will want to push the line? And then they will tell the patient what's the right surgical utilization rate. It might be. But it might not.

---

[17] It's a little known fact that 80 percent of physicians in the United States treat patients that are sicker than average.

[18] Wennberg, J., "Which Rate is Right?" *New England Journal of Medicine*, 30 (January, 1986), p. 311.

These distributions in health care are very complicated. They are best developed and best understood by those closest to the front lines—the providers. I tell physicians all the time: burn your own grass, run your own numbers, figure out your angle, and if you've got crummy outcomes, do something about them.

But there is a real fear—accountability. Still I would argue that you need to overcome the fear and burn your own grass *because your grass will be burnt for you by the managed care company, and they have worse data*, I can tell you that right now.[19] Hospitals and physicians have better data in their systems to measure things than an HMO *ever* will.

My message is the same to the nursing profession. You can benefit from exactly the same strategy. You can find and use data that will support any argument you may believe in with respect to the appropriate skill set. Is a higher level of nurse for a type of patient or care setting associated with better outcomes? Is a higher cost associated with better outcomes? What about a partial higher cost, but a lower aggregate cost? Many times it may be more expensive to use an RN in a specific situation, but if we get a half-day earlier discharge and that saves the hospital $600, it makes that RN day, compared with an LPN day, or an orderly day, start looking like a bargain.

The appropriate use of data is not easy. It takes a lot of work to collect and organize and analyze and demonstrate. But it's easy to convince someone once you have it. I think that ultimately, information and data are the real engines for the whole health care system.

No matter how disadvantageous you are in regard to cost structure—in a procedure, in an institution, *or even as a profession*—if you can figure out a way to demonstrate how that disadvantage equals something empirically better—better outcomes, better consumer appeal, higher patient satisfaction—you can use that information to position yourself in the market.

If information is the ammunition, a major battleground is going to be the internet. Just to re-establish my curmudgeon credentials once more before we get back to this topic, I want to remind you that I've been struggling with health care information-driven reform my whole career. I've seen the technology come and go. I remember CHIN,[20] the smart card, the EMR,[21] the Enterprise-Wide Client Server Clinical Data Repository.[22] I've been down the road, seen the movie over and over, and it usually has a really bad ending. But I'm excited now—because the internet *is* different.

Sure, there's a lot of hype about the internet.[23] We've all seen so many failures of information technology (IT), mostly because the HMOs or other payers don't install them. Why should they? Better IT just increases the ability of the payer to transact a claim faster. A lot

---

[19] Managed care entities are generally working with incomplete, truncated claims data.

[20] CHIN—Community Health Information Networks—a shared information base of patient care that many believed would be populated and used by different types of providers (often competing ones) to track patient care.

[21] EMR—Electronic Medical Record—a database within, or across, providers, designed to replace paper charts. They have not been widely accepted despite nearly ten years of attempts by software vendors to build and market them.

[22] A database of patient care built by combining data from multiple, unrelated, electronic systems.

[23] I'm not talking about the hype. (You do know that the internet is going to cure everything from world hunger to health care. Pretty soon, I'm told, you'll be able to deliver your babies over the internet.)

of the internet stuff *is* going to go down the same road as the CHIN and the EMR because there's no payback. In fact, there's a reverse payback for an HMO that invests in it. All they get is a bunch of happier providers. (Can you picture it? "Oh good," says the CEO of AETNA, "I'm going to use the web so I can pay claims faster!" Right.)

But here's the rub about the internet. The internet is different, because this time the patients are involved. CHIN failed, EMRs failed, and HEDIS[24] has failed miserably because the employee, the person seeking a good hospital, the person seeking a good doctor, or a good care system, never had access to any of the data. It was always treated as a secret, business to business. HCIA would build a data system, then the HMOs at hospitals would use the data to duke it out. The consumer was not involved. And as I have pointed out before, the consumer is the only stakeholder who really matters.

Remember the vaccine for pneumococcal pneumonia? The internet is the best place to tell someone about that new vaccine. The HMOs won't tell you. They don't want to pay for it. But the internet puts power in the hands of the consumer. Remember the quote from the old westerns? "God made man, but Colonel Colt made him equal." What's that mean? It means that in the Wild West if you were frail and short and couldn't run very fast, you were doomed—unless you got a gun and learned to use it. On the frontier, the gun changed the natural order of things, and the internet—with its almost unlimited access to medical information—is changing the "natural" order of health care. Whether it's the *Readers' Digest* or the internet, access to information changes the game.

I mentioned HEDIS data. HEDIS has been a total flop, a non-starter. HEDIS is basically this huge expensive attempt to gather information on whether health plans are doing a good job taking care of people. HEDIS' development was a huge effort, and we're currently in the third version. Unfortunately, it's estimated that only 12 percent of employers have ever looked at a HEDIS report, and less than 1 percent of employees have ever had access to one. Only one out of every hundred commercially insured persons, making choices about which health plan to select, has had access to data on the state-of-the-art, seven-year effort to measure health care quality. And you know why? Because employers don't want their people to see that they're buying a cheap plan. They don't want people to see that cheaper health care coverage is crummy health care coverage—that the HEDIS scores for the plan they selected are low. And that's the dirty little secret about HEDIS data.

Can we go on like this forever? I don't think so. Because tomorrow, someone will put up a website featuring HEDIS data. There's probably 10 of them being launched right now. Suddenly people have access to these data and they can see who has good scores, and they can go behind the scores and figure out who are the good providers. They already know about the ten things women doctors want them to know about their own primary care; they know what kind of care they need; and now HEDIS will tell them where to go and get that care. The internet really is the Wild West, where consumers can trump everyone standing in their way.

---

[24] HEDIS is an acronym for Health Plan Employer Data Information Set (currently version 3.0 or HEDIS 3.0). HEDIS is a standardized set of measures that assess the performance of managed care organizations.

The web can and should be used to implement every strategy in this talk—the branding, the managed care neutralization, the data gathering, and publicizing your positioning. It's certainly the best place to sell products with complex medical claims like blue corn flakes. You remember my physician friend, the gastroenterologist? Well he has his own website now—*dental-bridge-swallowers.com*. He has all of 25 users, so I guess it's time for him to go public and raise $150 million. But all kidding aside, the internet is not a fad. We've been though a lot of IT fads and a lot of them have failed because the economics have been wrong and the consumer wasn't involved.

Conclusions

I believe that the internet drastically changes the landscape of health care. I say "landscape" deliberately because a lot of people in my position who give these kinds of talks put these sort of "weather" maps up to predict next week's big, new "permanent" health care trend. And on the map there's a C that stands for capitation and an F stands for fee-for-service, and they stand there and say things like, "Oh, over Chicago, we're brewing capitation and we've got a heavy gust of capitation going through the Midwest, but out in the LA Basin we've got fee-for-service raining out across the desert." And people get tied into knots wondering what's really going to happen in health care.

It's so easy to get caught up in yesterday's bad news—easy to get caught up in the "weather" reports about health care. There's *a lot* of bad weather out there. Getting around it is tricky. As leaders, the hardest challenge that you face right now is keeping people focused on the landscape and not on the weather. Every time you open *Modern Health Care* to page three, it's a disaster. Bad news sells newspapers. The truth is that most of those failed business strategies made sense. They just take time. And it's not like it's easy. We're not talking about putting a Fed Ex pickup box in a yuppie neighborhood. It's complicated. We're talking about brain surgery here. And we're trying to do this at a point of what I believe to be maximum complexity in health care. We spend three-quarters of our time trying to deal with the fact that we're spending three-quarters of our time trying to deal with this. It's an infinite cycle.

Fixing health care is like highway construction. It's not hard to fix a lane on the Interstate. How hard is it to tear up a strip of asphalt and put in a new one? Not hard at all. You can do it in a day, right? So why don't they? *Because there's traffic on the road.* So they take the orange cones and the concrete dividers and they put them over here. Then they work for a while and then they take the orange cones and the concrete dividers and they put them over there. They spend seven-eights of their time in highway construction trying to cope with the fact that *the highway is still open.* And that's exactly what it's like trying to run a clinic, or a hospital group, or a staff of nurses, and trying to prepare them for a new world that's data-driven, where there's risk-based payment (which brings reward, but also brings a lot of downside) while you're still trying to operate in the old world.

That's the key message that I bring, particularly to providers whether they're hospitals, or doctors, or nurses. It's a 100-year problem, it's not going to be fixed overnight. Managed care is a solvent, and like most solvents it's hard on your hands—wear gloves. It's a

100-year problem and it's not going to be fixed in 10 years. The way we get out of this mess in one piece is to pay attention to the landscape and not the weather.

I'd like to close by going back to the forest fire story. Do you know what the real moral of the story is? Obviously, burning your own grass, seeing that the managed care fire is coming, and learning how to cope is an important moral of the story. But that's the obvious one. The more interesting and subtle moral is about leadership. Those 15 guys died for two reasons. First, they died because they were trying to do things in a panic. They tried to run, and that solution was inadequate and they perished. But even more importantly, they died because their leader—the guy who did burn his own grass—failed. He burned his grass and survived, but he was not able to explain and communicate to the others why he did that. And the other 15 guys perished as a result. And that's the real moral to that story. Burn your own grass, but explain why and explain how to the people you are leading. Ultimately, that's the way we'll thrive under managed care. To do that we need to keep our heads down. We need to pay attention to the landscape, not the weather. And, by the way, it wouldn't hurt to bring your raincoat.

PART THREE

Information Systems

We are in the information age, which has all kinds of implications. First, there is so much information that no one can keep track of it all. It is not humanly possible. Time is compressed. No wonder we feel like there is not enough time to complete everything we want to do! Information is not a big secret anymore. It is easy to access a lot of information, and our clients have become better informed. At times, they are better informed about their illness than we are.

Chances are, we health care providers have a knowledge deficit—it is not possible to keep up with all the current treatments, drugs, and research results that could improve our practice. This is where information systems comes to the rescue via some very dedicated librarians, discussed in Chapter 8, using the just-in-time concept to provide us with information as we need it, to more effectively care for our patients. In addition, the American Organization of Nurse Executives is "among the founding members of the National Alliance for Health Information Technology (NAHIT), a new coalition of health care providers, information technology vendors, and national health and technology associations who have come together to develop voluntary standards for health information technology" (AONE News Update, 2002, p. 2).[1]

Research indicates that care givers—both physicians and nurses—tend to go on doing what we were taught in school, even though there is current practice, or evidence based, information that indicates a better way to give care. Now we have information readily available right at the bedside as we give care. And, as many of us are not terribly computer literate, the librarians in Chapter 8 take us through the process step by step so we can successfully navigate the information highway.

---

[1] (August 12, 2002). *AONE News Update, 8*(11), 1–2.

Chapter 9 discusses what we administrators need to do when purchasing information systems. In fact, in our not-too-distant past, we would not have known what information systems personnel did. Purchasing systems can be fraught with difficulties. In fact, one big problem in health care presently is that one computer system is unable to communicate with another computer system; they are not integrated. Once again in this book, we advocate interdisciplinary involvement within an organization to deal with purchasing information systems, and the author advocates having an organizational information systems interdisciplinary committee to oversee this aspect.

CHAPTER 8

Knowledge Is Power:
Here's How to Plug In

Rick Wallace, MA, MDiv, MAOM, MSLS, AHIP

Martha Whaley, MSLS

What is the value of knowledge-based information in the health care setting? In some cases it may be worth only pennies, but in others it could be as invaluable as the life of a patient. Those who have information (or access to information) have a powerful tool, one which can give them the confidence to make wiser and more cost-effective decisions. In this chapter we consider the information needs of nurses from a patient-centric perspective, and we review various resources for locating health care information.

Information and Patient Care

We would like to begin with a bit of philosophy. Please do not change the channel. We promise we will get to the practical stuff.

The defining philosophy of health care librarians should be that our work begins at the point of care. The question, "What is best for the patient?" should take precedence over all other concerns. As "what is best for the patient" changes, the librarian must adapt to the new circumstances.

Many people think of libraries and information as nice to have, but ultimately non-essential. This is not true! Information is critical to providing the best health care. At our university, we host a camp for high school students who are considering a career as a health professional. These students are reminded that only one group of people can tell you to take your

> **IMPORTANT PRINCIPLE:**
> *Health care professionals need to learn more after graduation than before.*

clothes off or stab you with needles and knives and get away with it. The rest of us would be arrested if we did that. The difference between health care professionals and the remainder of the world is what is between their ears—their knowledge. This one group has mastered a body of knowledge that gives them special rights in society. Of course, that professional degree does not give the one who earned it permission to coast along the information highway.

Many studies detail the deterioration of health care professionals' knowledge over time. One study found that *a significant number of providers continued to use the treatment for hypertension that was standard in the year the provider finished formal training.* Other studies identified the gold standard of therapy for a disease. Then health providers were chosen randomly and asked how they treated the disease. The treatments varied greatly. Although these studies were done with physicians, the same assumption can be made about all professionals: Without frequent updating and retraining, knowledge and skill will decline over time. BOTTOM LINE: It is imperative for health care professionals to have the best information so everyone will get the best treatment.

In a study by Marshall (1992) done in Rochester, New York, 29 percent of clinicians who consulted the medical literature made a change in diagnosis. A total of 51 percent changed their choice of tests, and in 19 percent of the cases the patient experienced a reduced length of stay because of the information the clinician found in the literature. Also, an amazing 72 percent of the clinicians who consulted the literature reported a change in the advice given to patients based on what they learned from the literature. We have used similar surveys to judge services we have provided to rural health care professionals—doctors, nurse practitioners and nurses—and found similar results. Information is powerful.

Burke (1990), a practicing physician, noted several cases in her own practice in which lives were saved because she consulted the literature. She said that the value of the health sciences literature is difficult to document because,

> If a study is to be done documenting the effect of library services on improvements in patient care, the study would have to evaluate long term effects. This should include the effects of information obtained in one literature search and subsequently used to make a significant diagnosis in another patient, possibly several years later (p. 421).

This is why it is so shortsighted for administrators to reduce funding for libraries or eliminate them altogether. Libraries provide a benefit that is not always immediately evident. Pifalo (1994) stated that one physician believed so strongly in the importance of access to medical information by health care professionals that he said the federal government should make a law requiring hospitals to have access to a health sciences reference librarian! There is such a strong connection between good information and good patient care that a whole movement now exists—evidence-based practice (EBP)—to make sure that the best information gets into your hands. We will discuss EBP later in this chapter.

Another study examined medical residents and found that they had two information needs for every three patients they saw. They only looked up answers for 30 percent of the questions, mainly because of time constraints. Although study after study shows the great value of information in the clinical setting, nurses continue to underuse the literature. Blythe and Doyle, D. (1993) said, "Nurses, the largest group of health professionals, are not information literate. They visit libraries infrequently and rarely subscribe to research journals" (p. 433).

Exhibit 8–1 Healthcare Information and Patient Care

Study	Results
Marshall JG	Change in diagnosis, medications, advice given to patients by those who used the literature
Green ML, Ciampi MA, Ellis PJ	Medical residents had two information needs for every three patients seen, but sought answers for only 30% of the questions.

   This situation presents a great challenge to nurse managers who want staff nurses to stay informed of current trends so they can follow best practices. The nurse manager's role puts her in a unique position in which she must fight two battles. She must make sure that the institution's administration provides adequate information resources and that the staff nurses are adequately trained and involved in using these resources. Williams and Zipperer (2003) said, "Nurse administrators can establish partnerships with a medical librarian to help staff contribute to the safety of patients through improved access to the evidence" (p. 200).

Information and Money

"Show Me the Money," seems to be the theme song of health care today. Although it is difficult to quantify, we believe that information saves money for organizations. There is no denying that finding information can be expensive, but not finding it can also be costly. Consider the cost of a malpractice lawsuit brought on by using bad information. Recently, a participant in an asthma study at a prominent university *died because researchers failed to search the published literature before conducting clinical trials*. The volunteer, a healthy young woman, inhaled the drug being studied, which led to failure of her lungs and kidneys. Although the researchers had attempted to research the adverse effects of the drug, their search was apparently incomplete. The amount of the settlement from the resulting lawsuit was not made public, but the adverse publicity for the university was staggering. Malpractice lawyers frequently make extensive use of the literature to support their arguments.

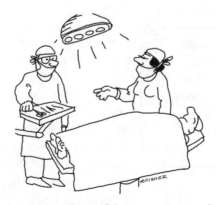

"Scalpel... MEDLINE Printout... Sutures."

Robin Fisher, Designer

Libraries save money and time because each individual does not need to buy information. Instead, the organization bears the expense and provides storage and/or access. It is also more cost effective to provide information than doing without. Doing without will eventually manifest itself in a lower level of patient care, which will eventually put you out of business. This is why JCAHO requires either ownership or access to "knowledge-based information." If a health care organization tries to save money by cutting out information services, then clinical staff can not keep up with new information and provide the best care. Ultimately this is unethical, because the patients do not receive the highest standard of care.

Klein, Ross, Adams, and Gilbert (1994) did a study that measured the costs of hospital stays by Diagnosis Related Groups (DRGs). Caregivers for one group of patients accessed the literature. The costs were compared to a control group whose caregivers had not accessed the literature as a part of patient care. The average savings per DRG for the group that used the literature were $7,379. The total savings across all DRG's were $250,871. The reason for this is:

> Not only does information serve to trigger new or different diagnostic tests or therapeutic maneuvers, but as studies have suggested, its usefulness also exists in halting procedures or therapies that have been shown to be ineffective in similar situations (p. 492).

Having best-evidence information gives caregivers the confidence to feel secure in diagnosis and treatment. These researchers even suggested that database searching could be billed to third-party payers. We have discovered in the hospital setting that a nurse or the education department, which is staffed by a nurse, most often consults the literature. Some caregivers have searched the literature and attached the resulting information to a patient's chart or medical record.

Griffiths and King (1993) also showed that information has economic value. They discovered that small facilities (small hospitals, nursing homes, free-standing clinics) might not have a critical mass of users to support a library. Therefore, these institutions might benefit from an outreach librarian. They demonstrated that in a period of time where a professional spent 121 hours acquiring information, if they had access to the staff of an information center, they spent only 27 hours gaining the same information. Therefore, they are saved 94 hours, which can, of course, be translated into both fiscal savings and more time for patients.

David Durenberger (2003) said: "If all physicians in the United States practiced as effectively as the top 10 percent, we would save enough money to add a drug benefit to Medicare and have funds to spare."

We like to use the following illustration to explain why we believe librarians are an essential part of the health care team (Holtum, 1999): While you may have learned some laboratory skills in school, you still send samples to a lab for analysis. It just makes sense to give a task to those who are trained and experienced at doing it. Libraries are similar. We hope you are good at finding information, but if a skilled professional is available to do it for you, then you can dedicate your time to what you do best—taking care of sick people. Griffiths and King also demonstrated that professional reading is directly related to speed of work, quality of work, productivity, and saving money. Griffiths and

Exhibit 8–2 The Economic Value of Healthcare Information

Study	Summary	Conclusions
Klein MS, Ross VR, Adams DL & Gilbert CM	Comparison in Detroit hospitals of cases by DRG where staff did and did not consult the literature for patient care	Savings shown where literature was used.
King D and Griffiths JM	Measure of the use of information by many types of professionals	High information users are more productive and save the organization money.
Durenburger D	Editorial	If all physicians in the United States practiced as effectively as the top 10 percent, we would save enough money to add a drug benefit to Medicare and have funds to spare.

King also documented that the average use of a library goes down based on geographical distance from it. People who were within one minute of the library used the library 4.24 times during the time studied. A potential library user, who was greater than 15 minutes away, only used the library 1.41 times. Because of this, health sciences librarians must continuously push health care information closer to clinicians, or it will not be used.

Oh, and one more thing. Please be an advocate for libraries in your institution. Librarians need your support when budgets are cut, because administrators often consider eliminating the library first as a simple cost-cutting measure. Most small hospitals and health care institutions do not have a library because of the cost. If this is your situation, you may want to consider contracting for the services of an outreach librarian. Of course, you can also contact a librarian by e-mail or by telephone.

OK. That is enough philosophy. Get up. Go to the bathroom. Get something to eat and drink. Rub the shoulders of the person closest to you. You can tell them we gave you permission. We are now going to delve into the nuts and bolts of finding health care information.

Consumer/Patient Health Information

This section will provide some practical tips that will help you be a better information seeker. These are our very best secrets and if broadly distributed could result in widespread unemployment of librarians. Therefore, you must promise to rip this chapter out and eat it before we allow you to proceed. Our whole professional future depends on the ignorance of others.

Here is a scenario to get us going: You work for a fertility specialist. A patient's husband says to you, "My wife has been coming to this office for one year now and she is not yet pregnant. I have heard that acupuncture can help with infertility. Do you know anything about this?" What do you do?

First, we would like to climb on our soapbox. Consumer/patient information is important, and most people are appallingly illiterate when it comes to health knowledge. This is well documented and sad. Conditions like diabetes and obesity could be greatly reduced if consumers were better educated about their health and if they would practice what they learn. We think it is a national crisis. (End of sermon).

Back to you and your patient. Where do you begin to find unbiased information that he can apply to his situation? Billions of consumer health information resources exist. Well, maybe not billions, but we could give you list after list of web sites, books, and organizations that provide consumer/patient health information. We have found this flood of information to be confusing to information seekers. What we prefer is to offer a limited, but manageable number of excellent resources.

Web Sites with Selection Policies Based on Evaluation Criteria

By using gateways that have already been evaluated by librarians, you can save time, energy and money. A good starting point for finding consumer/patient information is the database MedlinePlus® (http://medlineplus.gov). MedlinePlus is maintained by the National Library of Medicine® (NLM®), one of the National Institutes of Health (NIH) of the federal government. Often, this is the only place we go for answers. The information in MedlinePlus is grouped by topic and is easy to search. Some topics even have tutorials for those with poor reading skills as well as links to resources labeled "easy-to-read." The tutorials can be heard through computer speakers or through headphones while you watch a slide show which explains a procedure or condition. MedlinePlus is a good source of drug information, and includes directories and dictionaries as well. A Spanish version of the site is also available, and includes an excellent encyclopedia and Spanish-language tutorials. When you search by topic in MedlinePlus, you retrieve a list of links from other web sites that have been quality filtered. The National Library of Medicine continually updates, expands and improves the site. A typical screen looks like this:

Exhibit 8–3 MedlinePlus® Screen Print

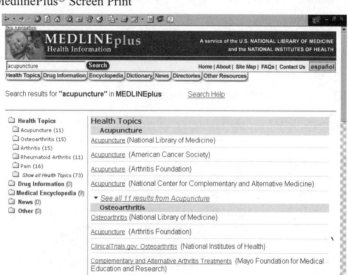

MedlinePlus, a service of US National Library of Medicine and National Institute of Health.

This is a screen from the Spanish version:

Exhibit 8–4 MedlinePlus® Espanol Screen Print

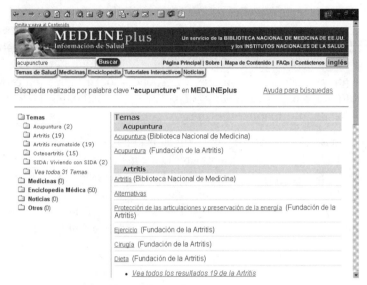

MedlinePlus, a service of US National Library of Medicine and National Institute of Health.

Another good choice for Consumer Health information is the New York Online Access to Health (NOAH). The address is www.noah-health.org. Here is the description of the origin of NOAH as found on the website:

> In 1994, four New York City library organizations joined forces to establish a single website to provide end-users a place on the World Wide Web to reach reliable consumer health information. The organizations: The City University of New York Office of Library Services (CUNY); the Metropolitan New York Library Council (METRO); The New York Academy of Medicine Library (NYAM); and The New York Public Library (NYPL) - later joined by the Queens Borough Public Library and the Brooklyn Public Library - had as a goal the development of a website which would provide health care information easily accessible and understandable to the layperson. The result was NOAH: New York Online Access to Health.

NOAH is much like MedlinePlus in that it is fairly comprehensive and easy to search. You only have to enter a term in the search field and click the search button. Like MedlinePlus, it has information in Spanish and it is easy to switch between English and Spanish.

Medem is a consumer health information web site located at www.medem.com. We like Medem because it is the joint product of various medical societies including the American Academy of Ophthalmology; American Academy of Pediatrics; American College of

Allergy, Asthma & Immunology; American College of Obstetricians and Gynecologists; American Medical Association; American Psychiatric Association; American Society of Plastic Surgeons and others. MedlinePlus topic pages often link to Medem resources as well as to pages from outstanding sites such as Mayo Clinic (www.mayoclinic.com).

If you cannot find an answer from the sites we have given you, we recommend that you use the Medical Library Association's Consumer and Patient Health Information Section (CAPHIS) site at http://caphis.mlanet.org. The people who maintain this site are the best of the best. They are professional librarians who spend a lot of their time providing consumer/patient health information on a daily basis. The group maintains a list of the top 100 consumer/patient health information web sites. According to CAPHIS:

> The purpose of the CAPHIS Top 100 List is to provide CAPHIS members and other librarians with a resource to use in their daily practice and teaching. Secondly, it is our contribution to the Medical Library Association so that the headquarters staff can refer individuals to a list of quality health web sites. Our goal is to have a limited number of resources that meet the quality criteria for currency, credibility, content, audience, etc., as described on our website.

Much fraudulent consumer/patient health information exists on the web. A site that exposes false and misleading health information on the web is Quackwatch (http://quackwatch.org). According to information found at the site, the mission of Quackwatch is as follows:

> Quackwatch, Inc., which was a member of Consumer Federation of America for 30 years, is a nonprofit corporation whose purpose is to combat health-related frauds, myths, fads, and fallacies. Its primary focus is on quackery-related information that is difficult or impossible to get elsewhere. Founded by Dr. Stephen Barrett in 1969 as the Lehigh Valley Committee Against Health Fraud, it was incorporated in 1970. In 1997, it assumed its current name and began developing a worldwide network of volunteers and expert advisors.

One final web site of interest to consumers is Healthfinder. This site is coordinated by the Office of Disease Prevention and Health Promotion (ODPHP) of the U.S. Department of Health and Human Services, in cooperation with representatives from other Federal agencies who include consumer health information specialists, librarians, and others actively engaged in the provision or use of online consumer health. Healthfinder links to more than 1700 health-related organizations. A topic search on Healthfinder will give you the name and address of national and regional organizations whose reliability has been carefully evaluated. These organization web sites, such as the American Heart Association and the American Diabetes Association, are rich sources of consumer/patient information.

Some print sources give an excellent overview of consumer health information. The *Consumer Health Information Source Book* by Alan M. Rees is the bible of consumer health information. Rees evaluates consumer health information clearinghouses, web sites, books, pamphlets, and Spanish consumer health information. A similar work is *The Medical Library Association Consumer Health Reference Service Handbook* published by the Medical Library Association through Neal-Schuman Publishers.

If you would like to help establish a consumer information library in your hospital, you may want to take a look at *Consumer Health Information for Public Librarians* by Lynda M. Baker and Virginia Manbeck. According to a *Library Journal* review by Margaret Allen, public librarians are the primary audience for Baker and Manbeck's guide, but all professionals providing consumer health information services will benefit from studying their work.

Exhibit 8–5 Web Sources of Consumer Information

Name of Resource	Web Address	Languages	Comments
Medline Plus®	Medlineplus.gov	English, Spanish	Produced by the National Library of Medicine. Excellent all-around site
NOAH	http://www.noah-health.org	English, Spanish	Produced by several New York libraries Like MedlinePlus, a good site for all questions
Medem	http://medem.com/pat/pat.cfm	English, some Spanish	A partnership of medical societies to provide consumer/patient information
Mayoclinic.com	http://www.mayoclinic.com	English	Expertise from the renowned Mayo Clinic
CAPHIS	http://caphis.mlanet.org	English	A list of 100 best consumer/patient health information sites maintained by the nations best consumer librarians
Healthfinder	http://www.healthfinder.gov	English and Spanish	Resource for finding the best government and nonprofit health and human services information

Exhibit 8–6 Print Sources of Consumer Information

Name of Resource	Publisher	Comments
Consumer Health Information Sourcebook	The Oryx Press, 2000, 6th ed.	The bible of consumer health information. Cost- $65
The Medical Library Association Consumer Health Reference Service Handbook	Neal Schuman Publishers, 2001	Another good print source for finding good consumer health information resources. Cost- $75
Consumer Health Information for Public Librarians	Rowman & Littlefield, 2002	Illustrates the need for quality consumer health resources. Cost- $45

Evidence-Based Practice

Recently a friend said she had just taught a library class for a group of nurses. She was startled to find out that the nurses were being told that everything they did should be evidence-based. All their work had to be supported by guidelines. How should they handle this edict? First, what does it mean if something is evidence-based? The formal definition is that evidence-based medicine (EBM) or evidence-based practice (EBP) is, "… *the conscientious, explicit and judicious use of current best evidence in making decisions about the care of individual patients*" (Sackett, 1996). EBP is an effort to filter out the best-evidence information.

Problem One: All information is not created equal. By this we mean that you may find a case study on hypertension based on one patient and in the same journal you may find a systematic review of ten large randomized controlled trials on hypertension. Which article do you think would give you the best answer to your question about care of your hypertensive patients? Different studies give different answers. What is to be believed? How do you know what is the truth?

The second problem lies in the amount of health care research being published. It is prolific and shows no sign of slowing down. Over 15 million bibliographic references are available in the National Library of Medicine's PubMed database. Out of this haystack of information, how do you find the needle that is the most reliable and valid?

A couple of essentials to remember when searching for the best evidence are that good questions must be formulated and the right type of study must be used. A mnemonic, PICO, has been developed to assist in clinical question building. PICO is an acronym for Patient/population, Intervention, Comparative intervention (if any), and Outcome desired.

So, a PICO question about hypertension might be written, "In elderly patients with hypertension (Patient/population) does drug A (Intervention) or drug B (Comparative Intervention) result in the greater reduction of morbidity and mortality (Outcome)?" The reason this exercise is necessary is that we too often make the mistake of searching for an answer from the literature without a clear idea of what we are actually looking for! It only follows that our search results will be unsuccessful.

As you read any type of study, you want to develop some critical skills. The most important question to ask is, "Is this something I need to know?" If not, use your time doing something else. If the study is important to you, you need to ask: "Were the correct statistical tests used? Were all the participants accounted for in the final results? Was the study randomized and blinded if a therapy study? Was a large enough sample used? Did a drug company finance the study, or does it have other potential sources of bias?"

> *PICO*
> *Patient/population*
> *Intervention*
> *Comparative intervention*
> *Outcome desired*

Well, now we have ruined your day. You probably thought you could just read the first journal article you found that was on your topic and that was sufficient. After all, aren't you reading this book to make your hectic life easier? Do you need a new layer of guilt about something else you are not doing well? Remember, in the literature you may find two studies on your research topic. One may be written based on experiences with just one patient (case study). The other may be based on dozens of well-done RCTs (randomized controlled trials) compiled into one systematic review. If they give conflicting advice, which would you want to use with your patients? As you can see, it is important to have discriminating skills so you can separate the wheat from the chaff in the literature.

SOURCES OF INFORMATION ON EVIDENCE-BASED PRACTICE

Do not worry if you feel you do not have the time or skills to make best-evidence judgments. You can turn to "secondary" or "translation" literature. This literature takes the raw studies and evaluates them for patient usefulness and methodological accuracy. So in the long run, evidence-based practice will make information searching easier for you as well as make the search more accurate. In the new world of information retrieval, you will not start with "raw" databases such as CINAHL® and PubMed®, (which we will discuss later), but will go to the evidence-based practice databases. These databases will have already filtered out the best evidence from the mountains of information that exist in the healthcare literature. Your search will result in highly relevant information that you will use to take care of your patients according to the highest standards.

One principle of evidence-based practice is that the randomized controlled trial (RCT) is the most accurate or "truthful" type of health information related to therapeutic topics. Randomized controlled trials are carefully designed. They are blinded or double-blinded so that neither the participants nor the administrators know who is getting the experimental treatment and who is in the control group. They are randomized in the sense that everyone who is in the population being studied has an equal chance of being chosen to be in the experimental group (arm) or control group. When many of these randomized controlled trials on the same topic are compiled, the result is termed a *systematic review*.

> *IMPORTANT PRINCIPLE*
> *A systematic review of randomized controlled trials is considered to be the best evidence on a therapeutic topic.*

Many areas of inquiry in nursing, however, do not lend themselves to being studied using the randomized controlled trial design. So, be sure to look for systematic reviews of other types of studies as well. Two wonderful resources for accessing these reviews are CINAHL® and MEDLINE®. They index the Cochrane Database of Systematic Reviews, which is part of a group of databases produced by the Cochrane Collaboration, based in Oxford, England. We highly recommend that you become familiar with Cochrane.

The Cochrane collection also includes the Database of Abstracts of Reviews of Effectiveness (DARE), which, unlike the systematic reviews database, covers topics other than therapy (such as etiology, prognosis, diagnosis, and economics). In addition, the Cochrane group of databases includes the Cochrane Controlled Trials Registry, which contains about one-third million reviewed randomized controlled trials. The summaries of the Cochrane databases and subscription information can be searched at no charge at www.cochrane.org. DARE can be searched at no charge at www.york.ac.uk/inst/crd/darehp.htm.

Comprehensive evidence-based practice databases which include the Cochrane Systematic Reviews are available. These can be purchased as an individual subscription, or as a license for a group. One such product is InfoRetriever (www.infopoems.com), which can be loaded onto a desktop computer or a handheld computer (PDA). A subscription to InfoRetriever allows access to the following:

- Cochrane systematic reviews
- A collection of practice guidelines
- A collection of summaries of clinically important journal articles (These articles are called POEMs, which stands for Patient-Oriented Evidence that Matters)
- Drug information
- An ICD-9 look-up
- Predictive calculators
- A daily summary analysis of a clinically important journal article (POEM) by email (This service is a great way to keep up with the extensive journal literature without reading hundreds of journals per month.)

Studies on the reading habits of health care professionals are alarming. Very little time is spent reading. This finding is not surprising considering the tendency of the health care system to put more and more work on fewer and fewer nurses. The daily email alert service alone is worth the price of InfoRetriever. The articles are "patient-oriented" because they measure outcomes that benefit the patient. They are "evidence that matters" in that they give the practitioner information which can improve the way he or she practices (Slawson and Shaughnessy, 1994). The health care literature is mainly filled with articles that are discussions of disease-oriented evidence (DOES). These articles do not help the caregiver because they have not been proven in populations of people. They are often just the tedious manuscripts of academics and researchers yakking it up with each other. In contrast, a POEM is important to the patient. It is information that has shown a positive benefit in a group of patients. Products similar to InfoRetriever are Clinical Evidence (www.clinicalevidence.com), DynaMed (www.dynamicmedical.com), FIRST Consult (www.firstconsult.com), and UpToDate (www.uptodate.com).

Types of studies in the literature other than randomized controlled trials are cohort studies, case control studies, and case studies.

A *cohort study*, on the other hand, is an observational study in which a defined group of people (the cohort) can be assembled in the present and followed into the future (a 'concurrent cohort study'), or identified from past records, such as medical records, and followed from that time up to the present (a 'historical cohort study'). An example of a cohort study is the famous Framingham study of heart disease, which has followed participant citizens of Framingham, Massachusetts since 1948.

Case control studies are retrospective in nature. They collect data from charts, data sets, and patient interviews. A good use of the case control study is for studies of harm. For example, we may choose patients with and without lung cancer, then examine the patients' records for a past exposure to a toxic substance.

A *case study* is a detailed analysis of a person or group from a social, psychological, or medical point of view. It involves one case, usually one that is unique. As we have mentioned, randomized controlled trials (or systematic reviews of them) are the best type of information to answer therapy questions and etiology questions. Prognosis questions are best answered by cohort studies. Questions on diagnosis issues are answered by cohort studies that compare the new diagnosis to the gold standard.

Guidelines are another source for evidence-based information. Be warned that not all guidelines are evidence-based; some guidelines are expert-based. The new trend, however, is for guidelines to support their recommendations with evidence. Systems have been designed to rank evidence on a one-to-five scale where a "1a" is a systematic review of homogeneous (the different studies were on similar population groups) randomized controlled trials, a "1b" is a systematic review of heterogeneous (the different studies were on dissimilar population groups) randomized controlled trials, a "2" is a cohort study, and so forth. An excellent place to search for guidelines is www.guidelines.gov.

> *For further information on evidence-based practice go to the Centre for Evidence-Based Medicine (http://www.cebm.net) or Centre for Evidence-Based Nursing (http://www.york.ac.uk/ healthsciences/centres/evidence/ cebn.htm).*

Definition

A *cohort study* is an observational study in which a defined group of people (the cohort) can be assembled in the present and followed into the future, or identified from past records, and followed from that time up to the present.

A *case control study* collects data from several sources and is retrospective in nature.

A *case study* is a detailed analysis of a person or group from a social or psychological or medical point of view.

The database PubMed, produced by the U.S. National Library of Medicine, has a clinical queries filter on the sidebar. When this filter is used, a special search strategy is implemented in addition to the terms you enter. These filters have been designed to find the best evidence in the literature—whether it is a question on therapy, diagnosis, prognosis, or etiology. For example, when you do a "therapy" search the filter adds additional terms such as "randomized," "placebo-controlled," and "blinded."

Just as many consumer/patient health sources are available, there are also many evidence-based nursing (EBN) sources available. For example, the *British Medical Journal* (BMJ) publishing group produces an online journal called *Evidence-Based Nursing* (ebn. bmjjournals.com) The product web site says:

> The general purpose of *Evidence-Based Nursing* is to select from the health related literature those articles reporting studies and reviews that warrant immediate attention by nurses attempting to keep pace with important advances in their profession. These articles are summarized in 'value-added' abstracts and commented on by clinical experts (British Medical Journal).

A good EBN site is the Centre for Evidence-based Nursing (http://www.york.ac.uk/healthsciences/centres/evidence/cebn.htm). The site lists its purpose as:

> The Centre for Evidence Based Nursing (CEBN) is concerned with furthering EBN through education, research and development. Evidence based nursing is the process by which nurses make clinical decisions using the best available research evidence, their clinical expertise and patient preferences, in the context of available resources (DiCenso A, Cullum N, Ciliska D. Implementing evidence based nursing: some misconceptions [Editorial]. Evidence Based Nursing 1998; 1:38–40).

The *Online Journal of Clinical Innovations* (www.cinahl.com/ceexpress/ojcionline3/index.html) is a peer-reviewed electronic journal published by CINAHL. It is "dedicated to harvesting new knowledge to be transformed into practice, and making sources of clinical innovation—new solutions or practices that solve problems—accessible to clinicians in varied roles and diverse settings." It is accessible by subscription, or you can purchase individual articles.

One more comment about evidence-based practice, before we move on to another topic. It has a direct bearing on patient safety. This was eloquently articulated in a recent article by Williams and Zipperer (2003):

> Efficient and timely access to evidence-based medical literature is an important element in providing safe patient care. This knowledge base exists in primary sources such as the medication administration records and patients' medical records, from colleagues, *and ideally, in the science reported in the biomedical literature* (italics added). Given the complexity and time constraints involved in care delivery, seeking out the right information at the right time is an increasingly difficult goal for many health practitioners to reach. Frontline nurses are no exception to this dilemma. A key role for management, therefore is to help improve access to evidence-based literature for nurses to enable them to interact more proactively for safety. Key to improving access to evidence from biomedical literature is the medical reference librarian or clinical librarian (p. 199).

Exhibit 8–7 Sources for Finding Evidence-Based Information

Name	Address	Comments
Cochrane Databases	www.cochrane.org	Database of systematic reviews of randomized controlled trials of therapy topics. Additional databases: DARE- has information other then therapy topics; Controlled Trials Database- 1/3 million validated RCTs.
InfoRetriever	www.infopoems.com	Cochrane's systematic reviews & POEMS plus guidelines, drug information and clinical calculators
Evidence-based Nursing	ebn.bmjjournals.com	Articles reporting studies and reviews that warrant immediate attention by nurses attempting to keep pace with important advances in their profession.
PubMed- clinical queries filter	pubmed.gov	Filters added to PubMed searches designed to find the "best-evidence" information for therapy, prognosis, diagnosis, and etiology queries.
Centre for Evidence-based Nursing	www.york.ac.uk/ healthsciences/centres/ evidence/cebn.htm	The Centre for Evidence Based Nursing (CEBN) is concerned with furthering EBN through education, research and development. Evidence-based nursing is the process by which nurses make clinical decisions using the best available research evidence, their clinical expertise and patient preferences, in the context of available resources
Online Journal of Clinical Innovations	www.cinahl.com/ cexpress/ojcionline3/ index.html	"Developed to provide up-to-date access to research reports and innovation implementation from conferences and communication with investigators and clinicians."

A Crash Course in Searching the Nursing Literature

First, we must apologize for the last section. That was a lot to swallow. So let's take another break. Get up. Walk around the room three or four times. Get out your cell phone (unless you are in an area where it would interfere with equipment) and call a friend. Be sure to get another snack (watch the carbs), and maybe a cup of coffee or hot herbal tea. OK. Here is a new scenario. Let's say you need to find information on staffing ratios. You want help from the literature in making a decision, so you will not be relying solely on your own experience. Where do you turn? Outstanding databases are available for situations such as this. The first one you should try is the online version (www.cinahl.com) of the Cumulated Index to Nursing and Allied Health Literature (CINAHL®). Another favorite of librarians is PubMed (no, not Club Med), the National Library of Medicine's free database of over 15 million journal citations (pubmed.gov).

To start a search in any database, clearly define what you want to find. Write it down. Think of synonyms for your concept. Then look at the database's indexing system. Databases that index the literature in a discipline, or citation databases, are compiled by professional indexers. Indexers read articles from the journals and decide what terms best describe them. Indexers are limited by a controlled vocabulary. The controlled vocabulary is necessary to prevent one indexer from reading an article and assigning the term "myocardial infarction" and then having another indexer read the same article and assign the term "heart attack." If this happened, and you used the term "myocardial infarction" you would miss all the articles indexed "heart attack." So, if you can determine the indexing term (also known as the subject heading) for the subject you are searching, you will have better success in your search, and you will find more of the articles you truly want and fewer of the articles that have little to do with your topic.

Another important searching concept is the use of limits. For example, *date* limits can be very important. In health care, as you know, information has increased exponentially. Articles that are only two or three years old may be outdated and, therefore, may be of little value or even harmful. Also, be sure to use *language* limits, particularly in PubMed®, which indexes articles from more than 40 languages. So, unless you read Azerbaijani, this is an important tip. *Publication type* is another useful limiter. For example, you may want to limit to clinical trials for therapy questions, or to guidelines or systematic reviews. You may want to eliminate letters to the editor or news and comments from your retrieval. In CINAHL® you can use the "Research and Systematic Reviews" publication type to limit your search.

Subheadings bring a tighter focus to your search. A frequent problem in searching is finding too much information. Subheadings help you focus on one aspect of a topic such as therapy, diagnosis, economics, or prognosis. For example in PubMed you may type the term "staffing" into the subject-heading index. Several choices are offered and you select "Personnel Staffing and Scheduling." You click on this term and notice that the subheadings are: classification, economics, ethics, history, legislation and jurisprudence, methods, organization and administration, standards, statistics and numerical data, trends and utilization. You choose the subheading "economics" because this is the type of information you need. Your retrieval of citations is more focused because you have chosen to eliminate articles with the other subheadings.

CINAHL® has over 3.3 million citations and abstracts more than 1200 journals. Its focus is nursing and allied health. It is a proprietary database, which means that it is privately owned and controlled. CINAHL® may be purchased from several vendors including ARIES Systems Corporation, Cinahl® Information System, Data-Star, EBSCO Publishing, OVID Technologies, ProQuest and SilverPlatter Information.

Exhibit 8–8 CINAHL® Search Screen. Note the use of the subject heading "RN Mix."

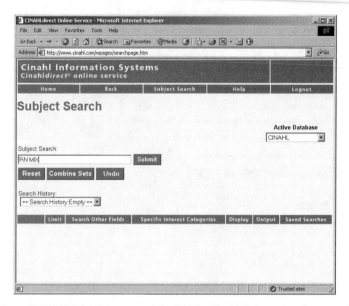

Source: Extracts from CINAHL® database, copyright ©2004 Cinahl Information Systems. Reprinted by permission.

Exhibit 8–9 CINAHL® Search Screen: The Search Narrows

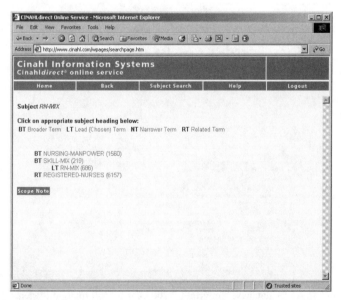

Source: Extracts from CINAHL® database, copyright ©2004 Cinahl Information Systems. Reprinted by permission.

Exhibit 8–10 CINAHL® Search Screen: The Search Is Further Refined

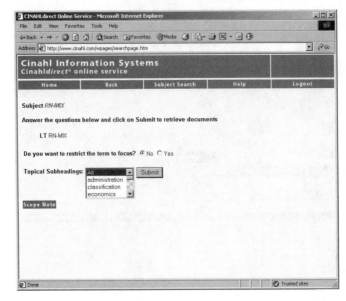

Source: Extracts from CINAHL® database, copyright ©2004 Cinahl Information Systems. Reprinted by permission.

Exhibit 8–11 CINAHL® Search Screen: The First Page of Results

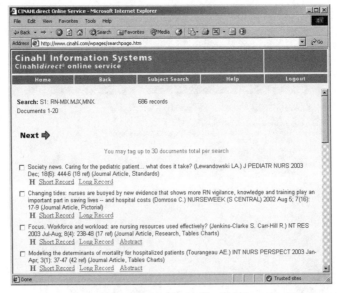

Source: Extracts from CINAHL® database, copyright ©2004 Cinahl Information Systems. Reprinted by permission.

Exhibit 8–12 A Record from the CINAHL® Database

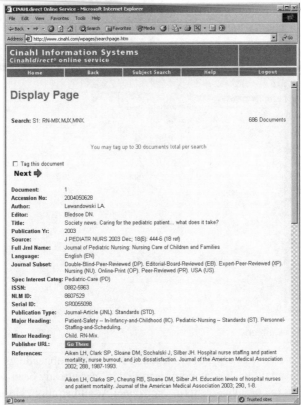

Source: Extracts from CINAHL® database, copyright ©2004 Cinahl Information Systems. Reprinted by permission.

Exhibit 8–13 The National Library of Medicine's PubMed® Database

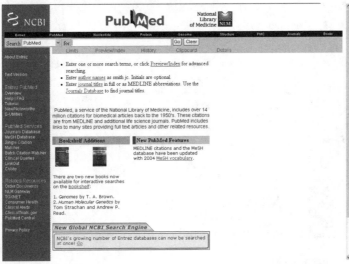

US National Library of Medicine.

Exhibit 8–14 This is the page in PubMed to search for a subject heading. PubMed calls its subject headings "MESH®" - Medical Subject Headings.

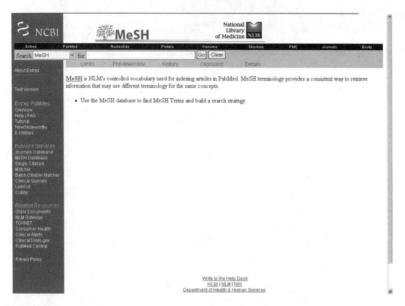

Source: http://www.ncbi.nw.nih.gov.

Exhibit 8–15 This is a view of a MESH® Heading. Notice the subheadings. The MESH heading "Nursing Staff, Hospital/legislation and jurisprudence" has already been selected as a search term. This will allow us to combine this term "Personnel Administration, Hospital" using the Boolean operator "AND".

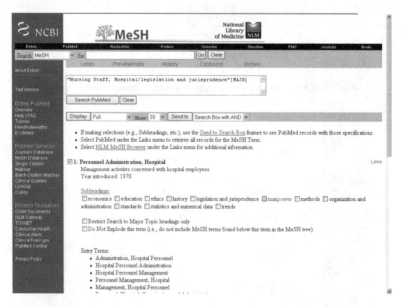

Source: http://www.nlm.nih.gov/MESH.

Exhibit 8–16 An Abstract Viewed Within PubMed®: It is in the Abstract Format.

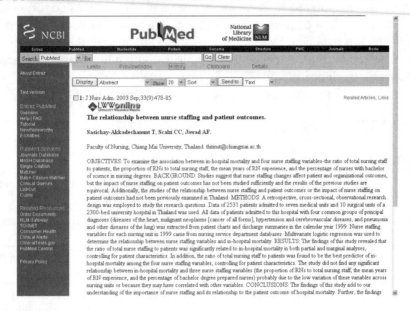

Source: http://www.ncbi.nw.nih.gov.

Exhibit 8–17 This shows the limit page in PubMed®: Notice Limits For Language, Date And Publication Type.

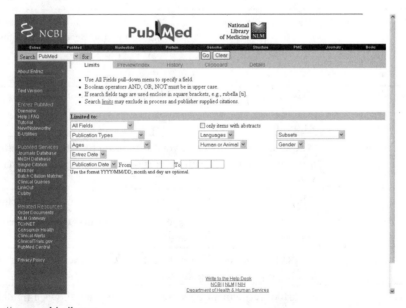

Source: http://www.ncbi.nih.gov.

PubMed® (Public MEDLINE) is produced by the U.S. National Library of Medicine and is free. Other information products we would encourage you to consider using (all proprietary) are MD Consult, a collection of medical textbooks, journals, and patient handouts; UpToDate, which is arranged by clinical topics that summarize the journal literature on that topic; InfoRetriever, an evidence-based information product that contains guidelines, critically-appraised clinically-important journal articles, drug information, systematic reviews, and clinical calculators; and StatRef, another collection of textbooks.

Exhibit 8–18 Summary of Databases Useful for Professional Nursing Information

DATABASE	Address	Comments
CINAHL®	www.cinahl.com	Citation database for nursing and allied health. Proprietary
PubMed®	Pubmed.gov	Citation database for all health sciences. Free!!
UpToDate	www.uptodate.com	Summary of clinical topics from the current literature. Proprietary
InfoRetriever	www.infopoems.com	Cochrane's systematic reviews & POEMS plus guidelines, drug information and clinical calculators. Proprietary
StatRef	www.statref.com	A collection of textbooks. Proprietary
MD Consult	www.mdconsult.com	A collection of medical textbooks, journals, patient handouts and drug information. Proprietary
Healthweb Nursing	www.healthweb.org	The nursing section contains an excellent collection of the best nursing sites on the Web. Free!!

Exhibit 8–19 Summary of Techniques for Successful Database Searching

Search Technique	Function
Subject Headings	Allows a sharper focus in your search. Increases recall (getting all the articles on your topic) and precision (not getting articles that are irrelevant).
Date Limit	Allows you to limit the time period in which you are searching.
Publication Type Limit	Very valuable for the advanced searcher. May want to restrict to clinical trials for therapy searches.
Language Limit	Particularly valuable for PubMed, which indexes articles in journals written in over 40 languages.
Subheadings	A further refinement of subject headings that allows a tighter focus. For example, instead of retrieving every article on hypertension you can limit to only therapy articles on hypertension.

Information Products and Salespeople (Vendors)

Suppose your Chief Financial Officer tells you that you may spend $5,000 on books and journals for the nursing staff. You work in a facility that has no librarian or outreach librarian service. So you are on your own. You will either buy excellent products which will lead your staff to the best health care practices, or you will waste the money on useless products and your staff will kill and maim thousands of patients because of their ignorance. (No pressure!) How do you proceed?

Since 1979 the "Brandon/Hill Selected List of Print Nursing Books and Journals" has helped nursing administrators and librarians select nursing literature that is most appropriate for their needs. The list is available at http://www.mssm.edu/library/brandon-hill, or by searching "Brandon Hill list" in your favorite web search engine. Unfortunately, the list is not being updated at this time, but it is still of value for selection of books and journals. Each time the list was revised it was also published in *Nursing Outlook*. If you choose to use the Brandon/Hill list in making book selections for a brand new library, keep in mind that it included only books that were available at the time of publication of the list, so you will need to consult earlier editions of the list or other sources for books that are considered to be classics in nursing literature. The introduction to the Brandon/Hill list explains the authors' rationale for their selections and suggests other sources, such as "Books of the Year Awards," which is published each year in the January issue of the *American Journal of Nursing*.

If you would like more information about books that you are considering for purchase, some easily accessible sources for book reviews are the large booksellers who list their inventory on Internet web sites. For example, Amazon (www.amazon.com) Barnes and Noble (www.barnesandnoble.com), and Books-a-Million (www.booksamillion.com) offer publisher and reader reviews. At this point, you may want to ask for input from your colleagues who will also be using the materials. And, of course, remember that hospital and academic medical librarians are always willing to dispense advice.

Now you know which books and journals you want, but where do you find them? And what format would be best for your needs? Should you purchase your selections in print or on CD? Or maybe you should purchase online access. But, you have heard that online access can get messy if the vendor requires a license agreement. Are there any simple solutions?

Good old-fashioned print books and journals offer the most uncomplicated access to information. To be sure, some information professionals regard print as old-fashioned and inadequate. It is, however, easy to store and maintain, and it is very accessible. These advantages may be more important to you and your staff than technological bells and whistles.

Some books and journals are also offered on CD. In this format they can be purchased for use on a single computer, or they can be purchased for use on a network, CD tower, or CD server. CDs can be updated more often than books, but, of course, if your computer or network crashes, the information will not be accessible. Many information professionals feel that CDs are even more outdated than books, because the hardware needed to access them may soon be unavailable.

Most medical libraries purchase books and journals through a vendor rather than buying directly from the publisher. The online book dealers mentioned above (Amazon, Barnes and Noble, Books-a-Million) allow purchase of books and CDs through corporate accounts by either purchase order or credit card. Some other vendors, such as Majors (www.majors.com) and Rittenhouse (www.rittenhouse.com), distribute only health care books. A major vendor of health care journals is EBSCO (www.ebsco.com).

Online databases of books and journals are now the preferred method of access to information, but if you decide to use them you will probably need to go back to your CFO to request additional funds. For example, Ovid (www.ovid.com) offers a variety of searchable nursing information databases with links to full-text articles and books. Gale Group (www.galegroup.com) provides a product called Health Reference Center - Academic, which gives full-text access to more than 700 sources, including nursing and allied health journals and reference books. EBSCO Information Services also offers full-text access to more than 400 journals and allows the user to link to full text from citations within CINAHL®. Your decision about which database to use will not be as simple as just finding out which vendor gives you the best price. Each vendor offers a different selection of titles, so your choice must be based on the information needs of your staff.

After you decide which online vendor to use, the vendor will send a site license or licensing agreement for your signature. You should read it carefully and your legal counsel should approve the agreement before it is signed.

Exhibit 8–20 Selected Information Vendors

Vendor:	Web Site:	Offers:	Comments
AddALL	www.addall.com	Books (including out-of-print)	"Searches for the best deal in books anywhere online"
Amazon	www.amazon.com	New and Used Books and Textbooks	"3 million titles in books, music and movies"
Barnes and Noble	www.barnesandnoble.com	New and Used Books and Textbooks	"Features a separate Medicine and Science section"
Blackwell's Book Services	www.blackwell.com	Books, Audiovisuals	"Market leader in combining traditional bookselling expertise with the latest developments in library technology"
Books A Million	www.booksamillion.com	New and Used Books and Textbooks	"Offers a Business 2 Business ordering department"
EBSCO Information Services	www.ebsco.com	Print and Electronic Journal Subscriptions	"World's most prolific aggregator of full text journals, magazines and other sources"
Gale Group	www.galegroup.com	Online and CD-ROM databases	"Serves the world's information and education needs through its vast and dynamic content pools"

Vendor:	Web Site:	Offers:	Comments
Majors Scientific	www.majors.com	Books, CD-ROMS, Monographic Series	"Started in 1909; largest distributor of health science books in the United States"
Matthews Medical Books	www.matthewsbooks.com	Medical Books, Multimedia Products	"Began as a retailer of health science books in St. Louis, Missouri in 1889"
Ovid	www.ovid.com	Online Journal and Book Subscriptions	"Offers a customizable suite of content+ tools+ services to fuel medical discoveries and patient care."
Rittenhouse Book Distributors, Inc.	www.rittenhouse.com	Books, CD-ROMS	"Provides access to products, services and information for health sciences, scientific and technical publishing."

Once you've decided on the best choices of both information resources and vendors, your books begin to arrive. How do you organize them? If you only have a few volumes, a simple arrangement by title or author may suffice. But if you decide that you want a bit more structure, you may want to classify the volumes and add a spine label with the classification number printed or typed on it. Classification numbers are included in the Cataloging in Publication (CIP) data that is printed on the back of the title page of most books. Librarians at the Library of Congress and the National Library of Medicine prepare the CIP information. You may use either the Library of Congress or National Library of Medicine classification numbers, but you must be consistent with whichever you choose. Large libraries that want to catalog current acquisitions may wish to contract the services of a company such as MARCIVE (www.marcive.com) or OCLC (www.oclc.org). These companies can provide catalog cards, book labels, smart barcode labels, and other bibliographic services.

You and the Information Technology Guy (or Gal)

You have carefully evaluated all the available databases, have made your decision, and have negotiated a reasonable price with a vendor. When your purchase order reaches the Office of Information Technology (or its equivalent), the IT (Information Technology) staff refuses to sign off on the order. (Hey, we just gave you $5,000 and now you can not use it. Welcome to the wonderful world of online information.) They maintain that the hospital's firewall will not permit the access you need. The database vendors require that port 210 be open. You also want to give access through a proxy server, so the nursing staff can access the information at home. Furthermore, you need a static IP address on the network for the computer at the nursing station. The IT folks will not allow any of this to happen, although the vendor promises you that the hospital's information system security will not be compromised. Furthermore, the vendor says that large hospital systems across the country use his product safely. What is your next move?

Beg? Cry? Resign? Purchase a billboard on the main highway in town that says, "IT STANDS FOR IGNORANT TOAD?" No, just take a deep breath and remember, IT folks are busy people, with great responsibilities who must please a diverse group of users. Above all, they are concerned with the security of the information system. Therefore, the cardinal rule when using information technology products is to learn to communicate with IT. If you are considering purchasing a technology product, let them know about it in advance. They can tell you if it will work with the existing system. Meet with them frequently. Let them know what your needs are. Perhaps they have a solution for you that you never considered. Take them out to lunch. Thank them for their efforts.

"Obviously, we have a problem with our firewall!"

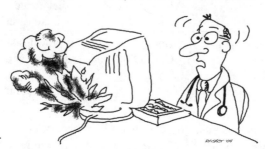

Robin Fisher, Designer

Now back to the problem at hand. First, what is a *firewall*? According to webopedia.com a firewall is:

> A system designed to prevent unauthorized access to or from a private network. Firewalls can be implemented in both hardware and software, or a combination of both. Firewalls are frequently used to prevent unauthorized Internet users from accessing private networks connected to the Internet, especially *intranets*. All messages entering or leaving the intranet pass through the firewall, which examines each message and blocks those that do not meet the specified security criteria.

A firewall is a mechanism to protect the security of your data. You do not need to be reminded of the utter importance this has in a health care setting. One word sums the importance of data security—HIPAA. The firewall is there to protect the network behind it. The network has ports that are, "in TCP/IP ... networks, an endpoint to a logical connection. The port number identifies what type of port it is. For example, port 80 is used for HTTP traffic" (webopedia.com). Data comes in and out of the network to your computer through ports, which are designated for different functions. Opening a port to outside users on the Internet opens the network up to the whole world and all the ugly things that can destroy an information system such as viruses. Therefore, IT staff is rightfully cautious about opening ports on the network.

The Internet was made possible by the development of the TCP/IP protocol. TCP/IP makes it possible for computers all over the world using different hardware and software and on different types of networks to communicate. Webopedia.com describes *TCP/IP* as:

> Abbreviation of Transmission Control Protocol, and pronounced as separate letters. TCP is one of the main protocols in TCP/IP networks.

Whereas the IP protocol deals only with packets, TCP enables two hosts to establish a connection and exchange streams of data. TCP guarantees delivery of data and also guarantees that packets will be delivered in the same order in which they were sent.

Your computer also has an address that identifies it on the Internet. An information vendor may need to recognize your computer by its address on the Internet or Internet Protocol (IP) address. Yet, usually IT has a pool of IP addresses that are assigned to you randomly each time you use the Internet. Therefore, your Internet address will change each time you use the Internet. (Can you imagine your home address changing every day and how difficult that would make it for the post office to send you a letter?) It is possible for IT to assign your computer an IP address that remains the same (static IP). Just remember, the number of static IPs is limited and therefore a static IP may not be possible to obtain.

Many information databases have an option that allows off-site access to the information through a *proxy server*. A proxy server is "a server that sits between a client application, such as a Web browser, and a real server. It intercepts all requests to the real server to see if it can fulfill the requests itself. If not, it forwards the request to the real server" (Webopedia.com). In our case it verifies that you are a member of your hospital or other healthcare organization when you are using the Internet at home or anywhere else outside

Exhibit 8–21 Dealing with Information Technology (from Webopedia.com)

Term	Definition
Proxy server	A server that sits between a client application, such as a Web browser, and a real server. It intercepts all requests to the real server to see if it can fulfill the requests itself. If not, it forwards the request to the real server.
IP	Internet Protocol. An IP address identifies your computer on the Internet, just like the address of your house or apartment identifies where you live.
TCP/IP	Transmission Control Protocol, and pronounced as separate letters. TCP is one of the main protocols in TCP/IP networks. Whereas the IP protocol deals only with packets, TCP enables two hosts to establish a connection and exchange streams of data. TCP guarantees delivery of data and also guarantees that packets will be delivered in the same order in which they were sent.
Port	In TCP/IP networks, an endpoint to a logical connection. The port number identifies what type of port it is. For example, port 80 is used for HTTP traffic.
Static IP	Generally refers to elements of the Internet or computer programming that are fixed and not capable of action or change. (In our scenario, a static IP is a computer using the Internet that keeps the same IP address.)
Firewall	A system designed to prevent unauthorized access to or from a private network. Firewalls can be implemented in both hardware and software, or a combination of both. Firewalls are frequently used to prevent unauthorized Internet users from accessing private networks connected to the Internet, especially intranets. All messages entering or leaving the intranet pass through the firewall, which examines each message and blocks those that do not meet the specified security criteria.

your organization's network. The proxy server then gives you access to information on the network just as if you were using a computer in the hospital. This is great, because you can then wear yourself out all day long on the floor and after that go home and read current nursing journals instead of watching Star Search on television. The problem with proxy servers is that they require ports on the firewall to be open and as we said earlier, IT is not going to hug you when you make this request to them. We hope this section has not sounded like "blah blah blah blah" to you. Our goal is to encourage you to communicate with IT and know some basic concepts of network computing.

Information and PDAs

You get a PDA for Chirstmas. What is a PDA? What do you do with it? A PDA is a Personal Digital Assistant or handheld computer. There are two major platforms or operating systems for PDAs—the PocketPC operating system and the Palm operating system. More products are made for the Palm system, which has been available for a longer time. The PocketPCs are closing the gap, primarily because of computer giant Dell entering the PDA market with a PocketPC system. PocketPC is a Microsoft operating system and works with Microsoft office products such as Word, Excel and PowerPoint.

Are PDAs just fancy calendar devices for geeks? No! The calendar applications are, however, very useful. They can be made to synchronize with the calendar on your desktop computer and store all the names, phone numbers, emails, and addresses of your contacts. PDAs have much more important applications in health care. They can be used for running health knowledge databases such as InfoRetriever, textbooks, drug databases, and just about every type of information resource that exists in print. Two sources for PDA health resources are skyscape.com and handheldmed.com.

Just a quick perusal of Skyscape shows that their best selling nursing texts for PDAs are RNotes (Nurse's Clinical Pocket Guide for Nurses), Davis's Drug Guide for Nurses, OncoRn (Oncology Nursing Drug Handbook) and RnIVDrugs (Nursing I.V. Drug Handbook). This gives you a taste of the type of information that can be used on a PDA in a clinical setting. A common product used by health care PDA users is ePocrates, a free drug database (www.epocrates.com).

Note: The National Network of Libraries of Medicine (NN/LM®) is a division of the National Library of Medicine (NLM). NN/LM has centers throughout the country. Each center has trainers who will come out to your town and teach classes on PDAs, consumer health, public health information resources, and NLM databases, just to name a few topics that are in their repertoire. The Web address for NN/LM is www.nnlm.gov.

Like desktop PCs, PDAs can be improved with accessories. You can buy keyboards and extra memory storage devices. The two most common types of memory expansion cards are Compact Flash (CF) cards and Secure Digital (SD) cards. These are the equivalent to floppy disks, zip disks, and CDs on your desktop computers. PDAs work with your desktop PC. A synching cradle is used to pass information between the two devices. Information is entered into the PDA with a stylus. This skill takes some practice to acquire.

It is necessary to learn a shortcut writing technique termed "graffiti" to enter data if you are using a Palm-based PDA. Graffiti is a character recognition method that converts stylus strokes on a PDA touch screen into data.

The folks at the University of Arizona have been leaders at compiling PDA resources on the Web. Their site is http://educ.ahsl.arizona.edu/pda/index.htm. Two nursing PDA sites are PDA Cortex (http://www.pdacortex.com) and Nursing Resources for the PDA (http://library.osfhealthcare.org/nursingpda.htm). Another site you will want to be sure to look at is Avantgo.com. Avantgo is a great site for digests that will update each time you synch your PDA. For example, you can sign-up for an abbreviated version of *USA Today*. Advantgo includes health care digest as well. This list is by no means exhaustive. It is just meant to give you a start at finding resources on some of the better Internet PDA resource sites. We encourage you to invest in a PDA. They bring information to the bedside, so you can bring better care to your patients.

Exhibit 8–22 PDAs

PDA Operating System	Comments
PocketPC	A Microsoft operating system, therefore works well with Microsoft products. Some companies that sell PocketPC-based PDAs are the Dell Axim, Compaq IPAQ and Hewlett-Packard. www.microsoft.com/windowsmobile/default.mspx
Palm	More software available with this operating system. Some companies that make Palm-based PDAs are Palm, Sony, and Toshiba. www.palmsource.com/palmos

Exhibit 8–23 PDA Resources

PDA Resources	Comments
Skyscape.com	Good source for buying electronic textbooks.
ePocrates.com	Free drug database for PDA.
library.osfhealthcare.org/nursingpda.htm	Nursing resources for the PDA
www.pdacortex.com	PDA Cortex
educ.ahsl.arizona.edu/pda/index.htm	University of Arizona
Handheldmed.com databases.	Like Skyscape, a good source for PDA texts and
Avantgo.com	Digests such as USA Today. Updated each time you synch.

Information Retrieval on the Web

Web Searching Resources

You need to find information on distance learning programs for one of your nurses who wants to do his/her BSN online. Not too long ago, this was the type of question for which you could not find an easy answer. That no longer is the case. Information is available, it seems, on every topic on the web. We often hear that *all* the information you need is free on the web. This is simply not true. Quality information products are usually sold through business entities, which exist to make money. Therefore, they are not going to give their products away. It is still worthwhile, nevertheless, for you to develop your skills as a web searcher, because much valuable information is waiting to be discovered by you. You should learn to use search engines such as Google, search directories such as Yahoo!, and meta-search engines such as Dogpile. A *search engine* searches a vast number of sites. A *search directory* is a categorized list and searches a smaller number (but a higher quality) of sites. A search directory yields higher precision (more of the retrieved sites are actually about your topic), whereas a search engine brings in a greater recall (finding more of the total number of sites on your query). A *meta-search engine* compiles the results of multiple search engines.

The consensus seems to be that Google is the search engine of choice, although other search engines have features not contained in Google. Take time to look around in Google. Under Google services, click on catalogs and browse through online catalogs of companies such as Lands' End or go to Froogle, which allows you to search by product (such as coats) across multiple companies. You may want to go to your neighbor's computer and click preferences in Google and set their retrieval to display in Klingon or Pig Latin. Or you may want to use the advanced search features to filter your retrieval if you are at home to keep the kids away from pornographic sites. Google News is a good site for news. The Google Images tab is a great service. It restricts your search to just images, so if you wanted an image of a pressure ulcer, for example, this would be a good place to look.

Exhibit 8–24 Web Searching Resources

Site	Address	Comments
National Network of Libraries of Medicine	http://nnlm.gov/train/supersearcher/resources.html	Excellent content on web search engines
Google	www.google.com	THE web search engine
Dogpile	www.dogpile.com	Meta-search engine
searchenginewatch	www.searchenginewatch.com	Lots of interesting stuff about search engines
Yahoo!	www.yahoo.com	Search directory. Have you Yahooed?

How to Evaluate Web Sites

The web has a tremendous potential for the delivery of health information. Never before has such an opportunity been available to deliver current information to such a wide audience. But, there is a downside. Much fraudulent health information exists on the web. You should keep several principles in mind when using web information. First, ask if it is produced by a reputable organization. What is the domain of the site? Is it an .edu (educational institution) or a .com (corporation)? A business corporation is in existence to make money, so have your "bias detector" turned on if you use a .com site. Often in health care an .edu or .org (an organization such as the American Heart Association) will have more reliable information. When was the site last updated? Is it current or out of date? There are certifications indicating the quality of health web sites such as the Health on the Net Foundation (HON) code. However, be aware that these approval seals are usually self-reported and any web page designer can copy the quality logo and paste it on his/her web page.

You should ask where the information originated and how it is selected. A good site will have a purpose statement and will clearly identify its funding and creators. Another thing to consider is how the site handles human interactions. Avoid a site that requires a lot of personal information before you are allowed to use it. Finally, although glitz and glamour do not equal a quality web site, a good site will be easy to navigate, be pleasing to the eye, and have a minimum of typographical and spelling errors.

Exhibit 8–25 Evaluating Web Sites

Principle

1. Who produced the site?
2. What is the domain?
3. Is the site updated regularly?
4. Does the site clearly state its purpose and how information for it is selected?
5. How does the site handle human interactions?
6. Is the site free from grammatical and typographical errors?
7. Is the site easy to navigate?

Information Need and Nursing

The literature is replete with studies on the concept of information need. Several of these reports are briefly summarized here. Christensen, Broadway, and Garbutt (1995) reported that, "when seeking medical information, most of the nurses, dentists, optometrists, orthodontists and pharmacists preferred verbal communication with colleagues (73 percent)... however, 53% of all respondents did express high interest in reading journals" (p. 60). Spath and Buttlar (1996) said, "Research and its application in the clinical setting result in improved patient care and provide a strong scientific knowledge base for nursing" (p. 112).

In their study 79.4 percent of nurses responding used professional journals as a source of information. Leckie, Pettigrew, and Sylvain (1996) reported that nurses have great information needs, but do not have great knowledge of information services. About physicians, they noted that information needs vary among specialties and that "use of library service increased with recency of training" (p. 169). Blythe and Doyle (1993) in a study on the information needs of nurses declared, "Nurses, the largest group of health professionals, are not information literate" (p. 433). Haynes, McKibbon, Walker, Ryan, Fitzgerald, and Ramsden (1990) said that "Physicians cannot keep all of the information they need in their heads, and even if they could, medical knowledge changes so rapidly that acquired information quickly becomes obsolete" (p. 78). Estabrooks, O'Leary, Ricker, and Humphrey (2003) said, "Nurses clearly lag behind other groups in workplace use of the Internet" (p. 80).

Hewins (1990) in her review of information needs and use studies said:

> Edward Huth, editor of the *Annals of Internal Medicine*, calls for better identification of the information needs of clinicians. He notes some barriers to the use of the medical literature such as 1) time and effort, 2) cost, 3) inconvenience and 4) inadequate personal libraries. He calls on the professional societies to design new systems to meet the information needs of physicians. [Nurses, too!] These systems must address the reasons why physicians underused the literature ... More importantly, he relates information use to physician competence, noting that the knowledge needed for medical competence can be related to information skills. (pp. 150–151)

Hewins stated that some have suggested that if physicians consult the literature their insurance rates should be reduced. The fact that several of these studies point out the information shortcomings of physicians underscores the obvious—that physicians do not know everything, and that because of their information gaps, nurses must be involved in finding best-evidence information for the good of the patient.

Lundeen, Tenopir, and Wermager (1994) in their information needs survey of health care professionals in Hawaii discovered "for all groups of personnel, journal articles were overwhelmingly the source that best met information needs, indicating the importance of access to journal indexes and collections or article delivery services" (p. 200). Tenopir (as cited in Lundeen et al., 1994) said that by far the source that best met information needs was the journal article.

A final reason why information services are needed by nurses in the clinical setting is because of the requirements of the Joint Commission on Accreditation of Healthcare Organizations (JCAHO). The JCAHO *2003 Hospital Accreditation Standards* gives the following definition of knowledge-based information management:

> Knowledge-based information management consists of systems, resources, and services to help health professionals acquire and maintain the knowledge and skills they need to maintain and improve competence; support clinical and management decision making; support performance improvement and activities to reduce risk to patients; provide

needed information and education to individuals and families; and satisfy research-related needs (p. 267).

The *Standards* also define knowledge-based information:

> Knowledge-based information refers to current authoritative print and non-print information resources, including current periodicals, indexes, and abstracts in print or electronic format; other clinical and managerial literature; successful practices; practice guidelines; research data; recent editions of texts and other resources; satellite television services; and on-line computer-linked information services via the Internet (p. 267).

The *Standards* go on to say that:

> All types of information do not have to be provided on site. A hospital is not required to have a library located in its facility. Services may be shared with other hospitals or community resources as long as information is accessible to the hospital's staff in a timely manner (p. 267).

Note that an onsite library is not required—only **access** to the stated resources.

Exhibit 8–26 Information Needs of Nurses

Study	Results
Leckie, Pettigrew, and Sylvain (1996)	Nurses have great information needs, but do not have great knowledge of information services.
Blythe and Doyle (1993)	Nurses, the largest group of health professionals, are not information literate.
Haynes, McKibbon, Walker, Ryan, Fitzgerald, and Ramsden (1990)	Physicians cannot keep all of the information they need in their heads, and even if they could, medical knowledge changes so rapidly that acquired information quickly becomes obsolete. This is obviously true of nurses as well.
Christensen, Broadway, and Garbutt (1995)	53% of all healthcare professionals expressed high interest in reading journals.
Spath and Buttlar (1996)	Research and its application in the clinical setting result in improved patient care and provide a strong scientific knowledge base for nursing.
Lundeen, Tenopir, and Wermager (1994)	For all groups of personnel, journal articles were overwhelmingly the source that best met information needs.
JCAHO	Requires either ownership or access to "knowledge-based" information.

Information and Ethics

Ethics is one of the hallmarks of professionalism. The Institute of Medicine (IOM) reported that there are one million medical errors and nearly 100,000 deaths from error each year (Homan, 2002). Information is critical to health care. Therefore, health sciences librarians should strive to provide information in a timely fashion and provide current state-of-the-art information to all stakeholders in health. This is not simply a job, but an ethical imperative.

One way information is ethical in nature is that it "empowers individuals by creating an information-rich atmosphere within which the patron can experience a sense of possibility and a belief that growth in personal autonomy is possible" (Alfino and Pierce, 2001, p. 481). Hawkins, Morris, and Sumsion (2001) argued that libraries provide external benefits to society, much like a public health department does. A person who uses the library is a more qualified individual, which benefits society. This shows the ethical benefits communities (such as the nursing community) derive from libraries. Other studies have shown that clinicians do not have time to find the information they need, and that therefore librarians are needed to find it for them. The point is that information is not just a neutral phenomenon, but instead a positive ethical value component of any community. Thus, libraries make a community an ethically richer place. Williams and Zippperer (2003) said, regarding patient safety (which is an obvious ethical issue):

> Access to information is essential to education which empowers nurses to become active participants in error-reduction strategies and to identify potential problems before harm occurs. Efficient access to the full range of biomedical literature means having searchable online access or, even better, building relationships with the gatekeepers to this knowledge base. Often this role is filled by a medical librarian (pp. 199–200).

Exhibit 8–27 Ethics

Information	Libraries
Reduces medical errors	Save time
Empowers people	Save money

Information and Libraries/Librarians

Hospital Librarians

You have three nurses out sick. Your census is up dramatically. You have more meetings than you have hours. You also to need to find some information. What do you do? Often, the information need goes unfilled. We have a better idea—use your librarian. Do not hesitate to "bother" your librarian if there is one in your facility. Librarians are one of the world's best kept secrets. Librarians will do literature searches for you when you do not have time. They can order articles for you that the library does not have. Some librarians are willing to come out to the clinical areas of the facility on a regular basis and interact with the clinical staff. A current trend is for the electronic delivery of information.

Librarians can find information and email it to you. One way, according to Reichel (1989), that librarians can meet the needs and obligations of the parent institution is by bibliographic instruction (BI) or teaching. Bibliographic instruction teaches library patrons how to locate and use library resources efficiently. Librarians are there to help you and they love to teach. Schedule classes for them to work with your nursing staff. They can explain the information resources available at your facility and teach your staff how to properly use them.

Outreach Librarians

You work in a rural long-term care facility. You want better information resources for your staff, but cannot afford a library in the facility. What do you do?

Jensen and Maddalena (1985) note that, "The results of our work show that small rural hospitals (100 beds or fewer) have extreme difficulty in maintaining adequate on-site library resources and services over a period of time" (p. 60). Pifalo's (1994) research discovered that "In the United States, only 43.1% of hospitals have libraries, and in hospitals with less than 200 beds, the figure is 28%" (p. 30). Given the financial crunch on small hospitals, it is safe to bet that the number is even less. Often, unfortunately, when a hospital makes spending cuts, the library is a victim. A solution for these hospitals may be to contract the services of an outreach librarian who would spend varying amounts of time there, depending on the size of the hospital and its information needs. The outreach librarian visits several key areas throughout the hospital including nurses' stations, the physicians' lounge, the emergency room, the pharmacy, or outlying clinics. In Gordner's (1982) experience with outreach librarianship, nurses were the largest users of the information service.

Many regions of the country have Area Health Education Centers (AHECs). AHECs provide library services, continuing education programs and many other services to health care professionals. AHECs are started with federal grant money and supported by user fees and state governments. You may have an AHEC librarian in your area who would be glad to provide library services to your facility. They may provide the service for free or in some cases may charge a reasonable fee to cover expenses. Fowkes et al. (1991) reported, " AHECs have demonstrated an ability to respond to current and emerging needs that distinguishes them from other institutions that have educational missions" (p. 219). AHECs responded better because they were more flexible than traditional academic bureaucracies and were more in touch with the communities they serve. Fowkes continued, "Having both academic and community roots, AHECs know the needs and resources of each and how to use them in a manner that benefits both, thus strengthening and balancing the partnership between school and community" (p. 219).

Librarianship in the Clinic

Florance, Guise, and Ketchell (2002) describe how Vanderbilt Medical Center librarians were trained in pharmacology, physiology, and biostatistics and are active participants in medical rounds. They not only gather information for clinicians, but also summarize it, appraise it, and offer commentary. This same practice could work with nurses. Williams and Zipperer (2003) said, "The occasional participation by the librarian in patient rounds with nurses and other clinical staff can engender trust in the relationship between the librarian and the clinical team" (p. 204). Your librarian could come on the floor once or twice every week. He/she could gather topics to be researched, meet new staff, update the staff about new developments in the library, and give one-on-one training. As a result, the nursing staff saves time and the librarian becomes an important part of the clinical team.

Exhibit 8–28 Libraries and Librarians

Title	Responsibilities
Hospital Librarian	Manages a collection of books, journals and electronic databases; does training; executes database searches; orders articles; is based in the local facility.
Outreach Librarian	Works from an academic health science center or other central facility to serve multiple healthcare facilities in a geographic region.
Clinical Librarian	A hospital or academic librarian who makes regular visits to clinical areas of a hospital, nursing home, etc to provide "on the spot" information services to the clinicians.

Specialized Information Resources for Nurse Administrators

As nurse managers you need specialized resources for your managerial role. An excellent source for business information is ABI/INFORM, a proprietary database. According to the vendor web site:

> One of the world's first electronic databases, ABI/INFORM has been a premier source of business information for more than 30 years. The database contains content from thousands of journals that help researchers track business conditions, trends, management techniques, corporate strategies, and industry-specific topics worldwide.

The *Journal of Nursing Administration (JONA)* is an excellent publication for nurse managers. It is published monthly (July/August combined) by J.B. Lippincott. Other first-rate journals are *Nursing Economic$*, *Nursing Management*, *Nursing Administration Quarterly*, and *Seminars for Nurse Managers*. General business journals such as the *Harvard Business Review* are also good sources as are generic business and administration textbooks. The Gale Group of databases is proprietary and has several business databases such as Business & Company ProFile ASAP; Business & Company Resource Center; Business & Industry; Business & Management Practices; and Business Reference Suite. Gale also has the health databases Health Reference Center Academic and Health & Wellness Resource Center. The Lexis/Nexis database is another proprietary database. It is an outstanding source of legal information and for news.

State web pages are a superb source of information. In many instances they will have the state code, health professional licensure verification, and rules and regulations from various state agencies. A good source of statistical information is The National Center for Health Statistics, produced by the CDC (www.cdc.gov/nchs). Another exceptional site for statistical information is "Statistical Resources on the Web" produced by the University of Michigan (www.lib.umich.edu/govdocs/stats.html).

Specific information on Medicaid and Medicare can be found at www.cms.hhs.gov/ at the Centers for Medicare & Medicaid Services (CMS). One useful database on the CMS site is "Nursing Home Compare". This is a searchable database to compare nursing homes in the United States.

Exhibit 8–29 Specialized Information Resources

Focus	Website	Resource
Nursing Administration Journals		The Journal of Nursing Administration (JONA), Nursing Economic$, Nursing Management, Nursing Administration Quarterly, and Seminars for Nurse Managers
Business	proquest.com/products/pt-product-ABI.shtml	ABI/Inform (proprietary)
Business	www.galegroup.com	Gale Group (proprietary)
Law	www.lexis-nexis.com	Lexis/Nexis (proprietary)
Statistics	www.cdc.gov/nchs/	National Center for Health Statistics
Statistics	www.lib.umich.edu/govdocs/stats.html	Statistical Resources on the web
Medicare/Medicaid	www.cms.hhs.gov	Centers for Medicare & Medicaid Services (CMS)
Nursing Homes	www.medicare.gov/NHCompare	Nursing Home Compare

Carol J. Galganski did a citation analysis of the nursing management literature. Recommendations she made other than the ones already listed are OCLC's ArticleFirst database (www.oclc.org/databases). Do not forget to use books in this electronic age. One trick is to search for a book on the Amazon.com web site. Copy the information and submit it to your librarian, who may be able to obtain the book on interlibrary loan. Please take time to search the online public access catalogs (OPACs) of large libraries. Almost all large libraries have made their catalogs available to search freely on the web. LOCATORPlus, the catalog of the United States National Library of Medicine, the largest medical library in the world, is available at http://locatorplus.gov. If you find a good title, ask your librarian to obtain it on interlibrary loan.

Summary

We have given you a lot of information. You are an official graduate of our crash course in access to knowledge-based health information. Congratulations! We hope we gave you enough exposure to different aspects of health information to know its value. We hope you can do a credible consumer search, a credible professional search, and a credible web search. We hope you understand the basics of best evidence information, the clinical value of PDAs, and the value of health sciences librarians. We hope you now can deal more fruitfully with information vendors and information technologists. We would like to conclude by taking this opportunity to tell you that it is a great privilege to serve you. The exemplary care and comfort you give the sick makes taking care of your information needs a joy. Our goal is for you to master the theoretical concepts and practical uses of healthcare information for your own personal growth as a skilled healthcare professional and for the benefit of the patients you serve.

The authors would like to thank Peg Allen, Martha Earl, Suresh Ponnappa, Janet Fisher, Robin Fisher, and Doug Driver for their assistance in the preparation of this chapter.

References

Alfino, M., & Pierce, L. (2001). The social nature of information. *Library Trends, 49*(3), 471–485.

Blythe, J., & Doyle, J. A. (1993). Assessing nurse's information needs in the work environment. *Bulletin of the Medical Library Association, 81*(4), 433–435.

Burke, L. (1990). The need for medical libraries in hospitals. *New York State Journal of Medicine, 90*(8), 420–421.

Christensen, S., Broodway, M. D., & Garbutt, H. (1995). Medical information needs and frustrations in a rural community. *Rural Libraries, 15*(2), 55–72.

Durenberger, D. (2003.) Inside-out, bottom-up healthcare reform. *Healthcare Financial Management, 57*(11), 66–68.

Estabrooks, C. A., O'Leary, K. A., Ricker, K. L., & Humphrey, C. K. (2003). The Internet and access to evidence: How are nurses positioned? *Journal of Advanced Nursing, 42*(1), 73–81.

Florance, V., Giuse, N. B., & Ketchell, D. S. (2002). Information in context: Integrating information specialists into practice settings. *Journal of the Medical Library Association, 90*(1), 49–58.

Fowkes, V. F., Campeau, M. A., & Wilson, S. R. (1991). The evolution and impact of the national AHEC program over two decades. *Academic Medicine, 66*(4), 211–220.

Galganski, C. J. (2004). Mapping the Literature of Nursing Administration. Unpublished manuscript.

Gordner, R. L. (1982). Riding the rural library circuit. *Medical Reference Services Quarterly, 1*(1), 59–74.

Green, M. L., Ciampi, M. A., & Ellis, P. J. (2000). Residents' medical information needs in clinic: Are they being met? *American Journal of Medicine, 109*(3), 218–223.

Griffiths, J. M., & King, D. (1993). *Special libraries: Increasing the information edge*. Washington, DC: Special Libraries Association.

Hawkins, M., Morris, A., & Sumision, J. (2001, September 16). The economic value of public libraries. *Australasian Public Libraries and Information Services, 14*(3), 1–8.

Haynes, R. B., McKibbon, K. A., Walker, C. J., Ryan, N., Fitzgerald, D., & Ramsden, M. F. (1990). Online access to MEDLINE in clinical settings. *Annals of Internal Medicine, 112*(1), 78–84.

Hewins, E. T. (1990). Information need and use studies. *Annual Review of Information Science and Technology*, 25, 145–172.

Holtum, E. A. (1999). Librarians, clinicians, evidence-based medicine and the division of labor. *Bulletin of the Medical Library Association, 87*(4), 404–407.

Homan, J. M. (2002). The role of medical librarians in reducing medical errors. Healthleaders. Retrieved November 8, 2002 from http://www.healthleaders.com/news/print.php?contentid=38058.

Jensen, M. A., & Maddalena, B. (1985). Implications of an AHEC library program evaluation: Considerations for small rural hospitals. *Bulletin of the Medical Library Association, 73*(1), 59–61.

Joint Commission on Accreditation of Healthcare Organizations. (1995). *An introduction to the management of information standards for health care organizations*. Oakbrook Terrace, IL: Joint Commission on Accreditation of Healthcare Organizations.

Klein, M. S., Ross, V. R., Adams, D. L., & Gilbert, C. M. (1994). Effect of online literature searching on length of stay and patient care costs. *Academic Medicine, 69*(6), 489–495.

Leckie, G. J., Pettigrew, K. E., & Sylvain, C. (1996). Modeling the information seeking of professionals: A general model derived from research on engineers, healthcare professionals, and lawyers. *Library Quarterly, 66*(2), 161–193.

Lundeen, G. W., Tenopir, C., & Wermager, P. (1994). Information needs of rural health care practitioners in Hawaii. *Bulletin of the Medical Library Association, 82*(2), 197–205.

Marshall, J. G. (1992). The impact of the hospital library on clinical decision making: The Rochester study. *Bulletin of the Medical Library Association, 80*(2), 169–178.

Pifalo, V. (1994). Circuit librarianship: A twentieth anniversary appraisal. *Medical Reference Services Quarterly, 13*(1), 19–31.

Rees, A. M. (2000). *Consumer health information source book*. Phoenix: The Oryx Press.

Reichel, M. (1989). Ethics and library instruction: Is there a connection? *RQ, 28*(4), 477–480.

Sackett, D. L., Rosenberg, W. M., Gray, J. A., Haynes, R. B., & Richardson, W. S. (1996). Evidence based medicine: What it is and what it isn't. *BMJ, 312*(7023), 71–72.

Slawson, D. C., & Shaughnessy, A. F. (1994). Becoming a medical information master: Feeling good about not knowing everything. *Journal of Family Practice, 38*(5), 505–513.

Spath, M., & Buttlar, L. (1996). Information and research needs of acute-care clinical nurses. *Bulletin of the Medical Library Association, 84*(1), 112–116.

Williams, L., & Zipperer, L. (2003). Improving access to information: Librarians and nurses team up for patient safety. *Nursing Economics, 21*(4), 199–201.

CHAPTER 9

Nursing Information Systems: Guide for Nursing Management

Sharron Rutledge Grindstaff, MSN, BSN, RN

Information systems have become an essential decision-support component for fiscal management, clinical management, and human resource management. In the hospital environment information systems (IS), clinical information systems (CIS), or hospital information systems (HIS), have become a critical link to the financial stability of health care organizations and systems.

The federal and state governments, in addition to other payers and health care consumers, are demanding quality care at less cost. This presents enormous challenges for health care management. Health care costs have increased at a rapid pace for several reasons: technological advancements in diagnosis and treatments, medication costs, shortages of health care providers, regulatory demands, and research, just to name a few. The Centers for Medicare and Medicaid Services reported that by the year 2013 health care spending is "projected to reach $3.4 trillion and 18.4 percent" of the gross domestic product (GDP) (www.cms.hhs.gov). In view of these figures, health care management must continuously strive to operate both more efficiently and more cost effectively while seeking a higher standard of care and practice.

Health care management must be in a position to make critical decisions to produce positive patient and staff outcomes. Information systems are an essential tool in the decision-making process. In addition to understanding the interpretation of information system data, nursing management must become actively involved and educated in the system selection, system capabilities, and system set-up. Nursing is in a unique position to use our clinical knowledge and expertise, and integrate it with the data-driven world of health care management. The following chapter provides an overview of the essential components that nursing management must consider in the use and management of health care clinical and nursing information systems (NIS).

Nursing Informatics

Nursing informatics was birthed as the use of computer and information technology has exploded into our lives. Hannah, Ball, and Edwards (1999) state that any time nursing uses information technology that is related to the "care of the patients, the administration of health care facilities, or the educational preparation of individuals to practice the discipline is considered nursing informatics."

The American Nurses Association Scope and Standards of Nursing Informatics Practice (2001) define nursing informatics as a

> specialty that integrates nursing science, computer science, and infor-
> mation science to manage and communicate data, information, and
> knowledge in nursing practice. Nursing informatics facilitates the inte-
> gration of data, information and knowledge to support patients, nurses,
> and other providers in their decision-making in all roles and settings.
> This is accomplished through the use of information structures, infor-
> mation processes, and information technology (www.ania.org).

It is fascinating to see how the field of nursing informatics has grown over the past two decades.

Nurses may obtain certification in nursing informatics through the American Nurses Credentialing Center (ANCC), thus recognizing it as a specialty. Information about this is accessible through their web site www.nursingworld.org/ancc.

The American Nursing Informatics Association (ANIA) defines nursing informatics as combining "nursing science with computer science together with information processing theory and technology" (www.ania.org). The ANIA provides members with the opportunity to network, and to obtain educational opportunities and resources related to health care informatics (www.ania.org). Other resources for individuals interested in nursing information systems are the *Online Journal for Nursing Informatics* (www.eaa-knowledge.com/ojin) and *Computers in Nursing* that provide current online journal articles and editorials regarding issues in nursing informatics.

Identification of Department Goals and Objectives

Since information systems have been introduced, it has become necessary for an organization or department to determine what information systems are needed. The best way to go about this is for administrators to identify specific department automation needs, and from that to develop short- and long-term goals and objectives (Kahl, et al., 1991). From this process, one can determine what information systems are necessary. An essential component involved in determining needs and selecting systems are the nurses who will be using the system, whether it is nursing management or staff nurses. This can be accomplished through a departmental information needs assessment.

For instance, if selecting a clinical documentation system, one important question to answer is, *will this system be used to create an electronic medical record?* If this is the case, *will the system be interfaced with the physicians' offices* in order to provide timely transmission and access of patient data to the physicians? The advantages of this capability include providing laboratory and radiology results as they are processed. Physicians can respond quickly and nurses can provide care based upon the revised treatment plans. Because treatment plans are changed more efficiently, patient care is timelier.

Patient demographic and health profile information are essential components of information systems. The majority of systems provide the capability of input of allergy data that, in turn, will be used to cross check medications or treatments to prevent adverse events. For example, a nurse or physician enters a pharmacy order in the system. If entered upon admission, or on a prior admission, the system will reference the allergy information and check this against the medications ordered. The system can recognize if there is a contraindication with patient allergies and a medication. This is a tremendous patient safety factor that could prevent a sentinel event or adverse outcome.

Selection of the Information System

Information Systems Committee and Implementation Team

The first step in the selection of an information system is to identify an information systems committee and implementation (pre and post) team. These individuals should be representative of departments that are either directly or indirectly impacted by the computerized functions. If an HIS or CIS is being evaluated, for example, for order entry, laboratory, and radiology results reporting, then representatives from nursing, medical staff, laboratory, radiology, pharmacy, admissions personnel, finance (billing), health information (coding), information systems, and administration must all be represented. Automating these functions not only creates various portions of the computerized medical record but are directly related to generating the patients' bill for care and services provided. If a department-specific information system is being selected, such as a nurse scheduling system, then representatives from the nursing and information systems departments, as well as departments that may be indirectly impacted, should be represented.

Selecting individuals who are able to define the functions and applications needed through a departmental needs assessment is essential to a successful selection and implementation. They must be able to identify the current workflow and issues to be able to address how the systems will either positively or negatively impact their departments (Newbold, 2004). When evaluating information systems, it is vital to work closely with the vendors. The vendors should work collaboratively with the team to conduct site visits. This will provide the team members the opportunity to talk directly to current users to evaluate the systems in a live setting. Through this process the team members can evaluate if the system would improve their current processes and decrease their documentation, or whether it would increase their workload.

Types of Information Systems

There are many information systems available, and more are introduced every year. Nursing management must continue to be aware of information system possibilities, and add them as appropriate. There are a variety of resources available for nurse administrators when searching for an information system. These include professional organizations and literature such as those published by the American Nurses Association (ANA), American Organization of Nurse Executives (AONE), American College of Health Care Executives (ACHE), and the Health Care Information and Management Systems Society (HIMSS) just to name a few. The state professional organizations and state hospital associations also maintain databases of vendors that provide a variety of services related to information systems. The internet also provides quick and easy access to contact information. Several examples are provided throughout this chapter. Some of the systems currently available are described here.

SCHEDULING AND ACUITY SYSTEMS

Staffing and scheduling are an important activity for nurse managers. The challenge to creatively balance organization or unit nurse-patient ratios while meeting the needs of the nurses can be difficult. Information system capabilities have expanded to include software that will assist in the development of schedules while factoring in the staffing and acuity needs of the unit. The systems require human resources to initially input the basic data to create staff and unit profiles. This data includes: employee names, skill level, full-time or part-time status, specific shifts, exceptions to days and/or shifts that each nurse can or cannot work, unit minimum skill mix requirements, and acuity/patient classification system data (Nygard and Hansen, 1991).

These systems may also allow coding for report generation, such as productivity management and turnover reports, if it is either interfaced or connected to the financial system. These systems can provide management information, and can be used for reports detailing the required (acuity-based) versus actual and budgeted staffing ratios by unit and shift. One example of this type of system is ANSOS/One Staff—A Nurse and Staff Scheduling Solution by Per-Se Technologies, Inc. that can function as a stand-alone system or be interfaced with the HIS (http://www.per-se.com/forhospitals/h_onestaff.asp). It is important to identify if the information system can accommodate the nursing acuity methodology. Nursing management can determine whether this process should be centralized or decentralized. The long-term benefits of an investment can not only positively impact the budget but provide invaluable data to assist in management decisions related to budgeting and staffing.

Another example of a scheduling and resource system is ORSOS by Per-Se Technologies. This operating room (OR) system provides the ability to computerize surgical case scheduling, staffing needs, staffing assignments, provide inventory control, surgeon-specific case information, and OR billing information (www.perse.com/forhospitals/h_orsos.asp). This type of system can provide management reports that can help to increase departmental efficiency, decrease costs, and provide data for performance improvement initiatives.

POINT OF CARE TECHNOLOGY

The advancement of technology has been partially driven by the demands of health care providers. As the acute care environment has placed increasing demands upon nursing to provide quality care in less time for an increasingly acute patient population, the increased demand for documentation has placed a greater burden upon the nurse. These demands have produced several options for nurses to input data close to the patient, more commonly referred to as the *point of care*.

Point of care (POC) devices help to increase productivity and are an efficient means of allowing the nurse to document while remaining close to the patient. Point of care devices can also be used to automatically record vital sign data at a frequency determined by the nurse and/or physician (Lower and Nauert, 1992). This is an important quality care and safety component that assures that this data is obtained at the intervals required.

Nursing management must consider several factors when assessing the needs of the patients and the nursing department.

The first question is to determine the basic needs.
- Will nursing use the device(s) to input vital sign data (blood pressure, pulse, temperature, venous pressure monitoring, and cardiac monitoring)?
- Will nursing input admission and shift assessment data?
- Will nursing use the system to enter information related to the plan of care, clinical pathways (care maps), medication administration, or physician orders?

Answering these questions will then help nursing and the vendors to determine what software and hardware devices will provide the necessary functions.

There are several hardware devices available, from small handheld devices to mobile personal computer devices (Picone, et al., 1991) and personal digital assistant devices (Newbold, 2004), that nurses can use. It is vital to include the front-line nurses in this decision-making process to assure that the devices are practical and can be easily used in the daily environment. Nursing management must consider whether the device(s) must meet federal and state requirements such as the Food and Drug Administration (FDA) regulations and safety requirements. Several devices are available on the market, but it is most helpful to research and try the devices. For example, the weight and durability of the device is an important ergonomic factor for nurses in their work environment. Others who use the system can provide useful information to the nursing representatives on the IS committee. This helps to determine if the mode of data input is "user-friendly," and whether it can be accomplished with ease in a minimal amount of time. Many vendors will state that their systems provide the capabilities, but, in reality, the process of data input may be cumbersome and time consuming. The primary purpose of point of care devices is to input quality data in a timely manner.

There are many different information systems available. Identifying the system that: has a history of being a successful, reliable system; provides on-going system support; provides regular upgrades for system applications; all at a reasonable cost, is a challenge. In addition to those previously discussed, the following, although not inclusive, list a few examples of systems that have been leaders in the health care industry:

Cerner   www.cerner.com

CPSI–Computer Programs and Systems, Inc. www.cpsinet.com

McKeeson Information Solutions   infosolutions.mckesson.com
Meditech   www.meditech.com
Siemens Medical Solutions   www.smed.com

PATIENT SAFETY

Handheld devices are becoming very common in hospitals mainly for the purpose of patient safety and the reduction of medication errors. *Bar code handheld scanners* are an example of devices that are used to identify patients by a "bar code identification bracelet" (Low and Belcher, 2002). The nurse is able to scan the patients' identification bracelet and reference the pharmacy database. This provides a process for verifying that the nurse is administering the correct medication and correct dose to the correct patient, at the correct time using the correct route (Low and Belcher). On February 25, 2004, the United States Department of Health and Human Service Secretary, Tommy G. Thompson, announced the "final ruling requiring bar codes" on "human drugs and biological products" (www.hhs.gov). This Food and Drug Administration ruling will also require "the use of machine-readable information on container labels on blood and blood components" (www.hhs.gov). This process will also provide automatic inventory refill as medication supplies are used.

Computerized physician order entry (CPOE) is another safety strategy being used in information systems. Though many physicians may resist this change, the first safety consideration is the issue of legibility. Medication errors comprise a large percentage of the medical mistakes each year (Low and Belcher). Many of these medication errors occur each year as a result of misinterpretation of physician orders. The other positive aspect of computerized physician order entry is the improved communication between the physician, nurse, and pharmacist (Cook, 2002).

Another patient safety example of innovation in medication automation and administration is the *Pyxis system* by Cardinal Health (www.pyxis.com). The Pyxis automated dispensing device helps to significantly reduce the incidence of medication errors. This device stores the patients' prescription with security controls that records the date and time the device was accessed by each individual, but, most importantly, will only dispense the correct medication at the correct time for the patient. This in turn will provide a mechanism for inventory control to assist in reducing costs and increasing efficiency.

Hardware and Software

Identifying the needed hardware for a new information system is one of the most important decisions in the purchasing process. There are several factors that must be considered. When function and needs are identified, the vendor can provide the options that are available. One vital question is to determine where the devices and hardware will be used and placed. If a point of care device is used, then this will generally be in close proximity to the patient. In regards to system hardware, what functions and capabilities are required? This will help to determine if, for example, a personal computer (PC) is required, and, if so, how many and where these PCs will be located.

It is very important to include the nurses in this decision process. These devices must be user friendly—not only factoring in the ease of the use of the device/hardware, but giving careful consideration to the work environment.

- Will the device require human data entry, voice activation, portable phones, or hand-held devices?
- Where will the hardware be located, how accessible will it be?
- Will it be housed within the unit or department, and/or the patients' room?

Give careful consideration to the physical location of the device. Questions to ask include:

- Will the device be located on a desk, table or portable cart?
- In order to use the device will it require the nurse to sit or stand?

The Information Systems (IS) Committee members should ask for input from the staff to determine the ease of use. This should include taking the hardware devices to the unit or department allowing staff to practice using the devices. The nurses' work environment is a very important factor in today's world. The ergonomic and safety factors must be carefully considered in the decision process.

Confidentiality and Security

In addition to the federal regulatory demands, such as the Health Insurance and Portability Act (HIPAA) (HIPAA is explained further in Chapter 6), the nursing code of ethics requires that the confidentiality of the patients be respected and protected. It is important to remember that "security is the protection of information from accidental or intentional access by unauthorized people, including accidental or intentional medication or destruction of data" (McConnell, 1999). The security of the information system is a priority in defining policies and procedures, and specifically identifying who is responsible for maintaining the system.

From a specific user perspective it is essential to evaluate whether the systems' security can be accomplished for each user, and to what level this can be accomplished, such as the protection of specific patient laboratory test results. This is generally accomplished through the use of user-defined security access codes for system sign on. These login codes not only provide system security, but allow for system security tracking, that helps ensure the integrity of the system. System security tracking tracks users by date, time, and specific information accessed.

In addition, system security procedures should include defining a time-out period should staff or a physician be signed on to the information system, and leave the work area for any reason. Defining a time-out period will decrease the possibility of another user or individual accessing patient data.

Other Important Factors

Important factors that many vendors will fail to communicate to the customers include the following:

1. Can one system accomplish the various requirements for nursing documentation? In actuality it may require different systems and/or devices from different vendors. It is not uncommon for one vendor to provide the primary hospital information system while another vendor provides the clinical and POC requirements. If this is the case, it is important to determine whether the two systems can be interfaced and at what cost.
2. Is there an interface written, or will one have to be written?
3. Do the systems require a backup, or separate backup? If so, what is the downtime of the system?
4. If more than one vendor is used, do they require separate downtimes?
5. What are the procedures during downtime and backup procedure, or during potential system failure?

It is vital that the vendor answer these questions in order to determine what the true costs of the system will be.

Determining the Information System Cost

Once nursing needs and the information system have been identified, there are several financial considerations that must be determined in the purchase of a system. It is very important to consider all costs involved. In addition to the hardware and software costs, these factors include:

1. The initial purchase price of the system,
2. IS Committee human resource time,
3. System installation including staff education,
4. Facility specific interfaces, and
5. The future maintenance requirements of the system.

System installation costs will also include the costs of the vendor on-site time, travel, food, and lodging. *System maintenance* includes the IS software, hardware, and system operations (McConnell, 1999). Future maintenance requirements can include: ongoing system maintenance costs, costs and frequency of scheduled upgrades, the costs and criteria for emergency maintenance, and additional costs for added features or capabilities. It is important to ask the vendor what fees are associated with each of the above named factors.

Staff Education

Staff education will be a major portion of the system budget. It is important that an IS Committee be formed to develop a staff education and implementation plan (McConnell, 1999a). Nursing management must carefully plan for both the number of nursing staff that will require training and education, and the numbers of hours needed for training. This includes pre-installation, system implementation, and future system maintenance. The length of educational time includes: the cost of individuals educating other staff, and the total number of staff to be trained and educated. The staff should be categorized by skill level to determine what level and amount of training is required based upon their job requirements.

It is important that staff education be considered an investment, not just an expense. Quality staff education in the initial phase can help to assure that the system is used to its full capacity, and can help to eliminate costly re-training in the future. A detailed educational plan defining the timeline and associated costs for education and training should be presented to the hospital executive team and governing body. The IS Committee should stress the fact that quality education and training on the front end will guide the success of the system. A successful implementation provides a return on the investment through confident and efficient users of the system while quality patient data is being communicated and synthesized in the system.

System Support

System support is an essential factor when considering which information system can meet the departmental and/or organizational needs (McConnell, 1999b). This includes system support pre-implementation, during implementation, and post-implementation. The vendor should provide the time frames available (times and days of the week) that system support is available. This can be accomplished through a "user help desk," "user hotline," or an identified support person.

System support is critical at each phase of implementation. This system support is vital through the vendor but the IS Committee must plan for on-going support and maintenance post-implementation. Human resources are a major aspect of implementation and individuals must be identified to fulfill these roles. It is helpful if the IS Committee can clearly define who is responsible for system support within the organization and define their role(s) and responsibilities. As technology and medicine evolve, the system will need to change.

Then there are the human resource needs post-implementation. A plan needs to be developed in collaboration with the system representative identifying ongoing system support needs within the department and/or organization. This includes who and what type of individual(s) is required to maintain the system. Will this include staff such as a clerical person, analyst, educator, and an Information Systems Department? It is common in large organizations that an Information Systems Committee is formed to provide internal ongoing support to maintain the system, as well as to provide future expansion and upgrades. For nursing, the identification of a nurse liaison and/or analyst role is essential to on-going development of the system.

Information System Implementation Phase

As nursing management is involved with the implementation phase of an information system, many of the factors already discussed will need to be implemented—purchasing the necessary supporting software and hardware, designating personnel assigned to serve as liaisons, analyzing building requirements, installing and maintaining the system for implementation and post implementation, identifying a pilot unit(s) to begin implementation, and determining who will provide both the education about the system and the release time for staff involved in the education.

This process should be clearly communicated to nursing management, nursing staff, hospital departmental staff, and hospital administration. Communication of the education plan, implementation plan, and timeline are essential components of a successful implementation.

During the pre-implementation phase create a flowchart of the current processes prior to the design of the new system (Faaso, 1992). The IS Committee should also carefully review the current procedures to determine revisions and additions for the new information system. Defining these processes will provide the IS Committee members with documentation of any revisions that may need to be made with the new information system, and will provide a basis for education of staff on the new information system.

Policies and Procedures

An important step in the implementation of any information system is defining the current and new procedures for order entry, reporting results, and any process involving data input and retrieving. Policies and procedures should include defining the new information system terminology for staff reference (Labuke, 2001).

Choosing information systems carefully is an important component of nurse administrator responsibilities and can have a long range effect in the health care organization.

References

American Nurses Association. (2001). *Scope and standards of nursing informatics practice,* Washington, DC: Author.

American Nurses Credentialing Center. (2004 February). Certification Exams: Informatics Nurse. Retrieved February 17, 2004 from http://www.nursingworld.org/ancc.

ANIA - American Nursing Informatics Association. (2004 February). Nursing Informatics. Retrieved February 17, 2004 from http://www.ania.org.

ANSOS / One Staff. (2004 February). Retrieved February 28, 2004 from http://www.per-se.com/forhospitals/h_onestaff.asp.

Ball, M. J., Hannah, K. J., Newbold, S. K., & Douglas, J. V. (1998). *Nursing informatics where caring and technology meets.* New York: Springer.

CMS - Centers for Medicare and Medicaid Services. (2004 February). CMS News. Retrieved February 22, 2004 from http://www.cms.hhs.gov/.

Cook, R. I. (2002). Safety technology: Solutions or experiments? *Nursing Economics, 20,* 80–81.

Faaso, N. (1992). Automated patient care systems: The ethical impact. *Nursing Management, 23,* 46–48.

Hannah, K. J., Ball, M. J., & Edwards, M. J. (1999). *Introduction to nursing informatics.* New York: Springer.

Kahl, K., Ivancin, L., & Fubrmann, M. (1991). Automated nursing documentation system provides a favorable return on investment. *Journal of Nursing Administration, 21,* 44–51.

Labuke, S. (2001). Online nursing documentation finding a middle ground. *Journal of Nursing Administration, 31*, 283–286.

Low, D. K., & Belcher, J. V. (2002). Reporting medication errors through computerized medication administration. *CIN: Computers, Informatics, Nursing*, 178–183.

Lower, M. S., & Nauert, L. B. (1992). Charting: The impact of bedside computers. *Nursing Management, 23*, 40–44.

McGonigle, D. (2004). OJNI - Online Journal of Nursing Informatics. Retrieved February 17, 2004 from http://www.eaa-knowledge.com/ojni.

McConnell, E. A. (1999a). Choose a successful clinical information system. *Nursing Management*, 65–68.

McConnell, E. A. (1999b). The freedom to roam. *Nursing Management*, 51–54.

Nygard, L., & Hansen, J. (1991). Making a computerized PCS work for psychiatric care. *Nursing Management, 22*, 40–44.

ORSOS. (2004 February). Retrieved February 28, 2004 from http://www.per-se.com/forhospitals/h_orsos.asp.

Picone, J., Wheatley, B., & Lewis, R. (1991). The hand-held, voice-controlled terminal: Medical information interface of the future. *Computers in Health Care*, 40–47.

Pyxis - Cardinal Health. (2004 February). Retrieved February 22, 2004 from http://www.pyxis.com/.

United States Department of Health and Human Services. (2004 February). News release. Retrieved February 28, 2004 from http://www.hhs.gov/.

PART FOUR

Budget Principles

Part IV provides the "bread and butter" information on budgeting. It is important that nurse managers, as well as other nurse administrators, have this basic knowledge.

Chapter 10 on Budgeting provides basic budgeting principles and terminology as well as giving an explanation of the "break even" budget strategy.

Before getting started on the budget journey, it is helpful to have some additional financial information about how budget information is organized within charts of accounts. Thus, we have included this information in Appendix A of Chapter 10.

Then Chapter 11, Budget Development and Evaluation, adds to the budgeting knowledge base to show a nurse manager how to both evaluate and develop a nursing expense budget. Certain principles should be followed as you develop a budget, including figuring nonproductive time, to be sure there is always enough staff.

Another very important budget responsibility for nurse managers, and other nurse administrators, is the ability to evaluate budget variances that occur. These are explored in Chapter 12. Some budget variances are not important, or will have occured due to circumstances one already has anticipated, such as staff training during the installation of a new clinical documentation system. But some variances can indicate that there are serious problems nurse managers can fix and avoid in the future. Although tracking is presented as an activity to do monthly, there are certain activities that the nurse manager will need to do on a daily basis to achieve maximum budget savings. Although there are a number of nurse managers that still do not have this kind of budget responsibility, especially in VA or long-term care freestanding settings, we recommend that such a process be consistently used all in settings.

Chapter 13, Comparing Reimbursement with Cost of Services Provided, reflects important budget responsibilities that have resulted since prospective payment was implemented. Here the nurse manager/nurse administrator, along with the rest of the administrative group, needs to examine actual reimbursements received and compare them with the actual costs of services provided. Examining reimbursements assures the facility is not spending more to provide service than the reimbursement amount will pay.

CHAPTER 10

Budgeting

R. Penny Marquette, DBA

Janne Dunham-Taylor, RN, PhD

Joseph Z. Pinczuk, MHA

Introduction

There are nurse managers who are not privy to budget information, but most nurse managers are both privy to budget information (at least in their area of authority), and *responsible* for budgets. While the extent to which nurse managers are involved in the budget process will vary by health care organization, most nurse managers will find themselves involved with budget preparation, holding spending to within budget limits, dealing with differences between the budget and actual performance (called budget variances), and identifying budget errors.

For most nurse managers, budgeting information and activities will be involved with *spending*. Having *revenue* information is not as common. On the revenue side, nurse managers may know the breakdown between private pay, Medicare/Medicaid, and non-paying patients. In some systems, the actual reimbursement amount will be shared with the nurse manager. Finally, the nurse manager is often involved with the entire area of case management which involves daily issues of determining whether an insurance plan will pay for services provided. Nurse managers must understand the vital link between the amount of money received from all insurance carriers (including Medicare and Medicaid) and the critical role of charting which supports the billing documents.

> **Definition**
>
> A *budget* is simply a financial plan for the future. Budgets are made for both spending and revenue.

> **Definition**
>
> A *Budget Variance* is the difference between estimated activity (the budget) and actual activity. *Variances* are calculated for many things including spending and revenues.

Budgets and Patient Care

Budget responsibility offers an opportunity for the nurse manager to be an advocate for patients. As the level of management closest to the services delivered to patients, a nurse manager with a firm grip on relevant budget information influences patient care, ensuring that the patient receives the best and safest services possible.

All managers are most effective when they are able to make sound decisions and defend those decisions with others in the organization. This is equally true for the nurse manager who needs *the skills and the vocabulary* to determine what financial information is available, acquire that information, and interpret its impact on patient care. Unfortunately, the nurse manager often must "ferret out" the data s/he needs to do this job. Data are often badly organized or even "hidden" from line managers.

Data Systems

Computer *systems* are becoming the norm in large health care organizations. By system, we mean integrated computer programs that can interface with one another.[1] For example, in an ideal situation, a nurse manager faced with staffing her unit for the coming week would have access to selected data from the finance department, the human resource (personnel) department, and the nursing department. With data from these sources, the nurse manager could know how much money is available in the budget for the unit, the salaries of cost center personnel, which employees have already worked this month, who has vacation scheduled, and so on.

If the patient classification system is also interfaced, the nurse manager would additionally have a description of the patients needing care, and the anticipated hours of care needed for each patient. With this information the nurse manager can evaluate whether the present staffing is adequate, too high, or too low to meet patient needs.

There are presently computer programs that do all of these tasks in isolation. The problem has been that the programs cannot "talk to each other." They are isolated programs, not computer *systems*. While the information may be available, it not easily retrieved and involves collecting data from many sources.

Nursing—A Big Budget Item

Nursing department costs often comprise 25–30 percent of the health care organization's budget. Because the nursing budget is so large, it often becomes the subject of close scrutiny. This makes it all the more important for nurse managers to have information available to quickly and effectively respond to such scrutiny with documented facts. Some questions to consider are:

- Do I have enough information about the nursing personnel? Data which the nurse manager might want quickly at hand would include starting dates; salaries and salary

---

[1] Interface can mean many different things. At minimum it implies the sharing of data. It can, however, also mean that when one system is changed, all related systems are also updated.

ranges, including ceilings for different classifications of personnel; sick, vacation, and personal time off (PTO) available and already taken; hours worked each week; shift(s) worked; and overtime paid.

- Do I have adequate information about the patient population served? Do I have a good handle on the type and severity of illness, length of stay or visit, satisfaction level, and method of payment?
- How productive are the personnel in my assigned area? How can I demonstrate the level of productivity which exists; could this level of productivity be improved?
- What changes could be made to reduce costs?
- How do selected cost changes impact the quality of service delivered?
- Is my organization and/or my area of responsibility financially viable?

Integrity

As with all aspects of health care, integrity is an essential component of the financial function. In the budget process, the nurse manager is faced with a choice. Does one ask for what is needed, or "pad" the budget request assuming that you will have to cut it later? "Padding" does *not* include reasonable slack. Things never go perfectly as planned. Leaving some slack in the budget is reasonable and prudent. "Padding," on the other hand, involves asking for more than you know you will need.

Remember first that your reputation is at stake. Once you have a reputation for padding your budget, every request you make will be examined with a fine-tooth comb. You will never be assumed to be accurate again. On the other hand, if you develop a reputation for prudence and accuracy, that reputation, once established, will support your requests in future years. The authors—representing nursing and finance—unanimously recommend that one choose to be truthful. "Crying wolf" will eventually be recognized. An honest relationship between those involved is *always* preferable for everyone concerned, including the patient.

Interfacing with the Finance Department

As they deal with their cost center budgets, most nurse managers will find themselves forced to interface with their finance department. We say "forced" because there exists an army of reasons why these encounters are generally stressful. Part of our goal in this book is to make those interactions work more smoothly.

Although there are budgeting and financial terms used throughout business, government, and nonprofit organizations, this terminology is not tightly standardized. Terms that mean one thing in a factory will mean something at least slightly different in a health care setting. To make matters worse, terminology is not standardized across all hospitals (or any health care facility), and is certainly not standardized across different health care environments. For example, a nurse manager who has worked at one hospital then moves to another will discover differences in terminology and budget forms, as well as distinct differences in terminology and budget organization going from a hospital to home care.

Finally, the financial people in the health care organization are likely to come from non-health care, business backgrounds. By looking at terminology from both a nursing and an accounting/finance perspective, the nurse manager will learn the links needed to communicate more effectively, and maximize mutual understanding of terminology, concepts, and issues when working with financial personnel.

We have one more important instruction before we begin to examine the budgeting process and the dictionary of budgeting terminology. When working with your financial people, and you seem to be at an impasse, skip the frustration stage and move on to *defining your terms*. Assume that you may be using a term differently. Once you understand the underlying concepts, you can simply ask, "How are you defining fixed cost? What are you including?" This approach can quickly move you beyond the stage where the finance person is looking at you as though you are an idiot, and you are getting ready to smack him or her with your unit's budget!

The Budget Process

To be most effective, budgeting should be an integrated function within the organization and all departmens should participate. Then, the nurse manager will be an integral part of the organizational whole.

Start with the Strategic Plan. The strategic plan outlines the programs and services to be provided for the upcoming year, including priorities and new opportunities to be pursued. Unfortunately, this process of strategic planning often does *not* include all the managers who need to understand the budget process. The nurse manager may not understand the goals of the organization, may not have seen the strategic plan, or may not have been involved in setting those priorities that specifically deal with the nurse manager's areas of responsibility. When this happens, the resultant budget will not be as accurate as it might be. For example, those developing the budget may not know that a surgeon has changed an operating technique, turning an inpatient length of stay into an outpatient procedure. This change (becoming increasingly common with micro-surgical techniques) will affect multiple levels of the budget, including most nursing costs. A few years ago, this type of procedural change occurred with gall bladder surgery. If finance department personnel

> **Definition**
>
> *Strategic Plans* are top-level plans which define the types of activities and goals an entity will pursue. They are, by definition, long-term plans from which all other plans will flow.

is unaware of such changes, both the revenue budget and the spending budget may end the year with major differences (called *variances*) between budget and actual.

Strategic plans need to take into account new surgical/medical/diagnostic advances that can require a different staff mix. For example, in long-term care, staff mix formerly included registered nurse coverage for eight hours a day with 24-hour coverage being provided by LPNs/CNAs. Now, with the increased complexity of the patient population, the staff mix has changed to 24-hour RN coverage and increased the licensed staff.

Another factor to consider if third-party reimbursement (including Medicare and Medicaid) is using the per diem payment method (further explained in Chapter 6), you must know what is included and excluded in the per diem. For example, if per diem includes all medications and the patient is placed on *Lovenox bid* at $80–$90 an injection, the budget is affected.

Generally there are separate budgets for each organizational unit. Units are defined as either (1) *cost centers* or (2) *profit centers. Profit centers have direct patient billing.* These include the operating room, X-ray, laboratory, outpatient and others. *Cost centers do not bill patients directly; instead, they support the profit centers.* Some cost centers have little direct relation to patient care. Payroll, custodial, purchasing, and senior management are examples of such cost centers. Other cost centers do support patient care, but do not bill patients directly for their services. These would include most nursing services, food service, and medical records.

Cost centers may be identified by their physical location (a floor) or by their function (all cardiology-related costs). Nurse managers are usually responsible for at least one cost center budget. As the manager's organizational responsibilities grows, so will the number of budgets for which the manager is responsible. When a nurse manager moves to a different organization, even at a similar health care entity, it is important to inspect the new budget, line-by-line, to get an accurate picture of how the budget is constructed. *A line item* may reflect salaries *and benefits* at one institution, *salaries alone* in another, and salaries, benefits and *overtime* at a third.

The Finance Department. Often the budget process begins with the finance department. This process begins at a specified time, perhaps six months before the new fiscal year.[2] The finance department generates a budget for next year based on actual spending during the current year. Major differences between the current budget and actual spending are investigated, and anticipated cost changes are factored in for such things as employee raises, supply and pharmaceutical cost increases, and the general rate of inflation. Hopefully, the system will include input from the nurse manager. For example, the nurse manager's cost center might be experiencing full census when the current budget

> **Definition**
>
> A *fiscal year* is a financial year that may begin on any month of the year. The *calendar year* is January 1 to December 31.

---

[2] In some organizations the fiscal year is divided into 13 months to reflect equal time periods, each 4 weeks in duration. This has some advantages over a 12-month fiscal year where the number of days per month will vary in length. With 13 identical, 28-day "months" it is easier for a nurse manager to compare staffing costs in February (when the census was up) with July (when the census was down).

The combination of fiscal and calendar years can be confusing. Often in health care, different calendar and fiscal years will be used. Usually the budget period will coincide with other financial reporting devices such as managerial reports, balance sheets, and profit-and-loss statements. It is not uncommon, however, to have federal government grants where the fiscal year (and thus the year for grant application, funding reports, and spending deadlines) correspond with the federal government's fiscal year of October 1 through September 30.

reflects 80 percent occupancy. If changes have occurred, the nurse manager must initiate a dialogue with finance department personnel.

Although budget figures are generally *annual* estimates divided by 12 (or 13), costs will not flow evenly through the year, and nurse managers should be prepared to explain short-term variations. For example, a clinic may anticipate an increased demand for immunizations in August before school starts in the fall, an orthopedic cost center may anticipate more fractures during ski season, or a psychiatric cost center may have a decreased census during the convention of the American Psychological Association because most of the admitting psychiatrists attend this meeting. Only front-line managers will understand these variations, which is another reason why nurse managers should help prepare the budget.

The value of those working *for* the nurse manager should also not be underestimated. This point in the budget cycle is a good time to talk with unit employees about budget issues. Staff can suggest how to provide patient care in a more cost effective manner while still achieving quality standards. It is also very helpful if administrators *from all departments* can meet and discuss changing circumstances and spending priorities.

Each Unit Submits a Budget to Help Achieve the Strategic Plan. The budget process starts at the top with the strategic plan, but once that is set, it moves back to the trenches and the budget is generally built from the bottom up. As each unit submits the costs (and/or anticipated revenue if in the OR or in a revenue-producing cost center) associated with achieving its portion of the mission, the *finance* or *cost and budget* department aggregates these costs into an overall, entity-wide budget. Clearly, the nurse manager must know what strategic goals are expected of the unit in order to determine the associated costs.

The Nurse Executive. Once the nurse manager has reviewed the next year's budget and provided feedback on changes, the budget is often sent to the nurse executive for further review. To negotiate successfully with the nurse executive, the nurse manager needs to consider the broader scope of responsibility that the nurse executive holds. Ask yourself what role the nurse executive holds in the organization's strategic plan and how your unit can help fulfill that role.

Developing Budget Numbers. Most budgets are based on either the prior years's budget, actual performance, or a combination of the two. It is typical for entities (whether business, government, or nonprofit) to simply take last year's plans, adjust for obvious errors in estimate, add on a little for inflation, and continue on. Called a *line-item budget*, this budgeting program clearly does not start with the strategic plan! Nevertheless, it is simple, and it is the most common approach to budgeting.

There is an opportunity here. If something has changed in the environment, this type of budgeting process allows the nurse manager to take the initiative and seek additional funding when the underlying circumstances have changed. For example, if the strategic plan of the hospital has changed to focus on patients with higher levels of acuity, the opportunity exists to argue effectively for a higher proportion of RNs or Nurse Practitioners. Unfortunately (or fortunately, if you are the one in hiding), activities are often funded long after they fail to support the strategic mission of the organization.

During the year. Throughout the year, the nurse manager must compare the budget (the plan) with actual results. The quality of reporting which supports this work will vary from organization to organization. In the best case scenario, the nurse manager will receive regular reports on a pay-period-by-pay-period basis, month-by-month basis and a *year-to-date* basis. The year-to-date numbers represent actual and budgeted numbers for the portion of the fiscal year that has passed. For example, if the budget year begins in January and it is now April, the budget report will include the actual and budget numbers for April, along with the actual and budget numbers for the four-month period that includes January through April. These year-to-date figures help smooth out minor fluctuations and help the nurse manager see if the unit is on target. Additionally, year-to-date numbers will also highlight *growing differences between budget and actual numbers which require immediate attention.*

Variance Reporting. In a well-run system, each unit will receive a regular monthly report showing the actual activity, the budgeted activity, and the difference between the two, called the *budget variance*. This report allows the nurse manager to focus in on those areas where things are not going according to plan.

The End of the Budget Year. As the end of the fiscal year approaches, the finance department often asks that purchases for the last month of the fiscal year be completed early in the month so that finance can more accurately reflect yearly expenditures by the end of the fiscal year. In fact, as the end of the budget period approaches, nurse managers are sometimes faced with the unusual problem of wanting to spend more money. Starting six months before the end of the fiscal year, nurse managers should begin examining their budgets (including grant budgets) to evaluate their remaining funds. The disposition of unspent funds varies from organization to organization and grant to grant. In the worse case scenario, unspent funds are returned to the administration *and* the following year's allocation is reduced by the same amount. (This is another place where budget "padding" can come back to haunt you.) In the next least attractive situation, the unspent funds are returned to the administration and you are commended for your careful control over organizational resources. In the best case scenario, you are allowed to retain (or *roll-over*) all or a portion of, your remaining funds.[3] It is the nurse manager's job to know how unspent funds are handled at the end of the fiscal year and plan accordingly.

Like our advice on honesty in the budget process, it is best to avoid spending money on things you really do not need. On the other hand, if you have been needing new patient beds for two years, and this year you have money left over, it would be a shame to lose it because you failed to plan ahead.

Fixed and Flexible Budgets. A *fixed budget* predicts a certain level of costs, ignoring the level of activity which occurs.[4] In reality, the cost of nursing services will vary greatly with census and acuity. Because the fixed budget is not too useful when activity is shifting,

---

[3] Even when it is policy to allow a roll-over of unspent funds, it is common for these funds to be "swept up" by the administration in years when financial results are poor.

[4] A fixed budget can be compared to planning for the cost of a wedding while ignoring the number of guests you invite. Of course, a fixed budget is appropriate *for some things*. The bride's bouquet, for example, will cost the same amount whether the wedding has 50 or 500 guests. Similarly, in a nursing unit with a nurse manager, the nurse manager's salary is the same whether the census is 50 percent or 100 percent. Most costs, however, will vary with volume.

> **Definition**
>
> A *Fixed*, line-item, *Budget* plans for the same amount of money regardless of the level of activity.

> **Definition**
>
> A *Flexible Budget* is a single budget that shows different amounts of cost for different levels of activity.

many organizations prepare a *flexible budget*. The flexible budget has different levels of cost based on levels of activity. The nurse manager may plan a flexible budget to cover different scenarios, for example a 100 percent census versus a census of 95 percent.[5]

Some health care systems have computer programs that automatically prepare flexible budgets. Sometimes, however, this is still a manual activity for the nurse manager. And, a note of warning: even when a computer program takes over the number crunching, the nurse manager should evaluate the assumptions underlying which costs will change and which will stay constant. A flexible budget provides guidance in anticipating cost increases when volume increases in terms of either census and/or acuity.

Optimistic–Pessimistic–Realistic Budget Estimates. Another approach that many organizations take is to have each manager prepare their budgets at two or more levels: optimistic (census or department activity levels are very high), pessimistic (census or department activity levels are very low), and realistic (department or activity levels stay the same as the previous year). First, this approach forces managers to consider which costs and services are absolutely essential; what can't the unit do without? Second, it forces the manager to consider the most attractive expansion of costs and services; what would you do if you were rolling in money? Even though these budgets may never be used, the thought process involved in their preparation helps the manager deal with changing realities.

Mid-Year Budget Adjustments. Cash receipts are often less than the amount expected, necessitating mid-year budget cuts.[6] It is best if the nurse manager has a plan for this possibility, rather than being forced to do budget cuts at the last minute.

Everyone Brings Something to the Table. Different groups in the organization have unique information crucial to the overall effectiveness of the budget. Nurses often do not know what revenues were generated last year (which the finance department does know), while finance personnel do not understand the myriad problems encountered in taking care of patients (which nursing personnel do know). The most accurate budget predictions are achieved when people from all departments contribute the unique information they have.

---

[5] A flexible budget is sometimes called a variable budget, but this term is not generally used by finance and accounting people. Accordingly, we are suggesting that the term *flexible* budget be used to describe a budget where costs vary according to volume (level of activity) or acuity.

[6] Shortfalls can be caused by changes in the census, problems with insurance reimbursement, lower-than-anticipated receipts from Medicaid and/or Medicare, or budget shifting, where one unit loses funds to compensate for over-spending in others.

Basic Cost Concepts—How Costs Are Defined

Cost accounting is an industrial invention. It comes from an environment where things are manufactured. Even today, cost accounting is not heavily applied to businesses which are *service* entities and provide services instead of goods.

Imagine a business that manufacturers surgical carts. They have certain requirements: a building, insurance, electricity, equipment, materials to make the cart (legs, wheels, shelves, handles, glue, sandpaper, paint), labor to take those materials and shape them into a cart, and finally labor to oversee the process and do the paperwork (accounting, payroll, insurance, and taxes).

> **Definition**
>
> *Cost Accounting* is the branch of accounting which works to determine what things cost to produce. That information then becomes an important *part* of deciding the price at which to sell goods and services.

We will go back to this simple example as we "cross-walk" nursing terminology for costs with accounting/finance terminology for costs and try to identify the places where misunderstandings are most likely to occur.

In manufacturing, there are three types of costs: direct materials, direct labor, and overhead.

Direct materials are materials which are large enough to be identified with a specific product. In the example of the surgical cart, the legs, the wheels, the shelves, and the handles would classify as direct materials. For a patient who comes into the hospital for the surgical insertion of a pacemaker, the pacemaker itself is clearly a *direct material*.

Indirect materials, on the other hand, are materials that cannot be associated with a specific product *in a cost effective manner*. These costs may or may not relate directly to the product, but it would be so time-consuming and expensive, there would be no overall benefit. *Indirect materials are part of overhead.* In the example of the surgical cart, the indirect materials would include items like glue, sandpaper, and paint. For the surgical patient, indirect materials would include things like antiseptic swabbing in the operating room, surgical gloves, and surgical masks.[7]

> **Definition**
>
> *Direct Material* can be identified with a specific product (ie, a wheel on a surgical cart or a pacemaker in a patient's chest). *Synonym:* Raw Materials

---

[7] Historically, because health care enjoyed "cost plus" billing, health care was far more willing to treat small costs as direct costs. If a cost could be identified with a patient or procedure, the hospital could bill the insurance company and receive reimbursement. Health care treated everything from aspirins to surgical trays as direct costs. With DRGs and capitation, the rationale for that type of detailed record-keeping has changed.

> ## Definition
>
> *Direct Labor* is labor which turns direct (or raw) materials into a finished product (i.e., the production worker who puts the wheels on the cart, the physician and surgical nurse who place the pacemaker into the patient's chest).

> ## Definition
>
> *Overhead*—All costs which are *not* either direct materials or direct labor. This includes indirect materials (glue on the surgical cart, and antiseptic in the OR), indirect labor (the custodians in both examples), and all other costs associated with making it possible to do the job.

Direct labor is the labor that actually turns direct materials (also called *raw materials*) into a finished product. In our surgical cart example, the direct labor would be the person who puts the cart together. In our hospital environment, floor nurses are direct labor. The physician who inserts the pacemaker is direct labor.

Indirect labor are those persons who do not actually turn direct materials into a finished product. In the industrial example, indirect labor would include the foreman, the person who runs the raw materials storeroom, the accountant, the custodian, the payroll clerk, and others. In our hospital, indirect labor includes all of these people, plus the housekeeper, the dietician, the medical records clerk, and many others. *Indirect labor is part of overhead.*

Overhead is composed of two things, the first of which you already know—indirect materials and indirect labor. These, however, are a tiny portion of overhead. The main overhead costs are often called the "costs to get ready to manufacture." In our surgical cart example, these costs include the building, insurance, electricity, and equipment. In our hospital example, overhead includes all these costs plus many others: insurance billing, kitchen staff, dieticians, medical records, accounting, billing, payroll, finance, and management.

Basic Cost Concepts—How Costs Behave

These definitions of types of costs (direct materials, direct labor, and overhead), interact with two important concepts of how costs behave: *fixed costs* and *variable costs*. Because health care environments are different from manufacturing environments, this is an area where misunderstandings can easily occur, and one where the nurse manager can play a role in educating finance and accounting personnel about the unique aspects of health care environments.

Fixed Costs. Fixed costs are those costs which stay the same regardless of the level of activity. The first example of fixed costs are those which would exist even if the organization were "shut

> ## Definition
>
> *Fixed Costs* are those costs which stay the same regardless of the level of activity.

down." In a manufacturing environment that would include such things as rent, insurance, taxes, depreciation on (the consumption of) buildings and equipment (although perhaps at a lower or higher rate than if the equipment and buildings were in use), a minimal level of utilities, and so on. Also fixed are those costs which stay the same whether the organization manufacturers one surgical cart or 10,000. Many overhead costs will fall into this category (manufacturing supervisors, accounting, billing, payroll, finance, and top-level management).

From a nursing administration perspective, fixed costs (including minimum staffing requirements), are the minimum costs that are always paid regardless of the volume of activity.[8] Regardless of patient activity, whether it is measured by patient visits, patient acuity, or patient minutes, hours, or days, certain costs are always present. Examples might include a cost center or department secretary working the day shift regardless of patient volume, telephone service, electricity, heating and cooling, staff development, quality assurance, dietary personnel, financial personnel, administration, infection control, and other cost center supplies that do not fluctuate with volume.

There is a subtle difference between the nursing concept of fixed costs and the manufacturing concept. As a profit-focused entity, a business would not consider the cost center secretary a fixed cost (s/he can be laid-off), and staff development is certainly not fixed and can be delayed or skipped entirely. Perhaps most importantly, the concept of minimum staffing will be alien to a finance or accounting person from a manufacturing background. (See Chapter 11, Budget Development and Evaluation.) In a health care environment where most financial managers come from a business background, the need to understand the *business* concept of *costs* is increasingly important. If finance department personnel tell you what your fixed costs are, have them explain how they have defined these costs. Generally, the nurse manager or nurse executive will need to educate finance department personnel about minimum staffing. You should be prepared to explain the concept of minimum staffing and present examples of actual minimum staffing requirements for your unit(s).

Variable Costs. Variable costs are those costs that change depending on the level of volume. In a manufacturing environment that is a simple concept—the more surgical carts we make the more costs we have. All *direct materials* tend to be variable costs. In manufacturing, *direct labor* may also be a variable cost because unneeded workers can be sent home (manufacturing has no

> ### Definition
>
> *Variable Costs* are those costs that change (vary) depending on the level of activity or volume.

concept of minimum staffing). Notice, also, that some elements of overhead are variable, including indirect materials, quantity of utilities used, and the amount of depreciation on buildings and equipment. In a health care environment, volume is a more complex concept. Volume includes not only the census numbers but also patient acuity, patient minutes/hours/days, and patient visits. Variable costs occur *in addition* to fixed costs to yield the organization's total cost:

> ### *Total Costs = Fixed Costs + Variable Costs*

---

[8] It is important to note that the definition of a cost as fixed or variable would change if, for example, a cost center or an entire institution were closed!

Staffing, beyond the minimum, is a variable cost based on the variable patient census. Other typical variable costs are forms used on a per-patient basis, medical and surgical supplies and both linen and food costs. While it is important to know these definitions, particularly when planning your budget, be aware that depending on the sophistication of your finance department's software, they may be unable to split out fixed and variable costs with a useful degree of accuracy.

Mixed Costs. Most costs are neither purely fixed, nor purely variable. They are what we call *mixed costs.* Utilities are a good example. Even if an organization shuts down, it still needs a minimum level of electricity to light the yard and heat the building in the winter. That level of utilities is a fixed cost. If the organization is up and running, however, it will need more electricity to run the equipment, for lights, and for higher levels of heat or air conditioning. So electricity is actually a mixed cost—part fixed and part variable. Staffing provides a similar example. There may be minimum levels of staffing (fixed cost), but as the census moves upward, or the average patient acuity increases, the staffing level rises as well.

In general, we do not attempt to split most costs into their fixed and variable components. Rather, we tend to classify them as either fixed or variable and ignore the area of overlap. In a health care environment, you may be best served by considering minimum staffing as a fixed cost, and other staffing as a variable cost. Remember that you may need to explain this unique aspect of health care costing to your finance department.

Exhibit 10–1 illustrates the relationship between fixed and variable costs over a *relevant range.*[9] The horizontal axis in **Exhibit 10–1** represents activity level.

Exhibit 10–1 Relationship Between Fixed Costs, Variable Costs, Total Costs
(Total Cost = Fixed Cost + Variable Costs)

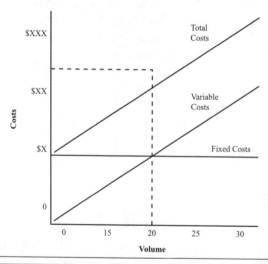

[9] All financial figures, including cost estimates, rely on the concept of relevant range. That is the range of activity over which your estimates (particularly estimates of fixed costs) remain reasonable. If, in our manufacturing example, we needed to go a second or third shift, almost all our fixed cost estimates (particularly indirect labor) would change. In a health care environment there will be a census or acuity level at which the underlying assumptions of the budget process will change. One needs to watch for that point to avoid outcomes that are very different from what was planned.

In our business that could be the number of surgical carts made, in a nursing unit it could be the number of patients, or patient days. The vertical axis represents *total* cost. The horizontal line *above the axis* represents fixed costs, staying the same regardless of the level of activity. The slanting vertical line represents the variable costs, increasing as the volume increases. The dotted line shows that at a census of 20 patients, this unit would have an average annual cost of $XX dollars. Notice that at shut-down, there would still be costs. Even with a volume of zero, the fixed costs remain.

Exhibit 10–1 not only illustrates the relationship between the different kinds of costs, *it is also a flexible budget.* This one diagram (**Exhibit 10–1**) can provide budget numbers, including both fixed and variable costs, for census levels from zero to 30 patients on a unit. Similar diagrams, or charts which move these numbers into columns for ease of use can be prepared for many kinds of individual costs, and for the overall costs of an organization. The important thing is to remember the names of the costs, the way they behave, and the manner in which they are put together.

Break Even Analysis

To stay in operation, the *minimum* long-run goal of any organization must be to at least *break even*. When one breaks even, the costs of operations exactly equal the revenues. There is no profit and no loss. More revenues will result in a profit, fewer revenues (or more costs) will result in a loss. When an entity operates below the break-even point, they must borrow or go into

> **Definition**
>
> *Break even* is the point at which the costs of operations exactly equal the revenues.

their savings from earlier periods when profits were made. Clearly these are short-term solutions, and when they are exhausted, the entity will be forced to close.

Break even can be shown graphically and it can be calculated mathematically. Both the visual and the mathematical approaches are based on the definitions of costs. Remember that there are two kinds of costs: (1) fixed costs and (2) variable costs. By adding a revenue line to **Exhibit 10–1**, we create **Exhibit 10–2**, a graphical representation of break even. In the following diagram, the *fixed cost* line has been eliminated to simplify the diagram. It has been replaced with a shaded area. Notice again that the *variable* costs begin to rise from the base of fixed costs—costs which continue even when activity drops to zero. The new element in **Exhibit 10–2** is the revenue line. The revenue line begins at zero—*no activity, no billing.* Thereafter, it climbs at a steady rate toward the upper right corner of the graph. The *slope* of the revenue line (the rate at which it climbs) is dependent on the rate of billing—bigger bills, steeper climb. Using the same measures on the horizontal and vertical axis as we used in **Exhibit 10–1**, our revenue slope would be based on the total revenue as it related to the average census or patient day. That is a crude measure, and there are many other measures which could be used. Nevertheless, at best, the break-even chart is a tool which will give you a rough idea of the activity level needed to remain solvent.

Exhibit 10–2 Graphical Break Even

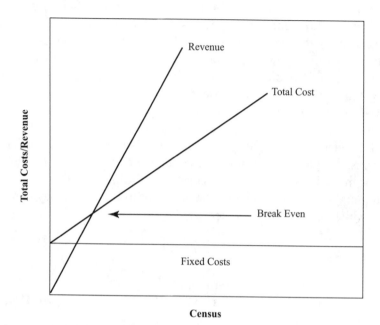

Census

Remember, the more detailed your cost analysis is, the better this tool will work for you. A break-even analysis for a *procedure* will be more accurate than a break-even analysis for a *unit* or *department*. Similarly, a break-even analysis for a *unit* or *department* will be more accurate than a break-even analysis for an *entire health care institution*. Unfortunately, at some point, the break-even point *for the organization as a whole* becomes the issue in question.

Mathematically, break even is calculated using the following formula. It indicates that one breaks even when the revenues equal the expenses. Since both revenues and variable costs are a function of activity level, in this case patient days, *we must know both the average cost and the average revenues as we add patients to the census.* Given that, break even occurs when revenues per patient day equal fixed costs plus variable costs per patient day. The question we want to answer is: *how many patients do we need in house, on average, to break even. What is the break even census?*

> **Break Even Occurs When:**
> **Revenues/patient day x census =**
> **Fixed Costs + Variable Costs/patient day x census**

Assume that the following data:

Revenue per patient day	$ 2,000
Variable cost per patient day	$ 110
Fixed costs per year	$ 1,000,000

> *Revenues/patient day x census = Fixed Costs + Variable Costs/patient day x census*
> *$2,000 x census = $1,000,000 + $110 x census*
> *(2,000 - 110) x census = $1,000,000*
> *Census = $1,000,000 ÷ 1,890*
> *Census = 529 per year*

You can verify your answer:

> *Revenues/patient day x census = Fixed Costs + Variable Costs/patient day x census*
> *$2,000 x 529 = $1,000,000 + $110 x 529*
> *$1,058,000 = $1,000,000 + $58,190*

Your answer may not be exact. First, *these are estimated numbers*. You can not be certain that your fixed costs will be $1,000,000, or that your average daily patient revenue will be $2,000, or that your average daily variable cost will be $110. What the break-even analysis has given you is a rough estimate. If, as you move into the year, you find that your estimates of revenues or costs are badly off target, or you find that your average census is only 475, you can go back to the drawing board and change the underlying realities or face a very bleak financial situation.

Similarly, *if your variable revenues do not exceed your variable costs you can never break even*. If, in this example, the revenues per patient day had been $2,000, but the variable costs per patient day had been $2,001, no amount of activity will result in a break-even situation. You will lose $1 per patient day and the harder you work, the farther in a hole you will find yourself. This understanding of the fact that variable revenues must exceed variable costs leads to an alternative way to think about the break-even calculation. This is not a change in either the concept or the calculation. It is simply an approach that avoids the manipulation of an algebraic equation and is easier for some people to remember.

Start with your fixed costs. They exist *whether* or *not* there are patients in the beds. To cover your fixed costs, you must make *more* revenue on the patients than you have costs *caused* by the patients. This "extra" revenue can then be used to cover your fixed costs.

Next, think about the revenues and the variable costs. These elements change with activity. In essence, if there were no patient in the bed, neither the revenue nor the variable cost exists. So a patient, in a bed, creates both a variable revenue and a variable cost. The term for the difference between these two is *contribution margin*. Contribution margin is the amount available to *contribute* toward covering fixed costs. When you have just enough contribution margin to cover fixed costs, you arrive at break even:

> *Break Even =* $\dfrac{Fixed\ Costs}{Revenues/patient\ day - Variable\ Costs/patient\ day\ x\ census}$
>
> *Break Even =* $\dfrac{\$1,000,000}{\$2,000 - \$110}$
>
> *Break Even =* $\dfrac{\$1,000,000}{1,890}$ *= 529 patients per year*

If one approach to calculating break even will work, so will the other. Perhaps the most important concept of break even is the understanding that some costs and most revenues are a function of activity. Some costs, however (perhaps most costs in a typical small health care institution), are fixed. and continue even after the shut-down point. When you consider actions which will improve profitability or reduce a loss situation, you must clearly identify which elements of cost and revenue you can best affect to improve profitability.

Alternate Ways to Organize the Budget

Thus far, we have been using a *line item budget*. Line item budgets are organized first by a cost center and then by the line items the cost center spends its money on. Line items include things like salaries, supplies, telephone, linen, and xerox copies.[10]

Another approach to organizing the budget is called a *program, performance, product-line,* or *community-benefit budget*. This budget is organized, not around a department or unit, but around a purpose. For example, a program budget might be organized around a product line in kidney care. The budget could include the transplant program, dialysis costs, outpatient care, and so forth. A program budget for cardiology might include cost center budgets for the operating room, recovery room, coronary intensive care, cardiac step-down, and cardiac rehabilitation services. While program budgets are conceptually appealing, they are not common. They are difficult to build, difficult to coordinate, and difficult to use as cost-control mechanisms. Perhaps the best way to get a picture of the overall cost of a program budget is to compile the program budget after the line item budgets are complete. A program budget for cardiology might include 100 percent of the costs associated with coronary intensive care, cardiac step–down, and cardiac rehabilitation services, along with some percentage of the costs for the operating and recovery rooms. Unfortunately, patients do not always fall cleanly within a product line. For example, when a cardiac patient requires kidney dialysis, it is unlikely that the cost will be picked up. Remember that budgeting is always an estimate; you will never have perfect data.When building a program budget, it is important not to miss the less obvious costs associated with such things as counseling cardiac patients and members of their families; training or ongoing education of staff; and recruitment and retention of staff.[11]

---

[10] The term *appropriations budget* is used by all governmental agencies, including governmental health care entities such as the Veterans' Administration Hospitals. The "appropriation" (short-hand for an "appropriation budget") has been passed by a governmental, legislative body and represents a *legal permission to spend* money on specified items. The unique aspects of appropriations budgets are that they are often very detailed in terms of *line items*. In a private health care institution, the ability to switch money from one line item to another line item (for example, from full-time salaries to part-time salaries) lies within the organization. With an appropriations budget, on the other hand, the organization may have to petition the legislative body in order to move money from one budget category to another. The second major difference in governmental budgets is that they almost always recapture unspent funds at the end of each budget period.

[11] Another term often heard is *zero-based budgeting*. With zero-based budgeting, the manager theoretically begins the budget cycle, not with last year's budget, but with a blank piece of paper. Every cost is then created and justified, building the new budget from scratch. While some variations of zero-based budgeting are used for small units and projects, zero-based budgeting is simply too time-consuming and costly to be routinely used. Where you do find true zero-based budgeting is during the creation of totally new programs and services. A hybrid of zero-based budgeting and program budgeting exists when programs are regularly re-evaluated to determine whether or not they should continue. This type of analysis, called a *sunset review*, is a practical addition to the line item budget and its tendency to always assume that last year's programs will simply continue with a slight increase in cost.

The purpose of a community-benefit budget is to identify specific costs allocated to meet social responsibilities in the community. These items include services for the poor and educational or outreach programs that enhance people's health in the community.

Capital Budgeting versus Operational Budgeting

Budgets can be divided into two major divisions: (1) the *Operating Budget* and (2) the *Capital Budget*. Most nurse managers will work primarily with the operating budget, which has been the focus of this chapter thus far. Operating budgets cover the day-to-day costs of a unit including such things as wages for regular and temporary workers, medical and office supplies, equipment rental, repair and maintenance, travel and education, and dues and subscriptions. Like all budgets, operating budgets represent the "best guess" for costs over a coming period.

The *capital budget*, on the other hand, covers the purchase of land, buildings, and long-lived (at least two years) equipment.[12] The capital budget is developed separately from the operating budget, and is often funded through separate sources such as capital campaigns, designated internal savings, and grants. Nurse managers are most often involved in capital budgeting when they request expensive, long-lived equipment for their units. In most organizations financial rationale must support the request for an item from the capital budget. The most obvious reasons for purchasing long-lived equipment are:

1. A necessary item is broken and must be replaced;
2. A newer, better piece of equipment exists which will provide better patient service or equivalent patient service at a lower cost; or
3. A new piece of equipment exists which will provide new patient services and help to generate new revenues.

The process of providing a rationale for capital spending is called *capital budgeting*. There are two fundamental differences in the way capital budgeting is approached in business (which may be your finance director's background) and in health care. First, from a *business* point of view, the underlying concept behind *capital budgeting* is that if: the future revenues, or the future cost savings from a new project or a new piece of equipment exceed the cost, then this purchase will increase the overall profitability of the organization. From a *health care* point of view, on the other hand, most capital purchases will be based on the requirements of quality patient care. Second, in *business*, if a project is deemed to be profitable, the funds to undertake that project will likely be borrowed if they are not available internally. In *health care*, on the other hand, funds are generally limited and capital projects will compete against each other for available capital funding.

---

[12] Because there are heavy record-keeping costs associated with equipment, most organizations will set a lower limit on the dollar amount of purchases to be called, and accounted for, as "equipment." This "threshold amount" may be $500, or $5,000. The larger the organization, the higher the threshold is likely to be. When long-lived equipment with a cost below this threshold is purchased, it will be treated as "*minor equipment supplies*" and expensed. Businesses handle low-value equipment in much the same way, generally using the term *small tools*. Thus, surgical scissors, which may last five years, but costs only $250, will probably be included as *minor equipment supplies* in the *operating* budget.

An OR nurse manager requesting a new autoclave, or a new computer system will often be faced with a set of forms from the finance department asking for a justification for the expenditure of capital funds. **Exhibits 10–3** through **10–5** are adaptations of the forms suggested by the American Hospital Association.

Sometimes when requesting capital funds it is necessary to give further explanation about why such funds are necessary. One possible format is given in **Exhibit 10–4**.

Assuming that the department has more than one capital request, the set of requests will be summarized on a capital requests work sheet similar to the one shown in **Exhibit 10–5**.

Exhibit 10–3 Request for Capital Equipment or Services

1. Department _____ Date of request _____
2. Equipment or service requested _____
3. Name of primary requestor _____
4. Type of request:
   - ○ Required by regulation or accreditation   ○ Replacement of existing service
   - ○ Expansion of existing service   ○ Addition of new service
5. Department priority: Priority number _____ out of _____ requests.

   _____

6. Brief description of general specifications (including major components) and possible vendors.

   _____

7. Brief description of use and capability.

   _____

8. List by name and/or job classification the hospital staff who will operate the requested equipment.

   _____

TENTATIVE cost information:

Number of units _____   Personnel cost/year _____

Cost per unit _____   Lease or buy recommended _____

Total equipment cost _____   Estimated useful life _____

Installation cost _____   Supply cost/year _____

Transportation cost _____   Maintenance cost/year _____

10. Optional comments. Describe the present system used to accomplish the same or similar function, why the present system is not adequate, and what other departments and areas will be affected or will support the project. Additional sheets can be used when necessary.

_____   _____

Signature of person completing form   Date

Exhibit 10–4 Problem and Solution Statement

Requesting department _____ Date of request _____

Project title _____ Accountable manager _____

PROBLEM STATEMENT

1. Description of the problem:

2. Which medical and hospital staff have helped define the problem?

SOLUTION STATEMENT

1. Briefly describe the proposed solution to the problem:

2. How will the proposed project resolve the problem?

3. What alternative solutions are available, and why were they rejected?

4. What are the standard uses associated with the project?

_____   _____

Signature of person completing form   Date

Exhibit 10–5 Capital Request Worksheet

	For Administrative Use			
	Referral to Medical Equipment Committee			
	Check Information Needed for Review**	R ▢ P-S ▢ N ▢ I ▢ C ▢ E ▢ F ▢	R ▢ P-S ▢ N ▢ I ▢ C ▢ E ▢ F ▢	
Estimated Acquistion Cost				
Unit Cost				
Quantity				
Check Appropriate Box	New			
	Expansion			
	Replacement			
	Required by law or JCAHO*			
Requested month of purchase				
Title of request and brief description				
Department Priority Number				

* If JCAHO standard is the reason for acquisition, complete the Needs Assessment section.

** Letters stand for R = Request Form, P-S = Problem and Solution Statement, N = Need Assessment, I = Impact Assessment, C = Clinical Assessment, E = Equipment Assessment, F = Financial Assessment

The trick to completing these forms is to ask yourself why you need the new equipment. Focus first on patient care needs, then on cost and/or revenue considerations. Remember to look at the "big picture." Failure to fix equipment or failure to acquire new equipment which is faster, more accurate, and/or less invasive, may result in patients choosing to go elsewhere for a wide range of associated services and thus a loss in revenue. If a piece of equipment is broken but the patient continues to come for patient services, there are often patient care issues (including possible negative patient outcomes), manpower costs associated with doing without that piece of equipment, and decreased revenues.

When you prepare your request, keep detailed copies of your notes and calculations *whether or not there is room for that amount of detail on the forms and whether or not it is requested*. Remember to:

- Make your calculations explicit;
- Label everything;
- Show every intermediate calculation; and
- Recopy when you are done and keep your notes where you can pull them up to justify your numbers.

Finally, remember to *be specific about your assumptions*. Your work as nurse manager will most likely be reviewed first by the nurse executive who will set priorities over the full range of nursing services. If the nurse manager requests additional information or clarification, the quality of your notes will be critical in supporting your request.

Generally, you can round your costs and savings to the nearest dollar. Remember that these are estimates and pennies are not generally accurate or helpful. Larger organizations may have you round everything to the nearest hundred dollars.

> *As we continue, where we provide examples with mathematical calculations, get out your calculator and work the examples along with the text. Pushing numbers is like any skill, practice makes (if not perfect) consistently better.*

Budgeting Revenues

Throughout this chapter we have focused on budgeting for cost control. Most nurse managers will work with costs, not revenues. Nevertheless, when you budget revenues, or set your own prices, there are additional things that you should know.

> ### Definition
>
> *Revenues* are the monetary value of services performed and billed to patients. The *money* will generally be received later. Perhaps much later, and perhaps not at all. *Synonyms: sales, income, professional fees, fees earned.*

Revenues versus Cash Flows

First, it is important to understand the difference between revenues and cash flows. *Revenues* are charges made to patients or other clients. When these charges are made, the health care organization believes that it is has *earned* the payment, and that it has a reasonable chance of receiving the money. Accounting (and finance) record a revenue *when it is earned, **not** when the cash is received*. When the revenue is earned, the accounting department bills the patient (or the insurance company) and records both the fact that the revenue is earned and the fact that the patient is obligated to pay. *This step of recording the revenue is called **recognizing a revenue**.*

An example may help to clarify the situation. Think of a department store at Christmas. December is a department store's biggest month of the year in terms of both sales (revenue) and expenses (various kinds of costs). *Yet very little money changes hands in December.* Most of the money associated with the Christmas season changes hands in January and February as people pay their charge account bills, and the department store pays for the merchandise it purchased for the holidays. Accountants call this *accrual accounting*—revenues are recorded when a sale is made and the seller has done the work, not when the cash is received. Similarly, most expenses are recorded when the organization has an *obligation* to pay, not when the cash changes hands.

Money (cash) is different from revenue. In health care settings, money is received long after the revenue is recorded (recognized). Although some procedures will involve direct payment from patients, money generally arrives when the insurance company, or Medicare or Medicaid pays the bill. To complicate matters further, when accountants and finance people talk about receiving money, they often say that they *realized* a revenue. *To realize a revenue is to receive the cash.* This situation is not helped by the fact that even accountants and finance people will occasionally get these terms backward! For this reason, when someone talks to you about revenues, it is often useful to clarify exactly what they mean.

If a health care organization has a very low population of indigent patients, then the difference between revenues and cash flows may be very small. Even in this case, however, the *timing difference* between when services are given and revenues are earned (recognized), and the payment date when revenues are received in cash (realized) may cause difficulties for the organization.

Nurses play a vital role in moving revenues from *recognized* to *realized* by charting. Every third party payer relies on the accuracy and detail of the patient's chart to validate payment. Until the charts are "clean" payment will be withheld. Poor paperwork can be a bottleneck that chokes off cash flow to the entire organization.

When a nurse manager enters any health care environment for the first time, whether that environment is a hospital, home health care, long term care, ambulatory center, or other, it is important to learn how patient billing works and develop an understanding of the time lag between submitting patient charges and receiving private insurance or government reimbursement.[13]

---

[13] Specific examples given for various health care environments are provided in *Health Care Financial Management for Nurse Managers: Applications in Hospitals, Long-Term Care, Home Care, and Ambulatory Care*. (2006). Janne Dunham-Taylor and Joseph Pinczuk.

Predicting (Budgeting) Revenues

Operating at a profit requires both revenues and costs to be carefully controlled. We attempt to control costs through careful budgeting. We attempt to "manage" revenues through careful price setting and by packaging a set of services that patients will want to buy and insurance companies will be willing to pay for. Revenues are predicted in the same manner as expenses. First you examine each major revenue source for the past two to five years and project the historical trend forward to next year. Next, carefully examine each revenue to decide whether there are reasons why it will behave differently next year than it did in the past. Finally, add any new "revenue streams" coming on line from new goods and services.

Pricing to Cover Your Costs

Pricing is done in several aspects. Beds and physical therapy services, for example, are priced on a per patient/per day, or per patient/per hour basis. On the other hand, procedures such as surgeries and laboratory tests are priced on a per event basis. Last, goods such as pharmaceutical supplies and prostheses are priced on a per unit basis. Regardless of the good or service we are pricing, in the long run, prices must cover *all* costs—direct labor, direct materials, and overhead. Thus, to set long-run prices, you must have a good idea of what your costs are. Prices are ***not*** based solely on costs, but *on average, costs will define the lower bound of pricing*.

For each individually priced good or service, you must try to identify the cost of all the direct materials, direct labor, and overhead associated with providing that good or service, and add them together to arrive at the cost—the *lower bound* of the price for that item. Some of these costs are reasonably easy to estimate. Others require enormous estimations. For the examples which follow, let's assume we have a good estimate of our average census for the coming year. We are estimating an average census of 500 patients per day or 182,500 patient days during the year:

> **500 patients per day x 365 days per year = 182,500 patient days per year**

Direct Materials and Direct Labor. Careful cost budgeting can provide you with reasonably accurate cost figures for direct materials and direct labor. Direct nursing labor is generally *applied*, or added to the cost of a patient day, based on average census figures or patient classification system data. Chapter 11, Budget Development and Evaluation, explains how to determine costs using a patient classification system. If we use only the patient census as an example, to arrive at a cost per day per patient for direct care nursing services, we would estimate our total direct care nursing salaries, wages, and benefits for the year, and then divide by 182,500 to arrive at a direct labor cost per day. Assume that the labor cost for direct nursing *on one unit* is $175,000 per year. The nursing cost to be added to each patient's daily bill is then $0.96.[14]

---

[14] With the increased incidence in 23-hour observation patients, we may want an hourly cost. To figure the hourly cost, just divide the daily figure by the 24 hours in each day to also get a usable figure for direct nursing cost per hour.

$\dfrac{\$175{,}000\ labor\ cost}{182{,}500\ patient\ days}$ = $0.96 labor cost per patient day

Developing the estimated cost for direct nursing services is a complex problem, which involves concepts of minimum staffing, staff mix (i.e., RNs versus LPNs versus Nurse Aides, and full-time versus part-time), and other elements such as shift differential. Detailed examples of direct labor budgeting are presented in Chapter 11, Budget Development and Evaluation.

Direct materials are easier to budget—the pacemaker is billed to the patient who receives it. Again, the cost of the pacemaker (or the bed-side wash kit, or the prosthesis), is the *minimum* charge for that item.

Definition

To *allocate* a cost (or a revenue) is to spread it. You may be spreading it over different departments, different DRGs, different product lines, or different months. The point is that while the cost (or revenue) is measured in one lump sum, it "belongs" to a larger number of causes.

Synonyms: spread, distribute, attach, apply

Overhead. Overhead is far more difficult to evaluate, and overhead is the reason that pricing is an art, not a science. Let's start with the easiest parts of overhead—indirect labor and indirect materials. Let's assume your *total* costs are calculated as *annual* costs, so you have an idea of the total cost for these items for the year. They can be calculated with some degree of accuracy for indirect labor, and indirect materials can be based on last year's costs. However, even if we knew total costs with absolute accuracy (which we rarely do), we still need to know how to *allocate* those costs to billable elements of patient care.

For example, if I know that a group of supervisory salaries cost $150,000/year, how do I *allocate* that cost to patient billings to ensure that the cost is recovered? The unfortunate answer is that you can never be absolutely sure.

You can, however, make a very good guess. For example, to spread the supervisory cost we might use our best estimate of patient days. Since we are estimating an average census of 500 patients per day during a 365-day year, we would spread our $150,000 salary cost over 182,500 patient days. Accordingly, we will "*attach*" $0.83 for this class of supervisory salaries to each patient's daily bill for room and board.

Step 1: 500 patients per day x 365 days per year = 182,500 patient days per year.
Step 2: $150,000 in supervisory costs ÷ 182,500 patients days = $0.822 per patient day. Let's round to $0.83 per patient day.

If we are exactly correct in our census estimate, we will *distribute* or *allocate* $151,475 and we will recover this cost from our patients and their insurance companies.

> *182,500 patient days x $0.83 per patient day = $151,475*

If our census falls short, we will have *under-applied* this class of overhead. For example, if our census only averages 490, we will apply only $148,446. If we actually spent the $150,000 we anticipated, then we have failed to recover $1,554 in supervisory salaries from our patients.

> **Step 1: 490 patients per day x 365 days per year = 178,850 patient days per year.**
> **Step 2: 178,850 patients days x $0.83 per patient = $148,446 recovered from patient billings.**

Alternatively, if our census is larger than anticipated—for example, 505 patients per day—we will have *over-applied* our supervisory salaries by $2,990. In other words, we will have realized an additional $2,990 more than anticipated.

> **Step 1: 505 patients per day x 365 days per year = 184,325 patient days per year.**
> **Step 2: 184,325 patient days x $0.83 per patient = $152,990 recovered from patient billings.**

When doing this type of budgeting vary your assumptions and see what happens. Called *sensitivity analysis*, this exercise allows you to check the outcome if your assumptions are wrong (and they always are). In this example, for instance, will you recover the entire $150,000 if your census is 497 instead of 500? How about 495? By testing several alternatives, you can pick a minimum price that provides a reasonable degree of comfort in terms of recovering your costs.

Indirect labor is, perhaps, the easiest example we can provide, although other indirect costs such as linen costs, utilities, and patient meals, can be budgeted in a similar manner. Notice that although linens and meals are direct costs in the sense that they directly touch each patient's time in the hospital, they are treated as indirect costs because it is not efficient to allocate them on a per patient basis. Linens and meals are like the paint on our surgical carts. Although not truly "overhead" (like the utilities and supervisory salaries), they are more easily and cost-effectively handled as indirect materials.

Definition

Assets are things you can use to make money in your organization. They include such things as cash, supplies inventory, medicines, land, buildings, and equipment. Note that you need *not own* an asset. Under certain circumstances it can be leased.

Fixed Assets are assets with long lives. In health care, fixed assets must have a useful life of at least two years.

Synonyms: Fixed Tangible Assets; Long-lived assets; and Plant, Property and Equipment (PPE).

For things like surgical supplies, we move beyond a per patient allocation and try to associate each kind of supply with the type of procedure that uses that item. We estimate the number of procedures, the quantity of supplies, the total supply costs, and then divide to arrive at a cost per procedure.

Allocating Long-Lived Assets. The hardest item to allocate is the "using up" of buildings and equipment. Land, buildings, and equipment are most commonly called either *fixed assets*, *fixed tangible assets*, or *plant, property and equipment*. These are long-lived assets (more than two years) and their cost is spread over the asset's useful life. The name of this cost is *depreciation* or *amortization*.[15]

In some cases, it might be possible to allocate the cost of a machine directly to patient care. For example, if you knew that a piece of surgical equipment would last through 200 surgical procedures and then be scrapped as no longer reliable, you could divide the cost of the equipment by 200 and *apply* the result to the cost of each surgical procedure. If we can do this, this element of depreciation is treated as a direct cost (one which can be directly associated with a specific element of patient care). Unfortunately, it is rare that equipment can be treated in this manner and it is virtually impossible to do it with a building. Here we need to make some *very big assumptions*.

> ### Definition
>
> *Depreciation* and *amortization* are the writing off of long-lived assets over their estimated useful lives. Technically, depreciation is used for buildings and equipment we own, and amortization is the correct term for buildings and equipment we lease. Land is *not* written off.

Assume we build a $20 million building. We need to recover that cost by charging patients for the building. The question becomes how much to charge per patient per day. If we are lucky, we financed part of the building with grants or a capital giving campaign. Nevertheless, when the building is "used up," we will have to replace it and we can not be certain that grants and donations will be available when the time comes to do that. Prudence dictates that we try to add the full $20 million cost of the building to patient charges over the building's useful life.

First, we need to estimate the useful life of the building. Assume it is 40 years.[16] Then we need to estimate the volume of activity which will go through that building each year for the next 40 years. Let's stay with our estimate of 500 patients/day. Remember, that was 182,500 patient days/year. In 40 years, that is 7.3 million patient days. That is $2.74 per patient per day to recover the cost of the building over its 40-year life.

> *Step 1: 500 patients per day x 365 days per year = 182,500 patient days per year.*
> *Step 2: 182,500 patient days per year x 40 years = 7,300,000 patient days over 40 years.*
> *Step 3: $20,000,000 building ÷ 7,300,000 patient days = $2.74 per patient day.*

---

[15] Technically, this should be called depreciation when you own the asset and amortization when the asset is leased. In practice, however, both words may be used interchangeably.

[16] There are published lists of estimates for the useful lives of long-lived assets. Sources include: the American Hospital Association (AHA) and the American Institute of Certified Public Accountants (AICPA). Ultimately, the best estimates depend on years of experience in a single environment (for example, health care).

Equipment is handled in the same way, but because its life is shorter than a building's our estimate of useful life is better. Remember, however, that in a high-tech environment like a hospital, most depreciation is not caused by physical deterioration, but by obsolescence. Our equipment might last five years, but if someone comes out with a new piece of equipment that performs the procedure with far less stress to the patient, we'll probably want to replace that equipment long before its five-year life expires.

Land is not depreciated, because it lasts "forever." It is placed on the list of assets and there it remains until you sell it.

What Did We Forget?

Doubtless, you have noticed that we have only scratched the surface. Even when we talk about spreading the cost of buildings and equipment we are ignoring things like repairs and maintenance. Hopefully, you never find yourself at the "top of the budgeting food chain," until you have had years of experience in health care—years to learn the ropes, budget a unit, budget a clinic, budget overall nursing services, before *you* are the person responsible for budgeting an entire entity and possibly setting its prices. But, in the meantime, you may have input into price setting, and some of the same ideas that matter in setting prices, help you understand the ways in which costs behave.

Reference

Dunham-Taylor, J., & Pinczuk, J. (2006). *Health care financial management for nurse managers: Applications from hospitals, long-term care, home care, and ambulatory care*. Sudbury, MA: Jones and Bartlett.

APPENDIX A

Charts of Accounts

R. Penny Marquette, DBA, CPA

Within the finance department, to have easy, orderly access to extensive cost information, one needs an organizing device. That device is called a *chart of accounts*. Most charts of accounts consist of two parts. The first is a listing of all *units of the organization* for which cost information should be gathered. In health care this might include laundry, rehabilitation therapy, infection control, housekeeping, operating room, X-ray, home health, physical therapy, separate nursing units, food service, finance, and others. The second part is a list of those *elements of cost* which occur in those cost centers. These elements of cost include such things as salaries, various fringe benefits, legal fees, pharmaceuticals, building supplies, grounds repair, equipment repair, oxygen, medical supplies, linen replacement, uniforms, xeroxing, advertising, postage, and so on. Some expenses will occur in only one unit of the organization, but most will occur in several places. By properly organizing our chart of accounts, we can compare similar costs across different units, and even compare costs of similar units across different health care institutions.

The typical format of a chart of accounts is a decimal system where a number representing the cost or revenue center of the organization appears before the decimal and the element of cost appears after. When such charts are first designed, the numbers are **not** *consecutive*. Gaps are left in the numbering so that new departments and new types of costs can be inserted in places where they best belong. For example, you would want to keep all kinds of salaries close together on the chart in order to help you find things quickly. (Unfortunately, the longer the list is in use, the more likely it is that you will run out of room in logical order and begin adding items to the end of the list.)

Before looking at the full chart of accounts recommended by the American Hospital Association (AHA), a brief example may be helpful. Assume an outpatient clinic with three departments: Respiratory Care, Laboratory, and Rehabilitation Services. Their chart of accounts might appear as shown here:

Account Name (organizational unit)	Department Charge Numbers (elements of cost)	
6170 Respiratory Care	.000	Salaries Supervisors
7091 Rehabilitation Services	.010	Salaries - R.N.'s
7010 Laboratory	.020	Salaries - L.P.N.'s
	.030	Salaries - Aides
	.160	F.I.C.A. (Social Security)
	.340	In-Service Training
	.360	Pharmaceuticals
	.420	Oxygen

.430	Solutions
.440	Medical Supplies
.441	Billable Supplies
.450	General Supplies
.480	Instruments
.490	Microfilming
.491	Minor Equipment

Using these data, we would have an account numbered 6170.480 to collect the costs for instruments purchased by the Respiratory Care Department. Account number 7091.480 would collect the same costs for Rehabilitation Services.

Comparisons of costs by Department can be facilitated by organizing data in the following table:

Cost Comparisons Using a Chart of Accounts			
Department Charge Numbers (elements of cost)	**Account Name (organizational unit)**		
	6170 Respiratory Care	7091 Rehabilitation Services	7010 Laboratory
.000 Salaries Supervisors			
.010 Salaries - R.N.'s			
.020 Salaries - L.P.N.'s			
.030 Salaries - Aides			
.160 F.I.C.A. (Social Security)			
.340 In-Service Training			
.360 Pharmaceuticals			
.420 Oxygen			
.430 Solutions			
.440 Medical Supplies			
.441 Billable Supplies			
.480 Instruments			
.490 Microfilming			
.491 Minor Equipment			

Data from the individual cells in this chart represent specific cost elements within specific health care units. These costs form the basis for many of the analytical financial tools used to measure health care entity performance.[17] In addition to the advantage of being able to compare costs across departments within a single institution, using a standardized chart of accounts allows health care entities to compare themselves with similar institutions in their own communities and elsewhere in the country.

---

[17] One such tool is ratio analysis, which compares one financial or performance element to another (for example, nursing cost per patient day, or in-service training cost per dollar of R.N. salaries). Another is a management technique called *bench marking*, where entities are able to compare their costs for an activity to the same costs for other, similar units.

American Hospital Association (AHA) Recommended Chart of Accounts

The following extensive list of departmental codes and cost element numbers is provided by the AHA. By using the AHA listing, health care entities will be better equipped to make use of published cost data to provide comparative information for their own institutions. Since no list is ever perfectly complete, it is likely that many health care entities will have either departments or elements of cost which do not appear on the AHA list. Often health care organizations use the AHA list and simply add those elements needed to make it work for them. Similarly, if they would have the most useful data by combining costs .780 and .790 (utilities, electricity and utilities, gas), they do that. You can still achieve comparative data with other institutions by calling your utilities-gas and electric by a different number (for example, 1785), and comparing that to the sum of .780 and .790 for other institutions.

Account Name (organizational unit)

6011	Nursing Staff	7170	Social Service
6012	In-Service Education	7181	Medical Records
6022	Med/Surg Unit	8050	Dietary
6080	Obstetrics	8060	Maintenance
6090	Nursery Unit	8076	Safety & Security
6120	Special Care	8090	Housekeeping
6151	Long-Term Care (Sub Acute)	8110	Laundry
6170	Respiratory Care	8210	Finance
6190	Delivery Room	8221	Patient Accounts
6210	Surgery	8231	Information Services
6218	Recovery Room	8311	Administration
6231	Emergency Room	8312	Volunteers
6232	Ambulatory	8314	Chaplaincy In-Service
6250	Central Supply	8315	Public Relations
7000	Occupational Health	8316	Infection Control
7010	Laboratory	8318	Risk Management
7020	Blood Bank	8331	Purchasing
7030	EKG	8332	Print Shop
7040	Radiology	8371	Personnel
7042	CT Scan	8410	UR & QA
7045	Mammography	8755	Outpatient Center
7052	Ultrasound	8757	Doctor's Offices
7055	MRI	8759	Prep Child Birth
7060	Nuclear Medicine	8901	Foundation
7070	Pharmacy	9609	Physician Office Support
7080	Anesthesia	9625	PSS - Central Services
7091	Rehab Services	9718	PSS - Medical Records
7093	Occupational Therapy	9806	PSS - Maintenance
7094	Speech Therapy	9807	PSS - Safety & Security
7095	Cardiac Rehab	9809	PSS Housekeeping
7150	EEG	9811	PSS-Laundry
7151	Home Health	9821	PSS-Finance

9822	PSS-Patient Accounting
9823	PSS-Information Services
9831	PSS-Administration
9835	PSS-Public Relations
9836	PSS-Infection Control
9838	PSS-Risk Management
9840	PSS-Materials Management
9841	PSS-Purchasing
9871	PSS-Human Resources
9880	PSS-UR & QA
9897	PSS-Employee Benefits

**Department Charge Numbers
(elements of cost)**

.000	Salaries - Supervisors
.010	Salaries - R.N.'s
.020	Salaries - L.P.N.'s
.030	Salaries - Aides
.040	Salaries - Secretaries
.060	Salaries - Technicians
.070	Salaries - Non-Technicians
.090	Paid Days Off
.110	Casual R.N.'s
.160	F.I.C.A.
.170	Unemployment Compensation
.180	Group Health Insurance
.185	Dental Insurance
.180	P/R Deductions
.190	Pension Plan
.200	Workers' Compensation
.210	Group Life Insurance
.215	Tuition Reimbursement
.219	Employee Service and Gifts
.220	Employee Physicals
.250	Professional Fees
.300	Other Professional Fees
.310	Consulting Fees
.320	Legal Fees
.330	Audit Services
.340	In-Service Training
.360	Pharmaceuticals
.361	Transfer Drug Costs Out
.370	Food
.375	Other Dietary Supplies
.380	Plumbing Supplies
.381	Electrical Supplies
.382	HVAC Supplies

.383	Building Supplies
.390	Grounds Repair
.400	Building Repairs
.410	PC Repairs
.420	Oxygen
.430	Solutions
.440	Medical Supplies
.441	Billable Supplies
.442	Sutures
.450	General Supplies
.452	PC Supplies
.470	Linen Replacement
.471	Uniforms
.480	Instruments
.490	Microfilming
.491	Minor Equipment
.540	Purchased Services
.550	Physical Recruitment
.560	Library
.561	Service Contracts
.580	Management Services
.590	Collection Fees
.750	Rental or Lease of Building
.770	Leased Equipment
.771	Equipment Rental
.780	Utilities-Electric
.790	Utilities-Gas
.800	Utilities - Water/Sewer
.850	Insurance
.870	Advertising
.880	Phone/Fax
.890	Dues/Books/Subscriptions
.910	Training Expenses (Info Serv Only)
.911	Cash - Over and Short
.919	Seminar/Meeting
.920	Travel Expenses
.921	Mileage
.922	Fuel
.930	Miscellaneous
.931	Administration Fees
.940	Bank Service Charges
.941	Interest
.950	Postage
.970	Gain/Loss on Disosal of Assets
.990	Transfer Non-Salaries Out
.991	Transfer Copier Costs In
.992	Transfer Dietary Costs In

Using this information, let's say that we are the nurse manager of a subacute long-term care unit. Our budget numbers would be 6151.030 for nurse aide salary costs, or 6151.360 for pharmaceutical costs.

CHAPTER 11

Budget Development and Evaluation

Janne Dunham-Taylor, PhD, RN
R. Penny Marquette, DBA

Introduction

Budget responsibilities usually include an evaluation of the adequacy of the budget and, at times, the development of a new budget. It is an important activity because a cost center budget may not have been *totally* evaluated for years. A piecemeal evaluation to add raises or cut the budget may have occurred, but is not sufficient in the overall budget evaluation process. What has been appropriate for the last ten years is not necessarily what is needed presently. This chapter is designed to help the nurse administrator determine whether the overall budget is appropriate and adequate to meet present patient needs.

Budget evaluation needs to occur on both a monthly and a yearly basis. The monthly evaluation is concerned with looking at the past month's expenditures and determining if budget variances are appropriate. This is discussed in Chapter 12 on Budget Variances.

The annual evaluation is more in depth and provides the nurse manager and nurse executive with data that either demonstrates the budget is appropriate and does not need to be changed, or that the budget should be specifically altered to better meet current program needs. This in-depth evaluation process is also appropriate when there are sufficient patient population or volume changes to warrant a budget reevaluation and possible mid-year budget adjustments. In this longer process, *question everything*. For instance:

- Are budget line items appropriate amounts for the patient population being served? Go through line by line and evaluate each category.
- Are we spending less than the reimbursement amount to provide the specified services? (Discussed in Chapter 13, Comparing Reimbursements With Costs of Services Provided.)
- Are there more efficient ways—staffing, facilities, other resources—to better meet patient needs? This is explained further in Chapter 21, Productivity. For instance, if everyone is working straight eight-hour or twelve-hour shifts, chances are the staffing is too heavy for certain times and may be too lean for other times. Or with facilities,

457

would a better physical set-up help save staff time? With resources, is there a computerized documentation system in place that helps save staff, especially RNs, time?
- Is the staffing plan effective? (Discussed in Chapter 20, Staff Our Most Valuable Resource.)
- Can staff productivity be improved? (Discussed in Chapter 21, Productivity.)
- Is the staff mix appropriate for the patient population served? See Chapter 20, Staff —Our Most Valuable Resource.)
- How could the leadership be improved? (If there are leadership problems, these need to be fixed as they cost a lot of money—discussed in Chapter 3, Quantum Leadership: Love One Another.)
- Are there unresolved organizational systems issues that are costing money unnecessarily for the organization? Are there organizational systems that could be streamlined? (See Chapter 4, Organizational Strategies.)
- Are there new safety measures, regulatory guidelines, or accreditation standards that will impact the budget?
- Does the new budget reflect cost inflation or anticipated raises?
- Are there new innovations or quality improvement strategies that have budget implications?
- What would increase patient—and patient family—satisfaction? Would these measures impact the budget?
- What would improve staff satisfaction and turnover?
- How will Medicare and Medicaid reimbursements, or other reimbursement discounts, impact the budget?

Have dialogue about these questions with all the nursing staff, physicians and other disciplines, and patients and their families. You can obtain invaluable input and find other approaches that better serve patient needs. Include the nurse executive in this process. The nurse manager must always have an accurate picture of the entire organization, understanding how unit issues fit with this larger picture. Many issues will need broader organizational involvement. In fact, some issues will necessitate the executive team or board action—the nurse executive will be more involved at this level. However, many issues, both on the unit and interdepartmentally, can be fixed by the nurse manager, or by the nurse manager working with other department directors.

We would be remiss here not to emphasize the importance of nurse executive expectations of the nurse manager—critical to overall organizational success. In the budget evaluation process, the nurse executive should expect monthly variance reports and annual evaluations of each cost center budget from the nurse manager. The reports should include recommendations and rationales for any budget changes needed for each cost center.

Additional Uses of Evaluation Data:
- *Determine and compare staff workloads.*
- *Measure outcomes.*
- *Provide quality of research data.*

The budget calculations presented in this chapter have additional uses. This data provides objective evidence to determine and compare staff workloads, to measure outcomes, and to provide quality or research data. In addition this data could be compared with benchmark data from other organizations.

Budget Terminology

Full-Time Equivalent (FTE)

Before evaluating a budget, it is necessary to introduce some additional budget terms that were not introduced in Chapter 10. First, the term *full time equivalent (FTE)* is used in all health care organizations. A nurse manager will be responsible for a specified number of FTEs. An FTE is a unit of measurement that represents one person who works a full-time position. In other words, a person working 40 hours/week will work 2,080 hours/year.

> **Full Time Equivalent (FTE)**
> *40 hours/week x 52 weeks/year = 2080 hours/year*[1]

However, one FTE can be filled by more than one person. Part-time employees will work less than one FTE. To figure out hours worked let's consider that an employee works 0.8 FTE. How many hours per week would this person work? Looking at this equation within the box, this employee will work 32 hours per week.

> *0.8 FTE x 40 Hours/Week = 32 Hours per Week*

See **Exhibit 11–1** for a listing of different FTE hours.

Exhibit 11–1 FTE Hours

FTEs	Hours per Week*	Hours per Year*
.1	4 Hours	208 Hours
.2	8 Hours	416 Hours
.3	12 Hours	624 Hours
.4	16 Hours	832 Hours
.5	20 Hours	1,040 Hours
.6	24 Hours	1,248 Hours
.7	28 Hours	1,456 Hours
.8	32 Hours	1,664 Hours
.9	36 Hours	1,872 Hours
1.0	40 Hours	2,080 Hours

*Based on an 8 hour day—this would need to be changed for a 7.5 hour day.

[1] Occasionally, in certain geographic areas, employees are paid 7.5 hours rather than 8 hours for a day's work. In this case, the work week is not 40 hours but is 37.5 hours; the year is 1,950 hours, not 2,080 hours. If this is the case in your facility, use 1,950 hours rather than 2,080 hours.

Definition

Unit of service–used by health care organizations to measure specific services a patient uses within a specific time frame (patient minutes, hours, days, visits, births, treatments, operations, or other patient encounters).
Patient days or *census*—the number of inpatients present at midnight.

A nurse manager responsible for 50 FTEs will most likely have 70–80 persons reporting directly to the nurse manager. This will include both full-time and part-time staff. An industry standard is that a nurse manager is most effective if responsible for less than 50 FTEs. In fact, ideally a nurse manager should be responsible for 25–35 people or 18–25 FTEs. When responsible for more than 50 FTEs there are too many people on direct report and the nurse manager will not be as effective. More legal and patient safety issues begin to occur when a nurse manager is responsible for too many FTEs.

Unit of Service

Unit of service is used by health care organizations to measure specific services a patient uses within a specific time frame, i.e., patient minutes, hours, days, visits, births, treatments, operations, or other patient encounters. *Patient days* are the number of inpatients present at midnight. One patient day is given for each day the patient is present on an inpatient unit. Sometimes terms are used such as *average daily census* (ADC). ADC may also be the average number of ER/home visits or outpatient treatments for a month or a year.

The patient day is used to determine the *length of stay* (LOS) or the *average length of stay* (ALOS). This averages individual patients' length of stay within a cost center or facility for a month or a year. Patient days are also used to determine the *occupancy rate*. If a long-term care unit has 50 beds and 40 are filled, a percentage is determined for the number of beds actually filled. So the long-term care unit would have an occupancy rate of 80 percent (40 filled beds ÷ 50 bed capacity = 0.8 or 80 percent).

Definition

Nursing Hours Per Patient Day (NHPPD)—nursing staff labor hours needed to provide care to a patient on an inpatient unit in 24 hours.
Synonym: Hours Per Patient Day (HPPD) may or may not have the same meaning.

Nursing Workload

Using the various units of service specified here causes a problem in that all patients do not require the same amount of nursing care. For instance, one treatment could take 1/2 hour while another could take 2 hours. Or one patient requires intensive care while another only needs the stepdown unit. Or a home care nurse could drive 30 miles to make a visit while other visits only required a 5 mile drive. So further unit of service specification is needed to accurately reflect *nursing workload* or the volume of work performed by nursing care givers.

One way to better specify units of service for nursing workload is to use *Nursing Hours Per Patient Day* (NHPPD) or *Hours Per Patient Day* (HPPD). NHPPD gives the number of nursing staff hours needed to provide care to a inpatient in 24 hours. NHPPD and HPPD are produced by patient classification systems.[2] NHPPD and HPPD most often have the same meaning, however, at times the definition is different.[3] For instance, if a health care organization uses a patient classification system to measure nursing hours per patient day, finance may use HPPD only using patient census data. In this case, the two terms are different and have different measurement. As discussed previously, this is an example where it is important to find out the definition/measurement of either the term NHPPD or HPPD. Since there is not a standardized definition for either term be sure to clarify definitions.

Another similar term is the *relative value unit* (RVU), used by reimbursement systems. On an inpatient unit, the RVU represents the complexity of a procedure.

> *Relative Value Unit (RVU) represents the complexity of a procedure.*

The NHPPD, a patient acuity factor, is produced from descriptors about a patient. In this process the nurse supplies the descriptors about the patient, the descriptors are entered or scanned into the computer, and the patient classification system assigns weights for each descriptor. Then the weight total is given. This weight total places the patient into one of several levels of nursing care needed on a 24-hour basis. Once the level of care is determined, the patient classification system can supply actual nursing care hours (NHPPD) needed that day. (See Chapter 19, Patient Classification Systems, for additional information.)

All levels of direct nursing care staff—RNs, LPNs/LVNs, and Nursing Unlicensed Personnel such as Technicians/Assistants/Aides—are included in the NHPPD. There is no standard for which specific nursing personnel are included in the NHPPD figure.[4] For example, the direct care nursing staff might include: registered nurses (RNs) and nursing assistants on one unit, and have RNs, LPNs, and Nursing Assistants on another unit. In some hospitals, the nurse manager is included. In other organizations the nurse manager is not included, or is only included if giving direct care.

> *There is no standard for which specific nursing personnel are included in the NHPPD figure.*

---

[2] Not all patient classification systems produce NHPPD or HPPD data. Prototype systems usually do not while other task-based or care interaction models usually do. (See Chapter 19, Patient Classification Systems.)

[3] In this chapter NHPPD will be used but HPPD could be substituted.

[4] When you are regulated by NHPPD rather than budget, nurse managers have the propensity to hire all RNs, whether you need them or not, because you are getting more for your money. It is easier to schedule, and it helps if the RN staffing is not sufficient otherwise, but it can be a misuse of RN time if the RNs are expected to do other tasks such as housekeeping.

Several issues need to be considered when using acuity data. First, *the NHPPD is not standardized between patient classification systems*. Thus there are differences in the hours of care for the same type of patient when using different patient classification systems.

> Cockerill et al.'s (1993) comparison study of four widely used nursing workload measurement tools (including GRASP) demonstrated that with different workload measurement tools there were significant clinical and statistical differences in estimated hours of (nursing) care. Discrepancies of up to 30% were noted in the costs associated with caring for exactly the same patients (Shullanberger, p.132).

> **The NHPPD is not standardized between patient classification systems.**

Second, even within the *same* patient classification system, the NHPPD *measurements* are not always standardized even when using the same classification system. In the factor evaluation classification systems, the nurse executive can choose the base hours of care given. At one hospital it might be 5.5 NHPPD, while at another the nurse executive might choose 6.0 NHPPD. Most likely this number will be higher for a tertiary care hospital or medical center and lower for a smaller, less acute general hospital that sends the more acute patients to the tertiary center. The classification system then uses this base number to compute the hours of care needed for most nursing care areas within that hospital. The acuity number would be higher for a critical care area and lower for a rehabilitation floor—all determined by the patient classification database.

> **NHPPD measurements are not always standardized even when using the same patient classification system.**

Third, it is very important that *reliability* (would two nurses rate the same patient in the same way) and *validity* (does the tool actually measure the appropriate activities that nurses are doing) have been regularly evaluated for the patient classification system. The first thing to examine is if the patient classification system has actual reliability and validity established. Some internal patient classification systems do not have reliability and validity established at all—and they may not take into account significant nursing staff time spent on such things as admissions, discharges, and transfers; also, they may not include such functions as an IV team, escort service, sitter, or orderly.

> **It is very important that reliability (would two nurses rate the same patient in the same way) and validity (does the tool actually measure the appropriate activities that nurses are doing) have been regularly evaluated.**

The second issue with reliability and validity occurs *within* the health care organization. Reliability needs to be evaluated regularly by having a nurse from a different unit rate the patient already rated by unit staff. Evaluation of validity is also necessary annually. For example, the classification system may say that nursing hours for orthopedic patients are 6.0 NHPPD. If the unit is long and narrow with supplies at one end of the unit, and charts in another area not as accessible for certain patient rooms, nursing staff may need slightly more than 6.0 hours to complete the care for certain orthopedic patients. Perhaps the system does not take into account that psychiatric nurses spend a lot of time teaching families as part of the RN role. In this case these nurses might be spending more hours of care with their assigned patients than the patient classification system reflects. (See Chapter 19, Patient Classification Systems, for more details about reliability and validity.)

Fourth, acuity data, if available, should be used instead of census figures, because census figures do not account for the acuity of the patient. If acuity data is not available, one could benchmark with like units.

There is another reason the NHPPD would more closely reflect actual nursing care hours than census data. Census data is gathered at midnight. Patients admitted and discharged within the same day may not be reflected by the midnight census at all. The patient classification system generally collects data around 11 AM, and may be done on a per shift basis. It is more likely to pick up short-stay patients as well as admissions, discharges, and transfers.

> *Acuity data, if available, should be used instead of census figures.*

While discussing the census issue, ANA supports not using census data. However, this is confusing because in the ANA staffing principles it actually says: "*There is a critical need to either retire or seriously question the usefulness of the concept of nursing hours per patient day (HPPD)* (p. 5)." They further clarify that:

> one size (or formula) does not fit all. In fact, staffing is most appropriate and meaningful when it is predicated on a measure of unit intensity that takes into consideration the aggregate population of patients and the associated roles and responsibilities of nursing staff. Such a unit of measure must be operationalized to take into consideration the totality of the patients for whom care is being provided. It must not be predicated on a simple quantification of the needs of the "average" patients but most also include the "outliers" (p. 5).

This statement seems to really mean using census data rather than acuity-based data.

Overhead

You may see a column called "overhead" on your budget sheets. Overhead items are indirect costs. *Overhead* includes benefits such as health insurance and Social Security (FICA); depreciation on buildings or equipment; nonproductive time (although sometimes this is mixed in with the labor budget figures). Overhead usually includes departments not giving direct care such as administration, housekeeping, maintenance, finance, medical records, and human resources. Overhead can be computed in several ways: administration costs may be divided by the census and billed to each inpatient unit in a hospital, housekeeping and utility costs can be computed by square footage, and linen by the pounds of linen used. Finance traditionally will use the same stepdown allocation for overhead as filed with the Medicare and Medicaid cost reports.

In most cases, overhead figures on the budget sheet are neither determined nor much effected by a nurse manager's efforts to save costs. Occasionally, such as with pounds of linen, the nurse manager could encourage staff to use linen more expeditiously and thus save on this cost. Responsibilities for the overhead figures generally are the responsibility of the executive team and determined by the finance department. However, the nurse manager should know how the overhead is determined, especially when the nurse manager is checking the budget for accuracy or building a budget from scratch.

Product Lines

Health care organizations may use a term, called *product line* or *service line*, that represents total services for a particular group of patients or similar patient diagnoses. For example, typical product lines may be cardiology, oncology, burns, or women's health. The product line can represent OR, inpatient, ambulatory, long-term care, and home care services for that product line and sometimes can serve as a "profit center" within the accounting system. Usually when using product lines there are administrators—including nursing—assigned to each line.

> *Product lines or service lines represent total services for a particular group of patients or similar patient diagnoses.*

Patients are often not clearly just needing treatment in one product line. This causes a problem because, for example, although a patient is admitted for knee surgery so is admitted into the orthopedic product line, the patient is diabetic, has emphysema, and has a cardiac arrhythmia. So treatment includes aspects not actually defined, nor costed out, by the product line.

Lost Leaders

There may be services that a health care organization considers a *lost leader*. These services do not make money—in fact lose money—but benefit the organization by bringing patients to the organization for services or gain potential patients as they see that hospital personnel are friendly, helpful people. Lost leaders can include such services as the ER and women's health programs.

> **Lost leaders** *lose money but* **benefit the organization by bringing** *patients to the organization* **for services.**

Another unit that often loses money but remains in general service hospitals is the pediatric unit. This establishes the full-service designation for the hospital even though it loses money. It also can help the community if there are no other pediatric inpatient units in the community. Minimum staffing is the issue here—there are so few patients that minimum staffing actually overstaffs the unit. To deal with this issue some hospitals have adopted strategies where additional patients are diverted to this unit, i.e., short stay patients, ill children of employees, day care patients, or even stationing pediatric outpatient services there.

Vertical Integration

In vertical integration, a hospital might want to add long-term care beds or home care services to increase profits but have additional options to save costs. For instance, it is cheaper to quickly move a post-operative patient into a SNF unit—a less expensive option than holding the patient on an inpatient unit for additional day(s). Or the hospital might start an HMO or PPO. They could even buy a medical supply company. All these additions are related services that expand the service options of the hospital and provide more stability.

> **Vertical integration *adds services to save costs.***

Financial Person for the Nursing Department

Many of the larger health care facility nursing departments will actually hire a financial person to:

- Work with the nursing budgets,
- Interface regularly with the finance department,
- Determine staff productivity,
- Forecast budget changes,
- Keep track of expenditures,
- Prepare financial statements for the nurse executive or other nursing personnel,
- Generate staffing reports,
- Shift funds to different accounts,
- Examine variances from budget statements,
- Educate nursing personnel on financial matters, and
- Provide date on financial planning for the next budget year.

This person is usually hired by the nurse executive but works with all the nurse administrators in the department. Even when such a person is present, the nurse manager must still understand and have the responsibility for cost center budget(s). The nurse manager provides the best link between budget decisions and actual patient care.

Annual Evaluation of the Cost Center Budget: Building a Nursing Expense Budget

Now we will evaluate a nursing expense budget. As we go through this process we will introduce additional budget terminology. Most often the nurse manager is given an established cost center budget. Yet changes continue to occur, e.g., the patient population changes, the acuity rises, a different staff mix is needed, the location or environment changes, or new reimbursement regulations occur. How does a nurse manager evaluate whether this historical budget accurately reflects current needs?

One way the nurse manager can determine whether the budget is adequate is to build a unit budget from scratch. This provides objective data that can then be used for the evaluation process. Too often a nurse manager tells the nurse executive, or financial personnel, that budget changes need to be made "for quality reasons," or "the patients are more acute," or "to meet accreditation standards." It is certainly important to meet accreditation or quality standards. And the acuity may have actually increased. However, the nurse manager is more effective when he or she backs up this statement with objective data, when the objective data is available. Building a budget from scratch provides objective data that then can be compared with the actual budget.

The nurse manager and nurse executive may need to either propose different budget amounts that more accurately reflect the services rendered, or within the same budget amount, reallocate how the money is used to better provide the needed services. When a change can be documented with objective evidence, it usually has the best chance of being supported by the nurse executive, the finance executive, and the executive team.

A hospital example will be given here. However, examples in long-term care, home care, and ambulatory care can be found in *Health Care Financial Management for Nurse Managers: Financial Applications in Hospitals, Long-Term Care, Home Care, and*

Exhibit 11–2 Building a Budget from Scratch by Calculating Direct Care FTEs

Step 1:   Average NHPPD x Patient Census/Year or # of Visits/Year = Average NHPPD/Year.

Step 2:   Average NHPPD/Year x 2,080 Hours = Total Nursing Direct Care FTEs.

Step 3:   Figure non-productive hours per FTE or get this figure from Human Resources.

Step 4:   2,080 Hours ÷ _____ Nonproductive Hours per FTE = _____ Productive Hours per FTE.

Step 5:   2,080 Hours ÷ _____ Productive Hours per FTE = _____ Actual FTEs.
(This step figures how many actual FTEs are needed to cover both productive and nonproductive time for each FTE.)

Step 6:   Take Total Nursing Direct Care FTEs determined in Step 2, and multiply times Actual FTEs determined in Step 5.
(Total Nursing Direct Care FTEs x Actual FTEs = Total Nursing Direct Care FTEs including both productive and nonproductive time).

Step 7:   Determine the percentage of each nursing staff category to give direct care (staff mix). Then multiply the percentage of each nursing staff category x the total Actual FTEs determined in Step 6, to calculate how many FTEs are needed for each nursing staff category.

Step 8:   Determine the cost of the nursing staff by actually putting in salary [or salary and benefit] amount for each nursing staff category. Total this amount for the total direct care cost for the division.

Step 9:   Determine the percentage of staff that will be appropriate by shift. Divide the number of FTEs needed for each nursing staff category calculated in Step 7 by the percentage of staff needed by shift to determine FTEs in each nursing staff category by shift.

Step 10:   Determine the part-time versus full-time ratio. Divide the FTEs determined in Step 9 by the part-time or full-time ratio. Then adjust the ratios to accurately reflect staffing needs.

Ambulatory Care (Dunham-Taylor and Pinczuk, 2006). Using the hospital example in this chapter, each step is defined in detail in the following sections, with the total process reflected in **Exhibit 11–2**.

Historical Data Sources of Services Rendered

To build a budget from scratch one needs to collect available historical patient data. Some possible hospital data sources include: historical census data (patient days) or visits per year; other volume indicators not on the census such as observation patients; admissions/discharges/ transfers—these may be already included in patient classification hours of care data but, if not, these activities take additional nursing staff time; and the nursing hours per patient day (NHPPD) or hours per patient day (HPPD)—that can be obtained from patient classification data. The patient classification data is most helpful and most accurate if reliability and validity have been established. If there is no patient classification system, or if the system does not have reliability and validity, one may have to use census data. If so, it still can be helpful to establish acuity levels for certain groups of patients by benchmarking with like units. The medical records department may have the most accurate data about short-stay or observation patients. Other sources may include the literature or an actual measurement of the amount of time it takes a nurse to perform certain tasks.

As a nurse manager looks at the available historical data, realize that this data will be totally inaccurate if major changes are occurring that are not reflected in the historical data. For example, perhaps a physician who is a large admittor is retiring and no one is taking his/her place. A nurse manager would then need to use data that would exclude that physician's patients. Or as technology developments occur—such as what happened with knee surgery—it might be possible to do a less invasive procedure that will change the data because the patient stay statistics will now be much lower. In this case the nurse manager would need to find out how many patients came in the previous year for this surgery, find out the care hours they required, and correct the data to reflect this new development.

Let's give an actual example of a nurse manager creating a budget and walk through this evaluation exercise together. You are the nurse manager of 4W, an orthopedic division. The orthopedic unit nurse manager figures the average NHPPD for the year is 6.6. (See **Exhibit 11–3**.) This means the direct care nursing staff will give an average of 6.6 hours of care in 24 hours to each patient on the orthopedic unit. This figure needs to be compared with the average hours of care for the previous year. If the figures are similar the current staffing level might be adequate. However, if the average figure is 6.4, the current staffing level might be inadequate.

The NHPPD figure can be further broken down into the individual classifications of nursing direct care givers, i.e., RNs give 3.4 hours of nursing care, LPNs provide 2 hours of care, and the nursing aides give 1.6 hours of care within 24 hours. The patient classification system specifies such information with established staffing ratios for the orthopedic unit.

Exhibit 11–3 Determining the Average NHPPD for the Previous Year

Month	NHPPD
January	6.7
February	6.5
March	6.8
April	6.5
May	6.5
June	6.4
July	6.6
August	6.7
September	6.8
October	7.0
November	6.5
December	6.4
Average for Year	**6.6**

Calculating Direct Care FTEs

> *Average NHPPD x Patient Census or # of Visits = Direct Care FTEs*

Once appropriate historical data has been collected, the nurse manager can begin the calculations to build the cost center budget. First, take the nursing hours worked in 24 hours and multiply by the patient census or number of visits. If patient classification system data is not available, then the nurse manager could actually compute direct nursing care hours worked by employee classification for the past year. Or the nurse manager might want to develop some data, i.e., we have had *n* patients who had 1/2 hour visits this past year and *n* patients who required an hour visit this past year. In long-term care, the Minimal Data Set (MDS) could be used.

Now let's go back to being the 4W nurse manager. The census data[5] for 4W shows that there were 6,800 patient days on 4W last year—or an average of 18–19 patients each day.

> *6,800 ÷ 365 = 18.63 patient days*
> *This means that there were an average of 18–19 patients on 4W each day.*

Historically, there is a patient classification system that is reliable and valid on 4W. The acuity data from the patient classification system indicates that:

---

[5] Make sure the census data includes all short-stay patients.

- 50 percent of the patients are at Level 3 receiving 8.0 NHPPD,
- 30 percent of the patients are at Level 2 receiving 6.0 NHPPD, and
- 20 percent of the patients are at Level 1 receiving 4.0 NHPPD.

Going back to the previous equation, to determine the nursing hours worked in 24 hours, the 4W nurse manager uses the patient classification system to determine the NHPPD or direct care nursing hours worked in 24 hours. The nurse manager computes the NHPPD as follows: (Remember that to multiply 50 percent, it becomes 0.50 in the equation.)

$$
\begin{array}{lll}
50\% \text{ Level 3 patients @ 8 hours/day*} & = 4.0 \text{ NHPPD} & (0.5 \times 8 = 4.00) \\
30\% \text{ Level 2 patients @ 6 hours/day*} & = 1.8 \text{ NHPPD} & (0.3 \times 6 = 1.80) \\
+ \quad 20\% \text{ Level 1 patients @ 4 hours/day*} & = 0.8 \text{ NHPPD} & (0.2 \times 4 = 0.80) \\
\hline
& 6.6 \text{ NHPPD} &
\end{array}
$$

*For 24 Hours

So the 4W nurse manager has determined that the average NHPPD for 4W is 6.6. Now the nurse manager is ready to finish the equation:

$$6.6 \text{ NHPPD} \times 6{,}800 \text{ patient days/year} = 44{,}880 \text{ NHPPD/year}$$

Continuing with this example the nurse manager is ready to compute the direct nursing care FTEs for 4W. She remembers that an FTE represents 2,080 hours/year. Now she is ready for another equation:

$$NHPPD/year \div 1 \text{ FTE} = \text{Total Nursing Direct Care FTEs}$$
$$44{,}880 \text{ NHPPD/Year} \div 2{,}080 \text{ Hours} = 21.58 \text{ Nursing Direct Care FTEs}$$

So 21.58 FTEs are needed to give direct nursing care for the 6,800 patient days the previous year. *There is a major flaw here. Do you see what it is?*

Productive/Nonproductive Time. The 21.58 FTEs includes *productive* time or actual time worked. This means that the budgeted FTEs do not cover anyone taking a holiday, going on vacation, or getting sick. The 4W nurse manager knows that employees receive paid time for: eight holidays/year, ten vacation days/year, ten sick days/year.[6] (Another term used in some organizations is personal time off, PTO, which combines sick and vacation time. If actually sick for more than a specified time, such as four days, the PTO time reverts to additional sick time.) In addition staff are given time off to attend two staff development days so this needs to be included in the 4W nurse manager's budget projection. The term for this is *nonproductive time* or time where an employee is paid but is not actually working.

---

[6] In some systems different categories of employees may have a different number of vacation days.

Usually the human resource department can give a nurse manager a nonproductive time figure. This figure is often for the entire organization. However, it is possible that this figure is not totally accurate for 4W. For example, if the 4W nurse manager has been an effective administrator and the retention rate is high, the 4W staff receive more vacation time than the organizational average. In this case the 4W nonproductive time average will be higher than the human resource department number.

For this 4W example, let's say that the human resource department does not have a figure for nonproductive time and, to simplify the equation, that all the direct care nursing staff have the same number of nonproductive days. To calculate the direct nursing staff nonproductive time the 4W manager uses the following calculation:

> *2 weeks vacation*   = *80 hours/year*
> *10 sick days*   = *80 hours/year*
> *8 holidays*   = *64 hours/year*
> + *2 education days*   = *16 hours/year*
> _____
>   *240 hours/year total nonproductive time*

Thus each 4W staff member has 240 hours/year of possible nonproductive time.[7]

Even though every employee does not always take all this time in one year, it is better to figure this total into the equation—unless at the end of employment unused nonproductive time is not paid back to the employee. Then one could use the average number of nonproductive hours taken per year by employees. Even then one has to be careful, i.e., if someone has a lot of sick time accrued and suddenly has surgery or an extensive illness they will use much more than the average number of hours for that year. This is another factor that the human resource department will consider with their nonproductive figure, i.e., the average number of sick days taken by all employees for the year.

Since each FTE represents 2,080 hours/year but part of these hours (240 hours in the 4W example) will be nonproductive time, the next step the nurse manager needs to compute is how many actual FTEs are needed taking the nonproductive time into consideration. One way of calculating this is:

> **2,080 Hours (1 FTE) - 240 Nonproductive Hours per FTE = 1,840 Productive Hours per FTE**

This means that out of 2,080 hours paid to a full-time employee each year, on 4W direct care staff will only *actually work* 1,840 hours annually.

---

[7] This assumes that all part-time and full-time employees will receive sick, vacation, or other nonproductive time. If part-time employees do not receive nonproductive benefits, include only their productive time. If employees do not use all their nonproductive time, we recommend that you still compute the full amount as this could possibly be used in the future.

Next the nurse manager needs to divide one FTE by 1,840 productive hours to determine the actual number of FTEs needed for the year:

> **2,080 Hours* ÷ 1,840 Productive Hours = 1.13 actual FTEs**
> **(*2,080 Hours = 1 FTE)**

This shows that for every 2,080 patient care hours, it is necessary to actually have 1.13 FTEs. One can translate the 1.13 figure into percentages—100 percent of the FTE (1 FTE) plus 13 percent of another FTE. This means that for every full-time FTE an additional 13 percent of an FTE is needed to cover nonproductive time. This figure is often approximately 15 percent.

Usually nonproductive costs are included in the division budget. This may include a factor for funeral leave or other such benefits where staff are actually paid for non-worked days.

Benefits. Other benefits such as social security, health care insurance, and worker's compensation are not included here as these cost extra money but do not effect actual work hours. Such benefits—and sometimes sick and vacation time are included with these figures—may be 20–25 percent in additional cost for a full-time employee. Such benefit costs may be included in a cost center budget or may be included in a different cost center such as a special human resource budget. Once again, there is not a standard for benefit costs and what cost center to put them in.

> **$40,000 x 1.25* = $50,000**
> **(*1.25 = 125%)**

Both nonproductive time and benefits can be expensive for the organization to provide. For example, an RN making $40,000/year, if 25 percent of the salary is needed for benefits, in addition to the actual salary, then the organization is actually paying $50,000 for each full-time RN. This means that an additional $10,000/year is spent for the benefits for this RN. Thus if writing a proposal for a new RN position, one needs to take into account that the actual cost for a new RN is $50,000—even though the actual budget statement only shows $40,000. The remaining $10,000 for benefits will be reflected in another cost center budget—most likely, human resources.

In the 4W example, the 240 nonproductive hours for the RN making $40,000/year actually costs $4,615.20/year.

> **$40,000/year RN salary ÷ 2080 hours/year = $19.23/hour**
> **240 hours/year nonproductive time x $19.23/hour = $4,615.20**

Other Personnel Cost Factors. Other personnel costs factors that need to be considered before having actual personnel costs are: holiday pay, shift differential, charge differential, overtime, on-call pay, cost of staff temporarily transferred to this cost center, PRN staff used including sitters, funeral leave, jury duty, orientation, or education costs, tuition reimbursement—if not already included in the cost center budget—and other costs such as differentials for having a BSN, for specialty or other certification, and for a specialty area such as critical care or operating room. Tuition reimbursement is another cost although this often is allocated to the human resource cost center.

A common practice in times of nursing or other interdisciplinary shortages is to pay extra to the staff experiencing a shortage. For example, one decides to pay a critical care differential. The message given to other nurses is that they are not as valued as a critical care nurse. Also, once a differential is started the personnel involved will be very upset if this is ever taken away. Once a shortage is resolved it can be tempting for administrators to dispense with the extra pay. It is the authors' recommendation to really think carefully about the implications if additional pay is given to a specific group based on a shortage. Quick fixes usually do not work and may end up being permanent. (See Chapter 4 that discusses *The Fifth Discipline* by Peter Senge.)

> *The authors do not recommend starting to pay differentials for certain groups of employees when there are staffing shortages.*

Direct Care Staff FTEs Needed. Our 4W nurse manager knows that the budgeted direct care FTEs must include both productive and nonproductive time. To compute actual direct care staffing FTE needs for 4W the nurse manager needs to multiply the productive FTEs by 1.13 FTE, which takes into account the nonproductive time. This figure, 24.4 FTEs, takes into account both productive and nonproductive hours of staff.

> *21.58 FTEs* x 1.13 FTE = 24.39 or 24.4 direct care nursing staff FTEs needed on 4W*

Determine the Staff Mix

Now another issue confronts the 4W nurse manager: What direct care staff mix is appropriate for 4W? The term *staff mix* is a marketing term that specifies what kind of direct care staff will provide optimum care within the available budget dollars. Because this is a medical-surgical division with a 6.6 average NHPPD, there is a need for an appropriate RN ratio. (See Chapter 20, Staff—Our Most Valuable Resource, for additional information as well as for the importance of setting up a staffing plan.)

When making staff mix decisions, start with the patient care requirements. In the 4W example, the patients are acute, post-surgical orthopedic patients, and therefore a higher ratio of registered nurses would be preferable. Other things to consider include nursing delivery system practices as well as structure and organizational issues. For instance:

- What is the division size?
- How are assignments made?
- What is the layout of the nursing division?

- Are there delivery system practices such as unit staff accompanying patients to X-ray, an IV nurse, or other off-unit responsibilities?
- What is the nursing department structure?
- Are there available support staff such an orthopedic technician or a float pool? (Sometimes the orthopedic technician is on another budget, i.e., an OR cost center budget.) If so, these people would need to be included in the staffing for the appropriate number of hours worked on 4W. Benchmarking data on staffing for other orthopedic units might be helpful as well.

In our example, the 4W nurse manager chooses to have a staff mix: 70 percent RN and 30 percent Nursing Assistant (NA). Thus for the 24.4 FTEs of direct care nursing staff needed on 4W, the nurse manager determines that 17.1 FTEs will be RN staff. We will continue to use this figure in this example. Fralic (2000) advocates creating a staffing plan based on a slightly lower number, such as 7.3 NHPPD or 7.4 NHPPD if the actual NHPPD was 7.5, to give some additional flexibility to the nurse manager. Then if the average NHPPD suddenly goes above 7.5 NHPPD, a staff member could be added on a shift without going over budget. In addition, this strategy could save money if less staff were actually needed on a shift.

> *24.4 FTEs Direct Care Nursing Staff x 0.70 RN Staff = 17.1 RN FTEs*

The remaining FTEs will be used for nursing assistants.

> *24.4 FTEs Direct Care Nursing Staff - 17.1 RN FTEs = 7.3 Nursing Assistant FTEs*
> *OR [It is always best to double check your figures.]*
> *24.4 x 0.3 = 7.32 or 7.3 [The 0.3 is from 30% Nursing Assistant staff mix.*
> *It is always best to round to the nearest tenth.]*

Indirect Nursing Staff

In the preceding section the direct care nursing staff requirements were computed. Now we will determine the indirect FTE requirements. Here one decides what indirect staff are necessary for optimal functioning of a cost center. Still using 4W as an example, the nurse manager knows that two unit secretaries are needed for each day and evening shift. (Staff work 8-hour shifts on 4W.) To compute the unit secretary FTEs, how many FTEs are needed to fill a seven-day-a-week position? If the unit secretaries work eight-hour shifts:

> *8 hours x 7 days/week = 56 hours/week*
> *56 hours/week ÷ 40 hours*/week = 1.4 FTEs per shift*
> *(*40 hours/week = 1 FTE based on an 8 hour day)*

To cover both day and evening shifts the 4W nurse manager would need 2.8 unit secretary FTEs.

As previously noted in the direct care nursing staff section, the 2.8 FTEs only reflect productive time worked. If there is a mechanism to replace the unit secretaries while they take vacation/sick time, such as a hospital-wide pool, costs for the nonproductive time could be charged to 4W when someone from this pool is actually used on 4W.

Another option to cover the nonproductive time would be to hire part-time unit secretaries that are willing to work extra shifts when the other unit secretaries are sick or on vacation. A budgeted amount reflecting up to 0.4 additional unit secretary FTE would be added to the budget to cover this additional time worked.

2.8 productive unit secretary FTEs x 1.13 productive and nonproductive time = 3.2 unit secretary FTEs

(3.2 unit secretary FTEs - 2.8 productive unit secretary FTEs = 0.4 unit secretary FTE nonproductive time)

Another choice that can be made is to not replace the unit secretaries when nonproductive time is taken. This presents a problem though because the division may have no unit secretary 13 percent of the time. This can be costly because the other RNs and nursing assistants will have to do the unit secretary duties—answer the phone, do the required paperwork, greet visitors—in addition to their regular duties. This can mean that expensive RN time is spent completing clerical functions. With the current nursing shortage, this is a waste of licensed staff time.

Perhaps a better option is to specially train certain nurse aides to also complete the unit secretary work and pay at a slightly higher level.

Occasionally, the unit secretary hours will be considered under direct care hours. The advantage to putting the unit secretary in the direct care hours is that when the census is low the nurse manager could replace the unit secretary with a care giver. The disadvantage to doing this is that the unit clerk could be counted into the NHPPD as a direct care giver, thus decreasing care giver hours. We recommend the unit secretary not be considered in direct care hours.

While considering indirect nursing personnel, the nurse manager FTE needs to be included. Going back to the 4W example, the nurse manager only had responsibility for 4W so one FTE would be allocated to the nurse manager position. An industry standard currently is that when the nurse manager takes sick or vacation time, no additional FTEs are allocated to cover this time. Often a manager on a nearby division will cover for the nurse manager who is off.

There are additional indirect nursing costs for the division. Indirect unit personnel costs might include: staff development, clinical specialist time, and/or assistant nurse manager time, if not included in the direct care staffing. Often staff development and/or clinical specialist time are found on other cost center budgets.

Total Cost Center FTEs

Continuing to use the 4W example, the nurse manager has now figured the total FTEs for the cost center personnel budget:

	1.0	*Nurse Manager FTE*
	17.1	*RN FTEs*
	7.3	*Nursing Assistant FTEs*
+	3.2	*Unit secretary FTEs*
	28.6	*Total FTEs for 4W*

Dividing FTEs into Shifts

The nurse manager now needs to determine the percentage of FTEs on each shift. As a general rule of thumb, as the patients are more acute, staff is more evenly distributed across shifts. Using eight-hour shifts on a general care division, the industry standard is that most direct care nursing staff are allocated to the day shift (40–45 percent) with a bit less for the evening shift (35–40 percent) and the fewest for the night shift (20–35 percent). A lot of this is determined by the actual patient population needs on the unit. Using twelve-hour shifts, the industry standard is that most direct care nursing staff are scheduled for days (50–60 percent) with the rest of the staff working the night shift. There is no absolute industry standard for shift allocations. This distribution relies on the judgment of the nursing staff and nursing administration.

On 4W the nurse manager determines that there will be 40 percent of the direct care nursing staff working day shift, 35 percent on the evening shift, and 25 percent on the night shift. This decision was made because the majority of medications happen on days and evenings, and most surgical procedures are scheduled on days. Also, days and evenings experience the most admissions and discharges. Now the nurse manager can determine the FTE distribution for each shift:

	Day Shift	*Check Your Figures*	
		RN	*NA*
17.1 RN FTEs x 0.40 = 6.84 or 6.8 RN FTEs		6.8	
7.3 NA FTEs x 0.40 = 2.92 or 2.9 NA FTEs			2.9
	Evening Shift		
17.1 RN FTEs x 0.35 = 5.98 or 6 RN FTEs		6.0	
7.3 NA FTEs x 0.35 = 2.55 or 2.6 NA FTEs			2.6
	Night Shift		
17.1 RN FTEs x 0.25 = 4.27 or 4.3 RN FTEs		4.3	
7.3 NA FTEs x 0.25 = 1.82 or 1.8 NA FTEs		+	1.8
		17.1	7.3

To check your figures, add them together. They should total 17.1 RN FTEs and 7.3 NA FTEs.

Determine Part-Time versus Full-Time Ratio

After determining the FTE distribution by shift, the nurse manager has another decision to make: What percentage of staff should be part time versus full time? One needs to make a thoughtful decision here as too many part-time staff mean that there will be a lack of continuity on the division. On the other hand, if there are too many full-time staff it will be impossible to cover weekends with adequate staffing. Ideally, a ratio of about 60 percent full-time personnel and 40 percent part-time personnel or 65 percent full-time and 35 percent part-time, is preferred. It allows for some flexibility in staffing yet achieves continuity.

Going back to the 4W example, the nurse manager decides to use the 60:40 ratio and figures the FTEs for both classifications of nursing personnel, checking the figures:

Day Shift	*Check Your Figures*	
	RN	*NA*
6.8 RN FTEs x 0.60 = 4.08 or 4.1 Full-Time RN FTEs	*4.1*	
6.8 RN FTEs x 0.40 = 2.72 or 2.7 Part-Time RN FTEs	*2.7*	
2.9 NA FTEs x 0.60 = 1.74 or 1.7 Full-Time NA FTEs		*1.7*
2.9 NA FTEs x 0.40 = 1.16 or 1.2 Part-Time NA FTEs		*1.2*
Evening Shift		
6 RN FTEs x 0.60 = 3.6 Full-Time RN FTEs	*3.6*	
6 RN FTEs x 0.40 = 2.4 Part-Time RN FTEs	*2.4*	
2.6 NA FTEs x 0.60 = 1.56 or 1.6 Full-Time NA FTEs		*1.6*
2.6 NA FTEs x 0.40 = 1.04 or 1 Part-Time NA FTEs		*1.0*
Night Shift		
4.3 RN FTEs x 0.60 = 2.58 or 2.6 Full-Time RN FTEs	*2.6*	
4.3 RN FTEs x 0.40 = 1.72 or 1.7 Part-Time RN FTEs	*1.7*	
1.8 NA FTEs x 0.60 = 1.08 or 1.1 Full-Time NA FTE		*1.1*
1.8 NA FTEs x 0.40 = 0.72 or 0.7 Part-Time NA FTE	+	*0.7*
	17.1	*7.3*

Now another challenge emerges as the nurse manager computes the full-time calculation. Several of the full-time FTE numbers are a *fraction*. A full-time person fills 1 FTE, not a fraction of an FTE. So the nurse manager must change several calculations. This first occurs on the day shift with both the RN FTEs and the NA FTEs. There are 4.1 full-time RN FTEs and 2.7 part-time RN FTEs. Here it is best to take the leftover 0.1 full-time RN

FTE and add it to the part-time RN FTEs. There are 1.7 full-time NA FTEs—one can either have 1 or 2 full-time NAs. In these cases one must think of the implications. The nurse manager could decide to have 2 FTEs be full-time with a resulting 0.9 FTE for part-time NAs on days. Alternately, the nurse manager could choose to have 1 full-time NA and 1.9 part-time NA FTEs.

There is no right answer to this dilemma; one must consider the implications of each. There probably will be less continuity with the second option, but it offers more flexibility with scheduling. The author, however, would choose to go with the first option due to availability of personnel. It can be very difficult to find nursing assistants who want to work part time. They do not make much more than minimum wage and prefer to have a full-time job with benefits.

Looking at the RN FTEs, on the evening shift the same problem occurs. Here there are 3.6 full-time RN FTEs. So the nurse manager must choose between three or four full-time RNs. In this case the author would choose to have four full-time RN rather than three. This is because if the RNs have every other weekend off, there will be two full-time RNs on every weekend. When one RN goes on vacation or is sick, there will still be continuity with another full-time RN available. So the nurse manager will plan to have four full-time evening RN FTEs and two part-time evening RN FTEs which totals six evening RN FTEs.

As one changes the budget figures, keep an ongoing tally of the changes as one adds or subtracts FTEs. In the end the tally should add to zero. In the following 4W example the nurse manager changes the FTE designations as follows and keeps a tally:

Had	*Change To*	*Day Shift*	*Tally*	
			RN	*NA*
4.1 to	*4 Full-Time RN FTEs*	*[4.1- 4 = +0.1]*	*+0.1*	
2.7 to	*2.8 Part-Time RN FTEs*	*[2.7 - 2.8 = -0.1]*	*-0.1*	
1.7 to	*2 Full-Time NA FTEs*	*Etc.*		*-0.3*
1.2 to	*0.9 Part-Time NA FTE*			*+0.3*
		Evening Shift		
3.6 to	*4 Full-Time RN FTEs*		*-0.4*	
2.4 to	*2 Part-Time RN FTEs*		*+0.4*	
1.6 to	*2 Full-Time NA FTEs*			*-0.4*
1.0 to	*0.6 Part-Time NA FTE*			*+0.4*
		Night Shift		
2.6 to	*3 Full-Time RN FTEs*		*-0.4*	
1.7 to	*1.3 Part-Time RN FTEs*		*+0.4*	
1.1 to	*1 Full-Time NA FTEs*			*+0.1*
0.7 to	*0.8 Part-Time NA FTE*			*-0.1*
17.1 RN FTEs and 7.3 NA FTEs or 24.4 Total FTEs			*0*	*0*

Once again, the nurse manager can double check the numbers. The part-time and full-time numbers should add up to the total FTE number for that position classification; the total direct care staff FTEs should still add up to 24.4.

The last action the nurse manager would need to do if using these numbers to actually staff the division, is to determine the number of actual part-time staff to hire. Using the 4W example, there are 2.8 RN part-time FTEs. In order to staff for weekends, it would probably be best to have at least four employees in part-time positions—two for each weekend if everyone gets every other weekend off. So the nurse manager could choose to make a couple positions 0.7 or 0.8 FTEs and two positions for less time. One option is to have two 0.8 FTE positions, and two 0.6 employees. Gear this decision by part-time staff availability and preferences. And be flexible and change the FTE designations if new staff prefer different numbers of work hours. The main goal is to stay within the 17.1 RN FTEs and the 7.3 NA FTEs.

There is no industry standard here. The FTE part-time designations are a result of personal preference, availability of potential employees, and good judgment. For example, if one had 2.6 part-time FTEs for a shift, one would not want all the part-time employees to be 0.4 FTE only working two days each week. Continuity would really be an issue if this were the case. On the other hand if one only has 0.8 part-time FTEs for a shift, it might be preferable to have two different people hired to allow more flexibility in staffing.

Calculate Nursing Care Hours Needed per Day

Now that we have figured productive and nonproductive time, let's go back to the 44,880 NHPPD given the previous year. Assuming that the average number remains the same for this current year, we can divide the 44,880 NHPPD by 365 days to determine the actual number of nursing care hours needed each day or 122.96 hours.[8] In the box provided one can see that on the day shift the nurse manager should have 34 RN hours and 15 NA hours; on evenings 30 RN hours and 13 NA hours; and on nights 22 RN hours and 9 NA hours. Full-time and part-time staff scheduled to work each shift should add up to these numbers.

4W Nursing Care Hours Needed Per Day

44,880 NHPPD ÷ 365 days = 122.96 nursing care hours needed each day

Skill Mix

122.96 hours x 0.7 RN = 86* RN hours needed over 24 hours

122.96 hours x 0.3 NA = 37* NA hours needed over 24 hours

*rounded to an even hour

---

[8] This assumes that the census and acuity remain at the average level determined by last year's figures. If you know other information that would change these numbers, one would use those figures. Increases or decreases in census or acuity would need to follow a staffing plan based on these numbers, as discussed in Chapter 20, Staff—Our Most Valuable Resource.

Shifts

86 RN hours x 0.40 day shift = 34*day shift RN hours
37 NA hours x 0.40 day shift = 15* day shift NA hours
86 RN hours x 0.35 day shift = 30*evening shift RN hours
37 NA hours x 0.35 day shift = 13* evening shift NA hours
86 RN hours x 0.25 day shift = 22*night shift RN hours
37 NA hours x 0.25 day shift = 9*night shift NA hours

*rounded to an even hour

If 4W has a staffing plan, the nurse manager could evaluate the staffing plan by comparing it with these numbers of staff per shift. In other words, when 4W has 18–19 patients with an average acuity of 6.6 NHPPD (these were the averages for 4W the previous year), the staffing plan should agree with the hours per shift designated previously.

Figure Actual Personnel Costs

To calculate actual personnel costs, one needs either actual salary costs of the personnel or average salaries for different personnel categories, i.e., nurse manager, RNs, LPNs, nursing assistants, nursing technicians, and ward clerks. Usually, this information can be provided by the department or by finance personnel. If available, use actual salaries and computer software programs (such as ANSOS/PerSe or finance department programs) to generate this data for the nurse manager or nurse executive. Additional costs such as shift differential, charge pay, on call pay, and other costs discussed earlier in this chapter may need to be included in this equation.

Other factors affecting personnel costs on a unit are such functions as an IV team, escort service, sitter, or orderly. Often these services are located within the centralized overall nursing department budget under a different cost center than the unit center. In some systems when these services are used by a cost center, the employee costs for that shift or service are billed to that cost center. If such functions exist and are regularly used on a unit, these costs would need to be added to the unit personnel costs. The same is true when regularly using replacement staff from another cost center.

Thus, using the 4W example, the nurse manager could calculate the actual salary costs as illustrated in **Exhibit 11–4**. In this example no other unit personnel have been identified. If such personnel exist and are necessary for the appropriate functioning of the unit, it would be important to include them in this budget.

There will probably be additional costs to figure into this equation. For instance, perhaps shift differential is paid for both the evening and night shift, holiday time is paid when employees actually work holidays, and on call pay is given. Pay raises or premiums are other possible costs. If per diem or traveling staff will be used, they should be added to the budget.

Exhibit 11–4 Calculate Actual Personnel Salary Dollars

1.0	Nurse Manager FTE (average Nurse Manager salary)	x $22.85/hour	x 2080 hours*	=	$ 47,528.00
17.1	RN FTEs (average RN salary)	x $17.89/hour	x 2080 hours*	=	$636,311.52
7.3	NA FTEs (average NA salary)	x $ 9.03/hour	x 2080 hours*	=	$137,111.52
3.2	Unit Secretary FTEs (average Unit secretary salary)	x $ 8.98/hour	x 2080 hours*	=	$ 59,770.88

Total Salary Dollars Needed $880,721.92

*2080 hours/year = 1 FTE

(Note: This calculation does not include additional benefits, differential, or bonus dollars)

Overtime—often meaning one is paid time and a half (1.5)—is another factor. One would assume that some overtime will be used. The industry standard is that overtime should not exceed 2 percent. One could look at what was actually used the year before and determine if this amount was reasonable under the circumstances. For example, if one nurse is on sick leave and two others leave their positions, accruing additional overtime could be a reasonable way to staff the unit to deal with this temporary situation. However, if overtime is consistently used by all the nurses to chart, other solutions may be necessary. Perhaps the workloads or skill mix needs to be adjusted. Maybe a computerized charting system would really save RN time. Maybe the nurse manager leadership needs to be examined because there is so much turnover on the unit. If additional money is paid for other reasons, be sure to add them to the budget if they seem realistic and reasonable.

The nurse manager may or may not have to include fringe benefits into these costs. Fringe benefits include health insurance, Social Security (FICA) payments, and other benefits. At times these costs are shown on the nurse manager's cost center budget, but often they are not and instead appear on the human resource budget. These are significant costs—20–25 percent—so the executive team will always need to include this expense when determining labor expenses.

Information Systems Technology

It is best to do budget calculations using a computer program. Certain programs, such as Per-Se ANSOS, allow the nurse manager to just sit at the computer and design staffing. Such programs can then schedule staff based on patient classification data, give staffing and variance reports, and compare what was actually spent with what was budgeted.

If such programs are unavailable, the next step would be to ask personnel in the finance department if they are using an existing program that could compute this data. Another option would be to use an existing spreadsheet software program. There are examples of spreadsheet systems given in the book *Health Care Financial Management for Nurse Managers: Financial Applications in Hospitals, Long-Term Care, Home Care, and Ambulatory Care* (Dunham-Taylor and Pinczuk, 2006).

Minimum Staffing

When evaluating the budget, you must understand another concept: *minimum staffing.* When the patient volume reaches a certain low level of service, it becomes a liability because more staff must be present than is actually needed to take care of the existing patients. This is because there are minimum staffing issues. Minimum staffing is a fixed cost. Remember from the Budget Chapter, fixed costs are those costs which stay the same regardless of the level of activity.

To figure minimum staffing let's begin with an inpatient example. For an inpatient cost center staying open every day of the year, the industry standard is that two personnel are available to care for patients regardless of the number of patients. Minimum staffing for an inpatient cost center are pictured in **Exhibit 11–5**. *Note that it is best not to include unit secretary time in the minimum staffing or fixed cost section of the budget, as this allows for more budget flexibility for the nurse manager.*

Exhibit 11–5 Inpatient Unit Direct Care Minimum Staffing for 24 hours

Day Shift	**Evening Shift**	**Night Shift**
8 hours = 1 RN	8 hours = 1 RN	8 hours = 1 RN
8 hours = 1 Aide/Tech/LPN/RN	8 hours = 1 Aide/Tech/LPN/RN	8 hours = 1 Aide/Tech/LPN/RN
16 hours	**16 hours**	**16 hours**

Add the hours from each shift:
16 hours + 16 hours + 16 hours = 48 hours/day

You may need to determine the actual salary dollars involved for your cost center. See **Exhibit 11–6** assuming an average salary amount per staff classification. Often the human resource department or finance department personnel have determined the average salary for each personnel category. Although this salary amount could be used to determine the fixed cost of minimum staffing, it may not be as accurate. For instance, if most staff RNs in a cost center have been there for many years, most may be at the top of the salary range. The human resource average staff RN salary figure may be lower. So it would be preferable to use the actual salaries rather than the human resource figure in this example.

Exhibit 11–6 Inpatient Unit Direct Care Minimum Staffing Cost/Day

Day Shift	Evening Shift	Night Shift
(8 hours = RN—Amy) @ $19/hour* = $152/day*	(8 hours = 1 RN—Bill) @ $18/hour* = $144/day*	(8 hours = 1 RN—Carol) @$17/hour* = $136/day*
(8 hours = 1 Nurse Aide—Robert) @ $9/hour* = $72/day*	(8 hours = 1 Nurse Aide—Sue) @ $8/hour* = $64/day*	(8 hours = 1 Nurse Aide—Tom) @$9/hour* = $72/day*

Add the salary rate from each staff member:

$152 + $144 + $136 + $72 + $64 + $72 = $640/day* (Minimum Staffing Cost/Day)

$640/day x 365 days = $233,600/year*

*Benefits and shift differential not included.

So far our minimum staffing example has included only the actual direct care nursing staff. Minimum staffing on an inpatient cost center also would include the nurse manager and other consistent cost center/department employees such as the cost center secretaries. To determine the fixed cost/day for the nurse manager, let's assume that the nurse manager is responsible for one cost center. Since the daily cost is based on seven days in the week, the actual daily rate for the nurse manager would be the nurse manager's hourly salary multiplied by 5.7 hours/day (a fixed cost/day).

Nurse Manager
40 hours/week ÷ 7 days/week = 5.7 hours/day
5.7 hours/day x $22.85/hour = $130.25/day

If a cost center secretary is always present on the inpatient cost center for a 12-hour shift, this would be added to minimum staffing. In this case the hourly rate of the cost center secretary would be multiplied by 12 hours/day.

Unit Secretary
12 hours/day x $8.98/hour = $107.76/day

Thus the minimum staffing would actually cost $878.01 per day or $320,473.65 per year (see **Exhibit 11–7**). So actually looking at the staffing budget for that unit, $320,473.65 would be a fixed cost.

The financial personnel may determine the fixed costs within the nursing cost center budget differently. Usually they understand neither what minimum staffing is nor how to measure it. If the finance staff tell you what your fixed costs are, be sure to have them define how they have determined these costs. Usually the nurse manager or nurse executive will need to educate finance department personnel about minimum staffing. The nurse manager/executive should both explain and show financial personnel actual minimum staff examples.

Exhibit 11–7 Total Inpatient Unit Direct Care Minimum Staffing Cost/Day

Direct Care Staff = $640/day*

Nurse Manager = $130.25/day*

Unit Secretary = $107.76/day*

Total = $878.01/day*

$878.01/day x 365 days = $320,473.65/year*

*Benefits and shift differential not included.

After determining the fixed cost of staffing—minimum staffing—the rest of the staffing budget would then be variable staffing costs. See **Exhibit 11–8**—Fixed (Minimum Staffing) and Variable Staffing—to see how this might actually look for a unit. If you remember, variable costs are those costs that change (vary) depending on the level of activity or volume. So staffing over and above the minimum staffing is a variable cost. Variable costs occur *in addition* to fixed costs. Thus the staffing needed above and beyond minimum staffing would increase or decrease as the patient volume increases or decreases. The volume determining the staffing would be related to the number of patient minutes/hours/days, patient acuity, or patient visits.

If a nurse manager were asked to prepare a flexible, or variable, budget (discussed in Chapter 10, Budgeting) giving alternative plans for different levels of spending, the nurse manager would have to figure both minimum staffing and variable staffing at different volume levels. In the book *Health Care Financial Management for Nurse Managers: Financial Applications in Hospitals, Long-Term Care, Home Care, and Ambulatory Care* (Dunham-Taylor and Pinczuk, 2006), Chapter 4 gives an example of a flexible budget presented on an Excel spreadsheet.

Systems differ when using a flexible, or variable, budget. In some systems this just means that there are two or more levels of spending (several fixed budgets at various occupancy levels) determined for different volumes of patients. In some systems variable budgets change as the volume of patients and the acuity of patients changes. For example, this budget could vary as the patient population changes throughout the day. A nurse manager in such a system could see what budget amount was available for the upcoming shift based on the current patient population. If there is a variable budget the nurse manager must discuss how finance department personnel determined the gradations in the variable budget

As the budget changes, it is important for the nurse manager to decrease variable costs in relation to the decrease in volume. When the census or acuity falls below the minimum staffing pattern, the nurse manager and nurse executive might consider closing/consolidating cost centers, or assigning patients in a manner that maintains a census on several cost centers that cover the fixed costs of minimum staffing.

Exhibit 11–8 Fixed (Minimum Staffing) and Variable Staffing

(Average HPPS = 6.5)

Patients		Days			Evenings			Nights		
		RN	LPN	NA	RN	LPN	NA	RN	LPN	NA
25		4	2	1	3	2	1	2	1	1
20		3	2	1	2	2	1	2	1	1
14		2	1	1	2	0	1	1	1	1
↓		1	1	1	1	1	1	1	1	1
9		1	0	1	1	0	1	1	0	1
8										
7										
1		1	0	1	1	0	1	1	0	1

Left vertical labels: Variable Direct Caregivers (25 through the blank row); Fixed Direct Caregivers and Minimum Staffing (9 through 1).

RN = registered nurse
LPN = licensed practical nurse
NA = nurse aide
UC = unit clerk

Equipment and Supply Costs

The nurse manager also needs to examine equipment and supply costs. These costs often include such items as: education, travel, standard office and medical supplies not used by specific patients, telephone costs, equipment lease/rentals, equipment repair, uniform allowance, books, and consulting charges.

Once again it is important to look at the historical data. If this data were accurate and reflected what is anticipated for another year, there is no need to change the data. However, most often the costs in these categories will have existed for years and not be totally accurate for present patient needs. Past experience can be helpful when looking at this data. If nurse managers have been regularly going over budget variances each month, it is often quite obvious that certain budget categories are insufficient to cover supply costs for the present group of patients while other budget categories may not be used as much or at all.

It is important to make sure that supplies are expensed to the proper line item to reflect adequate expenditures. If these expenditures are accurate, they may need to be adjusted each year to better reflect actual use. If they remain accurate, the nurse manager may not need to do much with this data.

In addition to the historical data, the nurse manager must anticipate what might change for the coming budget year. Will the unit purchase new equipment that requires a change in supplies? Are physician practice patterns changing? Are there anticipated inflationary costs to consider? How these are determined are discussed in the next section of this chapter.

For the evaluation process, the nurse manager needs to consider all changes that have, or are expected, to occur on the unit that might result in more or less being spent in equipment and supply costs. The nurse manager will need to provide additional documentation as to why the amounts need to be changed in certain budget categories. For example, if the cost center is treating a different kind of patient, the nurse manager might need to provide the number of such patients anticipated for the next year, and document typical supply needs required. Additionally, the nurse manager should specify any equipment and supplies that might be used less frequently.

Several additional factors need to be considered when evaluating the equipment and supply budget. The first problem is that personnel using supplies for particular patients are not careful about making sure such supplies are recorded as used for specific purposes. At times such expenses can be billable, [a sample charge form can be found in Crookston and Kirchhoff (1986)] and when this is the case, the organization could be losing money. Organizations have used different systems and strategies in the attempt to remedy this situation. Some have a bar code, sticker, or charge slip on all supplies, and expect staff to designate each supply used for a particular patient. Some have locked-up supplies, putting them in closed cart systems, (i.e., Omni cells). Staff have to key in both what they are taking and the patient's name. Many pharmacy systems, (i.e., Sure Meds, Pyxis), dispense medications by individual dose for specific patients. This not only helps to cost items to patients but to ensure patient safety.

Equipment can be similarly supplied. Specific equipment—such as IVACs, PLUMs, aquaK pads, or commodes—can be ordered from central supply in a specific patient's name. These can be charged by the day. The cost of daily use of such equipment is often set by the finance department based on the "average life" of the piece of equipment— meaning how long the equipment can be used before becoming non-functional or obsolete.

A second problem is that the finance department and/or the nursing department does not realize that certain items can be directly billed. It is so important for both the nursing administration and the finance groups to continue to share information with each other, as well as to network with peers and with professional organizations to find out how others are handling these costs.

A third problem is that nursing staff are being wasteful in using supplies. For example, if a nurse needs another catheter, he or she may open up the catheterization packet and take the catheter, throwing the rest of the kit away. Or an aide piles on Chux pads and uses 15 under a patient. Staff often do not realize the costs of their actions. Nurse managers can actually put labels where supplies are stored, giving the cost of each supply item.

A fourth problem occurs when staff squirrel equipment and supplies. For instance, every hospital has a problem with wheelchair availability. They are never where they are needed, so staff hide them somewhere. Meanwhile as others look, they cannot find one. When staff squirrel equipment, they do not realize how much money is sitting there, all they realize is that when they need the equipment, the equipment cannot be found. This is a systems problem in the organization that needs to be dealt with.

Measuring and Adjusting for Inflation[10]

Accountants and finance people adjust for inflation using a *price index*. The price index you are most likely familiar with is the *Consumer Price Index* which measures "the increase (or decrease) in the cost of living for an urban family of four" (U.S. Dept. of Labor Bureau of Labor Statistics). There are other price indices, including the *Wholesale Price Index*, which measure price changes in individual industries and sectors of the economy including a *market basket* of goods and services in health care.

All price indices are in the form of the "To/From ratio":

> **Prices in the period we are going "To"**
> **Prices in the period we are coming "From"**

To illustrate all price indices, let's look at the way the Consumer Price Index (CPI) is developed. First a panel of experts (usually economists) decide what items an "average urban family of four" spends its money on: food, housing, clothing, education, medical costs, entertainment, and so on. For the moment, assume that those are the only items on the list. The panel must now decide how to define one unit of food, or one unit of housing. These decisions can be pretty arbitrary *as long as they remain consistent from year to year*. That consistency, however, is actually impossible. How do you compare a unit of entertainment in 1945 with a unit of entertainment in 1999? Most of the things we do for entertainment in the 21st century did not exist at the end of World War II. The panel is simply left to do the best they can.

When the cost index is first created, the elements of the index are defined and priced. Let's assume the following elements with the accompanying costs.

Definition

Price Index—A ratio which represents the change in prices between two years.

Consumer Price Index or CPI—Perhaps the best known price index, the CPI measures the price of a "market basket of goods and services for an urban family of four."

Market Basket—a colloquial term, derived from the definition of the CPI, market basket indicates the change in prices for a set of goods and/or services. Price Indices, or market baskets, are measured for consumer prices, wholesale prices, and specific industries such as health care.

---

[10] The author of this section of the chapter, Measuring and Adjusting for Inflation, was R. Penny Marquette, DBA.

$6,000 = One year's rent
$3,000 = One year's food
$1,500 = One complete outfit (underwear to outerwear) for a man, woman, and two children
$600 = One year's costs for books and school lunches for two children
$1,200 = Two doctor's visits, and two dentist's visits for each of four people
One modest dinner and a movie for four people once each month - $1,250
The total cost of this "market basket" of goods and services is $13,550:

$$\textbf{\$6,000 + \$3,000 + \$1,500 + \$600 + \$1,200 + \$1,250 = \$13,550}$$

This $13,550 is the *base year cost*—the "From" in the "To/From" ratio. Next year, the panel will again *price the same basket of goods and services*. While the items may not be exactly the same, they will try to get as close as possible. Assume that the calculation above was done in 1995. Then 1995 is the base year. The chart below shows the market basket costs for the years 1995 through 2000.

1995	1996	1997	1998	1999	2000
$13,550	$13,984	$14,361	$14,691	$15,205	$15,631

To create a cost index, we select our base year (1995) and divide it into each of the other years. The *Price Index* is shown below in the third row:

1995	1996	1997	1998	1999	2000
$13,550 ÷	$13,984 ÷	$14,361 ÷	$14,691 ÷	$15,205 ÷	$15,631 ÷
$13,550	$13,550	$13,550	$13,550	$13,550	$13,550
1.00	1.03	1.06	1.08	1.12	1.15

Understanding the use of price indices can help the nurse manager in several ways. For example, what if the cost of supplies in your department has been rising steadily over the past three years. Your census is steady, but you have been using far more nurses aides and you wonder whether or not they may be less careful with supplies. The annual cost for supplies is shown in the table below:

1997	1998	1999	2000
$1,800	$1,836	$1,909	$2,203

We know that some of this is caused by inflation, but how much? We can use the price index to remove the effect of inflation and compare these costs on a *constant dollar* (a dollar without inflation) basis. While everyone knows that inflation exists, and everyone compensates for it to some degree, the ability to eliminate inflation from a series of numbers allows us to look at them in a far more realistic manner.

1997	$1,800 ÷ 1.06 = $1,698
1998	$1,836 ÷ 1.08 = $1,700 (+2)
1999	$1,909 ÷ 1.12 = $1,704 (+4)
2000	$2,203 ÷ 1.15 = $1,916 (+212)

Now we can see that there has been a large increase, but that it has happened entirely in the year 2000. The increases from 1997 to 1998 ($2) and from 1998 to 1999 ($4) are very small; both less than 1 percent over the prior year. The increase in 2000, however, is $212, a whopping 11 percent over the year before. This type of information allows the nurse manager to narrow her hunt for the cause of the increase and hopefully stop its continuation.

Another use of cost indices is to predict the amount of basic cost increase one will experience in the coming year. Price indices are predicted at regular intervals and can be used to estimate the effect of inflation for budgeting purposes. Unfortunately, these are predictions, and they are sometimes very wrong. If your own educated instincts tell you that inflation will be higher than the experts anticipate, follow your instincts, but be prepared to defend them with underlying facts. Remember that price indices are intended to cover a multitude of environments, and your environment has many special circumstances that no one knows better than you do.

Generally, the finance department personnel will indicate expected levels of inflation for different kinds of equipment, supplies, and pharmaceuticals. They get this information from the market basket index. If contracts for equipment and supplies change, it is important that the correct cost of these items be reflected in the budget.

Determining Variance between Historical and Newly Figured Budgets

Now that an accurate budget has been figured, it is time for the nurse manager to compare this data with the current historical budget. Do they agree? If so, the nurse manager can proceed with the budget planning process knowing that the data is accurate. However, if there is a discrepancy—or variance—between both budgets there will be some additional work the nurse manager will need to do. The first step would be to discuss this issue with the nurse executive, or the nurse manager's supervisor if the nurse manager does not directly report to the nurse executive.

By having computed the budget from scratch, the nurse manager has objective data to use when defining the problem and suggesting solutions. It gives the nurse manager actual *objective* data; finance department personnel are more likely to listen when presented with such data. It is easy to argue that additional staffing is needed for "squishy" reasons, such as this is needed to improve quality or to meet accreditation requirements. However, having objective evidence provides better documentation of actual patient needs, and will more likely be heard by the executive team. After all, it is the nurse manager who best understands and represents actual patient needs. *Patients will be more likely to receive needed services—and the nurse manager will have more success—when actual numbers can be presented to verify patient needs.*

If the *patient acuity/volume is higher*, this provides actual data that verifies additional staffing needs. Perhaps if the patient volume is higher, the nurse manager will suggest a different staff mix to better meet the needs of these patients. The nurse manager may propose opening a swing unit, available at times of peak census, or possibly the problem is that more staff are needed because nonproductive time was not taken into account.

If the *patient volume has decreased* within a cost center, other strategies can be considered. First, current staffing levels may need to be decreased. However, current staffing levels can only be decreased to the minimum staffing level. If below the minimum staffing level, other strategies could be to increase the patient volume on the cost center such as merging cost centers; alternately, one could close the cost center and send the patients to a similar cost center not at full patient capacity. This action is complicated by other issues such as medical patients with infections not being a preferable patient to divert to a surgical unit or labor and delivery area; and by staff cross training issues.

Be creative in thinking through the most appropriate strategy. Things do not need to be done the same way! Once thinking through such issues, and discussing them with the nurse executive, it may be necessary for the nurse manager to write a thoughtful proposal clearly defining the problem as well as discussing one or more potential solutions. See Chapter 14, Budget Strategies, for further information on proposal writing.

Other Ways Actual Cost Data Can Be Used

Cost data can be used in additional ways. Some uses are listed below.

Assignment Comparability. If this concrete cost data is available, when a staff member questions having a heavier load than other staff, the nurse manager can actually compare the acuity levels for assigned patients. This data can also be used for staff evaluation. If one staff member can *safely* care for a higher volume of patients, this staff might deserve additional merit pay. Or a staff member might need to be mentored and/or counseled as to how to safely care for a higher volume of patients.

Intra-Unit Comparability. Using our 4W example, the nurse executive or nurse managers on similar cost centers within this health care organization could compare staffing, skill mix, and budget information. For example, 4W was an orthopedic cost center. One might compare this unit with other surgical cost centers with similar acuity ratings. See **Exhibit 11–9**. Several surgical cost centers are illustrated. 4W, 6E, and Tower have fairly similar NHPPD. However, Tower has a higher number of patient days while 6E has fewer patient days. Each unit could be costed out to determine whether there was comparable staffing on each of these units. 2N has a higher acuity (8.0 NHPPD) so it may be best not to compare staffing with them. For the nurse executive, however, if the costing computation shows that 2N actually needs to have more staff assigned due to the higher acuity, this cost data would provide the statistics necessary to propose additional staffing dollars be assigned to this cost center.

Exhibit 11–9 Personnel Budget Sheet

General Hospital Personnel Budget
FY 200_

Surgical Cost Centers	NHPPD	Days	Direct FTES	Indirect FTES	Total FTES
4W	6.6	6,800	24.3	3.8	28.1
6E	5.8	6,200	22.2	3.8	26.0
2N	8.0	4,000	20.0	3.8	23.8
Tower	6.2	7,300	30.4	3.8	34.2

Benchmarking. The cost data can also be used to compare with other similar services across the country using available benchmarking data such as the Premier or VHA data for hospitals. Premier or VHA can give extensive data on skill mix, labor costs, overtime used, wages paid certain types of employees, and even provide the nurse manager a vehicle to network with peers from similar units nationally. When using such data, it is important to make sure that one is not comparing apples and oranges—one may think one is comparing like categories yet not be. For example, skill mix for a long-term care facility would be totally different than the skill mix on a critical care unit. It is important to get definitions of what is actually included for that category. To do this, we recommend that you contact a person at the facility to verify like activities.

Skill Mix Issues. Skill mix could be an issue. One could compare skill mix on similar units or with benchmarking data. The acuity could dictate the skill mix, i.e., an intensive care unit with higher acuity is generally staffed with more RNs than a general care unit. So it would be important to make sure that the units one is benchmarking are actually serving the same degree of patient acuity.

Full-Time/Part-Time Ratios. The ratio of full-time staff to part-time staff must also be evaluated. It is possible that there are constant staffing problems on weekends because the ratio of full-time staff is too high. Or if there are a lot of part-time staff working one to three days a week, it may become impossible to keep all staff informed as to changes as well as continuity of care being challenged. The cost data can provide helpful information to determine whether the part-time/full-time ratio is appropriate.

Establishing a Staffing Plan or Flexible Staffing Model. Another strategy for nurse managers is to establish ideal staffing levels—a staffing plan—for different volumes of patients when there are wide variations in patient acuity and/or numbers of patients served. When the volume is low perhaps part-time staff or specific full-time staff work fewer hours, or staff are floated to other cost centers. If volume is high, this is reversed. Part-time staff work more hours, full-time staff earn overtime, a float pool is available to supply additional staff, or additional agency staff are hired. It is always best to carefully plan various strategies that can be implemented when a certain volume of patients is present. Additional staff training is needed when staff are expected to work at different clinical sites. Planning for several scenarios ahead of actual happenings can help to eliminate stress for both staff and administrators, and maintain a continuity in quality of care. If staffing needs change, this staffing plan can be used as a flexible staffing model where a computer system—or the staffing personnel—automatically set appropriate numbers of staff at the designated staff mix.

Thus an annual evaluation of the budget can be helpful not only to determine that the allocated budget dollars are appropriate but for other staffing and supply/equipment issues as well.

References

American Nurses Association. (1999). *Principles for nurse staffing: With annotated bibliography*. Washington, DC: American Nurses Publishing.

Brink, J., & Gray, S. (June 1997). Cost modeling to justify technology acquisitions. *Healthcare Financial Management*, 72–76.

Crookston, B., & Kirchoff, K. (April 1986). A comprehensive charge system for unit supplies. *JONA, 16*(4), 31–34.

Dunham-Taylor, J., & Pinczuk, J. (2006). *Health care financial management for nurse managers: Applications from hospitals, long-term care, home care, and ambulatory care*. Sudbury, MA: Jones and Bartlett.

Fralic, M., Ed. (2000). *Staffing management and methods: Tools and techniques for nursing leaders*. Chicago: AHA Press.

Jenkin-Cappiello, E. (February 2000). Oh baby!: A labor and delivery staffing system measures patient census and acuity. *Nursing Management, 31*(2), 35–37.

Keeling, B. (September 1999). How to allocate the right staff mix across shifts, Part 1. *Nursing Management, 30*(9), 16–17.

Keeling, B. (October 1999). How to allocate the right staff mix across shifts, Part 2. *Nursing Management, 30*(10), 16–18.

Nursing's Report Card: A Study of RN Staffing, Length of Stay, and Patient Outcomes. (1997). Washington, DC: American Nurses Publishing.

Phillips, C., Castorr, A., Prescott, P., & Soeken, K. (April 1992). Nursing intensity: Going beyond patient classification. *JONA, 22*(4), 46–52.

Senge, P. (1990). *The fifth discipline: The art & practice of the learning organization*. New York: Doubleday Currency.

Shullanberger, G. (May–June 2000). Nurse staffing decisions: An integrative review of the literature. *Nursing Economic$, 18*(3), 124–148.

CHAPTER 12

Budget Variances

Norma Tomlinson, MSN, RN, CNA1

Introduction

Budgets are usually created several months before the beginning of the fiscal year. Annual budgets are based on assumptions about the types and volumes of patients that will be cared for over the coming year and the resources required to provide that care. The difference between the budget and actual performance is the *budget variance*. Well-researched and analyzed budget variance becomes a powerful tool in controlling cost while ensuring safe effective care.

A nursing unit or department is a *cost center*. Data comparing budgeted dollars to actual dollars is usually provided on a monthly basis by the Finance Department for each cost center. It normally shows data for the month and year-to-date. It is important, therefore, to be aware of the beginning of your fiscal year. If your fiscal year begins with January, and it is now February, the data for January and year-to-date will be the same since it includes only one month's data (January). If your fiscal year begins July 1 and ends June 30, in February the year-to-date (YTD) will include seven months of data (July through January).

The *cost center report* compares the *actual costs* with the *budgeted amount*. Often these reports show the percentage of the difference, or *variance*, between what was budgeted and what actually was spent. If it does not, you can calculate the percentage of variance by taking the difference between the actual and the budget, and then divide that number by the budget. For instance, using **Exhibit 12–1**, multiplying the difference between the budget and actual by 100 gives you the percentage of variance. Therefore the actual budget amount was 25 percent greater than the budgeted amount.

Often an operational report will show the data for the *prior year* for the same time frame that gives you an additional perspective to gage if you are doing better or worse than the same time last year.

Exhibit 12–1 Comparing Budgeted Amount with Actual Amount Used

Budget = $200

Actual = $250

$200 (budget) - $250 (actual) = -$50 variance

The difference between the budgeted amount and the actual amount is $50.

$50 (variance) ÷ ($200 (budget) = 0.25

0.25 x 100 = 25 percent (To get the percentage, one multiplies this amount by 100.)

Therefore the actual amount was 25 percent greater than the budgeted amount.

Types of Variance

The statistics, or types of variance, discussed here include: the volume or units of service, revenue, man hours, information about salary expense, benefit expense, and non-salary expense.

Expense Budget

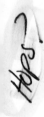

In an expense budget, units of service for inpatient cost centers are often broken into inpatient days for patients admitted and observation hours when the patient time on the unit was short enough that it did not qualify to become an admission. *It is important to capture all of your unit activity.*

If your report does not delineate these two types of patient days, it is very important to determine if the statistics includes both. The man-hours to care for a patient in observation status can actually be more time intensive per day, because admission and discharge activities have to be done within the same day (23 hour patient) or the next day. If the unit experiences many outpatient or observation days, and these are not included in the statistic for patient days, your data is skewed. It can appear that your hours of care per patient day as well as other costs are very high when benchmarked against other comparable nursing units that count all activity. (See **Exhibit 12–2**.)

If you are responsible for a unit that does not keep patients 24 hours per day, your volume statistic will be different. For example, if you are responsible for an operating room, an endoscopy suite, or a post-anesthesia care unit (PACU), your volume statistic will be patients or procedures. It is very important to understand which is being counted because a single patient may have several procedures done during the same visit.

- In obstetrics, the volume statistic may be patient days, both mother and baby, or it may be births. In obstetrics the volume of outpatient tests must be captured as well. That volume can involve a significant number of man-hours.
- In the emergency department (ED), the usual volume statistic measured is the number of visits. However, in these days of overcrowding, when patients can be held in the ED waiting for beds for more than a day, it is important to capture those hours beyond the time that the patient could have been admitted to an inpatient bed.

- Long-term care normally counts patient days.
- Home care counts visits. Some home-care organizations weight visits for productivity based on greater weight for opening or reopening a case because of the extensive documentation required to meet regulatory requirements.

It is very helpful when operational reports also provide data about full-time equivalencies (FTEs), average hourly rate, and a breakdown of data per unit of service. When looking at the data, you need to understand the meaning of brackets. In the examples provided in this chapter, negative variances (bracketed data) for *statistics* and *revenue* are favorable. Negative variances (bracketed data) on *expenses* are unfavorable.

In **Exhibit 12–2**, actual volume for patient days for both the month (735) and year (3,662) is higher than that budgeted (655 for the month and 3,354 YTD) and higher than what was experienced in the prior year (3,356). The actual observation days (15) for the month were higher (by one) than the budgeted days (14), but lower (by one) than the same month last year (16). Year-to-date the observation days are right on target to what was budgeted (68), but lower than last year (75). When combined, the total units, or total patient days, for both the month (750) and year-to-date (3,730) are higher than what was budgeted (669 for the month and 3,422 YTD), and what was experienced in the prior year (681 for the month and 3,431 YTD). The positive (higher) volume variance of 12.1 percent for the month and 9.0 percent year-to-date becomes very important later when analyzing the resources used to care for that volume of patients.

Exhibit 12–2 Example of a Monthly Report of Statistics for a Surgical Nursing Unit

Department Operations Report
For the period ending 11/30/200_
Main 7

	MONTH					YTD*		
Actual	**Budget**	**Var %**	**Prior**	**Statistic**	**Actual**	**Budget**	**Var %**	**Prior**
735	655	(12.2)%	665	Unit Patient Days	3,662	3,354	(9.2)%	3,356
15	14	(7.1)%	16	Observation Days	68	68	0.0%	75
750	669	(12.1)%	681	Total Units	3,730	3,422	(9.0)%	3,431

*YTD = Year-to-Date

Revenue Budget

Revenue is as important to monitor as expense. Looking at a revenue and expense budget, managers might think that their department is generating a very high profit margin, *even when it really is not*. Reported revenue reflects *charges* generated for the month and year-to-date by the department, *not actual dollars received for that care*.

> *Reported revenue reflects charges generated, not actual dollars received.*

In areas with a high population of Medicaid, Self-Pay, and Managed Care as the source of payment, the percentage of charges captured can be less than 50 percent. By multiplying the total revenue by the percentage of charges captured, you can identify the approximate amount of collectible revenue that will result from the care provided and billed. Subtracting the total expenses, which are actual dollars expended, usually does not leave a high profit margin, if any.

> *Total Revenue x Percentage of Captured Charges = Approximate Collectible Revenue*
>
> *Approximate Collectible Revenue - Actual Expenses = Net Revenue*

Example: The annual revenue budget for Main 7 is $4,119,257. That is the total amount of expected charges to be generated by Main 7 for the year. The budgeted annual expense is $1,816,255. Net revenue is those dollars remaining after expenses are subtracted from revenue. If the hospital received 100 percent of charges, the net revenue would be:
$4,119,257 - $1,816,255 = $2,303,002.

However, if the true capture of charges is 50 percent then half of $4,119,257 or $2,059,628.50 is all that will be collected. The net revenue then becomes:
$2,059,628.50 - $1,816,255 = $243,373.50.

$4,119,257	*Annual Revenue (from expected charges)*
- $1,816,255	*Budgeted Annual Expense*
$2,303,002	*Total Revenue (from expected charges)*

When charges were actually 50 percent of what had been anticipated:

$4,119,257 x 0.50 =	$2,059,628.50	*Actual Revenue*
	- $1,816,255.00	*Budgeted Annual Expense*
	$ 243,373.50	*Net Revenue*

That leaves a *narrow margin* for unexpected additional costs such as greater overtime dollars required, or the unanticipated cost of new sharps safety devices.

Before becoming depressed, keep in mind that other departments such as Pharmacy, Laboratory, Radiology, and Surgery, normally show much higher positive revenues for the same patients. Those departments would not see those higher profits if those patients were not receiving care on your unit.

Just as volume is reported for both inpatient and outpatient, the corresponding revenue is reported in the same manner. (See **Exhibit 12–3**.)

In this example, just as with volume, actual inpatient revenue is higher for the month ($355,501) and year-to-date ($1,794,790) than that budgeted ($318,724 for the month and $1,632,062 YTD). It is also higher than that experienced in the prior year ($286,985 for the month and $1,488,463 YTD).

Outpatient revenues for both the month ($5,469) and YTD ($23,482) are less than the budgeted amounts ($5,860 for the month and $28,464 YTD), and less than that experienced in the prior year ($4,436 for the month and $26,991 YTD).

Exhibit 12–3   Example of a Monthly Report of Statistics for a Revenue Budget

Department Revenue Report
For the period ending 11/30/200_
Main 7

	MONTH					YTD		
Actual	**Budget**	**Var%**	**Prior**	**Statistic**	**Actual**	**Budget**	**Var%**	**Prior**
(355,501)	(318,724)	(11.5)%	(286,985)	Inpatient Revenue	(1,794,790)	(1,632,062)	(10.0)%	(1,488,463)
(5,469)	(5,860)	6.7%	(4,436)	Outpatient Revenue	(23,482)	(28,464)	17.5%	(26,991)
(360,970)	(324,584)	(11.2)%	(291,421)	Total Revenue	(1,818,272)	(1,660,526)	(9.5)%	(1,515,454)

Outpatient or observation charges are usually not reimbursed at a very high rate. Therefore, the shift to higher inpatient charges when the patient stays long enough to convert to an inpatient stay, and experiences less outpatient charges, is positive.

Total revenues for both the month ($360,970) and YTD ($1,818,272) are greater than the budgeted amounts ($324,584 for the month and $1,660,526 YTD), and more than that experienced in the prior year ($291,421 for the month and $1,515,454 YTD). So this reflects the same pattern (increased amounts) as the volumes.

Man-Hours Budget

Because staffing is usually the most expensive resource in the provision of care, the amount and type of man-hours expensed to a nursing unit is very critical. The monthly operations report usually does not break down the man-hours by job classification such as RN, LPN, Nursing Assistant, and Unit Clerk. That information is normally provided in bi-weekly reports that show individual employee hours, and/or man-hours or FTEs by job classification. (See **Exhibit 12–4**.)

While bi-weekly reports may not correspond to the exact days, or the month, covered by the operations report, it will provide good data to monitor if your mix of staff corresponds to that budgeted. Man-hours are usually broken down into contract, productive, paid time off (PTO), overtime, education, orientation, and other (ETC).

Contract labor is usually the most expensive man-hours. Contract staff can be through local agencies or the more expensive "travelers" who are agency personnel assigned for several weeks or months at a time, and usually live in local temporary housing. While they may provide for better continuity of care than local agency staff, their costs include at a minimum: hourly rate, rent, food, travel, and car rental.

Productive man-hours are those hours where employed staff members provide care for patients. In the case of direct caregivers such as registered nurses, licensed practical nurses, and patient care technicians, it is the time they are assigned on the nursing unit actually providing hands-on care to patients. For indirect caregivers such as unit clerks, it includes the time that they spend on the nursing unit providing their specific indirect services, such as entering orders from the charts into the computer.

Exhibit 12–4 Example of a Bi-Weekly FTE Report

*Pay Period 0_   1/13/0_–1/26/0_*

Name	Classification	Productive FTE	Non-Productive FTE	Overtime FTE	Total FTE
T. Moore	Manager	1.0	0	0	1.0
Subtotal	**Manager**	**1.0**	**0**	**0**	**1.0**
A. Todd	Charge RN	1.0	0	0.1	1.1
S. Shaw	Charge RN	1.0	0	0	1.0
Subtotal	**Charge RN**	**2.0**	**0**	**0.1**	**2.1**
R. Barry	RN	1.0	0	0.2	1.2
J. Brown	RN	0.45	0.45	0	0.9
C. Collins	RN	0.9	0	0	0.9
R. Dix	RN	0.9	0.1	0	1.0
E. Fisher	RN	0.6	0	0	0.6
J. Robinson	RN	0.9	0	0	0.9
R. Smith	RN	0.45	0.45	0	0.9
Subtotal	**RN**	**5.2**	**1.0**	**0.2**	**6.4**
J. Edwards	LPN	0.9	0	0	0.9
R. Falls	LPN	0	0.9	0	0.9
E. George	LPN	0.9	0	0	0.9
T. Hall	LPN	0.6	0.3	0	0.9
Subtotal	**LPN**	**2.4**	**1.2**	**0**	**3.6**
J. Adams	PCT	0.9	0	0	0.9
N. Coates	PCT	0.6	0	0	0.6
T. East	PCT	0.9	0	0	0.9
Subtotal	**PCT**	**2.4**	**0**	**0**	**2.4**
A. Thomas	Unit Clerk	1.0	0	0	1.0
S. Vender	Unit Clerk	1.0	0	0	1.0
Subtotal	**Unit Clerk**	**2.0**	**0**	**0**	**2.0**
TOTAL		**15.0**	**2.2**	**0.3**	**17.5**

Note: These are fictitious names.

Non-productive man-hours include paid time off (PTO). Paid time off includes vacation, holidays, jury duty, sick time, and any other time off where the employee is paid by the organization but does not actually work during that paid time. It is an employee benefit. Paid time off may be expensed (charged) to the cost center at the time that it is earned, or at the time that it is taken.

The time at which PTO is expensed is important to know when analyzing the unit costs for the month.[1] If it is expensed to your department *at the time it is earned*, you will see it charged as an expense against your department based on the hours worked during that month. In this case it goes into a "bank" that the employee draws against when it is taken. Your department will not be charged for it again when the employee takes the time off because it was already expensed to you once. You will see it in the detail of what was paid to the employee on your bi-weekly report.

However, those dollars will not be added to the total on your monthly report. If you need to replace the employee to cover the man-hours required to care for the volume of patients, then you will be charged only for the hours worked by the replacement employee.

If, on the other hand, PTO is charged to your budget *only when taken* by the employee, you will see it included in the total on the monthly report. If, because of volume, you had to replace the employee to cover the man-hours required to care for the volume of patients, you will be charged for that employee's hours, as well.

In most organizations PTO is earned based on the hours worked. If you use part-time staff members more than their allocated FTE, they will earn PTO on those hours, as well. That will increase the non-productive time and dollars that will be expensed to your department.

Overtime is that time worked over 40 hours in a week if on a 40-hour work week. It can include, at the discretion of the organization, hours worked over a scheduled 8, 10, or 12-hour shift *even if less than 40 hours are worked in a week*. It can also include time designated as overtime at the discretion of the organization, such as any hours called in, and hours worked when on-call. While discretionary overtime pay can be a positive retention tool, it is also an added expense. It is important to know what the policy is in your organization regarding the designation of overtime.

On-call pay is a minimal hourly rate paid to staff who are not at work, but who have committed to be available to work on short notice. It is important to know if in your organization on-call pay hours stop when the individual is called into work. Some organizations stop on-call pay at the time the employee clocks into work. In this case, if they clock out before the end of their time on-call, the on-call pay picks up again when they clock out. Some organizations continue to pay the on-call pay in addition to any hours worked while on-call.

Education and orientation hours are those spent learning and meeting the competencies required for the employee's position. With HIPAA (further explained in Chapter 6) and other new regulatory rules, many hours of mandatory education are being added to the cost of staffing to ensure that all employees are educated about the rules.

---

[1] Remember the discussion in the Budget Chapter where we emphasize that budget terms are not standardized; it is important to find out the organizational description of what is actually included in that budget term.

In **Exhibit 12–5**, the data demonstrate a large increase in contract labor that has been utilized both for the month (344 hours) and year-to-date (1,840 hours). Year-to-date in the prior year shows only 284 hours of contract labor was used for the month.

Exhibit 12–5 Example of a Monthly Report of Man-Hours for a Surgical Nursing Unit

Department Man-hours Report
For the period ending 11/30/200_
Main 7

| MONTH | | | | | YTD* | | | |
Actual	Budget	Var%	Prior	STATISTIC	Actual	Budget	Var%	Prior
344	315	(9.2)%	258	**MANHOURS CONTRACT**	1,840	1,575	(16.8)%	284
5,759	5,267	(9.3)%	5,291	**MANHOURS PRODUCTIVE**	28,469	26,893	(5.9)%	26,860
611	570	(7.2)%	573	**MANHOURS PTO**	2,883	2,912	1.0%	2,988
192	270	28.9%	363	**MANHOURS OVER-TIME**	1,117	1,380	19.1%	1,627
764	750	(1.9)%	667	**MANHOURS ED/ORIENT/ETC**	3,392	3,825	11.3%	3,933
7,670	7,172	(6.9)%	7,152	**TOTAL MANHOURS**	37,701	36,585	(3.1)%	35,692
44.86	41.95	(6.9)%	41.83	**TOTAL FTES**	43.24	41.96	(3.1)%	40.94

YTD = Year-to-date

Note that:

- The budget of 1,575 hours YTD shows that the shortage of employed nursing staff was recognized and plans were made to use agency staff. However, due to the volume of patients and the shortage of regular employed staff, 16.8 percent additional contract hours were used in addition to what had been budgeted.
- Productive hours were higher than budgeted for the month (5,759) and year-to-date (28,469) as well.
- PTO was over by 7.2 percent for the month but 1.0 percent lower than budgeted year-to-date.
- Overtime was less than budgeted.
- Education/orientation hours/and other hours such as on-call were over for the month but under year-to-date.
- The total man-hours for the month were 6.9 percent greater than that budgeted for the month.
- The man-hours were 3.1 percent greater than budgeted year-to-date.
- The FTEs are based on conversion of the man-hours worked into FTEs (2,080 hours per year = 1.0 FTE).

Salary Budget

Salaries are normally the largest expense for a cost center. Salaries are broken down into the same categories as man-hours. The percentage of variance in salaries will not only reflect the number of man-hours used to care for a particular volume of patients, but also will reflect the mix of staff providing that care, such as RN, LPN, Nursing Assistant or Patient Care Technician, and Unit Clerk. Salaries for the department usually include the Unit Manager. If Nursing Education is decentralized, it may include a nursing educator for the unit. If the unit has a Clinical Nurse Specialist, that salary may be charged to the unit, as well.

In **Exhibit 12–6**, productive salaries are higher for the month ($85,670) than budgeted ($76,243) with the variance percentage being 12.4 percent over budget for the month. The same is true YTD ($424,059 actual against a budget of $381,320 and 11.2 percent over budget).

Exhibit 12–6 Example of a Monthly Report of Salaries for a Surgical Nursing Unit

Department Salary Report
For the period ending 11/30/200_
Main 7

| *MONTH* | | | | | *YTD* | | | |
Actual	Budget	Var%	Prior	SALARY EXPENSE	Actual	Budget	Var%	Prior
85,670	76,243	(12.4)%	80,107	**SALARIES PRODUCTIVE**	424,059	381,320	(11.2)%	399,027
9,125	7,601	(20)%	8,567	**PTO**	43,208	38,826	(11.3)%	42,621
4,547	6,701	32.1%	9,611	**SALARIES OVERTIME**	22,283	34,237	34.9%	42,610
18,319	8,734	(109.7)%	13,939	**CONTRACT SALARIES**	95,318	43,670	(118.3)%	15,357
900	2,070	56.5%	251	**SALARY/LUMP - SUM/RETENT**	1,982	5,988	66.9%	3,251
8,279	9,184	9.9%	7,119	**ED/ORIENT/ ON-CALL/ETC**	39,699	46,838	15.2%	48,424
126,840	110,533	(14.8)%	119,594	**TOTAL SALARY EXPENSE**	626,549	550,879	(13.7)%	551,290

Note in this example:

- PTO salary is 20 percent higher for the month ($9,125 actual against a budget of $7,601) and 11.3 percent higher YTD ($43,208 actual against a budget of $38,826) reflecting the additional PTO earned for the hours worked above budget.
- Overtime is under budget by 32.1 percent for the month ($4,547 actual against a budget of $6,701). YTD overtime is under budget by 34.9 percent ($22,283 against a budget of $34,237).

- The ratio difference between the variance percent of contracted man-hours to budget for the month of 9.2 percent in **Exhibit 12–5** is very different from the variance percentage of contracted salary-to-budget for the month of 109.7 percent in **Exhibit 12–6**. This reflects the extremely high cost of contracted labor. This will be explored further in this chapter when variance analysis and variance reporting are discussed.
- The salary–lump sum/retention is 56.5 percent below budget for the month ($900 actual against a budget of $2,070) and 66.9 percent under budget YTD ($1,982 against a budget of $5,988). This could reflect less use of this benefit by the staff in filled positions, or it could reflect open positions.
- Education/orientation/on-call/etc. is under budget for the month by 9.9 percent ($8,279 against a budget of $9,184) and under budget YTD by 15.2 percent ($39,699 against a budget of $46,838). This could reflect less orientation and/or less regular staff able to use the education dollars budgeted for the unit.

The percentages of the total salary expense line compared to the total units line (in **Exhibit 12–2**) can provide a "big picture" view to determine if your use of staff is in line with the volume of patients cared for during the month and YTD. In this case for the month, Main 7 was 12.1 percent above budget on volume of patients (from **Exhibit 12–2**); while salary expense was 14.8 percent greater than budget. YTD Main 7 was 9 percent above the budget for volume of patients but 13.7 percent over budget for salary expense.

When budgeting for the year, you should calculate each expense line based on one unit of service. This budget often is based on the cost per unit of service for the same expense line item from the previous year, plus information about changes that would impact that item. For example:

> *if last year the total cost of productive salaries were $941,757 to care for 8,488 patient days, the cost per patient day was $941,757 divided by 8,488 = $110.95 per patient day.*

> *$941,757 Total Productive Salary Cost ÷ 8,488 patient days = $110.95 per patient day.*

If this year it is anticipated that salaries will increase 3 percent, and that staffing mix and hours of care per patient day will remain the same, the expectation is that the productive salary per patient day will be 3 percent higher than last year or $110.95 X 1.03 = $114.28 per patient day. This becomes an indicator to use each month as you evaluate your costs.

In this specific instance:

> *$110,533 budgeted salary expense for the month ÷ 669 budgeted units for the month = $165.22 budgeted per patient day (from Exhibit 12–2).*
>
> *$126,840 actual salary expense for the month ÷ 750 actual units for the month = $169.12 actual expense per patient day (from Exhibit 12–2).*
>
> *$165.22 budgeted per patient day - $169.12 actual expense per patient day = - $3.90*
>
> *The negative number means that it actually cost $3.90 more per patient day than had*

The same can be done YTD:

> *$550,879 budgeted salary expense YTD ÷ 3,422 budgeted units YTD =*
>   *$160.98 budgeted per patient day*
>
> *$626,549 actual salary expense YTD ÷ 3,730 actual units YTD =*
>   *$167.98 actual expense per patient day*
>
> *$160.98 budgeted per patient day - $167.98 actual expense per patient day = - $7.00*
>
> *So it actually cost $7.00 more per patient day than had been budgeted YTD.*

This tells me that so far this year it has cost an additional $7.00 per patient day for salary above what was budgeted to care for patients on Main 7.

However, during the current month the $7.00 per patient day has been reduced to an overage of $3.90 per patient day. While not back to the budgeted salary expense, the salary expense to care for patients on Main 7 is improving from that experienced in previous months.

Benefit Expense

Benefit expense includes retirement, group health, flex benefits, and FICA. See **Exhibit 12–7**. Group health is the employers' portion of the cost for health insurance that can include dental, vision, life insurance, and disability. Flex benefits can be called many things. This can include special benefits such as dollars returned to employees who maintain specified health habits and physical parameters as an incentive to reduce health insurance costs. FICA stands for Federal Insurance Contribution Act. That is the law that covers Social Security and Medicare. The employer is responsible to pay half of the bill for the employee and it is charged to your department. Keep in mind that since FICA is based on earned income, if your salary budget is over or under budget, FICA will be over or under budget, as well.

Non-Salary Expenses

Non-salary expenses can include, but are not limited to: purchased professional services, patient non-chargeable supplies, instruments, implants, IV solutions, drugs, medical supplies, food service, department supplies, forms and paper, minor equipment, freight, maintenance contracts, repairs, equipment rental, dues and memberships, certification and re-certification, books and publications, and travel.

Purchased professional services can include fees paid to physicians contracted to provide services. This could include fees for medical director administrative services such as those paid to the medical head of a psychiatric department. It can also cover fees paid to other professionals who are not employees but who provide services where the hospital both submits charges and receives the reimbursement. An example would be for a

Exhibit 12–7 Example of a Monthly Report of Benefits for a Surgical Nursing Unit

Department Benefits Report
For the period ending 11/30/200_
Main 7

| | MONTH | | | | | YTD | | |
Actual	Budget	Var %	Prior	Benefit Expense	Actual	Budget	Var %	Prior
4,104	2,674	(53.5)%	3,011	**Retirement**	18,655	13,535	(37.8)%	15,212
10,342	11,533	10.3%	14,112	**Group Health**	51,174	58,551	12.6%	65,960
1,297	1,022	(26.9)%	1,007	**Flex Benefits**	6,977	5,172	(34.9)%	5,092
6,778	5,800	(16.9)%	6,325	**FICA/Taxes**	32,078	29,353	(9.3)%	32,099
22,521	21,029	(7.1)%	24,455	**Total Benefits**	108,884	106,611	(2.1)%	118,363

contracted group of psychologists who provide services to patients where the hospital bills for those services and keeps the revenue. There can also be purchased professional services paid to a physician specialty in short supply that does not receive adequate reimbursement for the services they provide. If these services are critical to the operation of the hospital, the hospital can, using fair market value to ensure compliance with legal parameters, provide a level of compensation in addition to what that specialty collects for billed services. Frequently Anesthesiologists are compensated in this manner in addition to what they bill and collect. This charge is usually budgeted under the Anesthesia cost center.

Patient non-chargeable supplies include items that are necessary to care for the patient but are items that cannot be charged directly to the patient. This includes items such as admission kits and syringes. It is important to know which supplies can be charged to the patient and which can not. Usually chargeable items have stickers or bar codes indicating that they can be charged to the patient.

The *instrument expense* can be very large in an operating room based on the cost of reusable instruments that wear out and require replacement on a regular basis. This would not be the case on a medical-surgical unit.

Implants can be a very large expense for items in the operating room such as joints for total knee and hip replacements, or for the cost of cardiac stents in a cardiac catheterization lab. This cost has become an even greater issue with the higher cost of drug-eluding stents.

IV solutions may be expensed to the department or may be expensed to the pharmacy. Usually IV solutions without medications added are expensed directly to the nursing units. IV solutions with medications added are usually expensed to the pharmacy.

Drugs are usually charged to the nursing unit only when patient charges have not been made, and when floor stock is used. The same occurs with medical supplies.

Be very aware of the expense your unit incurs for lost charges. That is, if patient chargeable items such as drugs or supplies like catherization kits are not charged to the patient, when the drug or kit is replaced, it is charged to the unit. If the staff is not careful about entering charges for patient chargeable supplies, expensive and unnecessary costs occur. More and more organizations have invested in drug and supply vending equipment that requires patient data to be entered before the door can be opened to get the drug or supply. This results in automatic charging of the item as well as providing automatic data to ensure inventory replacement to maintain par levels in the drug and supply vending machines.

Food service is not patient meals. It includes those items that are stocked on the nursing unit for patient use in addition to meals. This includes such items as sodas, crackers, sandwiches, and fruit. This is an item to watch carefully. If your kitchen is very easily accessed, visitors may be consuming food for patients. Although staff is usually aware that the food is for patients, staff may consume these as well. If you have special celebrations on your unit and have the dietary department provide the food, the cost of the food will be expensed to this sub-account.

Department supplies include office supplies such as ink cartridges for the printers, pens, and pencils. It also includes hand soap, paper towels, and other items that are necessary to care for patients but are not used specifically on a patient.

Forms and paper can be a significant expense. In departments such as OB there may be use of copyrighted nursing documentation forms from an outside vendor. Pre-printed physician orders and clinical pathways will need to be updated as evidenced-based practice changes and the forms must be changed to match. When policies change, the forms documenting the activity affected by those policies must be changed to match the new policies. Old printed forms may be wasted, or the organization may choose to wait months while stockpiles of the old forms are used before implementing the new policies. At the same time, the set up and printing of new forms can be a significant cost. Many organizations are moving to computerization of their forms and have put the forms online to be printed as needed. The forms are updated without waste of paper.

Minor equipment includes equipment that costs less than the level set by the organization to capitalize the equipment. It can include items such as opthalmascopes, video equipment, sphygmomanometers, and chairs. It is important to know when budgeting if the items you anticipate replacing or purchasing fall into minor equipment or capital purchases. It is not unusual to find that an item with a cost close to the line between minor equipment and capital that was put into the capital budget ends up costing less than anticipated. If it falls below the line for capital, it goes into the minor equipment sub-account even though not budgeted for it.

Dues and memberships include those dues and memberships that are paid for by the organization. An example is payment for the manager of an OR to belong to the local, state, and/or national AORN.

Books and publications include PDRs, other drug references, textbooks, and journals specific to the nursing care provided on the specific unit. Computer-based learning programs may also be included in this category.

Travel is a non-salary expense that can vary widely. This line item covers all of the expenses incurred when staff travels to educational programs, and includes airfare, car rental, hotel, and food. It also includes reimbursement for mileage when staff travels between locations on the job such as to meeting at another hospital within a system. In Home Care this can be a very expensive line item, because staff drive between patients' homes. It is very important in Home Care to teach staff to set up their route for patient visits on a given day based not only on services tied to specific times such as drawing fasting blood sugars, but also on the proximity of patient homes. Unnecessary mileage can be cut and staff productivity is raised by shortening the time spent driving between patients.

Other expense is a line item (sub-account) that should be used as little as possible and only when the item does not fit the description of any other sub-account. Most non-salary expenses will fit into one of the other line items and should have been budgeted accordingly. Expense charges to your department should be reviewed for accuracy. If a charge that was budgeted in one sub-account is charged to another sub-account, it is important to recognize and put the item into the correct sub-account. Otherwise one sub-account may appear under budget while another appears over budget. Also be sure that all charges to your department belong to your department. Many people enter charges to your department and errors can easily happen. By identifying and reporting errors, credits are made, and should be noted on the report the following month. Keep track of this month-to-month when reviewing your reports to ensure that credits have been posted properly.

Freight may or may not be a line item that is allocated to the nursing unit. Freight charges can be minimized with appropriate planning. The operating room, for example, may have high freight costs if needs are not well anticipated. Overnight charges for implants or supplies significantly increases the cost of freight. Some organizations expense freight directly to the nursing unit that special orders or uses an item. Some allocate freight charges according to a predetermined percentage of total charges to specific nursing units. Others keep freight charges as a single item in the purchasing department budget and charge it accordingly. Ask how freight charges are handled in your organization so that you will know how to respond to the data.

In **Exhibit 12–8**:

- *No purchased professional* services were budgeted or used by Main 7 during the month. However, YTD $250 was actually charged to this sub-account in a previous month although no money was budgeted for this purpose.
- The *patient non-chargeable* sub-account was over for the month by 160.9 percent. The actual YTD expense was $30,934 against a budget of $11,858. YTD this sub-account was over by 52.4 percent. The actual expense was $92,458 against a budget of $60,656.
- The sub-account for *drugs* was 100 percent positive for the month as no expenses were charged to the sub-account and $32 was budgeted. The same is true for YTD with no expenses charged to the sub-account but $165 was budgeted.
- *Food Service* was over budget for the month by 23.4 percent. Actual expense was $975 against a budget of $790. YTD Food Service was over budget by 21.8 percent. Actual expense was $5,252 although $4,313 was budgeted.
- *Medical Supplies*, like Drugs, was 100 percent positive for the month. No expenses were charged against the account although $68 was budgeted. YTD Medical Supplies was also 100 percent positive. No expenses where charged to the account but $349 was budgeted.
- *Department Supplies* were over budget for the month by 9.2 percent. The actual expense for the month was $2,038 against a budget of $1,866. YTD Department Supplies is 1.3 percent over budget with an actual expense of $9,668 against a budget of $9,546.

Exhibit 12–8 Example of a Monthly Report of Non-Salary Expense for a Surgical
Nursing Unit

Department Non-Salary Expense Report
For the period ending 11/30/200_
Main 7

| | *MONTH* | | | | | *YTD* | | |
Actual	Budget	Var %	Prior	NonSalary Expense	Actual	Budget	Var %	Prior
0	0	0.0%	0	**Purchase Professional**	250	0	0.0%	0
30,934	11,858	(160.9)%	14,338	**Patient Non Chargeable**	92,458	60,656	(52.4)%	59,995
0	32	(100.0)%	0	**Drugs**	0	165	100.0%	0
975	790	(23.4)%	1,068	**Food Service**	5,252	4,313	(21.8)%	4,736
0	68	100.0%	0	**Medical Supplies**	0	349	100.0%	0
2,038	1,866	(9.2)%	2,472	**Department Supplies**	9,668	9,546	(1.3)%	6,429
197	245	19.6%	264	**Forms and Paper**	1,024	1,254	18.3%	1,204
959	1,134	15.4%	47	**Minor Equipment**	5,148	5,670	9.2%	1,529
0	216	100.0%	0	**Equipment Rental**	0	1,080	100.0%	0
0	1	100.0%	0	**Dues & Membership**	0	5	100.0%	0
136	46	(195.7)%	0	**Books & Publications**	225	46	(389.1)%	40
228	207	(10.1)%	470	**Travel**	567	1,058	46.4%	1,325
0	82	100.0%	0	**Other Expenses**	0	410	100.0%	37
35,467	16,545	(114.4)%	18,659	**Total Non-Salary Expense**	114,592	84,552	(35.5)%	75,295

- *Forms and Paper* was under the budget for the month by 19.6 percent. The actual expense was $197 against a budget of $245. YTD Forms and Paper is under budget by 18.3 percent. Actual expense was $1,024 against a budget of $1,254.
- *Minor Equipment* is under budget for the month by 15.4 percent. The actual expense for the month was $959 against a budget of $1,134. YTD Minor Equipment is under budget by 9.2 percent with actual expense of $5,148 against a budget of $5,670.
- *Equipment Rental* was 100 percent positive to budget for the month with no expenses charged against a budget of $216. YTD was also 100 percent positive with no expense charged against a budget of $1,080.
- *Dues and Memberships* was 100 percent positive to budget for the month with no expense charged to a budget of $1. YTD the budget is also 100 percent positive with no expense against a budget of $5.
- *Books and Publications* was 195.7 percent over budget for the month due to the expense of $136 against a budget of $46. YTD Books and Publications is 389.1 percent over budget with the expense of $225 against a budget of $46.

- *Travel* is over budget by 10.1 percent for the month due to the expense of $228 against a budget of $207. YTD Travel is under budget by 46.4 percent with the actual expense of $567 against a budget of $1,058.
- *Other Expense* is 100 percent positive for the month with no expense charged against a budget of $82. YTD Other Expenses is also 100 percent positive with no expense charged against a budget of $410.

The *total* of Salary (**Exhibit 12–6**), Benefit (**Exhibit 12–7**), and Non-Salary (**Exhibit 12–8**) expenses is listed below the expense budgets as follows in **Exhibit 12–9**:

Exhibit 12–9 Total Monthly Salary and Non-Salary Expenses for a Surgical Nursing Unit

Total Department Expense Report
For the period ending 11/30/200_
Main 7

| | MONTH | | | | | YTD | | |
Actual	Budget	Var %	Prior	Total Expense	Actual	Budget	Var %	Prior
126,840	110,533	(14.8)%	119,594	**Total Salary Expense**	626,549	550,879	(13.7)%	551,290
22,521	21,029	(7.1)%	24,455	**Total Benefits**	108,884	106,611	(2.1)%	118,363
35,467	16,545	(114.4)%	18,659	**Total Non-Salary Expense**	114,592	84,552	(35.5)%	75,295
184,828	148,107	(24.8)%	162,708	**Total Expenses**	850,025	742,042	(14.6)%	744,948

Note in review of the sub-accounts under Non Salary Expense that one line item, patient non-chargeables, accounts for almost all of the budget overage both for the month and YTD. As with the total salary expense line, to get the "big picture" of non-salary expense, the total non-salary expense line should be compared to the total units line for both the month and YTD. In this case Main 7 was 12.1 percent (**Exhibit 12–2**) above budget due to volume of patients for the month. Total non-salary expense was up 114.4 percent for the month. YTD Main 7 was 9 percent above the budget for volume of patients and 35.5 percent above budget for total non-salary expense. This sounds terrible! However, before coming to this conclusion, further analysis is needed.

The *budgeted* non-salary expense per unit of service is the total budgeted non-salary expense for the month ($16,545) divided by the budgeted total units for the month (669 from **Exhibit 12–2**) = $24.73 per patient day. The *actual* total non-salary expense YTD ($35,467) divided by the actual total units YTD (750 from **Exhibit 12–2**) = $47.29 per patient day. The difference between the budgeted non-salary expense per unit for the month ($24.73) and the actual ($47.29) is $22.56.

This is quite a significant overage and will require appropriate analysis. The budgeted non-salary expense YTD ($84,552) divided by the budgeted YTD total units (3,422) =

> $16,545 (budgeted total non-salary expense for the month)
>   ÷ 669 (budgeted total units for the month)
>   = $24.73 per patient day
>
> $35,467 (actual total non-salary expense for the month)
>   ÷ 750 (actual total units for the month)
>   = $47.29 per patient day
>
> $24.73 (per patient day) - $47.29(per patient day)
>   = - $22.56 per patient day
>
> **So the non-salary expense is significantly over at $22.56 per day more than what was budgeted.**

$24.71. The actual total non-salary expense YTD ($114,592) divided by the actual total units YTD (3,730) = $30.72 per patient day. The difference between the budgeted non-salary expense per unit YTD ($24.71) and the actual YTD ($30.72) = $6.01 per patient day.

> $84,552 budgeted non-salary expense YTD
>   ÷ 3,422 budgeted YTD total units
>   = $24.71 per patient day
>
> $114,592 actual total non-salary expense YTD
>   ÷ 3,730 actual total units YTD
>   = $30.72 per patient day
>
> $24.71 per patient day - $30.72 per patient day
>   = $6.01 per patient day

This tells us that the $22.56 non-salary budget problem for the month is atypical since YTD the overage per patient day is $6.01. While not as significant as the problem for the month, it still requires understanding and a plan for correction if at all possible.

Variance Analysis

Variance analysis includes finding all of the pieces of the puzzle, putting them together, and understanding what the data is telling you about your operations. The pieces of the puzzle include all of the various reports that you are sent by the Finance, Materials Management, and Human Resources departments, as well as unit specific reports of daily or weekly activity that you create and track. These reports are uniquely named by the organization but include specific types of information. From Finance you should receive a monthly *Distribution Register*. This lists accounts payable payments made for your department. This can include items charged to your department by personnel in your department as well as from personnel in other departments. For instance, supplies required to repair broken equipment on your unit may be charged to your department by facilities management.

It is important to communicate effectively with support departments so that there are no surprises on this report. It will also save you time when preparing your variance report if you have made note during the month of special charges that will appear on your departments' report.

An *Accounts Payable Accrued But Not Invoiced Report* identifies items received on a purchase order but have not yet been invoiced. An example would be dollars you anticipate to be billed for "traveler" agency staff used during the month. Why not just wait until the bill arrives next month and explain it then? The reason is that you want to link expenses as closely as possible to what happened during the time frame that your variance report covers, which is this particular month. If you know that during the month you will be using 160 hours of "traveler" agency RN staff because of increased patient volume and open RN staff positions, you want the expense for that to show in the month where it happened. If you wait until the bill comes the following month and the volume is down during the following month, or you have filled the positions and are not using agency staff during the following month, it is much harder to reconcile and justify the expenses that appear to belong in that following month. It is better to tell Finance to accrue for the services you estimate will be used during the current month. When the actual bill arrives, it will be applied against what was accrued and already be explained.

A *Revenue and Usage Report* identifies charges by financial class and charge code. *Financial class* tells us if the patients were Medicare, Medicaid, Private Insurance, or Self Pay. *Charge code* tells us how many charges were made for specific services. In the case of a surgical unit, there should be charges for admitted patient days and observation patient days. In Surgery there will be charges for the initial minimum time for using an operating room.

Additional charges under a different code will show for additional increments of time beyond the basic charge. It is important to review this to see that it matches the activity in your department. If on a surgical nursing unit you know that you had 15 observation days but no charges show for those days, you will want to follow-up to determine why those charges did not get posted. These become lost charges unless caught before the patient bill is completed and sent out by Finance. It is important to find out from your Finance Department how many days post patient discharge late charges can be added so that the charges are not lost. Lost charges can be minimized if the Daily Department Log is reviewed on a daily basis and reconciled.

The *Daily Department Log* is an excellent tool to ensure that input errors are rectified before a patient's bill is completed. By reviewing this log you can tell if a patient in OB was charged for ten deliveries instead of one. Likewise, if you review the Daily Department Log against the log showing births, there is an opportunity to identify lost charges for a delivery that occurred in the last 24 hours that does not appear on the Daily Department Log. The charges can then be input within a timeframe that allows for capture.

The *Period Inventory Expense Report* lists expenses from Material Management. This is an important report to review to determine both if supplies are being used effectively, and if your unit was charged appropriately for what was ordered. If you note an increase in the number of intravenous catheters being used per patient day, you will want to investigate.

Do you have a bad lot of IV catheters resulting in multiple attempts by staff to start IVs? Did the hospital just change to a new safety IV catheter and the staff is in a learning curve? Did you order a certain number of boxes of IV catheters and got charged for that number of cases of IV catheters rather than boxes? Unless someone is checking this report, the problem would go unnoticed. By noting and investigating, you not only explain the variance, but prevent it from continuing. If it is a bad lot, Material Management may be able to get free replacements. If it is a change in product and a learning curve, select staff members may need re-education. If it is a charge for cases rather than boxes, and it is reported, you will receive a credit for it the following month bringing your year-to-date into line.

Payroll reports are bi-weekly reports that reflect hours by type being paid to each employee. These should reflect the hours worked by staff and should match the daily staffing plan actually worked. Regular hours, overtime hours, shift differential, education hours, and paid time off should be listed for each employee. Any special pay-by-type should appear as well. This could be added pay for being a preceptor for new employees, or other unique special pay categories. If you use an automated system for clocking in and out, you may receive individual employee reports from that system which allow you to make manual corrections prior to payroll being cut. Review of this data can identify if staff did not clock in or out appropriate to the hours the worked-unit-staffing plan reflects. It can also identify other errors that can be corrected to accurately reflect staff worked, or productive time. Recognize that bi-weekly reports do not exactly match to the hours worked, and charged, to a department during a given month.

For instance, as shown in **Exhibit 12–10**, if your work week is Sunday through Saturday, and the month begins on Monday of the second week of a pay period, that pay period will include eight days from the previous month as well as the first six days of the current month. The 7th through the 20th will make up the next bi-weekly report. If it is a 30-day month, the 21st through the 4th of the following month will make up the next bi-weekly report.

Exhibit 12–10 Calendar for Sample Month

Sun	Mon	Tues	Wed	Thurs	Fri	Sat
31	1	2	3	4	5	6
7	8	9	10	11	12	13
14	15	16	17	18	19	20
21	22	23	24	25	26	27
28	29	30	1	2	3	4

How then can you compare these reports to the hours and dollars charged to your department for the month? You can't. The important work is to assure that the hours and dollars charged to your department each pay period are accurate. Finance accrues expenses for the days that have not been covered in the current month, and reverses them the next month.

The important information to know is how the hours and dollars charged to your department for the full month compare to budget. If you are watching the bi-weekly reports closely, you will not have many surprises.

Unit Productivity Reports are important to watch, as well. Many organizations use national productivity products that compare the productivity of hospital departments to those in comparable hospitals throughout the country. It is crucial to ensure that the specific operations of your department are specified when building the base of organizations for comparison. If your surgical unit cares for orthopedic patients be sure to identify the type (orthopedics) to determine your comparison group. That is, if your unit cares for patients post-joint replacement and post-spine surgery, you will want to know that the base of hospital nursing departments that you are being compared to care for the same type of patients. If they care for some post-joint replacement, general surgery patients, and no spine surgery patients, the comparison may not be valid. You may have some unique differences that need to be added to the equation to have a valid comparison. For example, if your department includes a decentralized nurse educator, add it to the equation. The comparison groups may not have that position in their departments. Also determine if the productivity tool includes all man-hours, or if education and orientation hours are excluded. Once you have validated that your comparison groups are comparable, this becomes a very helpful tool for benchmarking.

National comparative productivity tools normally report data in quartiles of productivity. The budget should reflect the FTEs the hospital expects to be achieved for the quartile of productivity. For example, the FTEs budgeted for Main 7 are set for the 50th percentile of productivity compared to other comparative hospital units throughout the country. The staffing patterns scheduled should reflect that required to meet the productivity levels budgeted. One of the benefits of using a national productivity tool is that you have the ability to contact staff at other hospitals in your comparison group to network for ideas to improve productivity.

Turning to **Exhibit 12–11**, let's examine productivity measurement:

Exhibit 12–11 Example of a Monthly Comparison of Actual Productivity Performance to Comparative Midpoints for Actual Volumes Report

Main 7
Productivity

Name	Vol	Paid FTE Month	Paid FTE YTD	Mid	Actual Month	Actual YTD	Ed/Or % YTD	FTE Month	FTE YTD	Prod Index Month	Prod Index YTD
Main 7	750	44.86	43.24	8.791	8.393	8.425	9%	(2.2)	(1.9)	104.7	104.3

Note that:
- The volume corresponds to the actual patient days identified for the month for Main 7 in **Exhibit 12–2**.

- The paid FTEs of 44.86 for the month, and 43.24 for year-to-date correspond to **Exhibit 12–5**. Productive man-hours include man-hours contract (344) + man-hours productive (5,759) + man-hours overtime (192) = total productive man-hours (6,295).
- "Mid" stands for the comparative midpoint of productive hours/unit of service for the 50th percentile for comparative hospitals, derived from the national productivity tool.
- The actual productive hours/unit of service for the month were total productive man-hours (6,295) ÷ total volume (750) = 8.393. This is lower than the national midpoint.
- The actual productive hours/unit of service YTD were 8.425, also below the national comparative goal of 8.791 hours/unit of service.
- The 9 percent for Education/Orientation hours and earned PTO hours has been extrapolated from those identified as productive as these hours are not direct patient care hours.
- The next column reflects FTE variance from the comparative midpoint for the month of (2.2). This means that 2.2 less FTEs were utilized to provide direct patient care based on the units of service than the goal for the month.
- The next column reflects FTE variance from the comparative midpoint YTD of (1.9). This means that 1.9 less FTEs have been used to provide direct patient care based on units of service than expected YTD.
- The Productivity Index for the month shows that the staff worked at a productivity level of 104.7 percent compared to similar hospitals, and 104.3 percent YTD. The Productivity Index is calculated by dividing the national midpoint (8.791) by the actual productivity for the month (8.393) = 104.7 percent.

From a financial standpoint this is a very positive level of productivity both for the month and YTD. Review of patient satisfaction data and other quality data for the unit will reflect if this level of productivity is positive from a quality standpoint, as well.

If you do not use a national productivity tool to compare your department to others, then compare your monthly productivity to your budget by determining your budgeted and actual hours of care per patient day:

1. Subtract from the total man-hours those hours that are not for direct patient care. This would include PTO, education, and orientation.
2. Then divide the man-hour number by the total budgeted units of service.

Now we will give an example comparing actual to budget. This example will use the information for the month from **Exhibit 12–2** and **Exhibit 12–5**:

Use your productivity data to understand your variance. If your productivity was less than budgeted for the month, determine the reason. Did you have many staff in orientation but did not get their hours posted to the education sub-account? This would result in education hours being allocated to productive hours. Did you have many days with volumes that forced staffing to minimum levels? An example would be an oncology unit with a census of only four patients for five days. For patient safety it still required that two staff members be present on each shift, thereby resulting in a much higher number of hours of care per patient day than required for care of oncology patients. Understanding this data will help you to not only create the variance report for the month, but also will help you and your staff identify areas to explore for changes to improve productivity while ensuring quality of care.

> *Budgeted hours for PTO (570) + Budgeted hours for Ed/Orient (750) = 1,320.*
>
> *Total budgeted man-hours for the month is 7,172 - 1,320 (PTO/Ed/Orient)*
> *= 5,852 (direct patient care hours for the month).*
>
> *The total budgeted units of service for the month are 669 patient days.*
>
> *Divide the total budgeted direct patient care hours (5,852) by the total budgeted*
> *units of service (669) = 8.75 budgeted hours of care per patient day.*
>
> *Compare budgeted hours of care per patient day to actual hours of care per patient day.*
>
> *Actual hours for PTO (611) + actual hours for Ed/Orient (764) = 1,375.*
>
> *Total actual man-hours for the month is 7,670 - 1,375 (PTO/Ed/Orient)*
> *= 6,295 (direct patient care hours for the month).*
>
> *The total units of service for the month are 750 patient days.*
>
> *Divide the total direct patient care hours (6,295) by the total units of service (750)*
> *= 8.39 hours of care per patient day.*
>
> *Then subtract the actual hours of care per patient day from the budgeted*
> *hours of care per patient day (8.75 - 8.39 = 0.36).*
>
> *This is less hours of care per patient day than budgeted so it becomes a positive*
> *variance.*

Variance Report

The variance report is a summary of the major exceptions to the budget that are experienced during a given time frame and an explanation of why the exceptions occurred. Most organizations expect these reports on a monthly basis. This important report identifies opportunities to understand and control the exceptions, or variances to the budget. It is important not only for the manager to understand but also for the manager to help staff understand and become a part in controlling costs. Managers can use the monthly variance data to involve staff in identifying and planning the activities needed to make mid-stream corrections.

In order to focus on the items of most importance, only those variances that are large are noted in the report. You need to know what level of variance is expected to be included in your report. For purposes of this chapter, a variance of at least 10 percent for statistics and man-hours, and at least 10 percent and greater than $1,000 for the month for each line item reflecting dollars, will be included in the report. YTD information is only referenced to note overall trends for those variances reported on for the month. As a rule, review of the "total" line under each large category such as "Total Salary Expense" or "Total Non Salary Expense" will give you an idea as to the significance of that area's impact on the budget. Line-by-line review will point to specific areas for focused analysis.

Statistics

Refer to **Exhibit 12–2** on page 483. The actual volume of inpatient days for the month (735) was 12.2 percent above the budget (655), with the total patient days (750) 12.1 percent above the budgeted total patient days (669). This is data that you will use in your report to explain variance based on volume. In review of YTD data, actual inpatient days is above budget by 9.2 percent with YTD total units up 9.0 percent. In analysis it is determined that the addition of a new orthopedic surgeon has increased the volume of surgeries while the other surgeons are experiencing the number of surgeries expected from them. However, since the new surgeon started practicing at the hospital only three months before and has been increasing volume each month, this trend should be noted with a plan to ensure adequate staffing anticipating additional volume throughout the remainder of the fiscal year.

Revenue

Revenue, in ratio to the volume statistics, is also above budget. This information will also be used to explain variance for overages in specific line items that are related to the volume and subsequent revenue. Referring to **Exhibit 12–3**, the total inpatient revenue for the month of $355,501 is higher than the budgeted inpatient revenue of $318,724. Budgeted charges for Main 7 inpatient days can be determined by dividing the budgeted dollars ($318,724) by the budgeted volume (669) = $486.60. The same can be done for observation day charges. Budgeted charges for observations days are $5,860 ÷ 14 = $418.57. Admitted patient days are paid at a higher rate than observation days. Therefore, the higher volume in admitted patient days, and one less observation day than budgeted, results in positive revenue for the month of 11.2%, or actual ($360,970)—budget ($324,584) = $36,386. YTD revenue is up 9.5% from budget, or actual ($1,818,272)—budget ($1,660,526) = $157,746. There is a positive variance in revenue both for the month and YTD based on volume.

Man-Hours

Analysis of man-hours without analysis of salary expense information can be deceiving. In the example in **Exhibit 12–5**, the only variance significant enough to report is overtime, which is down 28.9 percent. That appears very positive. Overtime hours for the month were down by 78 hours from those budgeted (budget 270 – actual 192 = 78). Contracted man-hours were over only 9.2 percent, not enough to be reported. Contracted hours were over by 29 hours (actual 344 – budget 315 = 29). Productive man-hours were over only 9.3 percent, or 492 hours, (actual 5,759 – budget 5,267 = 492). PTO was over only 7.2 percent, or 41 hours, (actual 611 – budget 570 = 41). Education and orientation hours were above budget by only 1.9 percent, or 14 hours, (actual 764 – budget 750 = 14). The total man-hours were up only 6.9 percent reflecting 498 hours (actual 7,670 – budget 7,172 = 498). The total volume was up by 12.1 percent. The trend YTD is similar with total man-hours above budget by only 3.1 percent while total units is above budget by 9 percent. This looks very positive, but is it?

Salary Expense

This begins the line items to review for reporting purposes on the Monthly Variance Report. Referring to **Exhibit 12–6**, dollars do not correlate in the same ratio to man-hour statistics (**Exhibit 12–5**). Productive man-hours for the month were up by only 9.3 percent. The dollars represented by those man-hours were up 12.4 percent or $9,427 (actual $85,670 – budget $76,243 = $9,427). PTO man-hours were up by only 7.2 percent. The dollars reflecting those man-hours were up 20.0 percent or $1,524 (actual $9,125 – budget $7,601 = $1,524). The salary-lump sum retention was under by 56.5 percent, which sounds positive and very significant. In reality, it amounts positively to only $1,170 (budget $2,070 – actual $900 = $1,170). Education/orientation/on-call was also under budget. That positive variance of 9.9 percent reflects only $905 (budget $9,184 – actual $8,279 = $905).

Now compare the contract man-hour overage which was 9.2 percent and too small to report, to the contract salary variance of 109.7 percent. This significantly reflects the high cost of contract labor. The 29 hours over budget for contract labor resulted in a negative variance of $9,585 (actual $18,319 – budget $8,734 = $9,585). Added together, the positive and negative variances in salary expense result in a negative total salary expense variance of 14.8 percent or $16,307 for the month. This is far worse than the negative 6.9 percent of total man-hours.

To fully understand the variance in salary expense, it should be analyzed by dollars per unit of service. Referring back to the calculations made on page 466, the actual salary expense per patient day was $3.90 more per patient day than what was budgeted. In analysis you note that you have three full-time RN positions and two part-time LPN positions vacant. The good news is that you have hired three full time RNs who will begin orientation in two weeks. Also, because you have involved staff in understanding the negative impact that those open positions have on overtime, part-time RN staff has been wonderful picking up additional hours, thus keeping overtime down. The mix in staffing has changed resulting in RNs covering some of the hours of care per patient day that should have been covered by LPN staff. Contracts are coming to an end for two of the "traveler" contracted RNs that have been covering open positions and they will not be renewed. Given the expectation of continued higher volume of patients than budgeted, it will be important to fill the open part-time LPN positions to get the mix of staff back to that budgeted.

Discussions were held with the nurse recruiter to find two part-time LPNs. While the recruiter currently had no part-time candidates, she had one full time LPN candidate that has experience on a surgical nursing unit. Given the continued high volume and the fact that one LPN currently on staff is in school and wishes to work most weekends to be off for weekday classes, based on staff discussions you determine you could cover the schedule using a full-time LPN. You have scheduled the full-time LPN candidate for an interview. When this plan is fully implemented, the salary expense per unit of service should get back in line with the budget.

A review of Total Salary Expense YTD is similar to that for the month. YTD total salary expense is over 13.7 percent or $105,670 ($626,549 – $550,879 = $105,670). An ongoing review of YTD following implementation of the changes being made will be important. While by the end of the fiscal year you may not be able to get salary expense per unit of service to meet that budgeted, it should improve significantly from that currently experienced.

Benefit Expense

While benefits are an expense borne by the department, managers have little control over them. Retirement, group health, and flex benefits are based on choices that are made by employees. Analysis of benefit expense is useful for future budgeting purposes and to note the impact that it has on the department as a whole.

In **Exhibit 12–7**, the total benefit expense line shows that overall this category has little negative impact on the budget for the month. The variance to budget is a negative 7.1 percent, reflecting a negative dollar impact of only $1,492 (actual $22,521 – budget $21,029 = $1,492). While retirement and group health meet the reporting requirement for a line item by being over or under budget by at least 10 percent and $1,000, there is normally not an expectation that these will be covered in the variance analysis. Retirement is over budget by 53.5 percent, reflecting $1,430 (actual $4,104 – budget $2,674 = $1,430). Group health is under budget by 10.3 percent, reflecting $1,191 (budget $11,533 – $10,342 = $1,191). Flex benefit dollars, while 26.9 percent over budget, amounts to only $275 (actual $1,297 – budget $1,022 = $275). FICA Taxes Hospital portion while over budget by 16.9 percent reflects an overage of only $978. This overage is due to the increase in patient volume and the subsequent increase in taxed dollars paid to staff. The budgeted benefits per unit of service are actually below budget. This is calculated as for other unit of service categories or line items:

> *Budgeted benefits for the month ($21,029) ÷ the budgeted volume (669)*
> *= $31.43/unit of service.*
>
> *Actual benefits for the month ($22,521) ÷ the actual volume (750)*
> *= $30.03/unit of service.*
>
> *So the actual cost per unit of service was down*
> *($31.43 - $30.03 = $1.40) $1.40 per unit of service.*

A quick review of Total Benefit Expense YTD shows that YTD the negative impact of benefits to help absorb the additional hours used to cover the added patient days has been only 2.1 percent or $2,273 (actual $108,884 – budget $106,611 = $2,273).

Non-Salary Expense Analysis

In Exhibit 12–8, Patient Non-Chargeables are over by 160.9 percent for the month, reflecting an overage of $19,076 (actual $30,934 – budget $11,858 = $19,076). What is the difference per unit of service?

> *The budget called for $17.72/unit of service determined by dividing the budgeted dollars ($11,858) by the budgeted volume (669) = $17.72.*
>
> *Actual for the month was $41.25/unit of service*
> *(actual dollars $30,934 ÷ actual volume 750 = $41.25).*

This major difference creates a good point to test if the budget was logical based on prior year data. In review it is found that for the same month prior year there was $21.05/unit of service (prior year month actual dollars $14,338 ÷ prior year month actual volume 681 = $21.05).

To get an even better perspective, you go to the prior year YTD data and do the math:

- The prior year YTD actual dollars spent on patient non chargeables was $59,995.
- Divide this by the prior year YTD actual volume of 3,431 patient days and you find that the prior year YTD average cost/unit of service for patient non chargeables was $17.49.
- The budgeted cost/unit of service of $17.72 was somewhat aggressive considering the usual increase in cost of goods from one year to the next, and considering the prior year average YTD was $17.49, or 23 cents more than that budgeted for the current year.

However, it was known when budgeting that the hospital had engaged a new buying group that committed to reducing the cost of supplies as well as a plan to introduce an automated supply cabinet system.

Looking at recent months (not shown in this chapter), you determine that while the cost had been slightly higher than that budgeted, it was never over the prior year average of $21.03/unit of service. You know that during the month of November your department converted to an automated supply cabinet system that required switching out many patient non-chargeable items. Review of the last Inventory Expense Report from Material Management itemized all of the supplies added, but none of those removed.

A phone call to the director in Material Management finds that the credits, which should amount to $17,547 for those patient non chargeables removed, were not placed in time to be reflected in the November reports. He assures you that the credits will show in December, bringing the cost for patient non chargeables back in line with the budget.

Using this new information you determine what the actual budget should have been if the credits had been placed.

> *The actual for the month ($30,934) - the credits which should have been applied ($17,547) = $13,387.*
>
> *Therefore, the actual cost per unit of service was revised actual ($13,387) ÷ actual volume (750) = $17.85.*

While this is higher than budgeted, all of the changes with the new buying group have not been put into place. Therefore, the total decrease in the cost of goods has not been realized.

There are no other line items that meet the requirements for variance reporting. Armed with the information that you have, you are now ready to complete your monthly variance report for your cost center, Main 7. This will be done on an Excel Spreadsheet. See **Exhibit 12–12**.

Exhibit 12–12 Monthly Variance Report

Month and Year: **2-Nov**

Unit Name: Main 7

Reported by: N. J. Tomlinson

Unit # **7**

Account #	Description	Budget	Actual	Variance	Variance %	Explanation
1	Salaries Productive	$76,243	$85,670	$ (9,427)	-12%	Total Volume over budget by 12.1% (actual 750 - budget 669 = 81). New surgeon providing higher volume.
4	PTO	$7,601	$ 9,125	$ (1,524)	-20%	Additional PTO earned based on additional hours worked mostly by part time staff to cover volume and 3 FT RN & 2 PT LPN open positions.
9	Salaries Overtime	$6,701	$4,547	$ 2,154	32%	OT hours under budget by 28.9% (budget 270 - actual 192 = 78). OT salaries under budget based on 3 FT RN & 2 PT LPN positions being covered by contract labor, relief staff and PT staff increasing man-hours.
10	Contract Salaries	$ 8,734	$ 18,319	$ (9,585)	-110%	Using contract labor due to open positions and volume over 12.1%. Salaries/unit of service are over $3.90 due to use of contract staff. Have filled 3 FT RN positions to start in 2 weeks. Will not renew agency contracts.
	Total Salary Expense	$ 126,840	$ 110,533	$ 119,594	-15%	Productivity is 104.7% for the month & 104.3% YTD. YTD actual salary/unit of service is $7 more than budgeted. However, during the month that has been reduced to an overage of $3.90/unit of service. With filling positions and eliminating contract staff, this should return to budgeted levels.
26	Patient Non Chargeables	$11,858	$ 30,934	$ (19,076)	-161%	Volume up 12.1%. Credits for $17,547 for automated supply cabinet conversion not credited during month. Will be credited next month. With credits, cost/unit of service would have been $17.85. While not on budget, all changes with new buying group not completed.
	Total Non Salary Expense	$35,467	$16,545	$18,659	-114%	With credits the actual cost/unit of service is $17.85 against a budget of $17.72. This should be achieved with use of automated supply cabinet conversion and changes with new buying group.

Summary

The annual budget is based on assumptions based on experiences from the previous year, and what is expected to occur in a given department or cost center during the coming fiscal year. The difference between the budget and what happens is called the *variance*. When you compare the budget to what actually occurred each month and YTD, and analyze the variance, you have powerful data to understand what is happening on your unit. Given the multiple departments that can charge items to a given cost center, it also allows for review and accountability to ensure that items are charged correctly or credited in a timely manner. This also maintains the integrity of the data for future budgeting purposes.

Budget variance analysis that uses a line-item-by-line-item approach to determine cost per unit of service puts the information into an understandable context. It reflects the impact of volume and staff-mix changes, new technology changes, and other variables experienced throughout the year. Translating and sharing that information with unit staff allows for planning and implementation of measures to creatively manage fiscal resources required for excellence in patient care.

CHAPTER 13

Comparing Reimbursements with Cost of Services Provided

Patricia M. Vanhook, MSN, APRN,BC

Introduction

One very important question the nurse manager needs to answer is *whether the overall unit expense budget falls within the reimbursement amount.* The evaluation activity described in this chapter will help the nurse manager to recognize whether a service line is profitable, and to determine areas within the nurse manager's control that will influence profitability. To accomplish this the nurse manager needs to have a clear understanding of the different mechanisms of cost accounting used to reflect both services and reimbursement. This chapter will explain and provide examples of cost and reimbursement for acute care, hospital outpatient, ambulatory surgery, skilled care, and home health. It is imperative the nurse manager be well versed on this topic to understand, and respond appropriately to cost and reimbursement questions generated from the departmental operations reports produced by finance.

Reimbursement

Historical Perspective

Over the past twenty years hospitals, health care agencies, and primary care providers have moved from a cost reimbursement system based on "reasonable costs" (Cleverley, 1997), to a prospective payment system. Before prospective reimbursement, hospitals, home health care, rehabilitation, and skilled nursing facilities were paid retrospectively by total charges billed. This type of reimbursement fostered an environment of financial abuse and did not provide any incentive for health care agencies to control costs (Hoffman, 1984).

Health care costs escalated from $247.2 billion in 1980 to $1.04 trillion in 1995 (Durham, 2000). Van der Walde and Choi (2003) reported hospital care accounted for 31.7 percent of health care expenditures in 2001. Of these expenditures, Medicare and Medicaid accounted for $212 billion (58 percent), and private insurance paid $152 billion (42 percent). Home health care and skilled care costs also sky rocketed as skilled care facilities costs increased by 30 percent per year from 1990 to 1997. Home health[1] became the fastest growing health care industry with expenditures growing from $3.3 billion in 1990 to $18 billion in 1997 (van der Walde and Choi, 2003; van der Walde, and Lindstrom, 2003).

As health care costs soared, the old retrospective cost reimbursement method of payment was abandoned for an alternative method called prospective payment system (PPS). Prospective payment is based on median costs with adjustments made based on the local wage index (Sobun, 1999). Under prospective payment, the agency is paid a set fee regardless of the amount of resources used to provide the service (Division of Health Care Finance and Policy, 1998). This type of payment system creates some financial risk for the agency and keeps costs under control for the insurer, while also providing financial rewards for services provided at a lower cost. Should the agency be able to deliver services under cost and under the PPS reimbursement fee, the difference equates to profit for the agency. However, if services cost more than the reimbursement amount, it would result in a monetary loss. Therefore, prospective payment was an attempt to control rising health care costs through improved efficiency within the health care agency.

Prospective payment began in 1983 when the federal government initiated a calculated reimbursement based on diagnosis-related groups (DRG) for acute care (Sherman, 1994). In the early 1990s private insurers and employers implemented Health Maintenance Organizations (HMOs), Preferred Provider Organizations (PPOs), and Point of Service (POS) plans as additional forms of cost containment, which is further explained in Chapter 6.

As health care costs continued to rise, the federal government, being the largest health care payor, further decreased reimbursement through enactment of the Balanced Budget Act of 1997 (BBA). The BBA had a significant impact on hospitals, home health care, and skilled nursing facilities (Magnus and Smith, 2000; van der Walde and Lindstrom, 2003) because now prospective payment would be implemented in all agencies that cared for Medicare patients. Although hospitals were already under PPS for services other than pediatrics and psychiatry, reimbursement amounts were curtailed further to include all services. In addition, PPS for skilled care was initiated in 1998, implemented for home health in 2000, outpatient hospital services (same day surgery) in 2000, and was implemented in rehabilitation hospitals in 2002 (van der Walde and Choi, 2003).

Payors

Capitation (further explained in Chapter 6) is a mechanism used by insurers to contain costs by establishing a set payment amount for a population served by a defined health care service (Hoffman, 1984). With capitation, rates are negotiated between the provider and

---

[1] The home health industry costs, reported by the Center for Medicare and Medicaid Services (CMS), combined home health care, respiratory care, and infusion services.

the insurer under a contractual agreement for a year (Cleverly, 1997). Reimbursement rates may be for the all services offered, or for one specific service area, called a "carve out", such as laboratory. Within the health care setting, financial administration under a capitation system requires critical financial management and knowledge of the payors.

Thus it is important that the nurse administrator understands the various health care payors to appreciate the diversity of billing and reimbursement methods. The two types of payors for health care services are public and private. Federal and state are public payors, and include Medicare and Medicaid. The insured and uninsured are considered private payors, which are further explained in Chapter 6. Examples of types of private payors include Health Maintenance Organizations (HMOs), Preferred Provider Organizations (PPOs), Point of Service (POS) plans, indemnity, and self pay.

The difference between HMO, PPO, and POS is related to the reimbursement structure. HMOs strive to maintain the health of the participant, and provide "gatekeepers" who must authorize the need for additional services. Reimbursement is a set fee for all the participants of the HMO. The goal of the health care agency is to be the only provider of services for the HMO so it has sufficient numbers of inpatients and outpatients to generate revenue. The PPO is a discounted fee accepted by doctors and hospitals to provide care to participants. A POS establishes a "gatekeeper" to manage and direct care, evaluate the appropriateness of care including diagnostic studies, and either approve, or not approve, reimbursement. Last, indemnity is a traditional insurance plan in which the member pays a premium and must pay a deductible. When the deductible is met, the insurance pays a percentage of the health care expenses. In general there are not provider restrictions with this indemnity (http://ring.com/health/health/health.htm retrieved 11/8/03).

Reimbursement Sources

The majority of reimbursement for health care is governmentally subsidized. The *Acute Care Hospitals: Health Care Industry Market Update* (van der Walde and Choi, 2003) published by the Centers for Medicare and Medicaid Services, indicated 58 percent of hospital reimbursement was either federal or state funded. Private insurance commits 34 percent, and the remaining 8 percent comes from other sources of payment or from the uninsured. The home health or skilled care manager will also note a higher percentage of patients referred to their services that are covered by Medicare and Medicaid as these patient populations continue to be the highest users of acute, skilled, and home health care. Why is this important? It means the government sets the trend for reimbursement for other payors. The nurse administrator must understand the drivers of payment and how this affects the overall revenue for the unit and for the health care organization.

This payment pattern is further complicated because the mechanisms of reimbursement vary between acute care, long-term care, skilled nursing, and home health. Payment to the hospital and a long-term care facility is determined by the reimbursement structure the payor uses. It is important to note skilled care may be performed in a long-term care facility and is reimbursed by Medicare. However, Medicare does not pay for the services of long-term care. The residents' care are reimbursed predominantly by Medicaid and a few private payors (van der Walde and Choi, 2003). Different reimbursement mechanisms for services provided may be based on a per diem (specified daily) rate from private insurance carriers; a negotiated fee from managed care (HMO) or preferred provider organizations (PPOs); a perspective payment system (PPS) by assigned diagnosis-related group (DRG) or resource utilization groups (RUGs) from Medicare; or by the patient who is classified as self pay. Therefore, payment is not standardized and will vary by the type of reimbursement structure. The payment amount can differ within these structures as well. For instance, a different negotiated discount could be given to one PPO versus another PPO. The nurse manager can obtain a break down of payor categories and reimbursement amounts for the patients served from the finance or billing department.

Medicare reimbursement for skilled nursing care is based on PPS by assignment of the patient to one of the 44 RUGs (van der Walde and Choi, 2003). The concept of RUG is that there are conditions that require similar resources and services, and therefore reimbursement can be calculated based on the resources used by the skilled nursing facility patient. Routine services such as room, board, administrative services, nursing care, and therapy services are the three components of the RUG that are summed to determine the reimbursement. In addition, the Centers for Medicare and Medicaid Services do a "market basket analysis"[2] (further explained in Chapter 11) and the reimbursement is adjusted annually based on the inflation of prices of goods and services incurred by the facility (van der Walde and Choi, 2003). Later in the chapter, a case study will be presented to demonstrate how RUGs determine reimbursement.

Medicare payments for home health care ballooned from $3.3 billion in 1990 to $18 billion in 1997 (van der Walde and Lindstrom, 2003). The Balanced Budget Act of 1997 (BBA) was an attempt to counteract the rapid rise in home health care expenditures by reducing payments to the agencies. This caused over 3,000 agencies to close or to merge from 1997 to 2000.

The BBA allowed an incremental transition from fee for service to perspective payment from 1997 to 2000. During the transition to perspective payment home health agencies came under an Interim Payment System (IPS) that capped reimbursement at the 1993–1994 rates (Division of Health Care and Policy, 1998). In October of 2000 the transition to PPS was completed to "stabilize the industry" (van der Walde and Lindstrom, p. 3). Since that time the home health care industry has maintained profitability with some agencies shifting from insured patients under managed care contracts to Medicare, due to higher PPS payments. Van der Walde and Lindstrom (2003) report home health care spending reached $45 billion in 2001; $33 billion of this was directly contributed to home care services and $9 billion to respiratory and infusion care.

Reimbursement for home health varies by service. Each payor has fee schedules for the various visits as well as fee schedules for durable medical equipment (DME), and for respiratory and infusion therapy services. Van der Walde and Lindstrom (2003) report $33.2 billion[3] was spent on home health care in 2001 with 51.2 percent generated from Medicare and Medicaid. Under home health care PPS, reimbursement is determined by the standardized assessment tool, Outcome and ASsessment Information Set (OASIS), or negoti-

---

[2] Market basket is an economic term used to indicate a measure of inflation.

[3] Does not include respiratory care and infusion services.

ated fees from private insurance and HMOs. OASIS is mandated by Medicare. The tool was designed to measure quality of care and to assure appropriate reimbursement (van der Walde and Lindstrom, 2003). Again, under PPS, neither intensity of services nor supplies can be applied as additional charges. Instead the agency must try to maintain costs within the reimbursement schedule. In 2003 each sixty-day episode of home health care received $2,160 base payment per patient from the federal government. In 2004 the fee is increased to $2,230; that represents a $340 million increase in Medicare spending (van der Walde and Lindstrom).

Why do differences in reimbursement exist? Different payors use different strategies for payment of claims. Therefore a health care agency's reimbursement varies according to negotiated contracts and standard fees from Medicare or other insurers. Insurance companies and managed care organizations negotiate reimbursement with health care entities that provide services for their patients. Contracts are established for a period of time and renegotiated by the executive management team at contract end. Increases in cost of care for the patient population during the contract year are usually non-negotiable (Cleverly, 1997). The largest hospital payor, Medicare, reimburses by an assigned diagnosis-related group (DRG) code, or an assigned resource utilization group (RUG), with a fixed dollar amount for all services provided during the hospital, or skilled care stay. Therefore, knowledge of patient and payor mix is essential to understand the variation in reimbursement. Again the nurse manager may automatically receive this information, or may have to request it from the finance department.

Costs

Cleverly (1987) compared the costing of hospital care to that of manufacturing. Consider the patient as the beginnings of a car. The patient progresses through stages beginning with admission to discharge, much as a car begins with a frame and is complete at the end of the assembly line. The patient discharge is the outcome of the hospital stay. This is not to say each and every patient receives the same services, or that each and every disease process is the same. Yet each process contributes to the patient outcome, and must be accounted for, if cost information is to add value to managerial decisions (Cleverly). The nurse manager uses this thought process to identify all areas involved with the patient including administration, registration, laboratory, radiology, diagnostics, pharmacy, dietary, housekeeping, maintenance, materials' management, physician, building and utilities, and nursing with each contributing to the cost of the hospital, skilled care, or long-term care stay.

Hospital cost determination mirrors other businesses and industries with the exception that hospitals have high fixed costs (administration, depreciation, utilities, maintenance, etc.) and must attempt to cover these costs by increasing inpatient volume, adding services, using stringent contract management, and investing in capital to attract more business (van der Walde and Choi, 2003). Costs are calculated as direct or indirect, fixed or variable. The nurse manager should consider him/herself as both the CEO and CFO of their nursing unit or department and develop a good understanding of costs and revenue. How to determine nursing unit costs and manage the budget is presented in Chapters 10–12.

Skilled nursing care costs vary between hospital-based and freestanding facilities. The freestanding skilled facilities continued to decrease their costs after the introduction of PPS while the hospital-based costs continued to rise (United States General Accounting

Office [GAO], 2002). The GAO determined the increased cost for hospital-based skilled units was related to a higher acuity of patients and historical allocation of overhead costs plus an increased number of Medicare and Medicaid patients compared to the freestanding agency. The freestanding skilled facilities were able to offset Medicare and Medicaid losses by passing the costs on to the private insurers. The GAO also reported that the hospital skilled care unit reimbursement decreased 53 percent in 1999 under PPS due to payment being based on an average for all facilities versus payments based on the agency's own costs. Legislation was enacted in 2000 to boost the reimbursement to acute care facilities due to the extreme losses these agencies were experiencing by caring for predominately Medicare and Medicaid patients (van der Walde and Lindstrom, 2003).[4]

Historically, hospital outpatient services were reimbursed based on charges. The BBA created the 1998 Medicare proposed rules and regulations to establish a prospective payment schedule for hospital-based outpatient services and procedures in 2000. The Department of Health and Human Services designed an outpatient classification system entitled *Ambulatory Patient Classification (APC)*. "The composition of the APC groups is based on two premises: the procedures within each group must be similar clinically, and the procedures must be similar in resource and costs" (Department of Health and Human Services, p. 47,562).

The APC fee schedule was based on analysis of 1994, 1995, and 1996 outpatient claims. Relative payment weights were assigned by calculating the APC median cost, scaled based on a mid-level cardiovascular clinic visit that was found to be the most common outpatient service, and assigned a numerical value of 1.0. The assignment of each APC group relative payment rate was determined by dividing the median cost of each APC by the median cost for the mid-level cardiovascular visit.

There are two significant items the nurse manager must understand from this discussion. First, comparison of relative relationship of one APC to another, by knowing the median payment weight is 1.0, and understanding the reimbursement will be less, or greater, based on the variation from 1.0. Second, the hospital is reimbursed separately for each APC billed. Therefore a patient may have radiological and endoscopy procedures on the same day with each procedure reimbursed independently.

Home health cost determination varies somewhat from inpatient services. The home health agency manager considers different types of visit costs that are provided by a service line which includes nursing care, therapy services, and nursing assistance. The average cost per visit is calculated, much the same as acute care, by applying direct and indirect costs, and allocating for special fees such as accreditation services and other intermittent expected fees. The costs are averaged for the Medicare Cost Report and charges are set at an amount greater than the costs in order to recoup costs from high level care patients, and provide an established level for contract negotiations for private carriers that assure costs are reimbursed.[5]

---

[4] Further detailed information explaining the RUGs system can be found in *Health Care Financial Management for Nurse Managers: Applications in Hospitals, Long-Term Care, Home Care, and Ambulatory Care* (Dunham-Taylor and Pinczuk, 2006).

[5] More details about home care reimbursement are in *Health Care Financial Management for Nurse Managers: Applications in Hospitals, Long-Term Care, Home Care, and Ambulatory Care* (Dunham-Taylor and Pinczuk, 2006).

Clarifying the Cost Issue

Defining Costs, Charges, Payment

According to Finkler (1994), many studies have been published that have used the terms cost and charges interchangeably. Costs and charges are *not* interchangeable terms, and the nurse manager needs to understand the difference. *Costs* are determined by the organization's financial accounting system, which takes into account actual costs of supplies, manpower, facility, and administration for services provided (Cleverly, 1997). *Charges* are determined by the allocation of costs to the revenue-producing centers, and then projecting an amount needed to recover all the costs (Cleverly). Finally, *payment* is the amount the health care agency receives for the services provided. All payors will pay differing amounts for the same service depending on the type of payor and the contractual agreement between the agency and the insurer (Lane, Longstreth, and Nixon, 2001).

Projection of reimbursement is calculated by a payment-to-cost ratio that indicates the percent of costs that are covered by reimbursement. Medpac (2003) reported to Congress the Medicare payment-to-cost ratio was 99.4 percent, Medicaid 98 percent, uncompensated care 12.2 percent, and private payors 113.2 percent. Hospitals use the private-payor reimbursement as a cushion to offset the reimbursement from Medicare and Medicaid (Medpac) because it does not cover the full cost of the services provided.

The manager must remember that each private payor will negotiate fees contractually with the health care agency, and payment may or may not cover costs. **Exhibit 13–1** demonstrates a fictional example of charge, payment, and cost of a hospitalization. The hospital has calculated the costs of care to be $6,000 and determined charge to be $8,250 in order to capture any extended costs that may occur as well as to recoup losses that may be experienced from Medicare and Medicaid reimbursement. Contract negotiations between the hospital and the HMO and PPO have agreed on the reimbursement for the hospitalization to be $7,000. The last column represents the prospective payment from Medicare which equals approximately 99.4 percent of the actual costs incurred.

Cost of Service versus Reimbursement

What if more money is being spent on providing the service than is brought in by the reimbursement? In this case the executive team will need to determine an effective way to provide the service yet either cut the overall budget, decide to take a

---

Definition

Costs—actual costs of supplies, manpower, facility, and administration of services provided.
Charges—determined by the allocation of costs to the revenue-producing centers, and then projecting an amount needed to recover all costs.
Payment—the amount the health care agency receives for the services provided.
Projection of Reimbursement—calculated by a payment-to-cost ratio that indicates the percent of costs that are covered by reimbursement.

Exhibit 13–1 Comparison of cost to charge and payment*

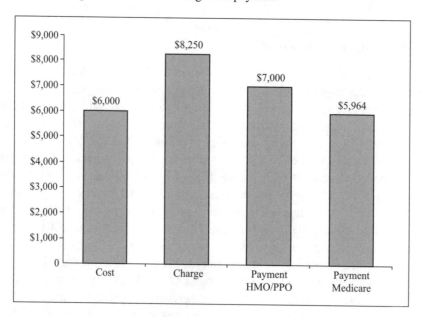

* Y axis represents whole dollars and X axis is the cost, charge, and payment information.

loss on the service, or stop providing the service. It is possible that we cannot answer this question because we do not know how much a service costs, nor do we know the actual revenue amount that is realized. In this section we will provide some helpful suggestions that can lead us to finding some answers.

The key financial question is: *Are we spending less than the reimbursement amount to provide the specified service?* A "yes" answer is desired. However, if the answer is either we are spending more than the reimbursement amount, or worse, that we do not know, immediate action needs to be taken by the entire management group—including the nurse manager.

Calculating the answer to this question is complicated because most often many cost centers—i.e., nursing, pharmacy, laboratory, dietary, medical records—will have been involved in providing the service. So to answer this question the interdisciplinary team needs to be able to figure *all the actual costs expended* to provide the specified service. This activity is sometimes called "costing" a service. This costing exercise should take place for all major services provided within the health care organization. Let's break this down into priority levels for the nurse manager. The first issue is determining cost.

Cost Determination Methods

There are four distinct methods of cost determination being used in health care today (Udpa, 2001). The first method is called the *cost-to-charge ratio* (CCR). Medicare specified this method be used to report annual costs. Thus most health care organizations today use this ratio as the primary source of all hospital costs and cost accounting information (Magnus and Smith, 2000). This report, called the Medicare Cost Report, is used by the Centers for Medicare and Medicaid Services to calculate and update reimbursement rates. Nationwide data is available as public information from the Healthcare Provider Cost Reporting Information System (HCRIS), and health care agencies use this information "to benchmark their costs and performance" (Magnus and Smith).[4]

The information contained in the Medicare Cost Report includes costs-to-charges ratios for inpatient, outpatient, departments, and functions such as medical education, utilization data, and financial statement data. The report is required for all Medicare-certified hospitals, skilled nursing facilities, home health agencies, and renal facilities. The ratio is determined by dividing the costs by the charges. **Exhibit 13–2** demonstrates the cost-to-charge ratio calculation. A ratio under 1.0 (equal costs and charges) is positive and indicates that the organization is making money on the service. A ratio over 1.0 indicates the organization is experiencing a loss—the costs are more than the charges (expected reimbursement). In the first example, the service is making money. In the second example, the service is losing money.

Using the cost-to-charge ratio, it is assumed that reimbursement (revenue) reflects the intensity of care, and therefore indirect costs (overhead) are assigned accordingly (Udpa, 2001). This method of cost determination does not allow for a full assessment of the true revenue production of a service, as all service areas are considered profitable if the health care agency as a whole is profitable. In addition, the higher the revenue generation, the higher the proportional allocation of overhead regardless of actual resource utilization. The nurse manager should be aware that CCR *could* lead to misrepresentation of cost when evaluating the profitability of a service (Udpa, 2001).

The second method of cost accounting is called *volume-based measures* (Udpa, 2001), which is much like it sounds. Here the indirect costs are assigned according to the volume (which may be visits, admissions, nursing hours per patient day), or machine hours (in

---

Exhibit 13–2 Calculation of Cost-to-Charge Ratio

Cost-to-Charge Ratios

Cost ÷ Charge = Cost-to-Charge Ratio

Examples:

(1) If costs are $50 and charges are $100:
$50 ÷ $100 = 0.5 cost-to-charge ratio (in the black)

(2) If costs are $100 and charges are $50:
$100 ÷ $50 = 2.0 cost-to-charge ratio (in the red)

---

[6] The HCRIS can be accessed at http://www.cms.gov.

radiology and the laboratory). A typical example of this measure is demonstrated (**Exhibit 13–3**) when the patient volume increases by 15 percent on a nursing unit and the nursing hours remain the same. The allocation of indirect cost is increased by 15 percent. Nursing hours did not increase to accommodate an increase of patient volume, yet the department is allocated higher overhead. It is difficult for the nurse manager to demonstrate increased productivity under this method of cost assignment. The nurse manager must understand the method of allocation of indirect costs in order to explain variation.

The next approach to cost allocation is called the *per-diem* approach (Udpa, 2001). This approach accumulates the indirect costs, divides by the number of patient days to determine per-diem costs, and allocates the indirect cost equally to all the nursing units. This method considers all patients the same regardless of intensity of care. In a facility that cares for varied types of patients, such as intensive care and obstetrics, this method of costing may also distort the departmental costs. For example, in one month a ten-bed cardiovascular intensive care has 100 percent occupancy and the thirty-bed obstetric unit occupancy rate is 55 percent. The indirect costs are distributed equally to the units when the per diem method of cost allocation is used. This means the departmental operations report for the obstetric unit and the cardiovascular intensive care unit will have the same dollar amount for indirect expenses even though the obstetric unit had fewer patient days.

The last method, *Balanced Scorecard and Activity Based Costing*, became a part of the industry in the 1980s but quickly lost favor due to the resources required to initiate and maintain this process (Easier than ABC: Will activity based costing make a comeback?, 2003). Over time, the advancement of health care management software technology has allowed health care to use Activity Based Costing (ABC) as a means of identifying true patient costs. This method of costing is more closely aligned with the true costs of caring for the patient (Udpa, 2001). ABC methodology also resembles performance improvement methods as processes and outcomes are evaluated. The complexity of "procedures and tests involved, the intensity of nursing care, the duration of an activity, and the intricacies of operative and post-operative care" identify the true costs (Udpa, p. 36). In this method, all areas and processes of patient interaction are identified and costs are allocated to the activity center.

Exhibit 13–3 Volume Based Cost Calculation

For an average daily census of 18:

Budgeted direct cost (salaries and benefits) for average daily census of 18 = $18,331

Budgeted indirect costs (professional fees, depreciation, and utilities) for nursing unit for average daily census of 18 = $5,781

For an average daily census of 21:

Average unit census per day for month X = 21

Actual direct costs for census of 21 = $18,331

Actual indirect costs for nursing unit for census of 21 = $6,648

The balanced scorecard adds the quality dimension to cost and reimbursement data. For instance, cost drivers outside the system, such as patient satisfaction, can be measured and reflected in the overall scorecard (Maiga and Jacobs, 2003). In this example, by combining these tools, the nurse manager will have an excellent overview of the financial aspects from cost, reimbursement, and patient satisfaction perspectives.

Exhibit 13–4 is an example of a balanced score card used by a hospital nurse manager to assess the unit performance against budget and revenue. This type of detail can be obtained from the finance department in a scorecard format if the agency uses this method of analysis. If the agency does not use a score card, the nurse manager can create one using information obtained from finance and spreadsheet software. In the example given here, the unit is under budget on expense and over budget on revenue, an excellent position. To truly determine if the unit is financially sound, the manager needs to clarify whether the revenue information is what was billed, or whether it was the actual amount received. The nurse manager must remember it is not possible to obtain this information in a timely manner because of delays in both billing and receiving the actual payment from payors.

The following studies have used the activity based costing (ABC) method through the hospital cost accounting system to both assess costs and to improve performance and patient care. Lester, Bosch, Kaufman, Halpern, and Gazelle (2001) were able to determine the actual inpatient costs of a patient undergoing endovascular abdominal aortic aneurysm repair. In their study, the direct costs were allocated to the individual units and the indirect costs were spread evenly among all departments. Time studies were performed and supply costs for each department were monitored. Surgery and radiology comprised 62 percent of the cost, with nursing contributing 22 percent, anesthesia 12 percent, and 4 percent attributed to an "other" category. The nursing costs reported in the study were allocated to the nursing unit on which the patient received post-operative care. While nursing costs were noted to contribute only a quarter of the costs, the surgical nursing costs were not separated from the total cost of the operative suite. By combining all nursing costs, it is assumed the total nursing costs would have represented a larger percentage than was presented in the study. However, the nursing costs, whether combined or separate, would continue to demonstrate a lesser percentage when compared to all other costs.

Popp et al. (2002) studied the cost of craniotomies to identify factors that affect the profitability of this procedure. The cost allocation method used was from a cost accounting system that used relative value units (RVU) to assign actual costs. The method to determine the RVU is based on the principle used by Medicare to reimburse physicians. Under physician reimbursement, RVU is the physician's subjective judgment of the time, skill, and resource costs that are required to provide services and procedures. The usual and common time, complexity, skill, and cost are assigned an RVU of 1.0 and all other services have some value above or below this baseline. For example, a weight of 2.0 is considered to be double the work of an RVU of 1.0. By assigning RVUs to tasks, the costs were allocated to different cost centers which included surgery, radiology, laboratory, pharmacy, anesthesia, physical therapy, rehabilitation, and room and board (nursing). Their findings also supported the Lester, Bosch, Kaufman, Halpern, and Gazelle study by identifying 80 percent of costs for a craniotomy were allocated into four major areas: operating room, room and board, pharmacy, and anesthesiology. In this study, room and board (nursing) contributed approximately 33 percent to the overall costs.

Exhibit 13–4 Performance Indicators

a.

St. Mercy Hospital
Somewhere USA

Year: FY 200_
VP: Nancy Nurse
Director: Perry Person
Dept: Medical

PERFORMANCE INDICATORS	NOV GOAL	JUL	AUG	SEP	OCT	NOV	DEC	JAN	FEB	MAR	APR	MAY	JUN	YTD TOT	YTD GOAL	FY04 GOAL
GROWTH																
Total Inpatient Unit	354	401	308	371	364	365								1,809	1,791	4,263
Total Inpatient Unit LYSM	322	361	346	363	377	322								1,789	1,789	4,370
Total Outpatient Unit	29	21	57	28	49	39								194	186	425
Total Outpatient Unit LYSM	47	28	25	37	42	47								179	179	396
Total Unit	393	422	365	399	413	404								2,003	1,977	4,688
Total Unit LYSM	369	369	371	420	419	369								1,968	1,968	4,756
COST																
Total IP Revenue per IP Unit	$506.13	$497.16	$491.94	$494.79	$494.65	$499.62								$495.78	$506.13	$506.13
Total OP Revenue per OP Unit	$324.59	$168.90	$388.28	$344.11	$377.10	$392.21								$356.10	$324.59	$324.58
Total Revenue per Unit	$492.73	$480.83	$475.75	$484.22	$480.71	$489.25								$482.25	$489.05	$489.67
Salary Expense per Unit	$157.61	$182.54	$169.73	$163.36	$158.81	$152.51								$165.44	$158.15	$159.32
Supply Expense per Unit	$9.56	$8.93	$8.46	$8.69	$8.35	$7.65								$8.42	$9.37	$9.16
Non-Salary Expense per Unit	$27.52	$25.50	$32.62	$26.09	$25.76	$25.32								$26.93	$27.50	$27.38
Total Expense per Unit	$185.13	$208.04	$202.35	$189.45	$184.57	$177.83								$192.37	$185.65	$186.70
Gross Margin per Unit	$307.60	$272.79	$273.40	$294.76	$296.14	$311.43								$289.88	$303.40	$302.97
PEOPLE																
Productive Manhour per Unit	8.1767	9.2633	10.3583	9.1105	8.7301	8.9210								9.2534	8.1746	8.1756
Total Manhours per Unit	8.9135	10.0061	10.8079	9.8303	9.4000	9.6263								9.9156	8.9114	8.9124
Overtime Hours	62	91	15	101	133	14								354	314	745
Overtime % of Productive Hours	1.94%	2.34%	0.40%	2.78%	3.68%	0.38%								1.91%	1.94%	1.94%
Total FTE's	19.88	23.97	22.39	23.01	21.98	22.75								22.82	20.26	20.09
Avg. Hourly Rate	$17.91	$20.63	$16.12	$16.69	$16.90	$15.84								$17.21	$17.97	$18.10
Contract Labor Costs	$2,431	$19,168	$468	$32										$19,668	$12,000	$28,705
Contract Labor Hours	44	488	102	17	1									607	217	520
Contract FTE Equivalent	0.25	2.77	0.58	0.10	0.00									0.70	0.25	0.25
VARIANCE																
Productive Manhour Variance	459	797	373	229	301									2,159		
Total Manhour Variance	462	692	366	201	288									2,010		
Productive FTE Variance	2.61	4.52	2.19	1.30	1.76									2.48		
Total FTE Variance	2.62	3.93	2.15	1.14	1.69									2.31		
Productive Salary Variance	$9,499.74	$12,842.59	$6,225.65	$3,870.07	$4,770.04									$37,154.12		
Total Salary Variance	$9,522.00	$11,153.20	$6,112.97	$3,403.53	$4,568.63									$34,583.98		

b.

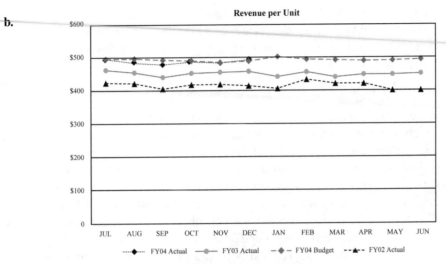

c.

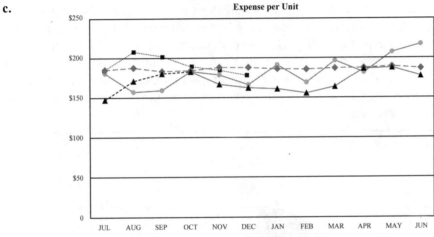

d.

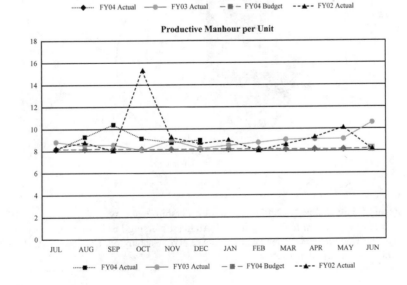

From the two studies presented, the nurse manager can begin to recognize, while total nursing personnel costs are the highest cost center of a hospital, the individual nursing unit contributes a quarter to a third of the overall cost of care for a hospitalized patient.

Nurse Manager's Role in Cost Control

The nurse manager usually has access to information that will assist with identification of global agency costs. Cost drivers that increase health care costs include salaries and wages, bad debt expense, depreciation and interest, supplies, and direct fringe benefits (see **Exhibit 13–5**). Understanding the relationship of these drivers to the total operating revenue provides guidance for the nurse manager, who can identify cost areas within his/her control. The median cost per hospital discharge in 2002 was $5,619 (The Advisory Board Company, 2003). **Exhibit 13–6** demonstrates the contribution of each cost component to the overall total cost for one hospitalization episode.

Kane and Siegrist (2002) report aggregated cost data for inpatient and outpatient care. Nursing comprised 33 percent of the cost for outpatient and approximately 50 percent of the inpatient cost. In 2002, salaries of health care workers increased by 6.1 percent due to workforce shortage (Carpenter, 2003). However, reimbursement rates did not increase to accommodate this increase in cost of providing care. Kane and Siegrist note that small increases in nursing costs will have a tremendous impact on the overall cost of hospitalization. The manager must be aware of this impact and plan the budget to accommodate annual performance evaluation raises.

Exhibit 13–5 Health Care Cost Drivers

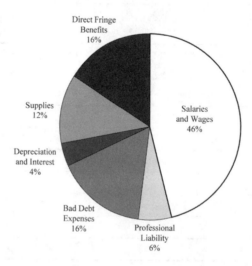

From: The Advisory Board Company (2003). Nursing Leadership Academy. *The fundamentals of nursing finance: a foundation for financial leadership.* p. 49. (Address: Nursing Leadership Academy, The Advisory Board Company, The Watergate, 600 New Hampshire Ave NW, Washington, DC 20037 202-266-5600 202-266-5700 (fax) http://academy.advisory.com/members.

Exhibit 13–6 Allocation of Cost for One Hospitalization*

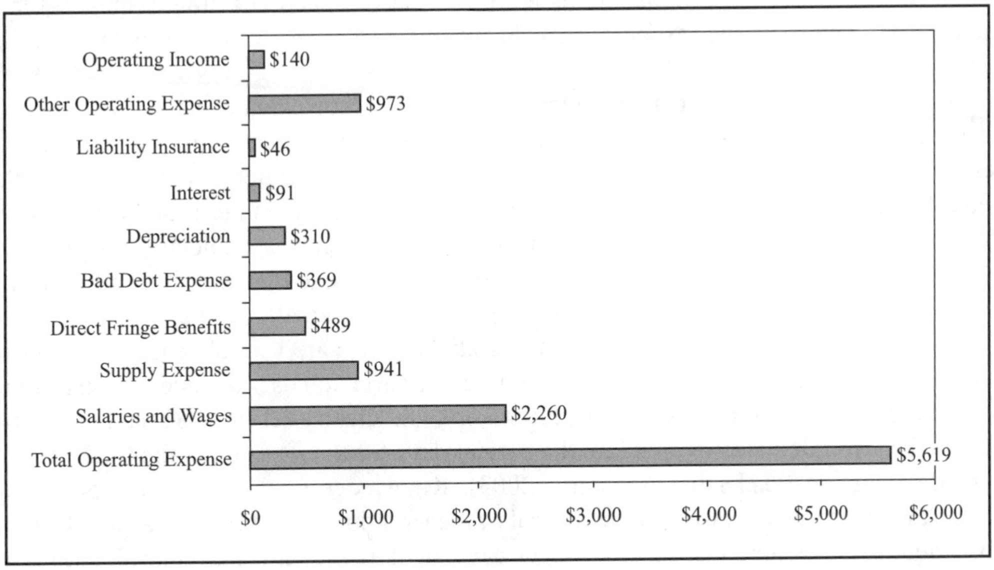

From: The Advisory Board, 2003. Nursing Leadership Academy. *The fundamentals of nursing finance: A foundation for financial leadership.* p. 48.

*Y axis represents direct and indirect drivers of cost. X axis represents cost of expense in whole dollars

The following will demonstrate what happens to a hospital nursing unit budget when a six percent across the board raise is given to RNs mid-fiscal year. This example came about to achieve nurse retention, and was based on local competition. A thirty-bed medical nursing unit has eighteen full-time RNs with an average salary of $22 per hour. The six percent increase raised the average salary $1.32 per hour, to $23.32. Since the raise occurred mid-fiscal year, the expected remaining hours of work are 1,040 for each full-time RN. The six percent raise increases the unit expense approximately $25,000. While $25,000 seems to be a small amount for one nursing unit, multiply this by all the RN FTEs within the hospital and the amount greatly increases the overall hospital costs of doing business. The nurse manager will be challenged to remain within budgetary compliance by identifying other areas to decrease costs.

Is the nurse manager able to control bad debt, depreciation, interest, or liability insurance? Of course not. Areas of cost the nursing manager cannot control need to be understood but are not the nurse manager's responsibility. Instead, the executive team must be concerned with these costs. Utilities, equipment expense, maintenance, and administrative costs are fixed costs that do not change as volume changes. (Of course, if the administrative team decides to take actions that decrease costs in these areas, the fixed cost amounts can change.) During the budget period the manager may be responsible for projecting these costs, or they may be supplied from the finance department. Whether the manager is given this responsibility, or the fixed costs are supplied by the finance department, the manager must assure allocations are made for unusual seasonal or billing issues that may increase or decrease the expense that has been noted by historical data (Nursing Leadership Academy, 2003).

For example, fees associated with accreditation may occur only once every two to three years and the cost of this service may be distributed among the nursing units under professional services. Another example is the expense of rental equipment such as specialty beds. The nurse manager is aware of increased use during the winter months because of the increase of ventilator patients. The astute manager, being a clinician, will not only assure this information is supplied to finance during the budgeting processes, but also will be able to provide sound rationale for the requested increased allocation.

Costs within the realm of nursing administrative control are variable costs. These costs vary in direct relationship to volume. Examples of variable costs include nursing hours, patient care supplies, pharmaceuticals, laboratory, and dietary services. Variable costs per patient day are calculated by dividing the patient days for the month into the total variable expense (Nursing Leadership Academy, 2003). Knowledge of the costs per patient day assists the nurse manager to improve control of the variation and be fiscally astute. **Exhibit 13–7** demonstrates how the nurse manager can calculate the variable (controllable) costs per patient day.

Exhibit 13–7 Calculation of Variable Costs

Cost per unit of service equals total variable expense divided by patient days.

($450,000 variable expense ÷ 500 patient days = $800 per patient day)

Managing Expenses with a Cost Accounting System

Under PPS it is crucial the health care agency know the exact costs of care in order to make responsible and accurate management decisions (Finkler, 1994). The cost of care on a nursing unit may be tracked through a financial cost accounting software system. Cost accounting software began to be developed after the implementation of prospective payment in the 1980s and has continued to be refined into a useful management tool (Durham, 2000). However, as Durham reported, less than 30 percent of health care agencies use cost accounting software because of the constant updates necessary to ensure information is current. The new manager should determine if the agency uses this technology as a means of financial assessment. If this information is available to you, then your job will be to diligently manage expenses.

Exhibit 13–8 is a fictitious example of a surgical services report generated from a cost accounting system. The report is for DRG 209 which is "major joint/limb reattachment" and includes hip replacement and fractures that use orthopedic hardware. This summary provides information regarding the number of orthopedic hip surgical cases, cost per case, and hospital charge per case for the operating room for supply items. Note this report does not include personnel costs as the nurse manager only requested supplies to evaluate this area for cost saving opportunities. For health care agencies with this type of software, the nurse manager can request a report customized to the unit and patient population.

Exhibit 13–8 Cases/Cost/Charge Summary for DRG 209 Surgical Services

Metrics	Cases	Cost/Case	Charge/Case
Perspective Clinical Summary			
Anesthesia Supplies	464	12	63
Anti-embolism hose/devices	359	96	184
Cath lab/angio supplies	1	124	234
Dialysis supplies	1	35	64
GI/Endo supplies	2	60	335
Implants ortho hardware	501	2,620	7,606
Med/surg supplies	522	2,332	9,840
Orthopedic soft goods	212	109	180
Ostomy supplies	39	6	11
Pacemaker/pacing supplies	2	57	130
Pulmonary/endo supplies	1	8	23
Respiratory supplies	494	35	190
Suction supplies	458	35	190
Urological supplies	440	24	45
TOTAL		**5,553**	**19,095**

Departmental Operations Report

What if you begin work as a new manager at an agency that does not have a cost accounting system? How do you determine the cost of care on your unit? The most efficient process is to determine the average daily census and review the departmental operations report from finance. **Exhibit 13–9** is part of a departmental operations expense report for November 200_ from nursing unit 5 North.

Exhibit 13–9 Departmental Operations Expense Report

Nov 200_ 5 North	Actual	Budget	Variance	Variance %	Favorable/Unfavorable
Expenses Total	87,121	106,305	-19,184	-18	F
Per unit	229.27	212.61	16.66	7.8	U

How do you, the new manager analyze this information? This is shown in **Exhibit 13–10**. The Actual and Budgeted Average Daily Census can be calculated by dividing the Actual or Budget Expenses Total amount by the Actual or Budget Per Unit amount. The Actual Average Daily Census (this might also be called the *average patient volume per day*) was 12.7 while the Budget had projected an Average Daily Census of 16.7 patients. While the total expenses were 18 percent less than budgeted (-18 percent variance that was favorable), the cost per individual patient was higher by 7.8 percent (7.8 percent variance that was unfavorable). The contributors of these variances may be linked to employee costs, supply costs, and how overhead is allocated to the department. The manager would need to investigate each possible contributing factor to identify opportunities to reduce expenses, or to explain the variation, that may in fact be due to a higher acuity of patient requiring increased nursing staff to provide safe, good quality care.

Exhibit 13–10 Calculation of Average Daily Census from Departmental Expense Report

Actual Expenses Total ÷ Actual Expenses Per Unit ÷ 30 (days in the month)
    = Actual Average Daily Census

   $87,121 ÷ $229.27 ÷ 30 = 12.7 Actual Average Daily Census

Budget Expenses ÷ Budget Expenses Per Unit ÷ 30 (days in the month)
    = Budgeted Average Total Daily Census

   $106,305 ÷ $212.61 ÷ 30 = 16.66 Budgeted Average Daily Census

---

Now, what if you do not have an operations report? Unfortunately in many health care organizations, costing does not take place at this level of detail. A usual mode of practice is to examine the overall bottom line for the organization, or to examine costing of a major service, represented by a product line or group of designated cost centers, i.e., cardiology or women's health. Here the total reimbursement is compared with the total expenditures. In this case, if there is an over-expenditure for one group of patients or services, there will need to be a savings accrued by another group of patients or services as the overall goal is that the bottom line is "in the black." Refer to **Exhibit 13–11**.

Exhibit 13–11 Comparison of Revenue and Costs of Two Strategic Service Units

Strategic Service Unit	Revenue (actual)	Departmental Cost (actual)	Variance	Variance %	Favorable/ Unfavorable
Cardiology	$650,980	$706,313	$55,333	8.5%	F
Women's Health	$325,987	$309,687	-$16,299	5%	U

The problem with this method is that the organization may not be aware that one service is losing money and another service is saving money. Using the hospital example, one

DRG may be delivered over cost (losing money)—while another DRG is costing less than the DRG (profit). So in a time when the reimbursements are not what were anticipated, services may be asked to cut equally, yet services for one DRG has been efficient while another has not. The nurse manager, working with the nurse executive, can use this data as an argument as to why cuts should not apply to the unit(s) coming in under costs.

The following DRG examples are used to further explain actual costs and reimbursement.

DRG Costing Example

Let's examine a hospital DRG to determine whether we are spending more or less than the reimbursement amount to provide the specified service. You are a hospital nurse manager/director/nurse executive responsible for an orthopedic cost center. A typical service provided on this cost center is DRG 209: Major Joint/Limb Reattachment Procedure, Low Extremities—No Complications (for Total Hip Replacement) and the Medicare reimbursement for this DRG is $9,269. Do you actually know how much you are expending to provide that DRG?

In this particular DRG there is a further complication: the costs of the prosthesis and direct supplies needed to do the total hip replacement may expend over 50 percent of the reimbursement dollars. So the amount of money left to provide all services this patient requires from admission to discharge must be low enough to stay within approximately 50 percent ($4,600) of the reimbursement amount. The question then is whether the service provided to a patient utilizing DRG 209 is less than $4,600. Or, in providing that service, is the service cost above that amount? If the latter is true, the organization is losing money on each patient having a total hip replacement. With profit margins as tight as they currently are in health care, it is very important that the nurse manager—as well as the executive team—know actual costs of the services provided.

It is interesting to note here that many hospital executive teams, not to mention nurse managers, cannot answer this question. Yet this is a key question that could determine the future viability of the organization.

Using the total hip replacement example, figuring out costs is further complicated because the reimbursement amount includes services and supplies delivered from several cost centers, i.e., operating room, laboratory, pharmacy, radiology, physical therapy, and orthopedic inpatient unit. So if the orthopedic nurse manager is working on the cost of this DRG, other cost center managers will need to provide their departmental costs of service assigned to each hip replacement patient in order to calculate the total DRG cost.

The following provides a specific example to demonstrate a case scenario for a patient admitted for a total hip replacement:

Jill Anderson is a 78-year-old female with severe degenerative arthritis of the right hip. She has been evaluated by the orthopedic surgeon who recommends a total hip replacement. Ms. Anderson agrees to the surgery and is scheduled for the procedure one week from the office visit. **Exhibit 13–12** is a representation of the hospital costs incurred for a three-day length of stay for a total hip replacement (DRG 209).

Exhibit 13–12 Costs for DRG 209 Total Hip Replacement

Day	Med surg	OR	Pharmacy	Pharmacy IV	Implants	Pathology	Lab	Supplies	Blood	Physical Therapy	TOTAL
1 (Adm)	480	2800	253	120	4,600	54	380	217	175	0	9,079
2	480		384				32			175	1,071
3	480		64				21			126	691
4 (D/C)			22	42			32				96
Total	**1,440**	**2,800**	**723**	**162**	**4,600**	**54**	**465**	**217**	**175**	**301**	**10,937**

As the manager can see, the cost of providing this service is greater than the reimbursement by $1,668 ($10,937 Actual Cost − $9,269 Reimbursement = -$1,668 Actual Loss) and an average case load of 500 total hips for the year would cost the hospital $834,000. This scenario is supported by a study Clancy et al. (1998) published, that concluded a loss of approximately $1,000 per patient occurred for DRG 209 and 210.

How can this procedure be profitable for the hospital? First, the interdisciplinary team must work aggressively to transfer the patient to another level of care, such as skilled care, as soon as medically indicated. The hospital will also generate additional revenue from the other services the orthopedic surgeon orders for the patient such as the surgical procedure, outpatient radiology studies, outpatient physical therapy, and referrals to a skilled nursing unit housed within the facility. By standardization of the hip prosthesis being used, the hospital can negotiate a contract with a supplier to be the vendor of choice, and thereby decrease costs. Also, the hospital may opt to purchase a prosthesis that costs less money. In addition, the volume of patients can be an important factor. We know that excellent patient satisfaction leads to the patient using the facility as their hospital of choice. As the manager can see, there are many global issues that are reviewed by management in deciding to provide a service line.

Now, let's take the same patient admitted to the skilled nursing unit. As you recall, the skilled units are reimbursed by resource utilization groups (RUGs) consisting of the costs for administration, room and board, nursing service, and therapy services. The length of stay on the skilled unit for Ms. Anderson is 11 days.

Ms. Anderson's RUG category is "ultra high" as her admission assessment indicated her need for nursing care, physical therapy, and occupational therapy (United States General Accounting Office, 2002). In the ultra high category, therapy must demonstrate Ms. Anderson received a total of 720 minutes of services in seven days (Medicare SNF-PPS Indices, 2003). The reimbursement and cost for the ultra high category is noted in **Exhibit 13–13**. As you can see, the skilled care facility is losing $800 per day of care and services provided to Ms. Anderson. In addition, as her therapy and nursing care requirements decrease as she improves, the reimbursement also decreases. After her seven-day assessment, the reimbursement for her care decreases to $296.15 per day.

Exhibit 13–13 RUG III Reimbursement for Ultra High Level of Care

Category	Nursing Care	OT, PT, Speech	Room, Board, and Administration	Total Rate per Day
Ultra high*	$142.32	$186.01	$55.88	$384.21
Actual costs	$444.03	$574.30	$165.77	$1,184.10
Difference	-$301.71	-$388.29	-$109.89	-$799.89

* Difference RUG rates obtained from http://www.cms.gov/providers/snfpps/snfpps_rates.asp. Actual costs calculated from historical data from a skilled nursing facility.

How does a health care agency afford to care for patients like Ms. Anderson? Van der Walde and Lindstrom (2003) report the free-standing skilled nursing facilities (SNF) have fewer Medicare, and more private pay patients, while a SNF in an acute care facility admits a higher percentage of Medicare patients. As their report indicates, the free-standing skilled nursing facilities (SNF) are profitable while skilled nursing facilities in an acute care setting are not profitable. Many hospitals have closed their skilled nursing facility due to the continued financial drain on the agency.

The next two examples demonstrate costs and reimbursement for a home health and same day surgery patient. As you recall, home health came under PPS October 2000 and outpatient surgery also began to be reimbursed by APCs (ambulatory patient classification) in 2000. The following case scenario was provided by a home health manager as a exhibition of the reality of home care:

Mr. Harold James is a 78-year-old diabetic, hypertensive African American with new onset atrial fibrillation, and survived a right hemispheric stroke (DRG 14). His deficits include left hemiparesis and speech difficulties, and he is discharged from a skilled nursing facility to home with a home health referral. Home health skilled nursing care will include medication management for diabetes and anticoagulation in addition to medication education. The following additional services will be used: physical therapy three times a week, speech therapy twice a week, and certified nursing assistant (CNA) visits three times a week. As Mr. James continues to improve the CNA visits will be discontinued, and occupational therapy will begin services three times a week. Medicare covers sixty days of home health service and a total of 66 home visits will be made during the sixty-day period (www.cms.hhs.gov/manuals/102-policy/bp102c07).

Since home health for this patient is primarily labor intensive, the manager can predict the cost of care by calculating the salaries and benefits for each team member, adding supplies and overhead, then multiply by number of visits, and finally multiply this number by two (average hours spent in the home by each care giver). **Exhibit 13–14** demonstrates this calculation.

In the past home health agencies tracked all costs and submitted these for Medicare reimbursement. However, now that prospective reimbursement has been implemented, our patient reimbursement is $6,098. Since the total cost for Mr. James is $6,428.80, the agency will lose $330.80 for this patient. $6,428.80 (total cost) − $6,098 (reimbursement) = -$330.80. For this reason, many home health agencies have limited the complex cases

Exhibit 13–14   Projection of Home Health Care Costs for 60 Days of Care

Salary/hr x Benefits (20%) + Supplies + Overhead x # Visits x Average time/visit = Costs

RN costs =	($18.79/hour x 0.2)	+ $37.45	+ $30	x 12	x 2	=	$2,160.00
PT costs =	($19.50 x 0.2)	+ $0	+ $30	x 16	x 2	=	$1,708.80
CNA costs =	($8.50 x 0.2)	+ $20.00	+ $30	x 16	x 2	=	$1,926.40
OT costs =	($19.00 x 0.2)	+ $0	+ $30	x 6	x 2	=	$633.60
Total costs =	$6,428.80						

they enroll in their service (van der Walde and Choi, 2003). The home health manager is also faced with the issue of the short-term home health admission. For example, a new diabetic may be ordered to receive home health visits for teaching. The visits are limited to three. The cost of admitting the patient to the service is $200 due to the time and intensity of the assessment as well as completion of OASIS. Our previous calculation indicates the cost of the two remaining visits (plus supplies of $25) is $155.10. The payor will only reimburse $90 for each visit ($270 total), and the agency again losses $85.10. While the manager may think this is a small amount, over time the agency will not be self sustaining due to losses from complex patients and short-term admissions. Therefore the home health manager must be creative and identify areas of savings such as decreasing supply costs that are not reimbursable, and set budget expenditures based on historical data that provides insight into payor reimbursements, as well as the types of patients admitted to the agency.

The same day surgery patient came under PPS in 2000. These services are reimbursed by codes called *APCs*, or *ambulatory patient classification* and are based on relative value units which are a measure of time and resources that are bundled into one of the 750 assigned categories (van der Walde and Choi, 2002). Many outpatient services have benefited from the APC process of reimbursement, more so from the private payors than Medicare. The following example (**Exhibit 13–15**) is a comparison of costs and reimbursement for a same day surgery laparoscopic cholecystectomy. The first example is a 42-year-old female with private insurance, and the second is a 70-year-old male with Medicare.

From the previous example, the manager has an understanding that the private insurance carriers truly offset the cost of caring for the Medicare patient. The manager, knowledgeable of payor mix, can determine the financial feasibility of the service that is provided by the same day surgery facility.

Other Factors Contributing to Reimbursement

Reimbursement is a complex issue. The information provided earlier in the chapter is from the broad perspective and can be generalized to health care agencies. Medicare participants are the largest user of health care services and in this section, additional information will be provided that will expand the previous information to include additional factors that

Exhibit 13–15 Same Day Surgery Cost and Reimbursement for Laparoscopic Cholecystectomy

51.23 Laparoscopic cholecystectomy	Charge code units (RVU)	Charges	Actual payment	Total Direct Costs	Total Indirect Costs	Total Cost
Private Insurance						
1662 Anesthesia	9	$1,658		$240	$77	$317
1665 Same day surgery	29	$4,514		$1,140	$927	$2067
1710 Central supply	6	$264		$131	$34	$165
1715 Pharmacy	12	$352		$96	$21	$117
1720 Pathology	1	$175		$12	$9	$21
1722 Lab	3	$91		$16	$6	$22
TOTAL Private Insurance	**60**	**$7,054**	**$4,573**	**$1,635**	**$1,075**	**$2,710**
Medicare Patient						
1662 Anesthesia	7	$1,384		$201	$64	$265
1665 Same day surgery	28	$4,546		$1,065	$866	$1,931
1710 Central supply	5	$255		$126	$33	$159
1715 Pharmacy	16	$469		$127	$28	$155
1722 Lab	5	$135		$26	$11	$37
TOTAL Medicare Payment	**61**	**$6,789**	**$1,767**	**$1,545**	**$1,002**	**$2,547**

contribute to Medicare reimbursement. The nurse manager can retrieve this information, in addition to the annual market basket updated fees for Medicare reimbursement, from the CMS website http://www.cms.gov.

Operating payments are an additional payment to the base DRG reimbursement, and vary from large urban (population over one million) to other urban and rural hospitals. In 2002 the reimbursement rate for the large urban areas was $4,157, while $4,091 was paid to other urban and rural hospitals (van der Walde and Choi, 2002). This amount is adjusted for the area market conditions and wage index.

St. Mercy Example

The following example demonstrates how the operating expense is added into the DRG payment for St. Mercy, a large urban hospital.

Capital payments are made for a portion of capital expenditures, and are adjusted also according to the local wage index. For fiscal year 2002 the large urban capital payment rate was $402, while it was $391 for other hospitals. Calculation of capital payments is the same as in Steps 1 and 2 below so that 70 percent of the reimbursement amount is allocated to labor costs and 30 percent to non-labor expense; the area wage index of 1.2045 remains the same.

Step 1: *Standardized reimbursement rate for fiscal year 2002 = $4,157.*
(The labor expense is 70% or $2,910, and $1,247 (30%) is allocated to non-labor expense.)

Step 2: *The labor-related portion is multiplied by the area wage index (1.2045), and added to the non-labor expense.*
$2,910 x 1.2045 = $3,505
$3,505 + $1,247= $4,752

Step 3: *The wage index adjusted amount is now multiplied by the RW (relative weight) of the DRG*
DRG 14 (stroke) RW = 1.2065
$4,752 x 1.2065 = $5,733 (Federal rate)

The amount paid to this hospital is $5,733 for DRG 14. However, this is not the ultimate payment.

Step 1: *Capital payment for fiscal year 2002 = $402*
(The labor expense is 70% or $281, and $121 (30%) is allocated to non-labor expense.)

Step 2: *The labor-related portion is multiplied by the area wage index (1.2045), and added to the non-labor expense.*
$281 x 1.2045 = $338
$338 + $121 = $459

Step 3: *The wage index adjusted amount is now multiplied by the RW (relative weight) of the DRG*
DRG 14 RW = 1.2065
$459 x 1.2065 = $554 (Capital Payment Rate)

The Capital Payment Rate ($554) is added to the Federal Rate ($5,733) and the reimbursement increases to $6,287.
$5,733 + $554 = $6,287

Now what if St. Mercy is affiliated with a medical school? Additional dollars are allocated to St. Mercy based on Direct Medical Education (DME) and Indirect Medical Education (IME) to underwrite the higher costs associated with resident training (van der Walde and Choi, 2002). The amount for DME and IME was established in the 1980s and has increased in proportion to inflationary factors. In addition, the amount allocated is dependent on the number of residents assigned to the facility. With only 1,154 teaching hospitals participating in Medicare, calculation of this amount is left to the finance and education department of those facilities and will not be discussed here.

Another component of reimbursement is based on the hospital providing care for the low-income and indigent patient. Hospitals with low-income and indigent care that exceed 15 percent of their volume are eligible for additional reimbursement and are called "Disproportionate Share Hospitals" (DSH). Hospitals caring for a large number of Medicaid patients are also noted to have a higher than average indigent patient and uncompensated care population. The DSH program was initiated through the Boren Amendment of the Omnibus Budget Reconciliation Acts of 1980 and 1981 (Coughlin and Liska, 1997). Through this legislation, states that demonstrated high Medicaid enrollment are eligible for federal financial participation dollars. These funds are then given to hospitals that qualify as a DSH provider. The DSH payment is greater than the cost of care for the Medicaid population, so hospitals receive some reimbursement for indigent and uncompensated care.

The following formula is used to calculate the threshold for inclusion in DSH payments:

$$\textit{Disproportionate share threshold (\%)} = \frac{\textit{Medicare patients eligible for SSI}}{\textit{Medicare inpatient days}} + \frac{\textit{Medicaid Inpatient Days}}{\textit{Total acute inpatient days}}$$

It is important to note there are different DSH payments for rural and urban hospitals. Rural hospitals under 500 beds are limited to a 5.25 percent DSH payment over costs while urban DSH hospital payments are not capped (van der Walde and Choi, 2002).

The most common additional reimbursement the nurse manager will experience is called *outlier payments*. As you recall, under prospective payment the DRG payments are based on the average cost per case. For the extreme cases of patients with complex disease processes that incur higher costs than the average, Medicare will make additional payments to decrease the hospital's financial burden for caring for this type of patient (van der Walde and Choi, 2002). The outlier payment is calculated by the cost-to-charge (CCR), which was discussed earlier in the chapter. To qualify for an outlier payment the cost must exceed the DRG payment and a threshold is established each year by the Centers for Medicare and Medicaid Services (van der Walde and Choi). CMS will then pay 80 percent of the costs of the case that is in excess of the DRG and the established threshold.

The following is an example of an outlier payment for our hospital, St. Mercy, for a patient discharged with a primary diagnosis of DRG 286—resection of a pituitary tumor. The patient developed complications and incurred hospital charges of over $90,000 with the assigned DRG payment only being $15,200. The Medicare fixed loss threshold for 2003 is $33,560. From this information we will calculate the expected reimbursement. The calculations used to determine base reimbursement used in this example are adopted from the appendix of *Health Care Industry Market Update: Acute Hospitals Volume II (2002)*.

This complicated process of calculating outlier payment is done by the Medicare financial intermediary when a facility requests payment for outlier cases. Why is this important for the nurse manager to know? The manager needs to monitor outlier patients and assure appropriate reimbursement is sought. Without this knowledge, outlier payments may not be sought and the nursing unit is out of budgetary compliance and the organization loses money.

Step 1: *The provider cost-to-charge ratio is 0.78 with 0.72 allocated to operations and 0.06 for capital costs*

Billed charges = $90,000 x 0.72 = $64,800 (Operating Costs)

Billed charges = $90,000 x 0.06 = $5,400 (Capital Costs)

Total case costs = $64,800 + $5,400 = $70,200

Case cost is greater than the assigned
$15,200 (DRG Payment) + $33,506 (Fixed Loss Threshold) = $48,760

Step 2: *Calculate the DRG payment*

Labor expense = $15,200 (DRG payment) x 0.7 (Operations Cost-to-Charge Ratio) = $10,640 for labor expenses

Non-labor expense = $15,200 (DRG payment) x 0.3 = $4,560 for non-labor expenses

Multiply wage index of 1.2045 for labor: $10,640 labor expenses x 1.2045 = $12,816 labor expenses

Add labor and non-labor: $12,816 + $4,560 = $17,376 operating expenses

Multiply by RW $17,376 x 1.32 = $22,936 total expected DRG reimbursement

Capital payment =$402

Adjusted = $402 x 0.7 =$281 (from labor expenses) x 1.2045 (wage adjustment) = $339 (total labor expenses) + $121 (non-labor expenses) = $459 (total capital payment)

Multiply total capital payment by capital payment rate: $459 x 1.32 = $606 total capital payment

Add the total expected DRG reimbursement to the total capital payment: $22,936 + $606 = $23,542 adjusted DRG payment

Step 3: *Calculate outlier payment which is 80% of the difference between DRG payment and the Medicare fixed-loss threshold*

$33,560 (fixed loss threshold) - $23,542 (adjusted DRG payment) = $10,018 x 0.8 = $8,014 outlier payment

Step 4: *Calculate full DRG payment + outlier payment*

$23,542 + $8,014 = $31,538 full payment

Revenue Budget

NURSING SERVICE DOES GENERATE REVENUE

In the health care organization—whether hospital, long-term care, home care, or ambulatory settings—nursing services provide organizational revenue. If you are a nurse manager on an inpatient unit you may hear a finance employee say your unit does not generate revenue. Technically on an inpatient unit, you probably do not have a revenue account—unless you have oncology services, O.R., or a service that can be directly billed. Instead nursing services on inpatient units are most often included in the room rate charge, and the finance department keeps the records of revenues. However, nursing care *does* generate and contribute to the revenue generation for the DRG payment in hospitals, and for the MDS reimbursement, or for other payments, in long-term care. In this example, revenue becomes muddy because so many disciplines are involved in the patient's care. Remember that patients always come to inpatient units because they need nursing care. Nursing services have traditionally been directly billed in home care as a separate line item. Two states, Maine and Maryland, have recognized nursing's contributions and have specified that hospitals take nursing service out of the room rate charge and list it as a separate item on the patient's bill. This could mean that more inpatient units will be considered profit centers and have a revenue budget.

There may be other services or items that can be directly billed such as O.R. procedures, ambulatory services, homecare services, drugs, supplies, educational programs, physical or respiratory therapy, consultation services, or wellness programs. In these programs, nurse managers usually will have a revenue budget; often called a *profit* center (profit centers are explained in Chapter 10, Budgeting). In this case, the cost center's services are directly billed to patients. In these settings the revenue budget is used to make sure that the organization/department/clinic remains viable.

Currently revenues are only occasionally reported on inpatient cost center budgets. If this occurs, the nurse manager must seek information to learn what these figures represent, are they billed dollars or are these dollars actually received? Are contractual allowances or discounts included in the revenue figures? Is the figure so unreliable, the nurse manager should just ignore it, or does it provide useful data?

When the nurse manager gets a revenue report for billable supplies or services, most often provided by the finance department, the nurse manager should check the accuracy of the figures and then compare costs and revenue.

The following **Exhibit 13–16** is an example of a detailed nursing unit operations report that includes revenues for inpatient and outpatient sources. Revenue in this type of financial report does not equal true reimbursement, but is a cost-to-charge ratio that is used in the Medicare Cost Report. The manager can also note from this report the distribution of payors for the department.

How is this information interpreted? The first column provides the payor source followed by the charge-to-cost ratio. Following the reimbursement are the budgeted dollars expected to be collected. The next column is the variance between actual charge-to-cost ratio and what was budgeted, or (actual - budgeted = variance). Percent variance follows next. This is the percent deviation between the actual column and the budgeted column. The last column shows whether the variance is favorable (F) or unfavorable (U). As you can tell from this report the revenue total for both in- and outpatient is below the budgeted amount at an unfavorable 4.7 percent.

The nurse manager must seek information to explain the variation from budget. For this unit, two areas were identified as reasons for the budget variation. First, the census was lower than expected by the budgeted amount, and second, there was decreased reimbursement from contractual agreements that went into effect in the previous month of October. Although, nursing management can not directly impact contractual agreements, nursing does have a strong influence on the census through providing high quality, safe care the patient and family value as well as by building a trusting relationship with physicians, patients, colleagues, and others in the organization. When everyone acts as an effective team, magic happens.

Exhibit 13–16 Monthly Nursing Departmental Revenue Report by Payor

			5 North	Nov-0_	
	Actual*	Budget	Variance	Variance %	Favorable/ Unfavorable
INPATIENT REVENUE					
Medicare	167,519	282,683	-115,164	-40.7	U
Medicaid	22,050	34,802	-12,752	-36.6	U
Managed care	29,578	44,515	-14,937	-33.6	U
Commercial	15,004	9,237	5,767	62.4	F
Self pay	27,293	5,294	21,999	415.5	F
Other	2,406	3,368	-962	-28.6	U
Inpatient Revenue Total	**263,850**	**379,899**	**-116,049**	**-30.5**	**U**
per unit	**782.94**	**796.43**	**-14**	**-1.7**	**U**
OUTPATIENT REVENUE					
Medicare	16,254	9,624	6,630	68.9	F
Medicaid	5,044	3,994	1,050	26.3	F
Managed care	3,388	6,913	-3,525	-51.0	U
Commercial	627	1,031	-404	-39.2	U
Self pay	1,533	587	946	161.2	F
Other	627	165	462	280.0	F
Outpatient Revenue Total	**27,473**	**22,314**	**5,159**	**23.1**	**F**
per unit	**639**	**970**	**-331**	**-34.1**	**U**
REVENUE TOTAL	**291,323**	**404,213**	**-110,890**	**-27.6**	**U**
per unit	**767**	**804**	**-38**	**-4.7**	**U**

* The *Actual* column represents gross revenue times the ratio of costs to charges from the Medicare/Medicaid report.

However, this variance is only a piece of the information the nurse manager has to consider. The manager must also compare the same period last year as well as the year-to-date financials to have the total picture of the unit financial performance. **Exhibit 13–17** provides the fiscal year-to-date financial information for 5 North. This nursing unit is generating 5.2 percent less than budgeted revenue for the fiscal year to date.

The challenge now is for the nurse manager to be knowledgeable not only of employee and supply expense but also the unit's primary admission and diagnoses, length of stay, complication rates, and reimbursement per DRG. Another area that impacts the financial performance of a nursing unit is the contractual agreements made between the hospital financial management team, a managed care organization, and a preferred price for supplies based on utilization.

Exhibit 13–17 Year-to-Date Nursing Department Revenue Report by Payor

	Actual*	5 North Budget	FYTD Variance	Nov-0_ Variance %	Favorable/ Unfavorable
INPATIENT REVENUE					
Medicare	1,120,051	1,358,542	-238,491	-17.6	U
Medicaid	205,504	167,253	37,801	22.6	F
Managed care	141,956	213,932	-71,976	-33.6	U
Commercial	67,857	44,392	23,465	52.9	F
Self pay	50,315	25,440	24,875	97.8	F
Other	12,824	16,187	-3,363	-20.8	U
Inpatient Revenue Total	**1,598,057**	**1,825,746**	**-227,689**	**-12.5**	**U**
per unit	**798.63**	**796.23**	**2.40**	**0.3**	**F**
OUTPATIENT REVENUE					
Medicare	88,162	47,653	40,509	85.0	F
Medicaid	18,805	19,776	-971	-4.9	U
Managed care	32,321	34,229	-1,908	-5.6	U
Commercial	3,615	5,106	-1,491	-29.2	U
Self pay	5,451	2,907	2,544	87.5	F
Other	4,117	817	3,300	403.9	F
Outpatient Revenue Total	**152,471**	**110,488**	**41,983**	**38.0**	**F**
per unit	**520.38**	**977.77**	**-457.39**	**-46.8**	**U**
REVENUE TOTAL	**1,750,528**	**1,936,234**	**-185,706**	**-9.6**	**U**
per unit	**763.09**	**804.75**	**-41.66**	**-5.2**	**U**

* The *Actual* column represents gross revenue times the ratio of costs to charges from the Medicare/Medicaid report.

The manager should review the DRG historical admission and discharge history of the unit. Then, the nurse manager can evaluate the unit patient population, and identify trends or changes in patient base that may require an expansion of nursing knowledge and skills. In addition, the manager should ask for the following information: length of stay by discharge diagnosis, list of secondary diagnosis, and complications. An analysis of this information will guide the manager to identify areas for improving care to decrease complications (which are costly and are not reimbursed), improve efficiency, decrease supply and manpower costs, and thereby improve the financial performance of the nursing unit.

Contractual agreements are negotiations between the health care agency and the health insurer or provider of services and supplies. Contracts may range from the amount paid by the insurer for a specific diagnosis to the amount of supply charges based on utilization.

The nurse manager does not have control over contract negotiations, but plays a significant role in providing information regarding changes in patient care that will influence negotiated reimbursement or prices. In addition, the nurse manager must be aware of the dates of contract renewals in order to recognize shortfalls during the budget planning process.

Exhibit 13–17 demonstrates an example of how changes in patient payors and contractual agreements impact the nursing units' budget. In this example, Medicare admissions decreased, private insurance decreased contractual reimbursement, and there was an increase in self-pay patients, which often contributes to indigent care services. The key factor that cannot be seen in the example is that the private insurance contract negotiations occurred after the budget had been set, and a lower reimbursement was negotiated by management as a means to increase patient volume by this carrier. The manager needs to continually evaluate admissions by payor to identify if the negotiated contract actually increased admissions for the nursing unit.

Predicting Financial Success

The case mix index has been used by hospital administrators to predict financial success since prospective payment was instituted by Medicare (Adams, 1996). The nurse manager can use this tool to predict financial success at the nursing unit level. DRGs are divided into 25 major diagnostic categories (MDC) which includes the following information: 1) the DRG number, 2) the narrative description, 3) relative weight, 4) geometric length of stay, 5) arithmetic length of stay, and 6) outlier threshold. The relative weight is an assigned number that is an indicator of the amount of resources needed to care for the patient with that particular disease process and includes all cost related to the hospitalization (Adams, 1996). The nurse manager should understand that the higher the weight, the more resources needed to care for the patient. The amount of resources needed to treat a particular disease process is the relative weight. A disease requiring many resources, such as total joint replacement, carries a higher weight than atypical chest pain. Using the DRG relative weight a simple calculation can be used to determine reimbursement for a specific DRG.

DRG relative weight x hospital payment rate = reimbursement
DRG 209 with RW of 2.2707 x $4,240.54 = $9,629

The case mix index (CMI) is an average relative weight over a period of time that indicates the patient's acuity and is used to determine reimbursement from Medicare and Medicaid for all patients admitted to the hospital. Adams (p. 31) uses the following example to demonstrate how the CMI impacts the overall reimbursement for a six-bed nursing unit:

Doe, John	DRG 89	RW 1.1211
Jones, James	DRG 143	RW 0.5159
Smith, Jane	DRG 127	RW 1.0302
Thomas, Harold	DRG 183	RW 0.5480

Williams, Timothy DRG 140	RW 0.6312	
Young, Mary DRG 14	RW 1.2065	
Total patients: 6	Total weights: 5.0529	CMI= 0.8422

From: Adams, T.P. (1996). Case mix index: nursing's new management tool. *Nursing Management*, 27(9). pp. 31–32.

To calculate the reimbursement for the unit, the nurse manager will need to obtain the Medicare median hospital payment rate. Then, take this rate and multiply by the case mix index (CMI) to get the total expected reimbursement rate for the unit. For example, say the reimbursement rate is $5,200. The total number of patients admitted to the unit for the week equaled six and the CMI is 0.8422:

$5,200 x 0.8422 x 6 = $26,277 (rounded to the nearest whole dollar)

From this information, knowledge of supply costs, and personnel expense, the nurse manager can be proactive in departmental financial management. Further, he/she will be able to alert the nurse executive and finance department about important reimbursement issues, i.e., lost revenues, higher expenses than revenues, and so forth. In addition to the case mix index, the nurse manager must realize the hospital's DRG payment rate is also contingent on geographic location, wage index, and patient mix.

The nursing manager should obtain the top ten DRGs for the nursing unit from the coding department (usually located in Medical Records). Then use the above formula to estimate the reimbursement, and multiply by the number of discharges by DRG for the month or year. This estimates the expected reimbursement. By knowing this information, the manager can influence reimbursement on the unit by assisting staff and physicians to document thoroughly for accurate coding. This then will increase the case mix index (Adams, 1996). The manager may choose to select one DRG that is costing more than the reimbursement, establish a multi-disciplinary team to evaluate processes of care that may impact patient outcomes and increase cost, and strategize to determine less costly ways to deliver the care safely and efficiently.

Nursing Management Decisions Impact Financial Outcomes

The nurse manager must be cognizant of unit expenses, including personnel and supplies. These are two key areas that nursing can affect to assure a positive bottom line. The flow of patients into and out of a service area determines the staffing and supplies needed. Nursing must have financial savvy and be creative to manage within this environment.

In long-term care, reimbursement for Medicaid patients is actually determined by the nurse and depends upon how well the nurse has completed the MDS.[6] The Balanced

---

[6] For further more detailed information on the MDS see Dunham-Taylor and Pinczuk, 2006, *Health Care Financial Management for Nurse Managers: Applications in Hospitals, Long-Term Care, Home Care, and Ambulatory Care.*

Budget Act of 1997 changed the format of nursing home reimbursement for both Medicaid and Medicare by allowing the states to set standard nursing home (Medicaid) reimbursement versus paying reasonable costs and establishing prospective payment for services covered by Medicare (Weech-Maldonado, Neff, and Mor, 2003). In addition, the prospective payment system for Medicare exposed the long-term-care facilities to an adjusted case mix index (Weech-Maldonado, et al.) as had been done in acute care for many years.

Usually though, to accomplish a detailed evaluation of cost versus reimbursement, the nurse manager can facilitate an interdisciplinary management team to determine and compare actual costs of the services provided with the reimbursement amount received for those services. The organization and participation in such a team can help all disciplines within the organization to become cognizant of the importance of rectifying systems problems that can contribute significantly to higher costs if left unidentified and unresolved.

Summary

Cost and reimbursement issues are difficult to understand, as there are many different aspects of how costs are calculated, and which payor is paying what amount. Hopefully, this chapter has assisted the manager to have an improved understanding of fiscal management for the nursing unit or department, and deems him/herself as the CEO and CFO of his/her area, now recognizing the power of the position in determining successful patient outcomes and a positive bottom line. Note that this chapter is concerned only with assisting the nurse manager in the financial aspects, not with other quality and ethical factors involved.

References

Adams, T. P. (1996). Case mix index: Nursing's new management tool. *Nursing Management, 27*(9), 31–32.

Carpenter, D. (2003 March). Soaring spending: No sign of a slowdown. *H & HN: Hospitals and Healthcare Networks*, 77, 16–17.

Clancy, T., Kitchen, S., Churchill, P., Covington, D., Hundley, J., & Maxwell, J. G. (1998). DRG reimbursement: Geriatric hip fractures in the community hospital. *Southern Medical Journal, 91*(5), 457–461.

Cleverley, W. O. (1987). Product costing for health care firms. *Health Care Management Review, 12*(4), 39–48.

Cleverley, W. O. (1997). *Financial environment of health care organizations: Essentials of health care finance* (4th ed., Rev., pp. 10–24). Gaithersburg, MD: Aspen.

Coughlin, T. A., & Liska, D. (1997 October). *The medicaid disproportionante share hospital payment program: Background and issues* (Series A, No. A-14). Washington, DC: The Urban Institute.

Department of Health and Human Services. (1998 September 8). *Medicare program: Prospective payment system for hospital outpatient sevices: Proposed rules* (42 CFR Part 409, et al.). Washington, DC: Health Care Financing Administration Office of Inspector General.

Division of Health Care Finance and Policy. (1998 April). Home health: An emerging challenge in health care. *Healthpoint*, 3, 1–4.

Dunham-Taylor, J., & Pinczuk, J. (2006). *Health care financial management for nurse managers: Applications from hospitals, long-term care, home care, and ambulatory care.* Sudbury, MA: Jones and Bartlett.

Durham, J. (2000 April). Healthcare's evolution in the technological universe. *Health Management Technology*, 91–92.

Easier than ABC: Will activity based costing make a comeback? (2003 October). *The Economist*, 369, 56.

Finkler, S. A. (1994). *Cost allocation: The distinction between costs and charges. Issues in cost accounting for health care organizations* (pp. 81–93). Gaithersburg, MD: Aspen.

Hoffman, F. M. (1984). *Prospective reimbursement. Financial management for nurse managers* (pp. 193–203). Norwalk: Appleton-Century-Crofts.

How to choose health care coverage. (n.d.). Retrieved November 8, 2003, from http://ring.com/health/health/health.htm.

Kane, N. M., & Siegrist, R. B. (2002, August 12). In *Understanding rising hospital costs: Key components of cost and the impact of poor quality*. Retrieved September 23, 2003, from http://www.selectquality.com/PDF/understand...ent%20costs.pdf.

Lane, S. G., Longstreth, E., & Nixon, V. (2001). *A community leader's guide to hospital finance.* Boston: The Access Project.

Lester, J. S., Bosch, J. L., Kaufman, J. A., Halpern, E. F., & Gazelle, G. S. (2001). Inpatient costs of routine endovascular repair of abdominal aortic aneurysm. *Academic Radiology, 8*(7), 639–646.

Magnus, S. A., & Smith, D. G. (2000). Better Medicare cost report data needed to help hospitals benchmark costs and performance. *Health Care Management Review, 25*(4), 65–77.

Maiga, A. S., & Jacobs, F. A. (2003). Balanced scorecard, activity-based costing and company performance: An empirical analysis. *Journal of Managerial Issues, 15*(4), 283–301.

Medicare SNF-PPS Indices [Data file].Washington, DC: Centers for Medicare and Medicaid Services. Retrieved November 24, 2003 from http://www.cms.gov/providers/snfpps/snfpps_rates.asp.

Medpac. (2003 March). *Report to Congress: Medicare payment policy.* Washington, DC: Medpac.

Nursing Leadership Academy. (2003 September). *Fundamentals of nursing finance: A foundation for financial leadership* (10889). Washington, DC: The Advisory Board Company.

Popp, A. J., Scrime, T., Cohen, B. R., Feustel, P. J., Petronis, K., Habinak, S., et al. (2002). Factors affecting profitability for craniotomy. *Neuorsurgery Focus, 12*(4), 1–5.

Sherman, K. R. (1994). Introduction of innovation in hospital cost accounting to Medicare rate setting for improved cost containment. *Hospital Cost Management and Accounting, 6*, 3–7.

Sobun, C. (1999). What does the future hold for Medicare and your reimbursement. *Health Care Biller, 8*(9), 1–4.

Udpa, S. (2001). Activity cost analysis: A tool to cost medical services and improve quality. *Managed Care Quarterly, 9*(3), 34–41.

United States General Accounting Office. (2002). *Skilled nursing facilities: Medicare payments exceed costs for most but not all facilities* (GAO-03-183). Washington, DC: U.S. Government Printing Office.

van der Walde, L., & Choi, K. (2003 July). *Health care industry market update: Acute care hospitals.* Washington, DC: Centers for Medicare and Medicaid Services.

van der Walde, L., & Choi, K. (2003 May). *Health care industry market update: Nursing facilities.* Washington, DC: Centers for Medicare and Medicaid Services.

van der Walde, L., & Lindstrom, L. (2003 September). *Health care market update: Home health.* Washington, DC: Centers for Medicare and Medicaid Services.

van der Walde, T., & Choi, K. (2002 November). *Health care industry market update: Acute care hospitals volume II.* Washington, DC: Centers for Medicare and Medicaid Services.

Weech-Maldonado, R., Neff, G., & Mor, V. (2003). The relationship between quality of care and financial performance in nursing homes. *Journal of Health Care Finance, 29*(3), 48–60.

Useful Websites

The Center for Medicare and Medicaid Services *http://www.cms.hhs.gov*

Social Security Online *http://www.socialsecurity.gov*

The Urban Institute *http://www.urban.org*

Agency for Healthcare Research and Quality *http://www.ahrq.gov*

United States Department of Health and Human Services *http://www.dhhs.gov*

The Henry J. Kaiser Family Foundation *http://www/kff.org*

Select Quality Care Library (SQC Library) *http://www.selectqualitycare.com*

PART FIVE

Budget Strategies

Budgeting strategies, and especially cost-cutting methods, are widely used today. Chapter 14 will cover a number of strategies, each of which works best depending on the setting. Organizational context is an important element because knowing and understanding the differences in parts of the organizational assessment may determine if we succeed in attaining our goals. Chapter 14 also examines the budgeting process and makes suggestions on how to both decentralize and streamline the process as presently in some organizations it can waste 30% of administrators' time. It is important for a nurse administrator to know how to write a proposal that includes the financial information along with what is needed. Thus at the end of the chapter, an appendix includes a sample proposal for a step-down unit.

Budget strategies need to be aligned with a larger issue: strategic management, which is discussed in Chapter 15. Systemic, objective strategic planning, along with the implementation of the plan, drives successful health care organizations. The key to successful planning is to make the process a part of the daily operations of the organization. Strategic management is a continuous process of revisiting the system and restoring balance.

Chapter 15 also describes the strategic management process that includes situation analysis, strategic formation, strategic deployment, and strategic management—which encompasses measurement, evaluation, and performance improvement. Directional strategies, mission, vision, values, goals and objectives provide needed processes for the organization to define and to implement in order to achieve the desired outcomes. Other tools and techniques, such as cost-benefit analysis, break-even analysis, and forecasting models are presented to help the nurse manager develop and support the strategic plan, as well to more effectively budget supporting the plan.

In Chapter 16 we turn to another budget strategy: Case Management. According to the American Nurses Credentialing Center (ANCC) case management is a dynamic and systematic collaborative approach to providing and coordinating health care services in a defined population. It is a process to identify and facilitate options and services for meeting individuals/ health needs, while 1) decreasing fragmentation and duplication of care; 2) enhancing quality; and 3) achieving cost-effective clinical outcomes. This chapter will deal with new models that link with-in-the-walls and beyond-the-walls models.

Mutual knowing between client and nurse enhances care including the client's ability for selfcare. This chapter describes three key certifications available to nurses, and discusses present trends that integrate and coordinate care as well as increased use of information technologies.

CHAPTER 14

Budget Strategies

Janne Dunham-Taylor, PhD, RN

Linda Legg, MSN, RN

Budget strategies, and especially cost-cutting methods, are used widely today. We will cover a number of strategies that we believe are important. This list is by no means complete as there are an infinite number of strategies that can be used. Please add to this list, and then share what works—and what does not work—with each other.

When thinking about strategies it is important to put them into an organizational context. We advocate *strategic thinking*, rather than across-the-board cuts. Strategic thinking takes into account which departments are already more cost conscious, and what services are strategically necessary to stay current in meeting patient needs. Strategic planning is further explained in Chapter 15, and organizational strategies are further explained in Chapter 4. It means staying ahead of the competition, and recognizing that the competition is much more than just what a similar facility is doing down the road. Competition can come from unlikely sources such as all the public interest in alternative therapies and vitamins, or the advanced technologies that are less invasive to patients, or a stand-alone surgery center.

Certain strategies will work more effectively in one setting, while not as well in another, because all of our facilities have particular quirks or differences that will affect the outcome. Knowing and understanding the differences is part of the organizational assessment that we need to consider before we actually decide to implement new approaches. Chapter 4 on Organizational Strategies explains how to do an organizational assessment. Having a total organizational assessment picture is part of the critical-thinking element in nursing administration. If our assessment is accurate, we can often guess how people in the organization will respond to changes. Sometimes we will be surprised by what happens. So it is important, when considering budget strategies, to think about where the organization presently is, and to choose strategies based on this assessment. Otherwise the chosen strategy may result in other more serious, unanticipated side effects.

Budget Cuts

Budget cuts have been happening regularly in health care for many reasons. A predominant reason is that government reimbursement for Medicaid and Medicare services only gives back cents on the dollar. This means that the reimbursed amount is less—as much as half—than that expended by the health care facility. Other insurance plans follow, taking similar measures, by asking for larger discounts.

Budget cuts can also result from poor business decisions such as giving too great a discount to insurance carriers, losing contracts with insurance companies such as Blue Cross, rescuing physician offices running at a deficit, providing poor leadership, or operating consistently at a loss yet never taking any measures to improve the situation.

What Is Our World View?

Our cost-cutting strategies are driven by our world view. This view creates silos and drives cost-cutting strategies. See **Exhibit 14–1**. The statement, *It's time to get out of the box*, is true for all of us, even when we think we are at the cutting edge of change!

Exhibit 14–1 Cost-Cutting Silos

Silos	Reality
• Resources are scarce.	• Resources are abundant.
• Doing things the way we have always done them.	• Change will always happen. We cannot escape it.
• One uses bottom-line thinking.	• The bottom line comes second, behind what the patient values.
• Financial decisions are separate from the rest of the organization.	• Financial decisions need to be made within the context of the total organization.

One silo is that *resources are scarce*. This is not surprising because, as we have discussed in previous chapters, accounting and financial theory are based on scarcity:

> Accounting and finance are applied areas of microeconomics. The theory of economics forms the foundations upon which all financial management is ultimately built. The essence of economics is that society has a limited amount of resources, with competing demands for them. The economic system attempts to allocate those resources in an optimal fashion (Finkler and Kovner, p. 4).

Correspond this way of thinking with quantum physics theory (further explained in Chapter 2), formulated more recently—or rather, it has probably been around longer (see the Ecclesiastes quote that follows). If you remember, in quantum physics, the description of the world is:

> A vast porridge of being where nothing is fixed or measurable.... [There are] dynamic patterns continually changing into one another—the continuous dance of energy.... The universe begins to look more like a great thought than like a great machine (Wheatley, pp. 31–32).

The same idea is found in the Bible:

> That which is, already has been;
> That which is to be, already is (Ecclesiastes 3:15).

Using quantum physics, one would say, *We need to be careful about our thoughts as they can create our reality*. If this is the case, we would much rather choose *abundance* than scarcity.

In fact, perhaps our present cost-cutting dilemmas have been caused by too many people thinking that there are *limited* resources! We probably would make different decisions if we thought resources were *abundant*! In this book, we choose abundance. Many financial people will have difficulty with this concept because their education and their work environment have always emphasized scarcity.

It is easy to get caught up into another box, or silo, as *we continue to do things the way we have always done them*. Staying with what is familiar is certainly more comfortable than change. However, if we never change anything, this will cause an organization's demise. Stasis equates to death. Regardless of our efforts to remain the same, everything changes. Thus, this effort can lead us into difficulties since *change* is our only constant. Does *everyone* in the organization realize this?

A third silo is *bottom-line thinking*. Throughout this book we have advocated that the core value, *what is best for the patient*, comes first with the *bottom line being second*. This is another guide for us when choosing a budget strategy.

Then there is the belief, another silo, that one can separate financial decisions from other organizational decisions when actually, *any action we take will affect the bottom line*. This means that *everyone* in the organization will need to be aware of, or actually making, the budget strategies.

How Do We Choose a Strategy?

What should guide us in choosing a strategy? The first thing, emphasized in Chapters 3 and 4, is the importance of getting everyone in the organization to agree to commit to a basic core value such as, *we will always do what is best for the patient*. This means we will do what the patient wants or values. As we are considering budget strategies, everyone needs to be constantly vigilant as to what is right for the patient, and try to accomplish this in a cost effective way. This means that every decision we make, including the choice of budget strategies, needs to support this value.

Within that core value, patient safety has become an enormous issue. The Institute of Medicine's (IOM, 1999) report, *To Err Is Human*, suggests that more than a million injuries and as many as 98,000 deaths each year are attributed to medical errors. These errors are costly, not only in human suffering, but also in dollars and cents. We are in need of a new system with better safeguards right as we are dealing with budget cuts and becoming more efficient.

When making budget strategy decisions, it is important to use the The Institute of Medicine's (IOM) safety/quality guidelines. In fact, regardless of budget, IOM proposed that every health care organization, purchaser, regulator, and educational institution focus on and align their environments toward providing care that is:

- *Safe:* Avoiding injuries to patients from the care that is intended to help them.
- *Effective:* Providing services based on the best available scientific knowledge to all who could benefit and refraining from providing services to those not likely to benefit...
- *Patient-centered:* Providing care that is respectful of and responsive to individual patient preferences, needs, and values and ensuring that patient values guide all clinical decisions.
- *Timely:* Reducing waits and sometimes harmful delays for both those who receive and those who give care.
- *Efficient:* Avoiding waste, including waste of equipment, supplies, ideas, and energy.
- *Equitable:* Providing care that does not vary in quality because of personal characteristics such as gender, ethnicity, geographic location, and socio-economic status (Shortell, pp. 7–8).

The Budget Process—Is It Flawed or Is It Effective?

Then we need to examine the budget process that is used. In our interconnected world, the best budget process will involve everyone in the organization—including patients, families, and physicians. This process is participative but extends beyond just participation. The process is most effective when all involved are equal partners, using dialogue (both sharing information and listening to others). This approach is much more effective than an authoritarian, or top-down, method of communication.

Therefore, everyone from the housekeeper or nursing assistant through the physician and the board chair is involved in the decision-making process, with the patients and their families being the pivotal, or most important, part of this process. Physicians have to be included because physician practice patterns can have a direct effect on increasing or decreasing the budget.

We recommend being *honest* about budgets (see Chapter 10, Budgeting). The problem with dishonesty is that once you have been found out, your believability is gone. Trust, once lost, is extremely difficult to gain again, or realistically, is probably never gained again! Obviously, it is best if *all* are expected to be honest in an organization. *Integrity*, discussed in Chapter 3, is the essential core value of prime importance. After all, when integrity is not present, lies beget more lies.

Honesty can become a problem in an organization where *everyone else* is playing games. If you, a manager, have been honest, and have been diligent about holding down costs, yet no one else has been held accountable, when there are budget cuts, you may be expected to cut the same percentage as those who have not been accountable. Your unit then becomes penalized for being more effective! Thus it is very important to stress with your supervisors right from the start, that you are holding down costs; and ask them to promise that your unit will not be penalized if there is a budget cut. In certain organizations it is important to get this in writing.

Historically, a flawed budget process has been used. This process started in the 1920s when large companies used the process "as a tool for managing costs and cash flows" (Hope and Fraser, p.113). Then in the 1960s:

> companies used accounting results not just to keep score but also to dictate the actions of people at all levels of the company. By the early 1970s, a new generation of leaders schooled in the finer arts of financial planning had begun to rely on financial targets and incentives—in lieu of such benchmarks as productivity and marketing effectiveness—to drive performance improvement (Hope and Fraser, p. 113).

This caused serious problems in the 1980s and 1990s when companies started paying more attention to sales targets than to satisfying customers. Suddenly money was running the game, rather than supporting it.[1]

BUDGET GAMES

When dishonesty is prevalent and is allowed to continue, serious problems result all through the organization. This includes the budget process. Hope and Fraser (2003) report that budgeting can take up to *30 percent of management's time*! This time commitment becomes even *more* overwhelming when mergers and reorganization occur. *This is expensive time that does not really accomplish much in the way of outcomes.* In fact, many harmful games can result. Consider the following from Jensen (2001) in the *Harvard Business Review*:

> CORPORATE BUDGETING IS A JOKE, and everyone knows it. It consumes a huge amount of executives' time, forcing them into *endless rounds of dull meetings and tense negotiations. It encourages managers to lie and cheat, lowballing targets and inflating results, and it penalizes them for telling the truth.* It turns business decisions into *elaborate exercises in gaming.* It sets colleague against colleague, creating distrust and ill will. And it distorts incentives, motivating people to act in ways that run counter to the best interests of their companies.
>
> Consider... the recent debacle involving a big beverage company. The vice president of sales for one of the company's largest regions dramatically underpredicted demand for an upcoming major holiday. His motivation was simple—he wanted to ensure a low revenue target that he could

---

[1] A book coauthored by Tom Johnson, called *Relevance Lost: The Rise and Fall of Management Accounting*, describes all this.

be certain of exceeding. But the price for his little white lie was extremely high: The company based its demand planning on his sales forecast and consequently ran out of its core product in one of its largest markets at the height of the holiday selling season....

The sad thing is, these shenanigans have become so common that they're almost invisible. The budgeting process is so deeply embedded in corporate life that the attendant lies and games are simply accepted as business as usual, no matter how destructive they are....

As soon as you start motivating unit and department heads to falsify forecasts and otherwise hide or manipulate critical information, you undermine the salutary effects of budgeting. Indeed, the whole effort backfires. You end up with uncoordinated, chaotic interactions as people make decisions on the basis of distorted information they receive from other units and from headquarters. Moreover, since managers are well aware that everyone is attempting to game the system for personal reasons, you create an organization rife with cynicism, suspicion, and mistrust.

When the manipulation of budget targets becomes routine, moreover, it can undermine the integrity of an entire organization (Jensen, pp. 96–97).

Another similar perspective is presented by Hope and Fraser (2003):

Budgeting, as most corporations practice it, should be abolished.... Companies... cling tenaciously to budgeting—a process that disempowers the front line, discourages information sharing, and slows the response to market developments until it's too late.... In practice, they marshal the power of computer systems to uncover mind-numbing levels of detail and, using the budget as a benchmark, demand to know why a sales team has rung up higher-than-normal telephone charges, for instance, or why it has underspent the quarter's entertainment allowance. And where is 'all the authority of the chairman' when the team finds it can't meet the budget's sales targets? Fearing the consequences, the team will lean on customers to order goods they have every intention of returning. And if by some chance the team thinks it will exceed its targets, it will press customers to accept delivery in the next fiscal period, delaying valuable cash flows.

In extreme cases, use of the budget to force performance improvements may lead to a breakdown in corporate ethics. [They then discuss several failed companies where, for example, employees had to be 2 percent under budget with nothing else being acceptable.] Other failed companies had tight budgetary control processes that funneled information only to those with a 'need to know.'

A number of companies have recognized the full extent of the damage done by budgeting. They have rejected the reliance on obsolete data and the protracted, self-interested wrangling over what the data indicate about the future. And they have rejected the foregone conclusions embedded in traditional budgets—conclusions that render pointless the interpretation and circulation of current market information (pp. 108–109).

Bart's research (1989) on gamesmanship found there were several games that managers played: understating volume estimates; not declaring/understating price increases; not declaring/understating cost reduction programs; and overstating expenses for advertising, consumer promotions, trade-related issues, and market research. These budget manipulations resulted in "*'cushion,' 'slush fund,' 'hedge,' 'flexibility,' 'cookie jar,' 'hip/back pocket,' 'pad,' 'kitty,' 'secret reserve,' 'war chest,'* and *'contingency'* funds" (p. 286). This occurs because usually senior management does not have the time to find the cushions, or because others were not as familiar with the product so did not realize the true costs.

Another game that is played with budgets is the *spend it* or *lose it* mentality that goes on at the end of the budget year. In this game, a manager knows that any money left in the budget will be lost at the end of the fiscal year. So the manager decides to find things to spend the money on just before the fiscal year closes.

Bart's research also examined companies where games were not played. Here "there was a good deal of *trust* between senior management and product managers" (p. 290). Honesty was valued. In fact, trust and honesty were so important one manager said,

> The moment I betray my… manager, I've had it in this company. My bosses will be angry with me for being unfair. And [people reporting directly to me] will never take my word at face value again. They'll start to play games with me and I'll have to try and catch them… and that sure can waste a lot of time! (p. 291).

WHAT CAN WE DO TO SOLVE THE BUDGET PROCESS PROBLEMS?

Today, more participative, customer-oriented processes for employees to use in organizations are being developed. This process is resulting in flatter structures; rapid responses to market changes; and staying close to the customer—emphasizing public relations; empowering workers to make appropriate decisions as they do their work; and sharing information, including information about budget expenses and revenues. Yet, by still using the cumbersome, flawed, historical budget process, we do not achieve any of these objectives. In fact, we hamstring employees, rather than enhance our systems to help employees have all the tools present so they can do their job most effectively.

That is why we advocate a different process that includes dialogue and honesty. For instance, consider the following:

Do Away With The Budget

Some companies have done away with the budget and the budget process. Instead they use the following method:

> Alternative goals and measures—some financial, such as cost-to-income ratios, and some nonfinancial, such as time to market—move to the foreground. And business units and personnel, now responsible for producing results, are no longer expected to meet predetermined, inter-

nally selected financial targets. Rather, every part of the company is judged on how well its performance compares with its peers' and against world-class benchmarks.

In companies using these standards of performance, business units become smaller, more numerous, and more entrepreneurial. Strategy becomes a grass-roots endeavor. The aggregate result of many small teams exploiting local opportunities is a much more adaptive organization.

But that's not to say these companies abandon their high expectations. They don't naively assume that everyone who is given more autonomy will improve his or her performance. In fact, they require employees to do something much tougher than meet a fixed target. They ask them to chase a will-o'-the-wisp, to measure themselves against how well comparable groups inside and outside the company will turn out to have done in the same period, given the economic conditions prevailing at the time. Because employees won't know whether they've succeeded or by how much until the period is over, they must use every ounce of their energy and ingenuity to ensure that their performance is better than that of their peers. Business units,... can measure their progress against comparable units within the company through the use of a few key financial measures. In order to measure themselves against external peers, they can use operational benchmarks based in industrywide best practices....

Abandoning budget targets... frees a business to give a wise variety of emerging information its due.... This shifts the emphasis from meeting short-term promises to improving our competitive position year after year. The result is much more accurate interpretation of our results (Hope and Fraser, pp. 109–110).

Replace the Traditional Budget with Rolling Forecasts

Hope and Fraser (2003) report that the focus has shifted from detailed budget plans to trend analyses and three-month rolling forecasts for five to eight quarters. Managers, along with the finance department, are expected to constantly revise the forecasts. Instead of the cumbersome, detailed traditional budget approach, these forecasts only include "key variables, such as orders, sales, costs, and capital expenditures, which means they can be compiled relatively easily and quickly, sometimes by a single person in a single day" (p. 112). This way the budget information is constantly updated, and takes the latest economic trends and customer usage patterns into account. Information is open to all in the organization. Playing budget games becomes difficult, and everyone receives more accurate, updated information for appropriate strategic planning information.

> Here's how rolling forecasts usually work. Let's say that in the middle of March 2003, a company creates a five-quarter forecast that covers the period from the beginning of April 2003 through the end of June 2003.

From the moment it is completed, new data start coming in. Once three months' worth is in hand, the process begins again. A new five-quarter forecast updates the projections for the period covered by the previous forecast and creates a brand-new projection for the quarter farthest in the future, July-September 2004.

Volvo relies on several types of rolling forecasts. Every month, it orders up a 'flash' forecast that looks three months ahead, informing managers about current demand and helping them determine whether, for example, price promotions should be introduced or curtailed. Every quarter, a 12-month forecast updates the managers' working assumptions about customer behavior and economic trends. And every year, two additional forecasts—one looking four years ahead, one looking ten years ahead—help managers assess the company's market positioning and determine schedules for phasing out old models and phasing in new ones (p. 112).

Companies using this approach have discovered that they can save up to 95 percent of the time they originally spent going through the historical budget process. For those of us that are used to having budgets, this can be a difficult change to picture. Instead of anticipating the budget for the next year, longer-term goals, often rolling forecasts that project for the next couple years, are identified. Then the manager reviews the forecasts every quarter. The quarterly review helps managers to continually assess the action plan, and to change it as new developments occur. Elements measured include both hard and soft performance data such as profits, cash flows, cost ratios, customer satisfaction, and quality. The organizations became radically decentralized and needed a much smaller corporate structure to support the front-line managers. Hope and Fraser (2003) describe companies that use this method:

> In an empowered organization, people are free to make mistakes and equally free to fix them. Managers have wide discretion in making decisions; as a result, they can obtain resources more quickly than in traditional companies and without having to document need quite so elaborately, partly because they are accountable for the profitability of their units and can therefore be expected to shed any excess in the event that demand falls.... And employees, because they don't require much supervision, don't need the extensive central services that most organizations provide. Eliminating those services has a dramatic effect on a company's cost structure....

> Without budget expectations to worry about, staff members can do something with the nonconforming customer and market information they collect—other than hide it. The reporting of unusual patterns and trends as they unfold helps the business avoid shortages or overages and formulate changes in direction. Instead of being imposed from above, strategy seeps up from below (pp. 110–111).

Margin Management

A similar solution was reported in 1987 by Posner. Determining that the budgeting process had become too cumbersome, McManus, a CEO, changed the budgeting approach in the company he had started. He found that the final budget, arrived at during a painful, traditional budget process, was "based on assumptions that may or may not bear any resemblance to what will actually happen in the next 11 months" (p. 117). So what could be done about this time waster?

Luther, one of his managers, suggested doing away with the historical budget process and, instead, move to a margin management way of doing budgeting. McManus decided to try it. In a margin management system, out of every dollar generated, 15 percent pays corporate overhead expenses and pretax profits. Then the manager would take over from there, determining how the rest of the money will be spent to accomplish the work. This turned the whole budgeting process around. Managers were careful to only spend money on what was necessary, and all employees began to really watch expenses. Managers were now planning budgets with input from staff based on what was actually occurring, and then making the decisions on how the money was spent.

The article stressed how this was a much more effective process than having the CEO make the budget decisions, because the CEO was so removed from the day-to-day issues that employees faced. This worked very well for normal business and they suggested using three guidelines: 1) agree on the overhead amount; 2) empower managers and employees to make the budgeting decisions, rather than having the executive group make the decisions; and 3) add incentives for both managers and employees to benefit from revenues they generated.

There were two times when this strategy did not work—in new start-ups when people did not have any idea as to actual costs and revenues, and with very unstable businesses.

BUDGET STRATEGIES

Once the budget process is examined, and changed if necessary, other budget strategies can be considered. The first priority with budget strategies is that they effectively manage costs yet give quality service; and, as we said at the beginning of the chapter, it is important to put the budget strategies into an organizational context as most often the strategies will effect more than one department.

ADMINISTRATIVE LEADERSHIP

A first priority within an organization is to identify and rectify poor administrative leadership. Effective leadership is discussed in detail in Chapter 3. Some clues to look for are issues like: administrators who focus too much on the bottom line; those who give lip service to core values yet their actions do not support the values; or those who lead from their own selfish motives, not what is best for others. Another problem that can occur is that an administrator may not realize how various actions or decisions impact others. For example, when the president is preaching that everyone else needs to be cost effective and make budget cuts, and then proceeds to purchase expensive new cherry office furniture. Or, when administrators never make rounds, never deal with patients or patient issues, yet continue to make budget decisions and pull wonderful salaries.

As previously noted, poor administrative leadership results in higher direct costs, such as more patient complications and other patient safety issues, an increased need for service or increased length of stay, expensive staffing, more patient care delivery problems, or patients and physicians choosing to go elsewhere for services. There are also large indirect costs such as high staff turnover with new staff needing to be hired and oriented; more legal fees due to more patient lawsuits; more service that is not reimbursed; and more dissatisfaction on the part of the remaining patients, staff, and physicians. The spiral continues downward.

Contrast this with effective leaders who are doing daily rounds, can identify many issues that can be fixed as they occur, can encourage staff to take action on problems, and will have a more realistic picture of the organization—what staff and patients are experiencing. In this case, chances are the unit or organization is using effective teamwork; patients are satisfied with their service and may even rave about how helpful certain people have been; physicians enjoy unit staff and know the patients will be taken care of properly; and direct and indirect costs will not get out of hand while revenues continue to come in.

FIXING SYSTEMS PROBLEMS

Besides the leadership problem, *incredible cost savings* can be realized by examining and fixing systems problems. For example, it is amazing how many *things we continue to do that no one really needs to do anymore*. Take our admitting procedure. Perhaps there are 120 steps that need to be done to admit a patient and only 75 of them are necessary presently, yet we go on doing all 120. Or on an inpatient service, the bed may not need to be changed daily. Or certain administrators never deal with problematic behaviors with staff or physicians—directly causing more budget costs that could be saved.

Then there is *duplication*. For example, we may have five or six people all getting histories and physicals from the same patient. Or, we do not use the history and physical already completed in the facility that just transferred the patient to us.

It is possible that there are staff *that are very busy for a certain period of time, but do not have enough to do at other times*. Yet we continue to schedule them in the same way and do not add to their responsibilities.

Huge problems can occur when we, as administrators, implement a *quick-fix solution* that actually compounds the situation and results in more problems than had previously occurred. Quick-fix solutions are discussed further in Chapter 4 on Organizational Strategies. A common example occurs when suddenly the executive team, or the financial officer, determines that drastic cost cuts are necessary. Then everyone gets into the frenzy, and quick-fix cost cuts are made such as:

- Cut the education budget, travel costs, and positions—and then wonder later why there are more safety issues occurring;
- Have every department take the same percentage cut, not taking into account which departments might be more efficient already, or which departments need to contract or expand due to environmental changes; and/or
- Suddenly restructure—which generally translates into losing some positions with no pre-planning.

Another strategy is to give the patient care in the least expensive setting, i.e., move a surgical patient quickly from the recovery room, to ICU, to general care unit, to skilled nursing unit, to home with home care. This saves money but can result in less continuity for the patient.

A big time-waster is the time spent finding care givers. For instance, sometimes a nurse will call or page the physician who is unavailable at the time. Then the physician calls the nurse but it is hard to track down the nurse. Having documentation systems linked between the practice setting and the physician office can facilitate this communication. Another example is a family member who wants to talk to the nurse but the nurse cannot be found. Some facilities are using a tracking device that the nurse wears so the nurse can easily be found.

Costs Associated With Reengineering, or Rather Restructuring, Redesign, or Reengineering/Layoffs

Reengineering "is the fundamental rethinking and radical design of business processes to achieve dramatic improvements in critical, contemporary measures of performance, such as cost, quality, service, and speed" (Hammer and Champy, 1993, p. 32). Reengineering was meant to happen in a carefully crafted way, following dialogue by many of the staff in an organization. Instead, it was often bastardized and called various terms such as redesign, restructuring, or reorganization, to accomplish "slash and burn," frenzied budget cuts that do not represent careful crafting and dialogue. Is it any wonder that in the frenzy there are additional costs incurred that were not considered?

> It is both obvious and worthy of emphasis that if we are going to improve cost and service performance in [health care organizations], we must begin by looking at how we use our employees—how many there are, what kinds, what we ask them to do, how we organize them, and how in reality they spend their time and the institution's resources.... For [health care organizations], the value added is the sum of all personnel-related expenses.... Not all costs are created equal.... What was needed was a framework that recognized the differences between costs and the different strategies to which each might or might not be susceptible. As a result, operations strategists devised a conceptual model for thinking about costs: the cost performance hierarchy (Lathrop, pp. 24–27).

This hierarchy is contained in **Exhibit 14–2**. Thus, depending on the question being asked, strategies and cost performance could be measured for the categories contained in the table. For instance, if one is starting with the basics, at the *inherent level*, one would ask, "*What* is done?", and one might measure census or location. If one wanted to find out structural issues, one would ask, "*How* is it done?", and one might measure skill mix or physical size and layout. And if one were in the execution phase, one would ask, "*How well* is it done?", and one might measure productivity levels.

Two common ways to restructure or reorganize are: 1) inpatient bed consolidation by reaggregation of the patient population, and/or 2) by downsizing and cutting present staff positions. Either can have drastic effects on both the remaining work force, and on effi-

Exhibit 14–2 Operations Performance Hierarchy

Category	Composition
Inherent Level: "**What** is done?"	Census and admission rates
	Variability of demand (external)
	Intensity of care required/severity of illness
	Quality of care objectives
	Service offerings
	Location
Structural Level: "**How** is it done?"	Organization structure
	Management processes
	Operating policies and systems
	Capacity management
	Physical size and layout
	Equipment deployment
	Skill mix
Execution Level: "**How well** is it done?"	Productivity levels
	Work pace
	Skill level

From: Lathrop, J. (1993). *Restructuring health care: The patient-focused paradigm.* San Francisco: Jossey-Bass, p. 28.

ciency in general. Most often, the result is inefficiency, realized in elevated costs and other costly short-term and/or long-term effects.

A *short-term effect* of redesign is that the "survivors" need an orientation to assume the duties of displaced personnel. This means that a less effective, less efficient staff are not only dealing with the acquisition of new duties—and the resultant creation of more patient safety issues—but are also experiencing "survivor sickness." Burke (2002) describes "survival sickness" as having the following characteristics: "low morale, decreased commitment, and increased cynicism, mistrust, and anger. Affected caregivers may question the effectiveness of their facility's functioning, describe their work environment as deteriorated, and believe that this deterioration threatens patient's well-being" (Burke, p. 41). These are the short-term effects. However, it may not stop there.

How well the organization supports staff during times of restructuring will directly impact retention of the remaining staff. So a long-term effect, along with additional costs, may be that there will be a subsequent increase in staff turnover rates resulting from restructuring. Sometimes it is easier to be the person who is displaced than be one of the remaining staff on a unit/department. Based on these facts, it is very important for the nurse leader and other health care organization officials to provide support for the "survivors."

Actually, providing survivor support is a tall order. It is best if administrators are continually communicating with staff about the changes that will take place as well as why these changes were necessary. Once staff trust is lost, it is very difficult to regain. In addition, staff morale will suffer when layoffs or restructuring occur; and teamwork may be affected within and between departments. Burke (2002) advocates taking the following steps to improve staff involvement dealing more effectively with survivor issues:

- Create focus groups or hold employee meetings to discuss the restructuring, particularly what went right and solutions for what went wrong [note here that it would have been better to do focus groups and employee meetings as part of the planning process for redesign in the first place];
- Develop education programs to help employees adjust;
- Identify employee concerns through surveys [or do rounds!];
- Formulate new communication strategies; and
- Reevaluate jobs to better reflect new responsibilities (Burke, p. 41).

There is an important *long-term* financial effect. People who advocate "slash and burn" cost cutting would do well to heed some research published in *Harvard Business Review*. "Companies with few or no layoffs performed significantly better than those with large numbers of layoffs" (Rigby, 2002). In addition the research found that companies with similar growth rates that *did not* downsize were found to consistently outperform those that downsized. Aside from all this, there were costs associated with lay offs:

- Severance packages;
- Temporary declines in productivity or quality; and
- Rehiring and retraining costs (Rigby, 2002).

Are the costs associated with downsizing and restructuring in health care that much different than those listed above in other businesses? Something to think about…

Thoughtless approaches are implemented without considering future consequences. This research shows that *greater cost savings are realized by dealing with the more knotty organizational and leadership problems*, and that downsizing and layoffs can actually be more expensive in the long run.

Focusing on the Budget with Patient Safety in Mind

While discussing patient safety issues, there is always a current, newly identified issue that can have costly implications, such as when we needed to start wearing gloves for everything. The current issue is achieving the six patient safety aims identified in the Institute of Medicine (IOM) report, which recommends that care is: safe, effective, patient centered, timely, efficient, and equitable. This is a major redesign issue for health care organizations in all settings, and needs to be implemented at the point of care that includes the home and the health care giver's car in the case of home care.

To achieve this redesign, Shortell and Selberg (2002) suggest four main environmental areas that should be targeted for improvement:

- **The infrastructure that supports the dissemination and application of new clinical knowledge and technologies.** When we are focused on providing evidence-based care, we will significantly improve quality. As nursing executives, we must provide the latest and greatest in tools for clinicians to use to adopt best practices. With the growing number of elderly in the US, which in turn increases the population of patients experiencing chronic illness, healthcare teams with best knowledge and best practices will provide the most improvements in patient care (p. 7).

- **The information technology infrastructure.** Automation is a must. From automated drug order entry to the automated patient record, a paperless system with its integrated documentation provides less errors and better quality. When improvements in quality are noted by consumers/patients, The Institute of Medicine committee believes that confidence in the healthcare system will return (p. 8).

- **Payment policies.** Financial incentives must be built into the system to provide for the alignment of care based on best practices with the achievement of better patient outcomes. This change in the environment directly affects the budget process. These incentives would be built in up front. The Institute of Medicine is suggesting that "all stakeholders in the system reexamine payment policies to develop methods that provide fair payment for good clinical management of the types of patients seen" (p. 8).

- **Preparation of the healthcare workforce.** Today's healthcare workers will need new skills to accommodate the aims of the 21st-century healthcare system as set forth by The Institute of Medicine. Because systems thinking will be a cornerstone of a transformed health system, its workers will need skills to transfer best practices to other parts of the organization. Administrators at all levels must also learn to work closely with clinicians so that there is less separation between medicine and management (pp. 7–8).

Several major healthcare systems have achieved national recognition in implementing the IOM recommendations in Health Care in America's *100 Top Hospitals* study. For example, Exempla Healthcare—a Denver-based healthcare system—was named as having one of the top intensive care units in the nation. They implemented the IOM strategies in their strategic plan, making quality their key priority. This achieved improvements in quality and in collaboration with the medical staff, by becoming a system-oriented, rather than a process-oriented, institution (Shortell and Selberg, p. 8).

Exempla first started with a protocol, for example caring for a surgical patient, and, using a systems perspective that accounted for both processes and the interdependencies of care givers, evaluated and redesigned the protocol from admission to discharge. Responsibility was then assigned in this larger entire systems context, rather than with just one process within the system. This integrated approach achieved a common framework with a common goal (Shortell and Selberg, p. 10).

In this example, Exempla's first priority was the patient; the IOM strategies were achieved; but the redesign also achieved a better profit margin. (The bottom line did not drive the change, but was an effect of the change.) It is an example of how improved healthcare quality provides improved outcomes—for the patient, for the organization, and for the bottom line.

Progressive Care Units

Progressive care units, also called swing units, have been established to provide care for patients who are waiting for an available bed for admission, i.e., from the emergency room, or have been in an ICU and are waiting for a stepdown bed. It may be an overflow unit, or may be designated for certain kinds of patients, such as cardiopulmonary or neurological step-down units. Generally criteria are established for admission. This prevents the bottlenecks that occur when patients have not yet been discharged, yet other patients already need those beds (Meyer, 2002).

Benchmarking Hospital Lengths of Stay

As prospective pay and managed care became a reality, it was suddenly necessary to make hospital lengths of stay as short as possible. Inpatient stays were directly linked with resource use. As hospitals benchmarked length of stays for specific DRGs with other hospitals, using averages was somewhat useful but did not capture enough information about distributions to make the data as meaningful as it could be. Histograms have proved to be more helpful to picture this data [an example of a histogram is on page 569]:

> Histograms are bar graphs which employ relative heights of each bar to identify relative numbers of patients generating particular stays. Histograms thus take the form of collections of bars where peaks identify stays with the largest numbers of discharges and valleys indicating stays with the lowest numbers of inpatients. They provide more information than simple median lengths of stay in identifying the compactness of the distribution of stays and more information than mean stays in identifying numbers of outlier cases. Outlier cases are also more clearly pictured with histograms (Lagoe, Arnold, and Noetscher, p. 76).

Benchmarking has aided hospitals to decrease the length of stay by using multidisciplinary approaches, like case management and critical/clinical pathways, as discussed in previous chapters. For instance, case management departments use benchmark data to identify the costs and efficiencies associated with their care practices. Improvements can then be made to these practices and to deal more effectively with outliers.

Holding Down High Costs of Inpatient Care by the Employment of Advanced Practice Nurses and Hospitalists

Recently, *advanced practice nurses* have been employed in health care organizations in an attempt to become both more effective and more cost efficient. Nurse practitioners are often involved in primary, and less often in tertiary, care roles where they can do an initial assessment and history. They also follow up with chronic, or typical acute, patients while the physician is involved with the care of more acute or complicated patients. Nurse anesthetists (CRNAs) are often found in the OR, thus achieving a cost savings for less complicated surgeries. Clinical nurse specialists can be found in hospitals helping nursing staff take care of more complicated patients and/or having an education role with nursing staff with an end result that patient outcomes improve and length of stay is reduced (Rosenfeld, 2000). In psychiatry, clinical nurse specialists have patient practices in the community. In some states, nurse midwives (CNMs) are delivering babies in both hospital settings and in the home.

Advanced practice nurses can be employed by hospitals, long-term care facilities, physicians, or can freelance on their own. When employed by hospitals they are credentialed along with the physicians. Some physicians feel that advanced practice nurses help them care for chronic patient conditions, freeing physicians to treat more complicated patients; other physicians feel that advanced practice nurses have a negative impact on physician income. Advanced nursing practice varies in practice act definitions from state to state.

Another recent addition on the hospital scene is to hire *hospitalists*. Hospitalists are physicians that treat inpatients of all ages only during a hospital stay—admission through discharge.

> Managed care and the Balanced Budget Act are propelling the shift to hospitalists, an emerging subspecialty of internal medicine which is devoted to improving the efficiency of care for hospitalized patients. Intensive, on-site care management by hospitalists can produce substantial savings.... Studies show that inpatient specialists can reduce length of stay by more than 30 percent, and hospital costs up to 20 percent.
>
> ... The reasons for these dramatic improvements in costs per case and length of stay are not hard to find:
> - No delays of treatment after admission,
> - Volume-based experience of hospitalist enhances diagnostic speed, facilitating earlier start of treatment,
> - Vigilant attention to changes in patient condition on a 24x7 basis, e.g., new lab data, nursing observations,
> - Minimal patient down-time in waiting for care, testing results, or specialty consultations,
> - Continuous, rapid fine-tuning of therapeutics over the course of hospitalization,
> - Ready availability of hospitalist to patient and family improves communication and facilitates their approval for changes in treatment,
> - Hospitalist knows 'how to get things done around here' to facilitate timeliness, improve efficiency in use of the hospital's resources,
> - Greater confidence in early discharge from ICU, recovery room, to more appropriate (and lower-cost) levels of care, and
> - Discharge planning begins at start of admission (Coile, p. 8).

The downside of hospitalists include: less continuity of care for the patient, as the patient returns to the regular physician when discharged; the patient does not know the hospitalist so does not have a relationship with him/her; some primary care physicians want to continue to follow the patient; and at times the hospitalist can order more tests and drive up costs rather than decrease them.

Marketing

Budget strategies can include activities that will increase business. Over the past twenty years, marketing has become commonplace in the health care arena. Competition continues to intensify, and many find that reimbursement remains insufficient. Reaching a specific market segment with the latest and greatest is becoming more and more important as new endeavors are undertaken by health care facilities.[2]

"The goal of marketing efforts is to enable the organization to determine what customers want or need and to develop and offer those goods or services"(Woods, p. 190). Such a simple definition, or is it? Effective marketing translates into *going beyond*, or giving *more*, than the customer expected. This occurs when everyone goes the extra mile and *"delights"* the patient. Disney, Southwest Airlines, and Marriott built their market share on this premise. The only way to achieve patient "delight" is for *each* staff member in an organization to perform their daily tasks as best they can. On a personal level, it means that everyone is evaluating the patient experience and personalizing approaches to best meet patient needs. On an organizational level it involves improving environmental processes, and enhancing structural capabilities.

Examples of customer delight might include special "helps" that are available to patients such as not having to walk long distances to get to an appointment (this is especially helpful for the frail elderly but is useful for anyone coming to the facility); not having long waits for service; and providing someone to help fill out all the insurance paperwork. The sky is the limit on ideas here...

The most effective marketing that an organization can achieve is the marketing that is done by "word of mouth" from satisfied clients/patients. If processes and procedures are in place to assure that patient care is delivered in a manner pleasing to the patient, and supportive of good patient outcomes, this will speak for itself. Having satisfied clients is much more effective as a marketing tool than all of the high tech market research that can be performed. In fact, much of the marketing budget is wasted if service is poor.

Everyone in an organization contributes to the marketing effort, not just the person or department that is labeled as having the marketing responsibilities. It is possible that another silo can exist if marketing personnel do not realize the importance of staff contributions, or if staff themselves do not realize their marketing function. After all, "if marketing is about meeting patient needs, who better than the nursing staff to make informed marketing decisions" (Wood, p. 190)?

---

[2] Some good references on health care marketing include Berkowitz (1996), Cooper (1994), Alward and Camunas (1991), or Hillestad and Berkowitz (1991).

As discussed in Chapter 4 on Organizational Strategies, departments and functions within an organization are all integrated. Marketing is really everyone's responsibility. Thus it is important that nurse administrators and staff work collaboratively with marketing colleagues to develop and implement strategic marketing programs. Our role as administrators is to make sure that staff understand the marketing role, along with the strategic plan.

> To excel at meeting the needs of those you serve, and to do so profitably, you must exert your influence to ensure that the whole organization is knowledgeable and market driven. By understanding the broad strategic principles of marketing, and making them a part of your strategic planning, you can better position your organization to become the market leader. When you are questioned about why there is any need to market healthcare services, you can reply with confidence, 'It ensures that we meet our patient needs' (Woods, p. 194).

Although many people define marketing as being advertisements or promotion, it actually has a much broader definition. It actually involves the entire strategic planning process discussed in Chapter 15, Strategic Planning: Facing the Future with Confidence. This process is most effective when the following issues are identified about the customers being served:

> *Who* do you want to serve?
> *What* are their needs?
> *How* can their needs be met (Woods, 2002)?

The strategic planning process is most effective when everyone in the organization contributes, understands, and supports the strategic plan. Once the plan is determined and implemented, it is important to measure its effectiveness. Has market share increased? A continual evaluation of market effectiveness is very important in an organization. This information, along with dialogue about how services can be improved, changed, or added to better meet market needs must be shared across the organization.

TREND SPOTTING

Effective strategic planning requires health care executives' expertise in identifying the trends occurring in the health care market. There are some resources available that help to identify current trends, including the 1998 edition of *Setting Foundations for the Millennium: An Assessment of the Health Care Environment in the United States*, published by Deloitte & Touche and VHA. This document reflects data collected from nearly 60 sources and identified eight trends:

- Upward Cost Pressures (health care spending will climb as the population ages)

- Efficiency and Productivity of the Health Care System Increases (mergers continue, care continues to get passed on to less costly settings)

- Managed Care Growth Continues Apace (true capitation is still rare but will become more common)

- Consumer Voice Is Getting Louder (Desire for better service, choice, and availability; more will want alternative therapies; more information will be accessed electronically)

- Government Captures Savings and Offers Choice (Will curtail spending, but may expand coverage, i.e., to children.)

- Doctors Remain a Wild Card (Some aren't feeling the pinch; some are taking stronger governance roles; public funding for MD education will decrease)

- Technology Investment Grows

- Quality Takes Center Stage

Other sources for possible trends surround us. We will find them by having dialogue with patients and families; health care workers; physicians; the public at large; professional organizations; the internet, books, journals, magazines, television; and so forth.

One trend is that consumers are not just accepting the "norm" or "usual" as being the "best" practices. Instead, there is a well-informed public relying on the information and knowledge available through the Internet. Many times, patient/customer satisfaction depends upon the amount of influence, and input, they have over making their own healthcare decisions. Healthcare organizations are awakening to the interests of consumers. Focusing on the latest trends, and providing for customer/patient satisfaction, can provide the edge for a healthcare system, individual specialized department/unit, or service to remain viable (Solovy, pp. 60, 64).

MARKET RESEARCH

Market research can be a source of information necessary to enhance the organization's chances for success. It allows organizations to improve the quality and usefulness of their offerings and can guide decision making. Market research is the science of listening. All employees have the opportunity to add to the market research, especially when they have regular contact with patients.

Data collection concerning the numbers of procedures performed, or number of patient visits for a specific diagnosis, can be very beneficial in determining the direction for future service development. It can reveal trends in patient usage. This can provide direction for the strategic plan.

According to Gershon and Jackson (2003) there are five steps involved in the market research process, regardless of what it will be used for or who is conducting it. They are as follows:

1. *Defining objectives.* With this first step, the end result that needs to be achieved is identified. For example, are we conducting the research to get a better understanding of customers' perceptions of our current services and products, or is the reason to determine the

level of customers' interest in the new offerings?

2. *Developing the sample.* This step asks us to determine the composition of the research group, or who can provide us with answers. For example, if our objective is to find out if enough physicians are serving a particular community, we have to figure out whom to ask. Should we be asking physicians, residents of the community, or both?

3. *Developing questions.* This step lays out the questions that will help us obtain information without biasing the results. Clearly, structuring these questions should be scientific to prevent the questions from leading the respondents to particular answers.

4. *Collecting data.* This step allows us to choose the method for listening to our customers. These methods include face-to-face interviews; focus groups; and mail, telephone, and web-based surveys. The choice is influenced by a variety of factors, including the research objectives, cost, and timing.

5. *Analyzing results.* This step is all about understanding and interpreting what the collected data revealed. Analyzing results can be as simple a providing a basic summary of major themes discovered or as complicated as developing a variety of cross-tabulations (p. 153).

Good market research can be used to educate oneself on a proposed target market. Successful organizations, whether they provide soft drinks, computers, or health care, invest ample resources into staying in tune with their market. What better source for tuning into the market than the nurses who care for patients every day, the secretaries who set up patient appointments, the housekeeping staff who talk to patients, or the finance staff who deal with patients calling about the bill? A feedback loop should be established so these people can relay their information to others in the organization—including the marketing staff.

MARKET STRATEGIES

Before identifying various market strategies that can be used, we need to be aware that there are several anomalies with marketing in health care. First, the physician is a powerful health care supplier, and certainly influences whether customers use a health care facility. Second, there are third-party payers and employers that can influence a patient's choice in providers. Third, health care is not something that a customer looks forward to using. We usually do not save our money and look forward to having a hospital experience.

Fourth, the typical rules of supply and demand do not apply in health care. The economic rules of an efficient market are:

- Whoever demands a service pays for it directly;
- Whoever supplies a product, bears all costs associated with supplying it; and
- Customers have full information about what they are buying (Woods, 2002, p. 154).

When dealing with the health care setting, the first two rules do not apply and the third is often questionable. In the health care market, the patient may demand a service but be prevented from getting it, i.e., rationing health care services by gatekeepers in managed care. As for the second rule concerning who bears the cost, the majority of services are only partially paid for by the customer/client. Instead, third party payers and employers assume the larger part of the payment.

As to the third rule, customer knowledge about the service they require is not always there. This is changing as there has been a beginning groundswell of customer sources of knowledge—such as the internet—available to the public concerning their illnesses, as well as an increased awareness and knowledge about what achieves and maintains health. But, even then, we do not necessarily know what will happen when we purchase health care because it is a service industry, and interactions with people can differ.

Because of these differences in the healthcare market, one needs to give careful thought to setting the strategic direction. Positioning (focusing on significant differences between your product and another organization's product), market segmentation (only serving a group with certain specific characteristics), and product differentiation (explaining how your product differs from other organization's products) are the three closely interrelated

---

Exhibit 14–3 The Interrelationship of Positioning, Differentiation, and Segmentation

Positioning	"The act of designing the company's offering and image to occupy a distinctive place in the target market's mind."
	Example: *Creating the perception that your healthcare system is the luxury leader in the market. More than just saying so, this requires product differentiation such as offering exclusively private rooms, excellent meals, and premium décor.*
Product Differentiation	"The act of designing a set of meaningful differences to distinguish the company's offering from competitors' offerings. Differentiation is not dependent on segmentation."
	Example: *Earning Magnet status, having an inhouse children's hospital, or highest percentage of certified specialty nurses.*
Segmentation	"A merchandising strategy by which products are adjusted to serve a particular group of users. Segmentation cannot be achieved without differentiation."
	Example: *Offering comprehensive culturally adapted services for Spanish-speaking patients. The market segment is Spanish-speaking patients and the product differentiation required might include a full complement of bilingual nurses and physicians, patient education materials in Spanish, and concentrated outreach into the Hispanic community.*

From: Woods, D. (April 2002). Realizing Your Marketing Influence, Part 1. *JONA*, 32(4), 189–195.

---

cornerstones of marketing strategy. **Exhibit 14–3** provides a quick reference to these concepts and how they relate to one another.

When marketing health care for positioning, one might consider promoting a new procedure that is not as invasive to the patient, or the fact that because your organization performs more procedures, it is safer. If one decides to use the market segmentation strategy, one might consider advertising birthing rooms to a population who has health insurance benefits and can choose to come versus choosing a competitor. For product differentiation, one might say that various alternative therapies are available along with more traditional health care services.

Other terms used to help define marketing strategies focus on the manipulation of the four Ps of the marketing mix—product, price, place, and promotion—found in **Exhibit 14–4**.

In this table, the four Ps are corresponded with the four Cs (Marketing Mix)—customer solutions, customer cost, convenience, and communication—that occur in the health care market. For example, the product is often a solution that one offers to resolve a customer problem; the customer cost (price) involves what the patient actually pays as well as what insurance(s) pays; the place is most effective when it is convenient to the customer; and the promotion effort communicates the offered services to the customer.

Therefore, marketing is an integrated function that contributes to the viability of the organization. It affects the bottom line, but the most important aspect of marketing is staying in touch with the basic value, *what the patient wants or values*.

Keeping a constant focus on the health care market is very important in maintaining a hospital budget. The health care market is in continual flux as new technologies and services are developed. Being on the cutting edge of these advancements, and redesigning the organization accordingly to provide inclusion of the latest, most up-to-date services may be the deciding factor on whether or not an organization remains viable. At the same time, other services may need to be discontinued, and environmental influences may impact the services offered. Obviously, this has a great impact on the budget.

OPERATING ROOM EXAMPLE

Let's examine a specific department, the operating room (OR), as we explore what happens as the market changes, environmental influences impact services, and the strategic plan remains dynamic and changing. With its high overhead and crucial status as a revenue generator, the OR is a prime target for process improvement that will lead to margin improvements. Changing services in these areas can have a large impact on the overall financial status for an organization.

Examples of OR environmental conditions that will affect costs and necessitate change are as follows:

1. Staffing shortages, whether nursing staff, anesthesiologist, or other specialties, create and impact services in the OR. As for the nursing impact, the costs generated by the time required to both find and hire staff, and for intensive specialized training needed by these nurses, is an issue. Retention and recruitment for this area is of high priority.

2. Another environmental issue is that competition from increasing numbers of ambulatory centers, as well as in other hospital facilities, may draw patients from the

Exhibit 14–4 The Four Ps and Cs of the Marketing Mix Applied to Health Care

Four Ps	Four Cs	General Description	Health Care Applications
Product	Customer solution	Product Variety	Product/service lines
		Quality	Patient outcomes
		Design	Service quality
		Features	Physical plant
		Packaging	design/decor
		Brand name	Hospital "name"
			and reputation
Price	Customer cost	List price	Cash prices
		Discounts	Contract prices/
		Allowances	reimbursement:
		Payment period	PPO
		Credit terms	HMO
			Medical groups
Place	Convenience	Location	Health care system
		Coverage	location, including
		Assortments	clinic or other service
		Inventory	branches
		Channels	Adjacent medical offices
		Transport	Ancillary services on site
			Referral relationship with
			physicians, medical
			groups, insurance
			providers, etc.
			External patient transportation
			such as vans, taxi
			vouchers, etc.
Promotion	Communication	Sales promotion	Physician relations
		Advertising	Advertising
		Sales force	Community events and
		Public relations	outreach
		Direct marketing	Media relations
			Direct mail

From: Woods, D. (April 2002). Realizing Your Marketing Influence, Part 1. *JONA*, 32(4), 189–195.

facility. In addition, facility charges in an ambulatory center may be lower than a larger full-service facility.

3. Service lines may change due to medical advances, new procedures, and development of new drugs which decrease the requirements for procedures. One example is open-heart surgeries.

4. Increasing costs of malpractice insurance is affecting the numbers of physicians in the specialty areas, such as obstetrics, gynecology, and neurosurgery. With these numbers decreasing, facilities may not have the resources to offer these services profitably. In fact, it may be necessary to focus on other specialty areas in order to stay viable in the market.

5. Population influences are coming into play. For example, ORs will see increasing numbers of joint replacement and other procedures as baby boomers come to require these services.

6. Issues such as prompt start times for OR cases can really affect costs in the OR. Delays do not only cause frustrations for staff and physicians. First and foremost, they create patient discomforts that can affect customer relations. Patients who have their needs met in a pleasing manner are much more apt to return for any further treatments required. All these factors affect costs.

Purchasing high-tech gadgets and powerful software, which is revolutionizing care in surgery suites, is a large OR budget item. This expenditure is a must, yet can be very costly. Thoughtful strategic planning is needed to balance the budget yet provide services in the best way for the patient (Haugh, pp. 51–54).

Staffing Expenses

The largest cost within the expense budget in health care organizations is the employee budget. Because this is a service industry, more people are needed to give the care the client receives. Chapter 20 provides strategies on staffing. However, one bears repeating here: *budget savings can be realized by hiring a higher number of RNs rather than to hire a higher number of nursing assistants or LPNs.* For a person oriented to the bottom line as first priority, this may be hard to fathom. You will hear, "But nursing assistant salaries are less than an RN salary. How can this be true?" Chapter 16 shows how expenses are *lower* using higher RN ratios, having enough support staff present to facilitate the RN function. This is true across the health care continuum.

Another factor with staffing is making sure that the staff is there when needed, and not there when there is less to do. (See the example of this in Chapter 21, Productivity.) Effective scheduling is essential. *Actually, we need to get out of the box on this one.* Think about how rewarding it would be to see someone in the hospital, follow them through a SNF unit, and then see them in their home for home care. And the patient would love the continuity. Think of the cost savings achieved with the larger bonus of both patient and staff satisfaction! We need to break down the barriers!

Along with staffing by actual needs, some hospitals have given RNs the responsibility to restrict admissions. One system used at the Mayo Clinic's Luther Midelfort Health System in Eau Claire, Wisconsin follows:

> At least three time a day staff nurses or clerks on each unit fill out a simple form via the hospital's Intranet indicating the Unit's current patient volume and staffing situation. The computer assigns a numerical value to "anecdotal data," entered by the unit staffer and generates a "traffic light" color—red, orange, yellow, or green—signaling the unit's capacity. The unit's assigned color is posted on the Intranet's "status board" and is immediately available to nursing supervisors. Nurses have the ability to override the assigned color if they disagree with the computer's assessment. Each unit designates its own nurse or nurses to evaluate the computer-generated assessment; very often the charge nurse or another direct-care nurse with a leadership role is given the assignment. The nurses' "capping trust"—the authority the system grants them to restrict unit admissions—cannot be overridden by doctors or administrators....[This] has not only improved throughput... but also contributed to increased job satisfaction among nurses and a percent drop in the hospital's RN vacancy rate (Connoly, 2002).

Martha Jefferson Hospital in Charlottesville, VA, implemented a program where they provided a nurse refresher program to inactive nurses, and then hired them as admission-discharge-teaching nurses, to help with this function throughout the facility. This was another win-win situation because the patients got better care, hospital stays were shortened, and staff morale improved (Blankenship and Winslow, 2003).

Another cost strategy used with employees is to either provide a wellness program, or to get employee discounts at local facilities that will enhance employee health and well being.

Streamlined Documentation/Computerization/Enhanced Reimbursement

> Knowledge traditionally has been viewed as something that one possessed. Today, however, it is viewed as a utility—something not possessed but accessed. People who want to use knowledge should know how to access it, how to use it, and when to let it go (Porter-O'Grady and Malloch, p. 30).

Achieving complete and accurate documentation is another large expense with a lot of potential cost savings. Streamlined documentation is a vital necessity in the overall medical records process to provide accuracy and ease of access to the required records to justify insurance payments, to document the time and cost of nursing care, and also to meet regulatory guidelines (Hensley, pp. 38–40). It has become even more critical today as reimbursement has dwindled. There are several strategies being used to achieve this objective:

- Computerized documentation provides ready access of the patient's medical record for all members of interdisciplinary care teams.

- Effective case management of patient care requires a seamless method of documentation. New interdisciplinary forms have been developed by interdisciplinary task forces in most hospital facilities in an effort to further reduce duplication of information, to save precious nursing time, and to provide efficiency in patient care delivery.

- Billing and coding of patient's records is more efficient when electronically billed. In fact, reimbursement priorities are given by most insurance companies, including Medicare, to those using electronic billing—with payment lags given to providers who still use the paper method.
- Avoiding duplications. Now that patients are being transferred to different units and facilities through an episode of illness, it is important to not repeat histories, physicals, and other medical information needed for effective care.

One might wonder if streamlined computerized care is of such importance, why hasn't there been a fast and furious shift to this method of documentation at all health care organizations? Well, cost has been a major factor. Computerized systems are expensive, and with the lack of financial resources in the health care industry, the electronic medical record has not been purchased as rapidly as one would have expected. The issue of maintaining security and confidentiality of computerized patient information has also been a factor in slowing the progress to paperless systems.

It is now becoming evident that the advantages outweigh the disadvantages. The upfront cost of purchasing and implementing computerized charting is offset by the cost efficiency it provides. Take coding, for instance. In a paper system, a lot of time is spent searching through mounds of paper to obtain coding information. Computerized charting decreases the turn around in reimbursement for hospital stays by providing a fast, efficient retrieval of the pertinent coding information.

Another advantage is the growing competition. For example, HMOs now cover some 67 million Americans. Kaiser Permanente, the nation's largest HMO, spent $1 billion for information technology that will achieve better care as well as document that the care was given (Schonfeld, p. 111). Then they marketed this to employers to show that their care would be safer because of this technology. This was prompted when employers, such as General Motors and Xerox, started ranking health plans by cost and quality in order to give their employees the best possible health care. To give an HMO the edge in the saturated market, low cost care was not enough. Higher standards and quality of care must also accompany the lower cost.

Information technology also makes it possible to achieve better management decisions and patient safety. There is so much knowledge available that it is impossible for a physician or nurse to know all the information needed when caring for a patient. Davenport and Glaser (2002) describe efforts to improve knowledge sharing and retrieval designed by Partners HealthCare (the Boston-based umbrella organization that includes Brigham and Women's, Massachusetts General, and several other hospitals and physician's groups). Their approach is "to bake specialized knowledge into the jobs of highly skilled workers— to make the knowledge so readily accessible that it can't be avoided.... The most promising approach is to embed it into the technology that knowledge workers used to do their jobs" (p. 109).

For example, as the physician logs onto the computer to order a medication, the computer program is linked with both the patient's medical record and a clinical database system. This system can alert the physician about potential allergies, side effects, and contraindications related to the medication being ordered, putting it into context with the patient's history:

> Imagine that a patient with a history of sleep apnea is prescribed a narcotic to mitigate pain after surgery. Narcotics can cause people with sleep apnea to go into respiratory arrest, but, as long as the history of sleep apnea is noted in the patient's medical records, the system will alert the physician to that potential problem. It also takes into account the patient's age, likely metabolism, probability of renal failure, maximum allowable lifetime amounts of a chemotherapy agent, and hundreds of other factors.
>
> The logic engine and knowledge base… are used more during order entry than at any other time. But they are used increasingly during normal review of patient medical records as well. For example, the system alerts the physician, as he or she reviews Mrs. Smith's record, to follow up on her marginally abnormal mammogram or to recheck her cholesterol levels. In addition, it may remind a physician that a particular patient should receive a call or schedule a follow-up appointment.… [It] alerts a physician when a hospitalized patient's monitored health indicators depart significantly from what is expected. The physician is notified through a pager and can then visit the patient directly or call in a new treatment. Minor variations are routed to the nurses' station, and the nurse can decide whether to call in the physician.
>
> The power of knowledge-based order-entry, referral, computerized medical record, and event-detection systems is that they operate in real time. Knowledge is brought to bear immediately without the physician having to seek it out. In some situations, physicians can consult with other experts in real time, via teleconferencing and other technologies (pp. 109–110).

See Chapter 8 for more information on the internet links for best practices available to practitioners in real time. In this case a nurse, physician, or patient can look at the latest research on a specific disease or problem, the latest treatments being used, and the efficacy of various possible treatments, right at the time the information is needed to care for a patient.

BARCODING

Barcoding is another recent information technology tool implemented by the health care industry. It accomplishes several purposes:

- Decreases the incidence of medication error,
- Improves patient identification processes,
- Improves medical supply inventory,

- Achieves a more accurate charge for treatments and supplies, and
- Provides for more automation of the electronic medical record.

Barcodes were first developed in the railroad business to keep track of which cars went with which engines. The barcodes were imprinted on the side of railway cars that went with a particular railway system. As their use increased across various industries, barcodes were used for cataloging items, "tagging" people, or "tagging" items. The health care industry has been slow to make use of this technology. Then the patient safety issue emerged.

This prompted the Food and Drug Administration (FDA) to propose that by the end of 2003, barcoding would be mandated on all single-unit packages of prescription drugs, over-the-counter drugs commonly used in hospitals, vaccines, and biologics such as blood. With barcoding, a three-way match is required before drugs can be administered. Patient safety has driven the implementation of this technology. With this change the FDA estimates that 50 percent of all medication errors will be intercepted, resulting in 413,000 fewer adverse events in a 20-year period. "In today's dollars, that would save $41.4 billion, and hospitals would save as much as an additional $7.6 billion in record-keeping and reporting costs, not to mention the savings in litigation associated costs, according to the FDA" (Becker, p. 7).

CODING ACCURACY USING CHARGEMASTER

Coding[3] has become a part of information technology necessary for prompt patient billing. It is easy to overlook possible charges that could be made, and miss out on revenue because of denials from inaccurate coding, missed charges, and incorrect use of modifier codes. It is helpful to standardize costs, and provide frequent updates on line and in the Chargemaster. This can be very confusing because, as outlined in Chapter 6, reimbursement varies depending upon the service. Sometimes specific costs can be directly billed such as in some outpatient and surgical services, and then sometimes, such as with DRG and with RUG reimbursements, the costs cannot be billed separately because an overall reimbursement amount is paid for a specific patient stay.

It behooves the nurse administrator to understand how billing should occur for areas of responsibility. If costs can be directly charged, and if no one realizes this, the facility could lose considerable money. Usually the finance department is cognizant of what can be directly billed and what cannot, but sometimes nurse administrators have discovered that additional items should be billed. So, the nurse administrator needs to have accurate knowledge of billing nuances. There are several sources that can be very helpful, besides a discussion with the finance department, i.e., professional seminars or networking with peers across the country who are responsible for similar specialty areas.

> Nurses not only document provided services and supplies, they also play
> an active role in the process of generating an accurate and timely bill. To
> that end, it's critical that managers offer feedback and expertise regarding

---

[3] Coding is explained in detail in Chapter 10 of Dunham-Taylor and Pinczuk (2006) *Health Care Financial Management for Nurse Managers: Applications in Hospitals, Long-Term Care, Home Care, and Ambulatory Care.*

a pivotal financial tool—the charge description master [CDM]. A CDM serves several critical functions:

1. **Compliance**, offering a consistent approach to regulations and billing requirements.

2. **Support**, creating the database to support the billing and collection of legitimate revenues.

3. **Accounting**, providing the detail to accurately account for services and support financial planning. . . .

The charge description master (CDM) automatically bills for high-volume services—a process often referred to as 'hard-coding.' The CDM supports an automated process that exposes departments to coding and billing errors, especially if the finance department and department directors don't review and make adjustments for the frequently occurring coding and billing changes. . . .

A hospital CDM computer file or database stores thousands of entries. It's critical to update the CDM because a small error can significantly decrease potential revenue. For example, a $12 dropped charge for a code that's used 2,000 times a year equals a $24,000 shortfall in revenue. Additional financial loss occurs if coding errors stop or slow the processing of these 2,000 claims (Contino, p. 16).

The chargemaster contains information to correctly identify patient charges, which in turn is posted on the patient's bill. One major advantage of the chargemaster is that it can streamline and simplify the patient's bill. Patients are much more likely to pay their bills on a timely basis when they understand the items listed on the bill. Turn-around time on receiving payment is lessened if correct charges are listed. Therefore, having patient-friendly bills can speed up the whole charge/payment process. Listing these charges in an easy-to-read fashion also speeds up this process.

TELEHEALTH

Telehealth can provide health services more conveniently for patients as well as provide another cost-saving approach.

Telehealth is defined as the 'removal of time and distance barriers for the delivery of health care services and related health care activities through telecommunication technology.' Telehealth broadly encompasses computers, including the internet, satellite, video, or telephone usage. Besides providing direct services or health information to people in their homes, offices, or schools, it can be used to: provide consultations between health care providers, register and schedule patients, charge insurers or have other payment applications, and provide data that can be used for research purposes. An advantage of this approach is that it saves time, providing service promptly at the site where the information is needed (Blouin and Brent, p. 292).

One of the most exciting new uses of telehealth is in the form of telemergency services, including triage services, which brings the benefits of fast and efficient emergency care to underserved rural areas. Electronic or telephone links can connect patients at distant sites with physicians and nurse practitioners for care. As this has gained in popularity it has become evident that the healthcare providers need additional computer skills and competencies, and educational programs are needed. Another issue is confidentiality and privacy of the patient record, particularly with HIPAA regulations (HIPAA is further explained in Chapter 6).

Besides emergency medicine, "telephone health consultation accounts for up to 25% of patient encounters in internal medicine and even more in pediatrics" (Simonsen-Anderson, p. 117). Phone consultations can save as much as $50 to $240 per member, and also save the customer's time. Often services are provided by nurses who have physician back up. Telephone nursing service does not come without a significant organizational cost upfront. Setting up an in-house service requires a large amount of financial resources in the beginning months. The usual in-house location for these services requires renovation or construction costs. Installation of telephone lines, office supplies, and office cubicles to afford privacy for the nurse answering calls are examples of these costs.

> Staffing costs are also a major up-front, as well as ongoing, cost.
>
> Safe, effective telephone health assessment depends on solid initial training and education of the RNs fielding calls, as well as ongoing monitoring and feedback. Professional nurses with varied and broad experience, as well as excellent communication and interpersonal skills, are best prepared to address the challenges of a fast-paced telephone health consultation service (Simonsen-Anderson, p. 41).

Nursing salaries must be comparable with others possessing similar qualifications in the immediate vicinity. Usually there is competition with area healthcare facilities when recruiting staff for the service.

Purchasing integrated, database systems that are capable of handling what we have been describing are expensive. Health care organizations will need to figure out how to fund this type of real time technology because the technology achieves so many benefits—better patient outcomes, more accurate billing, and saving on costs that could have been avoided. Smaller organizations may need to develop partnerships with other organizations for such purchases. Some of this data capability, however, is available through library links as described in Chapter 8, that only require internet access and a computer. For smaller organizations or physician offices, library links serve as a starting point that does not require a large capital outlay.

Cost Savings through Efficient Use of Supplies

Supply costs, rising daily in healthcare, also need to be examined. These costs are second only to the cost of staffing. One way to decrease supply costs is by exercising more reasonable use of supplies by nursing staff. Nurse managers responsible for creating and maintaining their unit's fiscal budgets can provide substantial decreases in costs by controlling supply expenditures. An overall decrease in the organization's fiscal budget may be realized as each individual unit's supply budget is trimmed for efficiency.

CREATING A COST-CONSCIOUS ENVIRONMENT—IT'S EVERYONE'S RESPONSIBILITY

As we become more conscious of supply costs as managers, it is important to involve staff in this issue.

> We must also communicate to patients, nurses, and physicians that [health care organizations] no longer can afford to give things away. Someone always ends up paying. Nurses are trained to help people, to be generous and giving. For example, a nurse may give a patient a bunch of sterile pads rather than instructing him to go to the local pharmacy. Even those who mean well can put a [health care organization] out of business (Lefever, p. 30).

Inefficiencies mount up. For unit-based cost savings to occur, staff should be involved in the formulation of the department's fiscal budget and know the overall organization's financial targets. Staff then have a better sense of how they are contributing to either cost inefficiencies, or to cost containment, without compromising quality. After all, practice behaviors can affect the cost of delivering patient care.

Another strategy to maximize efficiency of supply usage by staff is to provide an educational approach to the issue. Krugman, MacLauchlan, Riippi, and Grubbs (2002) report a successful multidisciplinary financial education research project taken by a Western tertiary teaching hospital. In this project nurses, resident physicians, pharmacists, and nursing students integrated fiscal knowledge into practice. This study measured baseline financial knowledge regarding charges, reimbursement, and regulatory issues prior to implementing several initiatives. The team then developed a variety of initiatives to target knowledge deficits. A logo was created and used as a symbol for identifying financial articles published quarterly in the hospital newsletter. Subcommittees addressed the institution's financial problems. Efforts began with various educational activities, such as videos and the purchase of a financial software program for nursing leadership.

The post-survey showed that the subjects' financial knowledge improved. Targeted educational interventions proved successful. Financial outcomes included an increase in captured patient charges, improved documentation of services rendered, and decreased materials loss/wastage. This study was indicative of the positive affects that can be realized from awareness campaigns and educational activities involving staff and physicians (Krugman, et al., p. 277). An additional finding was that often nurses had negative attitudes related to cost effectiveness, associating these with staffing reductions, pay cuts, longer work hours, and diminished resources. Because of these negative attitudes, nurses may not be as cost effective in their nursing practice.

INVISIBLE COSTS

Invisible costs for unused supplies from packs and trays, obsolete and slow-moving inventory, pilferage, giveaways, and uncontrolled usage create waste and are a prime target for nurse managers wishing to correct supply budget variances. First, a nurse manager must determine how and where the major waste is occurring. This may be done by reviewing the unit's present inventory of supplies and determining if there are opportunities for efficiency in areas where practice creates costly waste. An example of this may be when there are supplies requested by physicians who no longer have patients in the department where they are kept. Correcting this waste may be as simple as revising or providing standardization of supplies and of supply usage. Decreasing this type of stock will not only decrease the number of dollars required for the department's supply budget, but will also provide more space for pertinent supplies.

STANDARDIZATION OF SUPPLY USAGE

Standardization of supply usage can also provide cost savings. For example, the standardization of items placed in sterile trays and packs for labor and delivery procedures on obstetrical units, in emergency rooms, or in surgery departments may be warranted.

Meeting with the physicians up front to elicit their input on the design of the new trays is a must. The changes need to satisfy their needs as well as provide efficiency. Otherwise, more waste could occur.

Sales representatives from supply vendors, who are providing the most efficient contracts for their supplies, may be especially helpful in the design of these new packs and trays. Attending health care supply trade fairs may also provide the nurse administrator with excellent information concerning the newest, and most efficient, items available to be placed in the packs. Price wars from vendors may be your best bet in acquiring the most items of quality for the least amount of money. In other words, cost comparison is a must.

JUST-IN-TIME APPROACH

One common purchasing approach has been to only have supplies delivered as they are needed: the just-in-time philosophy. The idea behind this is to save money by not stockpiling; the idea is to avoid having too much already present at the facility. In health care, a service industry, where one is not making the same widgets every day, it can be difficult to anticipate which patients with which medical or surgical problems will need supplies each day. It is difficult to anticipate emergencies. So it is best to be more moderate with this approach.

HOARDING SUPPLIES, LINEN, AND EQUIPMENT

As the financial resources available for purchase of supplies, linen, and equipment has dwindled due to low reimbursements, there has been more hoarding of supplies and equipment. While hoarding provides staff with immediate access to the resources they need for patient care, staff do not realize that they add to their supply and equipment problems overall. Overstocking costs money. Tying up financial resources for purchase of more and more supplies due to stockpiling can actually build to a point where the whole facility is not efficient in the management of materials. For example, hoarding of linen (or IV pumps, monitors, or wheelchairs) only creates the need to purchase more linen for the facility. The linen hoarded is the equivalent of money not able to be used for other purposes. This "lost" inventory of linen would be less costly if left in circulation throughout the health care organization.

DEALING WITH SUPPLY SHORTAGES—AN INTERDISCIPLINARY APPROACH

In actuality, the shortage problem is a symptom of a larger systems problem. Instead of hiding and storing up more linen for the unit, it would be much more cost efficient to bring together a group of representatives from appropriate departments to work out a better solution. Efficiency is the key. For instance, perhaps they would decide to take inventory of where the shortages occur in the facility, and increase the linen counts for those areas to reflect volume fluctuations for various shifts, weekends, and holidays. The solution needs to have the right numbers at the right times in the right place.

This systems strategy is also a useful way to examine supply and equipment fluctuations as patient volume changes. For instance, if the patient census, or acuity, has decreased, the nurse manager, as well as other appropriate departmental managers, could check to see if the inventory usage has also decreased. A periodic survey and inventory of all nursing units in a facility can help with these issues.

In addition, nurse administrators can periodically review overall monthly budget costs for linen, supplies, and equipment. Sudden variances in this budget could indicate that there is hoarding going on, creating the need for purchases to counteract the decreases in certain areas. Close interaction with departments, such as the laundry, central supply, and materials management, could shed light on areas of concern. Educating staff concerning supply costs so they can adjust inventories to meet patient demands is extremely important. The staff should realize that they have a direct responsibility to achieve efficiency, and if something is not working, to express their concerns to the appropriate managers so problems can be fixed. Everyone, including the nurse manager, needs to be involved in achieving better efficiencies.

SUPPLY SOURCES, PURCHASING TRENDS, COOPERATIVE STRATEGIES

Because the cost of medical supplies and equipment is one of the major costs associated with health care, it is imperative for nurse administrators to be knowledgeable in the latest trends affecting the purchasing of these supplies. Having knowledge and being able to "talk the talk" with purchasing managers is essential for nurse managers to have an influence on the buying practices for their units and the institution as a whole.

The Future of Purchasing and Supply: A Five and Ten Year Forecast was compiled in 1998 by the National Association of Purchasing Management (NAPM). This research was completed by the Center for Advanced Purchasing Studies, A. T. Kearney, Arizona State University, and Michigan State University. (In *Nursing Management*, February, 2000, pp. 41–42). They identified eight direction-setting processes that would shape the purchasing and supply profession over the next five to ten years.

1. **Improvement in supply chain**

   Having a seamless supply chain throughout the healthcare organization will improve efficiencies within departments, between departments, with suppliers, and eventually spread process improvements along the entire supply chain. With a seamless supply chain as their top priority, purchasing managers will focus on recognizing where to improve. When dealing with your purchasing manager, keep this objective in mind. To optimize the supply chain, organizations will need to:

- see the broader picture and long-term strategies,
- identify areas where they can reduce duplication or improve processes,
- enhance integrated relationships with supply chain partners.

2. **Improvement in purchasing strategy development**

   Competitive advantage may be achieved when organizations develop key supplier partners and time is spent focusing on strategies to improve purchasing practices. Organizations may implement procurement strategy boards comprised of key purchasing and supply managers from each of the organization's departments. These boards actually make the purchasing decisions with input from frontline managers. Major cost savings can be achieved.

3. **Relationship management**

   Improvement in the relationships between organizations and their suppliers benefits everyone involved. Purchasing managers will need to analyze supplier relationships. From this focus, the purchasing agent can identify improvements needed in purchasing processes and supply usage. Having an open communication and relationship with the supplier increases the information sharing from both directions. Nurse leaders can support that relationship by helping purchasing managers get the data they need from nursing departments.

4. **Global supply development**

   Expansion of the supply chain now extends to far reaching global proportions due to new internet technology and increased use of multinational sourcing (purchasing goods from other countries). These expansions will have a definite effect on purchasing and pricing efforts as new frontiers in manufacturing are included in the supply chain.

5. **Third-party purchasing**

   The trend is emerging to implement third-party purchasing in order to achieve cost efficiency. Third-party purchasing may be used in the form of master contracts, outsourced purchasing operations, or consortiums. It is mainly effective for high volume, low-value, non-strategic purchases. When this model of purchasing is implemented, it must be done with caution and constant, ongoing, financial analysis by the purchasing manager.

6. **Virtual supply chain**

   Researchers write that, "The creation of virtual supply chains is a secondary trend that will continue over the next 10 years." Organizations will need to form short-term alliances, without the legal entanglements of complicated mergers or long-term contracts. This will require many supply chains to have partners and perform tasks that consolidate efforts. This will take a broader vision to accomplish and put in place in an efficient manner.

7. **Strategic supplier alliances**

   As evidenced in many larger healthcare organizations at present, these alliances are forming. Suppliers and healthcare organizations are joining together to place employees from the suppliers on site to work hand in hand with the materials management department to assure cost reductions, product improvements, and or better service. Nurse executives can achieve cost efficiency in their departments by building relationships with these persons. Together with these representatives from the suppliers, they can share knowledge and determine the best products to meet their unit's supply needs.

8. **Complexity management**

   The trend of using complexity management of materials involves cost-reduction methods, such as standardization of supplies or systems used in departments to achieve cost-efficiency. An example would be if the purchasing manager or purchasing board decides to use the same equipment, such as wireless phones, throughout the organization. The supply of accessories and stationary phones would also be purchased through the same vendor. By doing this, the purchasing manager is managing several links of the supply chain at once. Nurse managers who understand this complexity management can assist purchasing by assuring that he/she has gone through proper supply channels in materials management to assure that standardization may be maintained rather than separately purchasing items from other suppliers. Clear communication between materials management and nursing management must exist to assure that these purchasing standardizations are upheld.

Writing a Proposal

Because budget strategies can result in making changes, and especially if it will alter the way money is spent, the nurse manager must be able to effectively express needed changes in an organized, professional fashion that emphasizes not only *what* needs to happen but the *costs* of this change. Thus we have included this section on writing proposals. A proposal is also known as a business plan.

Proposals may request a needed piece of equipment, explain a different way of implementing patient care, or be more extensive such as designing a new service. This proposal may simply be given to a supervisor, go to the nurse executive or director of nursing, or, after consultation with the nurse executive, it may go to the finance department personnel, the executive team, or even to the board.

The proposal should present actual data and costs as well as provide a thoughtful rationale for the solutions. It should be readable and concise—executive team members like one-page executive summaries. However, the first step is to prepare a thoughtful proposal for the nurse executive, and this is what will be discussed here.

Generally, a proposal reflects changes in the way services are delivered and involves a shift in the way money is spent. Alternately, the proposal may request that the budget reflect different monetary amounts within certain categories based upon changes in the patient population. However, the proposal may be more extensive and ask for several different, or more updated, pieces of expensive equipment needed to provide a service—such as new cardiac monitors—or the proposal may request a new technology such as a new system for computerized charting for the entire facility or system. And, because nurses are involved with patients, the proposal may even suggest a new, innovative service that the nursing staff and the nurse manager have realized is not presently provided.

A proposal has more credence if it is typed neatly using word processing software such as Word Perfect or Microsoft Word, and can often be illustrated more effectively using Power Point, or other graphic computer programs. The proposal needs to be carefully thought out and lead the reader through understanding a problem, being given the proposed solution to effectively deal with the problem, and presenting the reasons why this proposed solution is the best way to solve the problem. At times, it may be best to actually present several solutions that may cost different amounts of money, giving the pros and cons of each solution.

Think of to *whom* the proposal will go. What is their perspective about the situation to which your proposal refers? What information will they need to know? What background information might be helpful to include in the proposal? Be clear about what is requested and what the impact or effect will be on the whole organizational system. Be organized in the delivery and present a reasonable solution to the problem.

Proposals should include:

- *Title*—The person's name who wrote the proposal followed by appropriate background information.
- *Definition*—Define the proposed item, change, service, or program.
- *Rationale*—Why is it needed? Why is this the best item, or way, to do the service? Here you may need to outline other alternatives you considered.
- *Implementation Plan*—Specify what needs to happen. Provide timelines.
- *Costs/Benefits*—Show the actual costs and, if appropriate, how this will change existing costs. This can often be presented more clearly using a spreadsheet, table, pie chart, or bar graph.
- *Evaluation Plan*—How will you evaluate the effectiveness of this proposed item or service?

A sample proposal, authored by Velvet Vanover, MSN, RN, can be found in the following Appendix. In this proposal she requests a new neuro/surgical stepdown unit be established in a hospital setting.

References

Alward, R., & Camunas, C. (1991). *The nurse's guide to marketing.* New York: Delmar.

Bart, C. (November 1988). Budgeting gamesmanship. *The Academy of Management Executive, 11*(4), 285–294.

Barry-Walker, J. (February 2000). The impact of systems redesign on staff, patient, and financial outcomes. *JONA, 30*(2), 77–90.

Becker, C. (June 2003). Scanning for higher profits. *Modern Healthcare,* 6–16.

Berkowitz, E. (1996). *Essentials of health care marketing.* Gaithersburg, MD: Aspen.

Blancett, S., & Flarey, D. (1995). *Reengineering nursing and health care: The handbook for organizational transformation.* Gaithersburg, MD: Aspen.

Blankenship, J., & Winslow, S. (January 2003). Admission-discharge-teaching nurses: Bridging the gap in today's workforce. *JONA, 33*(1), 11–13.

Blouin, A., & Brent, N. (2000). Happy y2k. New and old challenges for the nurse administrator. *JONA, 30*(6), 292–294.

Burke, R. (February 2002). The ripple effect. *Nursing Management, 33*(2), 41–42.

Clifford, J. (1998). *Restructuring: The impact of hospital organization on nursing leadership.* Chicago: American Hospital Publishing.

Coile, R. (December 2000). Hospitalists redefine the future of inpatient medicine. *Cost & Quality,* 8–11.

Connolly, (5/17/02). Luther midelfort: Granting rns authority to restrict admissions streamlines patient flow. *Boston Business Journal.*

Contino, D. S. (October 2002). Take charge of your chargemaster. *Nursing Management,* 16–18.

Cooper, P. (1994). *Health care marketing: A foundation for managed quality.* 3rd ed. Gaithersburg, MD: Aspen.

Davenport, T., & Glaser, J. (July 2002). Just-in-time delivery comes to knowledge management. *Harvard Business Review,* 107–111.

Dunham-Taylor, J., & Pinczuk, J. (2006). *Health care financial management for nurse managers: Applications from hospitals, long-term care, home care, and ambulatory care.* Sudbury, MA: Jones and Bartlett.

Finkler, S., & Kovner, C. (2000). *Financial management for nurse managers and executives.* 2nd ed. Philadelphia: W. B. Saunders.

Hammer, M., & Champy, J. (1993). *Reengineering the corporation.* New York: Harper.

Haugh, R. (March 2003). The future is now for surgery suites. *Hospitals and Health Networks,* 51–54.

Hensley, K. (November 2002). Form and function, streamline documentation during the admission process. *Nursing Management,* 38–40.

Hillsted, S., & Berkowitz, E. (1991). *Health care marketing plans: From strategy to action.* 2nd ed. Gaithersburg, MD: Aspen.

Hope, J., & Fraser, R. (February 2003). Who needs budgets? *Harvard Business Review*, 108–115.

Jensen, M. (November 2001). Corporate budgeting is broken-let's fix it. *Harvard Business Review*, 94–101.

Krugman, M., MacLauchlan, M., Riippi, L., & Grubbs, J. (2002). A multidisciplinary financial education research project. *Nursing Economic$, 20*(6), 273–278.

Lefever, G. (August 1999). Visible savings. *Nursing Management*, 29–32.

Lagoe, J., Arnold, K. A., & Noetscher, C. M. (1999). Benchmarking hospital lengths of stay using histograms. *Nursing Economic$, 17*(2), 75–85.

Lathrop, J. (1993). *Restructuring health care: The patient-focused paradigm.* San Francisco: Jossey-Bass.

Meyer, M. (June 2002). Avoid pcu bottlenecks with proper admission and discharge criteria. *Nursing Management*, 31–35.

Nursing Management. (February 2000). Purchasing influence. Top trends that support your stance. Reprinted with permission from the publisher, the National Association of Purchasing Management, D. R; "Trail blazing," *Purchasing Today, 4*(10), 45–52, 1999.

Page, D. (April 2003). Dial-up care. *Hospitals and Health Networks*, 21–22.

Porter-O'Grady, T., & Malloch, K. (2002). *Quantum leadership: A textbook of new leadership.* Sudbury, MA: Jones and Bartlett.

Posner, B. (February 1987). Margin management. *INC.*, 117–118.

Rigby, D. (April 2002). Look before you lay off. Downsizing in a downturn can do more harm than good. *Harvard Business Review*, 20–21

Rosenfeld, B. (December 2000). A remote possibility. *Cost & Quality*, 38–39.

Schonfeld, E. (March 1998). Can computers cure health care? *Fortune*, 111–116.

Shortell, S., & Selberg, J. (January/February 2002). Working differently: The iom's call to action. *Healthcare Executive*, 6–10.

Simonsen-Anderson, S. (June 2002). Safe and sound. Telephone triage and home care recommendations save lives-and money. *Nursing Management*, 41–44.

Solovy, A. (March 1998). Trend spotting. *Hospitals & Health Networks*, 60.

Valanis, B., Moscato, S., Tanner, C., Shapiro, S., Izumi, S., David, M., & Mayo, A. (April 2003). Making it work. Organization and processes of telephone nursing advice services. *JONA, 33*(4), 216–223.

Wheatley, M. (1992). *Leadership and the new science.* San Francisco: Berrett-Koehler.

Woods, D. K. (April 2002). Realizing your marketing influence, part 1. Meeting patient needs through collaboration. *JONA, 32*(4), 189–195.

Wellmont Health System
Bristol Regional Medical Center

Proposal for
Neuro/Surgical Step-Down Units

Prepared by
Velvet Vanover, MSN, RN, CCRN
Clinical Manager, Wellmont Health System

December 10, 2003
Wellmont Health System
Bristol Regional Medical Center

Proposal for Neuro/Surgical Step Down Units

History: The three intensive care units (30 beds total) are remaining full at all times. Intensive care patients often have to wait either in the emergency department or on a medical/surgical unit for a patient to be transferred out before they can be admitted to the Intensive Care Unit. This causes delays in patient treatment, increases nursing demands on the medical/surgical unit, and increases length of stay.

Proposal: **Formation of two - 4 bed Neuro/Surgical Step-Down Units to be located on the existing nursing units of 2 East and 2 West. Creation of these step down units would allow patients to be moved out of the intensive care units.**

2 East

The four existing, camera monitored, beds would be upgraded to become a full Neurological/Surgical Step Down Unit. The primary patient would be the complex neurological/surgical patient that no longer meets the criteria of a critical care unit, but requires more intensive observation, intervention, and treatment than can be offered by a medical/surgical floor.

2 West

The four existing beds currently utilized as step down beds would be upgraded to become a full Surgical Step-Down Unit. The primary patient would be the complex surgical patient that no longer meets the criteria of a critical care unit, but requires more intensive observation, intervention, and treatment than can be offered by a medical/surgical floor.

The development of two step-down units would increase both the efficiency and quality of care presently offered to patients at the hospital. Other advantages include: decreased length of stays in the SICU, smoother transitions to Medical/Surgical areas, supported "fast tracking" for discharge home, and increased patient/family satisfaction. In addition, there would be increased physician satisfaction by providing additional options and alternatives for the most appropriate patient care.

The purpose of each of the Step-down units would be to provide specialized care for neurological/surgical patients who require close clinical and technical observation with rapid interventions. Patients may require continuous monitoring of one or more of the following: Cardiac, NIBP, pulse oximeter, A-line, and/or CVP line.

The Step-down units will be staffed on a nurse (RN) patient ratio of 1:4.

In addition, Patient Care Technicians will be assigned to assist in patient care.

They will be responsible for assisting with the collection of vital signs to include temperature, pulse rate, respiratory rate, and blood pressure. The RN will be responsible for monitoring vital signs more frequently than every 4 hours.

Patients

Three patient types would benefit from these step-down units.
1. Patients that are currently admitted to an intensive care unit but do not fully meet the requirements of an ICU. These patients require closer observation than a medical/surgical unit can offer.
2. Patients admitted for elective surgical procedures that require multiple care units. These patients would benefit by avoiding the surgical intensive care unit. They could be admitted and return post-operatively to the same room. This would result in increased patient satisfaction, increased communication, and ultimately may decrease the length of stay.
3. Patients that have had appropriate lengths of stay in the surgical intensive care and no longer require the same level of care. At the same time this patient still requires more care and observation than is offered on a medical/surgical unit.

Physicians

Physicians have voiced many concerns regarding the current patient flow. Among those concerns are: the costly delays in transfers from the surgical intensive care unit; the skill levels of nurses on the medical/surgical floors; and the nurse/patient ratios. Specific specialties concerns are:

1. Neurosurgeons feel additional education is needed for nursing staff to include close observation and assessment for rapid patient changes. In addition, they would like to have access for cardiac and pressure monitoring of the neurosurgical patient.
2. Surgeons site concerns over delays in transfers out of the intensive care units; consistency in the nurse/patient ratio; lack of cardiac monitoring in the current step-down area; and inability of staff to do basic critical drips and arterial lines.

Staff

Both nurse managers on 2 East and 2 West feel that a staffing nurse/patient ratio of 1 to 4 would be possible without increasing the current FTEs on those units. There would need to be assurance of an assigned nurse for those beds without overflowing into the other medical/surgical beds. Additional needs for staff would include:

1. Education in both cardiac and arterial line monitoring.
2. Education in critical thinking.
3. Education in assessment and observation of the neurological and surgical patient.

Benefits of Developing Step-Down Units

Improved Patient Outcomes

- Increased continuity of care through same caregivers and decreased transfers.
- Increased patient satisfaction and compliancy through consistent patient teaching.
- Increased observation and assessment for quick interventions.
- Increased family participation consistent with Planetree.

Improved Operating Efficiency

- Increased and appropriate use of intensive care units by eliminating admission or allowing earlier discharge from those units to step-down units.
- Financial savings by having step-down beds to move patients to when order for transfer is written.
- Increased telemetry monitoring capabilities.
- Increased rate difference on 2 East and 2 West for monitored beds.
- Increased use of present staff at higher level of care.

Improved Physician Relationships

- Fulfillment of request by physicians for step-down areas with guaranteed staffing patterns.
- Increased physician satisfaction by providing competent, quality patient care.

- Increased relations with neurosurgeons by meeting patient acuity needs.
- Increased loyalty for patient admissions to Wellmont-Bristol Regional Medical Center.

Enhanced Market Shares

Development of two, 4-bed step-down units would increase patient flow and allow increased market shares in the neurological patient and intensive care patient. Additional step-down beds would free up intensive care beds that are often in short supply. This would eliminate the need for possible diversion to another facility. An increase in the number of neurological surgical patients would occur because of the additional beds available as well as increased care levels.

Financials

Initial Investment

4 Monitors	$ 55,712.10	
Rewiring	$ 1,000.00	
Education	+ $ 17,145.60	(16 hrs educ x $17.86 avg hourly salary x
Subtotal	$73,857.70	60 nurses = $17,145.60)

Step Down Charge	$607.50
Average Room Rate	− $370.00
	$237.50 increase per room per day

8 beds at $4,860.00 per day
    (Step Down Rate)
8 beds at   − $2,960.00 per day
    (Private Rm. Rate)
               $1,900.00 per day

$1,900.00 x 365 = $69,350.00 increased revenue per year

Salary Comparison

SICU salary cost per pt. day (2:1 ratio)	$857.28 per day*
SDU salary cost per pt. day (4:1 ratio)	$428.64 per day
Salary Savings	$428.64 per day
8 patient beds per day	$857.28 per day Salary Savings

*Fixed cost of Manager, Clinical Educator, and Unit Coordinator approximately same for all units. Ergo, does not influence salary cost.

Reimbursement Issues

Case Mix of Patient Population: 65% Medicare/Medicaid/TennCare
                                       35% Managed Care*

*Self pay/Worker's Comp and other payers included in Managed Care %.

A. Medicare/Medicaid/TennCare
Pays at flat rate per stay. Savings to be achieved by providing the service at a lower cost to WBRMC would be seen in saved salary dollars.
$857.28/day Salary Savings x 365 days x 65% Payer Mix = $203,389.68 year savings.

B. Managed Care
Pays at per diem rate or % of charges rate. Per diem rate change would result in loss of charges to organization. Changing from ICU rate to step down rate equals $528.00 loss per day.
$528.00 loss per day x 8 beds x 365 days per year x 35% payer mix =
                                       $539,616.00 loss per year *

*This would only be if all 8 patients would have been in ICU.

Impact: $ 539,616.00 Loss
                                     − $ 203,389.68 Savings
                                       $ 336,226.32 Loss per year to Organization

Total Financial Impact   Initial Investment $ 73,857.77
                              + Loss Revenue $ 336,226.32
                                                      $ 410,084.09 Loss

1st Year Increased Revenues $ 69,350.00
Salary Saving Per Year   + $ 312,907.20
                                                      $ 382,257.20

1st Year =   Loss of $27,826.89
After 1st year =   Revenue of $23,319.12 per year

TITLE: ADMISSION AND DISCHARGE CRITERIA NEURO/SURGI-
      CAL STEP-DOWN UNIT

PURPOSE: To facilitate the increased care of the complex neuro/surgical
      patient requiring continuous observation, assessment, and interven-
      tion but not requiring intensive critical care.

OBJECTIVES: To deliver safe, effective, quality care to acutely ill neurological
      and/or surgical patients.
      To participate in collaborative interdisciplinary healthcare teams.
      To maintain a competent, highly trained nursing staff to provide
      acute care utilizing the nursing process.

GUIDELINES:

Medical Staff Management:

The attending physician will retain authority and responsibility for the admission,
transfer, and discharge of the patient except where special problems are designated to
the care of consultants.

Nursing Management:

The nurse manager of the 2 East and 2 West units will have (24 hr) responsibility for
each of their 4 bed step-down units.

Admission Criteria:

Admission to the surgical step-down unit will be based on the following criteria:
 a. The acuity status of the patient based upon the patient classification system.
 b. Technology required for monitoring the patient.
 c. The needs of the patients requiring the following:
  1. Ongoing observation and assessment.
  2. Monitoring of NIBP, Cardiac Rhythms, Temp, Arterial lines, and/or CVPs.
  3. Frequent monitoring of vital signs.
  4. Administration and monitoring of intravenous drips**:
   Dobutamine
   Low-dose Dopamine
   Lidocaine
   NTG
   Nipride
   Neosynephrine
   Cardizem
   Labetolol

**Levophed, Epinephrine, and High-dose Dopamine should only by used in the ICUs.

Adult Admission/Discharge Criteria

Patients may be admitted to the Step-down Units by members of the WBRMC medical staff based on the priority of each patient's needs and the specialized care provided.

GUIDELINES IN DETERMINING INDICATIONS* FOR ADMISSIONS INCLUDE:

1. Post-operative patients requiring assessment > every two hours following recovery from anesthesia in the Post Anesthesia Care Unit. Patients should meet the following criteria prior to transfer.
   A. Aldrete score of 9 or 10, or meets or exceeds pre-operative score.
   B. Successfully extubated with oxygen saturation maintained at or
      above 90%.
2. Patients requiring vital sign monitoring every two hours or more frequently.
3. Post-arterial surgery patients who require neurovascular checks every hour for 12 hours.
4. Patients of multiple traumas requiring frequent assessment and observation.
5. Neurological patients with ventriculostomies in place.
6. Neurological or surgical patients requiring invasive arterial line or CVP line monitoring.
7. Neurological or surgical patients requiring cardiac monitoring.

*Patients requiring ventilatory support or more intensive care are ineligible for admission to the step-down units.

Specific Admission and Discharge Guidlines follow:

1. **Anterior Cervical Fusion**

   Admission

   a. Potential airway compromise secondary to hematoma formation.
   b. Potential dysrhythmias.
   c. Potential neurological impairment.
   d. Labile blood pressure.

   Discharge

   a. Airway stable without compromise.
   b. Rhythm stable without ectopy.
   c. Neurologically stable.
   d. BP within acceptable range without IV vasoactive drugs.

2. **Craniotomy/transphenoidal hypophysectomy**

   Admission

   a. Potential neurological impairment.
   b. Potential dysrhythmias.
   c. Impaired gas exchange.
   d. Ventricular drainage.
   e. Labile BP.
   f. Unstable temperature.

g. SIADH.

Discharge

a. Neurologically stable.
b. Rhythm stable without ectopy.
c. Airway stable.
d. External ventricular drain out for 24 hours.
e. BP within acceptable range without IV vasoactive drugs.
f. Temperature not > 100.8 F PO within past 24 hours.
g. Urinary output > or = 30 cc./hr. for past 24 hours.

3. **Spinal surgery with or without spinal instrumentation.**

Admission

a. Potential neurological impairment.
b. Potential dysrhythmias.
c. Impaired gas exchange.
d. Unstable temperature.
e. Decreased urinary output.

Discharge

a. Neurologically stable.
b. Rhythm stable without the use of IV antiarrhythmic agents.
c. ABGs acceptable.
d. Temperature < 100.8 F PO for 24 hours.
e. Urinary output > or = 30 cc/hour for 24 hours.

4. **Trauma**

Admission

a. Potential neurological impairment.
b. Potential dysrhythmias.
c. Impaired gas exchange.
d. Ventricular drainage.

Discharge

a. Neurologically stable.
b. Rhythm stable without the use of IV antiarrhythmic agents.
c. ABGs acceptable.
d. External ventricular device out for 24 hours.

5. **Carotid Endarterectomy**

Admission

a. Potential neurological impairment.
b. Potential dysrhythmias.

c. Potential airway compromise secondary to hematoma formation.

d. Hemodynamically unstable.

Discharge

a. Neurologically stable.

b. Rhythm stable without the use of IV antiarrhythmic agents.

c. Airway Patent.

d. BP stable without the use of IV vasoactive drugs.

e. ABGs acceptable.

6. **Fem-Fem/Tib/Pop Bypass**

Admission

a. Potential dysrhythmias.

b. Potential graft occlusion.

c. Potential neurological impairment.

d. Labile BP.

Discharge

a. Rhythm stable without the use of IV antiarrhythmic agents.

b. Graft patent per doppler auscultation.

c. Neurologically stable.

d. BP stable without the use of IV vasoactive drugs.

7. **Gastric Bypass**

Admission

a. Potential airway compromise.

b. Potential dysrhythmias.

c. Potential impaired gas exchange.

d. Labile BP.

Discharge

a. Airway patent.

b. Rhythm stable without the use of IV antiarrhythmic agents.

c. ABGs acceptable.

d. BP stable without the use of vasoactive agents.

8. **General Vascular Surgeries**

Admission

a. Potential impaired gas exchange.

b. Potential dysrhythmias.

c. Potential neurological impairment.

d. Labile BP.

Discharge

   a. ABGs acceptable.

   b. Rhythm stable without the use of IV antiarrhythmic agents.

   c. Neurologically stable.

   d. BP stable without the use of vasoactive agents.

ASSURANCE OF APPROPRIATE ADMISSION/TRANSFER TO THE STEP-DOWN UNIT

A. Patients whose condition does not appear to meet the guidelines for admission to the surgical step-down unit, will be clarified by the Acute Care Nursing Director (or her designee) with the attending physician.

B. If requests for admissions exceed the number of beds available, the acuity of the patient's condition will determine the priority for available beds. The Acute Care Nursing Director (or her designee) will consult with the attending physicians who have patients in the unit, to determine which patient can be transferred out, using established admission/discharge criteria.

CHAPTER 15

Strategic Management: Facing the Future with Confidence

Sandy K. Calhoun, MSN, RN, CPHQ

Strategic Management

> You got to be careful if you don't know where you are going, because
> you might not get there (Quotations Page, "Yogi Berra," 2004).

Effective decision making is the primary task of management. Seemingly justified by time constraints and the mistaken assessment that issues are minor, decisions are often made without essential information. By chance, the nurse manager may be successful in the short run, but in the long run, the use of intuition without planning can lead to disappointment. The delivery of health care devoid of a systematic process for planning forces managers to "fly by the seat of their pants"—relying on their own intuition and experience. Strategic planning shifts decision making from intuitive information gathering to systematic and objective investigation. Thus, the task of strategic planning is to generate accurate information for decision making. In the midst of chaos, as the volume and pace of change in health care accelerates, managers may declare they have no choice but to spend their time and resources "putting out fires." Gelatt (1993) observed that change itself has changed. He describes the chaos in which we work as *white water change*, because it has become so rapid, complex, turbulent, and unpredictable. It is amazing that psychologically normal people are overwhelmed by change after years of colliding with it. Nevertheless, the dynamic and complex nature of health care mandates managers not forsake planning and strategic management if the organization is to be positioned for long-term success. Strategic management fulfills the need for knowledge of the organization, the market, and the competitive situations health care leaders face, and provides the ongoing, dynamic changes in the plan when appropriate.

Dr. Henry Mintzberg (2000), an authority on strategy, notes that strategy is the art of crafting a unique position in the market. Strategy need not change often; however, when there is a need to rethink the organization's position, the change should emerge from the ideas and actions of the people in the organization. Nurse managers, situated in the organization between the front line staff and senior leaders, are in a unique position to recognize the need for change. Successful organizations understand the need to modify or change its strategic plan based on feedback from customers. Nurse managers may be the first to recognize that strategies that have been successful in the past are no longer. Innovative ideas are better conceived if the entire organization, not just senior leaders, put their intellect to the task.

Even though everyone in the organization should be encouraged to come up with new strategic ideas, it is the responsibility of senior leaders to make the final choices. Organizational leaders must choose which ideas will be pursued; otherwise the result is chaos and confusion. Strategic planning allows health care leaders to meet the future proactively rather than responding to the internal and external environment in a haphazard manner. While strategic planning will not eliminate all challenges, the process can drive innovation, integrate the system, and align resources to enable the organization to face the future with confidence.

Systematic, objective planning is the key to the development and implementation of plans that drive successful health care organizations. How do organizations get beyond large binders with numbers, graphs, charts, and jargon? Can organizations use this dense documentation to improve organizational performance? The answer is "yes." Why do many organizations have separate plans for performance improvement, education, recruitment, and retention? Silo thinking is effective to prepare and sustain war or missile sites, and needs to be able to stand alone. However, in health care organizations departments must work together to assure the long-term success of the organization. The key to successful planning is to make the process a part of the daily operations of the organization rather than a task to be completed during the planning cycle in preparation for the budget. Strategic planning is a continuous process of revisiting the system and restoring balance.

Health care organizations must focus on patient satisfaction as well as patient retention and loyalty. What is the status of the organization's market share? Are new markets emerging? These aspects are key factors in competitiveness, profitability, and success of the organization. Choices organizations made five to ten years ago may no longer be valid, and must be continuously questioned. In the past, being decisive was an essential talent often thought to be reserved for those in leadership positions. The health care environment of today has replaced the skill of making up one's mind with a new essential skill of the future—learning how to change one's mind (Gelatt, 2002). Technologies, customer preferences, and competitors are ever changing and the organization must be flexible. Successful organizations question past choices to determine if change is necessary. The heart of strategic planning is to devise a systematic, well-balanced process that allows the organization to fit in the environment.

Strategic planning must be objective. The necessity for objectivity was cleverly stated by the 19th century American humorist Artemus Ward, who said, "It ain't so much what people don't know that hurts as what they know that ain't so" (Artemus Ward, Creative Quotes, 2004). Thus, the facilitator of the strategic planning process must be detached and impersonal rather than engaged in biased attempts to prove preconceived ideas.

According to Mintzberg, strategy is nothing more than answering three simple, yet difficult questions:

1. Who should the organization target as customers and who should they not?
2. What should the organization offer these customers and what should they not?
3. What is the most efficient way to do this?

Organizations that do not have clear answers to these three questions will drift aimlessly until they eventually fail. Team members need clear parameters to guide their actions; these three dimensions help provide the autonomy they need to focus on the key tasks at hand. Without clarity of these three dimensions, organizational efforts will be disjointed, as no common understanding of the strategies, actions, and goals of the business exist.

According to the 2004 Baldrige National Quality Program, "Health Care Criteria for Performance Excellence," strategic planning criteria stresses patient-focused quality and operational performance improvement (National Institute of Standards and Technology [NIST], 2004). These key strategic issues are fundamental to the organization's overall planning. Patient-focused quality and health care performance provide a strategic view of quality, focusing on patient satisfaction, patient loyalty, patient health status, and health care service improvement. The ultimate test of quality is customer satisfaction, and it carries significant weight among the award's criteria—40 points for "Patient, Other Customer, and Health Care Market Knowledge," 45 points for "Patient and Other Customer Relationships and Satisfaction," and 75 points for "Patients- and Other Customer Focused Results" (NIST, 2004). Although the term "customer" was not used often in health care until recent years, twenty-first century health care leaders recognize the primary customer to be the (formally called) patient. Areas to consider are those important to the patient such as speed, responsiveness, and flexibility. Improvement in operations contributes to short- and longer-term productivity, cost containment, and the overall well being of the organization.

The Tennessee Center for Performance Excellence (2004) proclaims that customers are the judge of the organization's quality and performance. Since strategic planning focuses on operational performance and quality as judged by the customer, we will examine first the notion of customer-driven quality. Who are the customers of health care? Customers of health care are both internal and external to the organization. Internal customers include patients and families, physicians, visitors, team members, and volunteers. The employment of physicians has changed physicians from external customers (supplier of the patients we served) to both internal (employee) and external (supplier) customers. This dual role may conflict when organizational priorities are unclear or when organizational and personal goals are incongruent.

The primary external customers of health care are quite complex and consist of suppliers (insurance companies, physicians, labor markets, and donors), consumers (the general public and research community), and interfacing organizations (medical profession, teaching hospitals, board of directors, health insurances, and drug and supply companies). Additional external influences include licensing, governmental, and regulatory agencies, in addition to other health care facilities (Bennis and Nanus, 1985).

Determining the measures customers use when they assess and judge the quality of our services is an important process. Our perception of quality may be vastly different from the customer's perception. We may feel sure that zero defects are priority, when, in fact, timeliness is what is most important to the customer. Various listening strategies, aimed at assessing how the customer perceives quality, will be discussed. Listening to the customer provides baseline knowledge. Once opportunities to improve are identified, leadership, through strategic planning, must assess and drive improvements. Thus, the Joint Commission on Accreditation of Health Care Organizations (JCAHO) holds leadership accountable for strategic planning as well as for performance improvement (JCAHO, 2004).

Why do our customers choose our services? Providing quality care does not guarantee success; customers must perceive that we add value. We may have an erroneous perception that our services are superior in design and service. If, in fact, our services are inefficient or out-dated, innovation and advances in the market will produce customer dissatisfaction with our endeavors. Customer satisfaction is paramount to the success of the organization, and capturing this information encompasses a major expenditure. This is true whether the data is captured internally or through an outside vendor such as Gallup or Press Ganey.

Are patients and families qualified to assess health care quality? The answer is an astounding, "Yes." The internet has eliminated the time-honored adage, "We know what is best, after all we have years of education" and ushered in the age of informed consumers. No longer is it acceptable to lecture the patient, "Just do as I say." or "The doctor knows best." Patients often seek health care after an extensive Internet search on the diagnosis in question. Patients and families often arrive for care with an array of scientific literature— indeed often better informed than the clinician.

An organization's commitment to performance excellence should not be measured by cost, but by investment. Organizations purchase equipment to improve processes and cycle times. An organization that makes a similar investment in their team members receives a much higher return. Successful health care organizations recognize and reward team members with an appreciation of the link between team member satisfaction and patient satisfaction—rarely is the latter realized without the reality of the former. If team members are expected to meet the needs of customers, their needs must be met *first*.

The second notion related to strategic management stressed by The Tennessee Center for Performance Excellence (2004) examines operational performance. What are the short- and longer-term goals of the organization? How does the organization maintain cost competitiveness? Operational capabilities such as speed, responsiveness, and flexibility contribute to the organization's competitive fitness. The strategic plan must align work processes with the strategic direction of the organization by embedding improvement and learning in work processes. This alignment assures that priorities for improvement and learning reinforce the priorities of the organization. Comprehensive strategic planning establishes the organization's strategy (the plan for achieving the desired end result), and plan of action (what the organization must do to get there). Of key importance is the deployment of the plan of action to all business units and identifying how accomplishments are measured and sustained. JCAHO requires leaders to engage in short- and long-term planning. This includes data measuring the performance of the processes and outcomes of care, treatment, and services (Comprehensive Manual for Hospitals [CAMH], 2004).

While the business sector has successfully used strategic planning for the past 50 years, strategic planning has only been used in health care since the 1970s, and then only sporadically (Zuckerman, 1998). According to Ginter et al. (2002), the concept of strategic planning was broadened to strategic management during the 1980s when business transformed planning and budgeting beyond the traditional 12-month operating year and began to understand the importance of strategy implementation and control.

The strategic management process described in this chapter will trace the following map: 1) situation analysis, 2) strategy formation, 3) strategy deployment, and 4) strategic management, which encompass measurement, evaluation and performance improvement. **Exhibit 15–1** outlines the strategic management process.

Exhibit 15–1 Strategic Management Process

Situation Analysis	Strategy Formation	Strategy Deployment	Strategic Management
External environmental analysis: • Opportunities • Threats	Directional strategies: • Mission • Vision • Values • Goals and Objectives	Culture	Goals and Objectives
Internal environmental analysis: • Strengths • Weakness	Adaptive strategies	Structure	Measurement • Balanced Scorecard
• Mission • Vision • Values • Goals	Market entry strategies	Resources	Evaluation standards
	Competitive strategies		Performance Improvement

Situation Analysis

Situation analysis, the initial stage of strategic planning, is the process of determining the current state of the organization. While historical data is an asset in determining the current state, leaders should resolve to avoid the trap of focusing on the analysis of past performance. Zuckerman (1998) describes this phenomenon as "analysis paralysis," a serious problem that can bog down the strategic planning process. Undue emphasis on past performance can result in loss of focus and momentum. Key players may become disinterested and buy-in may be lost. Leaders must focus on results not "busy work." There will always be those in the group who insist on more and better data; however, profiling key business drivers for the organization should be captured and analyzed on an ongoing basis, thus negating the need for over-analysis of historical data. Rarely will data be needed beyond the past five years. Key issues to consider include which factors are within the control or influence of the organization, and how external forces will affect the competitive position of the organization. Understanding and analyzing the current situation is accomplished through three interrelated processes: external environmental analysis, internal environmental analysis, and the development of the organization's mission, vision, values, and goals. These processes are not separate and distinct, but rather overlap, interact with, and influence one another.

External Environmental Analysis

The first process, *external environmental analysis*, focuses on determining the current position of the organization within both the general environment and the health care environment. This profile is the beginning of a forward-looking process that considers market trends and forecasts (Zuckerman, 1998). To understand the external environment, the organization must look outside its boundaries (beyond itself) to identify and analyze issues taking place outside of the organization. These issues represent opportunities and threats, and assist in identifying "what the organization should do." Opportunities and threats influence strategy formation and represent fundamental issues that can directly impact the success or failure of the organization. It is insufficient to simply be aware of these issues; health care managers need to understand the nature of the opportunities and threats *before* they affect the organization. The organization must have an effective method for scanning the external environment for pertinent information. Factors to be considered include: legislative/political changes, economic modifications, social/demographic shifts, new technology, and competitive/market changes (Ginter, et al., 2002).

Review of legislative, political, and regulatory trends is necessary to determine any major environmental influences that may affect the future performance of the organization. Regulatory and legislative changes in both public and private health care organizations will continue as these entities struggle to ensure health care access, patient safety and privacy, and cost management. Major trends should be profiled for the past three to five years. Forecasting, using alternative scenarios, should be identified and discussed (Zuckerman, 1998). What should be done to minimize negative impacts? What can be done to maximize potential benefits?

Economic trends and forecasts should be exercised with caution; avoid over analysis. Only the broadest trends and variables that impact the organization should be considered. Nevertheless, shifts in the national economy cannot be ignored, as the impact will be realized at the local level. Although minor shifts in economic performance are of minimal consequences to the strategic planning process, local trend analysis may identify geographic segments with potential for future penetration (Zuckerman, 1998).

Demographic changes, such as an aging population and increased life span, must be considered because these factors directly impact health care organizations. Major population shifts may indicate geographic areas that may be targeted for future market growth. Social trends, such as a more ethnically diverse and better-educated population, impact the provision of services as well. Critical shortages of nurses, pharmacists, physical therapists, and other health care professionals necessitate a focus on retention and recruitment efforts.

Technology needs continue to escalate. As health care organizations become "wired," system integration (radiology, nursing, laboratory, pharmacy, and other ancillary departments) become a logistical nightmare. No one system has "one stop shopping"; while one system excels in a key feature, it may be deficient in another. Furthermore, the software competitor probably excels in a different key aspect of an integrated system. To be more efficient, practitioners no longer complete laborious manual record reviews and "paper and pen" documentation. Those facilities that do not keep pace with emerging trends in technology will become dinosaurs in short order. Health care organizations need to leave the chisel and stone technique with comic characters such as Fred Flintstone.

Primary market research is completed by focusing on competitive and market changes external to the organization. This information helps to determine the organization's competitive position in the market. Market research is completed through interviews, focus groups, and surveys. Targets of this research include senior leaders of competitor organizations, community leaders, primary employers, and those knowledgeable of the market situation. The primary task is to generate information, thereby decreasing the uncertainty that comes with the managerial art of decision making. Research means literally to "search again," a process whereby one looks at the data to understand all that needs to be known about a subject (Zikmund, 2003). While caution must be exercised so that this aspect of the process does not take an undue amount of time and resources, and is not overemphasized, leaders must know the market. At times, research reveals information not readily apparent and key to success in the market.

> The secret of business is to know something nobody else knows (BrainyQuote, "Aristotle Onassis," 2004).

A parallel matrix is helpful when examining the external analysis. This matrix allows visualization of competitively relevant threats with external opportunities. **Exhibit 15–2** provides an example matrix.

Exhibit 15–2 External Environmental Analysis

Nurse's Heaven Medical Center
Strategic Plan 2004
Opportunities and Threats

Opportunities	Threats
No competitors offer wound management services.	Increased competition from larger hospital serving the same population.
Physician offices are needed to attract new physicians.	Customers expect specialized care that the organization cannot afford to offer.

Internal Environmental Analysis

Available resources, competencies, and capabilities, influence success in the external environment. *Internal environmental analysis* involves an extensive review of internal processes, culture, structure, and technology in order to reveal strengths and weaknesses.

Gelatt (1993) offers caution regarding "info-mania." He described info-mania as the idolizing of information. "Info-maniacs" worship facts. There is sure to be at least one member of the leadership team that demands more and more facts even when the team is drowning in information. Exactly how many admissions did Dr. X have three years ago? Four years ago? Five? Focusing only on facts leaves little room for innovation. Generating more information than the human mind can process is dysfunctional. Health care leaders must understand the competitive relevance of these issues. Weaknesses require strategies to minimize the vulnerability of the organization, while strengths must be optimized to maximize their impact. This information provides a foundation for strategy formulation (Ginter, et al., 2002). Plotting strengths and weakness on a parallel matrix (example, **Exhibit 15–3**) provides a visual for evaluating the competitive advantages relative to strengths and the competitive relevance of weaknesses.

> The real voyage of discovery consists not is seeking new landscapes, but in having new eyes (Quotations Page "Marcel Proust," 2004).

Exhibit 15–3 Internal Environmental Analysis

Nurse's Heaven Medical Center
Strategic Plan 2004
Strengths and Weaknesses

Strengths	Weaknesses
Convenient ground level parking	Resistance to change by many team members
Patient-oriented team members	Lack of well-defined management succession plan

Zuckerman explains that primary market research serves to gather information regarding the organization's strengths and weaknesses as it relates to its competitors, and to involve leadership in the strategic planning process. Leaders should begin by reviewing any recent market research that is available and gathering information through interviews, focus groups, and surveys. Primary targets groups for market research include: board members, physicians, health professionals, management staff, and other key stakeholders of the organization.

Many organizations use focus groups to solicit stakeholder input (Morgan, 1993; Krueger, 1988). Focus groups incur significant cost (time and money), thus priority is given to key customer groups such as patients, families, team members, community members, and physicians. A focus group consists of a small group of individuals (six to ten), usually with similar interests, who participate in an unstructured, free-flowing interview with a skilled facilitator. The facilitator begins by introducing the topic with the goal of uncovering core issues related to strategic planning. A recorder documents key statements for management to consider in strategy development. Caution must be used, however, as focus groups may not represent the entire population.

Drenkard (2001) documented the success of the Inova Chief Nurse Executive (CNE) team in using large group interventions to convene and engage nurses across a large health care system in northern Virginia. This method involved the entire system, and used a key mass of people affected by the change. This critical mass participated in: 1) understanding the need for change, analyzing the current state, and deciding what needed to be changed, 2) generating ideas about how to make the needed changes, and 3) implementing and supporting the change. The CNE team sponsored six large group events to engage the several hundred nurses in the work force. These sessions provided time for interaction, development of the strategic plan, and networking for the involved nurses.

Mission, Vision, Values, Goals

The mission, vision, values, and goals of the organization ultimately affect the strategy that is adopted. According to Ginter et al., the organization's *mission* is the articulation of the external opportunities and threats and the internal strengths and weaknesses. The *vision* is the view of the future based on the understanding of the forces. Chapman (2003) notes our mission needs to matter. It must not be just tired words framed on the wall. Likewise, health care organizations need volcanic vision statements that eliminate old patterns of mediocrity. He describes three elements of effective mission and vision statements: clear and easy to remember, a call for dramatic improvement in the lives of others, and proclamation by leaders who, through example, demonstrate a passionate commitment to making the statements come alive.

The *core values* (the organization's purpose and core values are explained further in Chapter 4, Organizational Strategies) constitute the fundamental truths that the organization holds dear and reflect the philosophy of the organization. Examples include: honesty, integrity, customer service, commitment to excellence, and so forth. *Goals* specify the major direction of the organization and provide actionable linkage to the mission. The mission, vision, values, and goals are considered a part of the situation analysis because they are influenced by both external and internal environmental analysis.

Strategy Formation

The first step in the strategic planning process, situation analysis, involves data gathering. *Strategy formation* involves using this data for decision making. These decisions are critical to the success of the organization, as they become the organization's strategy. Ginter et al. (2002) describes four types of strategies: directional, adaptive, market entry, and competitive.

Directional Strategies

While the mission, vision, values, goals, and objectives are part of the situation analysis, they are also part of strategy formation; they provide the broadest direction for the organization—*directional strategies*. Common mission, vision, values, and goals indicate what the organization wants to do. These strategies reflect the critical success factors within the particular service category, in this case, health care. Critical success factors are applicable to all competitors and take into account the external environment. In other words, they define what the organization must accomplish to stay in business. These strategies provide initial direction for the organization, and guidance when making key organizational decisions. The reciprocal relationship (adapted from Ginter, et al., p. 177) of directional strategies may be viewed in **Exhibit 15–4.**

Exhibit 15–4 Directional Strategies

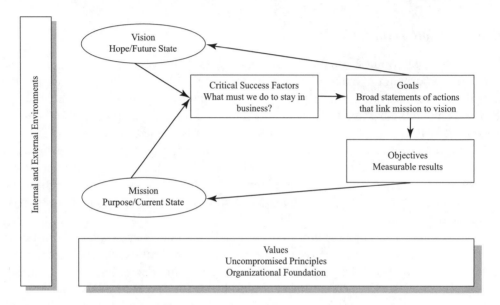

Adapted from: Ginter, P., Swayne, L., & Duncan, W. (2001). *Strategic management of health care organizations* (4th ed.). Malden, MA: Blackwell.

MISSION

The organization's *mission* should articulate the organization's purpose or reason that it exists. It describes what makes the organization distinct and reflects the expectations of stakeholders, those who have an interest in the business. In short, the mission defines the organization and describes what it does. The mission statement must be more than an attractive wall hanging. The mission must be communicated with and lived by all team members in the organization, especially to team members who work directly with customers.

VISION

The organization's *vision* describes the optimal future state of the business. The vision should create a mental picture of what the organization will be when leaders and team members accomplish their mission. It describes the hope for the future—what should the organization be five years from now? Time and effort link the mission (what the organization is today) and vision (what will it be in the future)? The vision should be stated in clear, simple terms that provide a challenge, and leaves no doubt as to the importance of the vision. Stakeholders should be able to understand the vision and commit it to memory. The vision should be inspiring, and is generally not stated in quantitative terms. Though the vision should stand the test of time, it should be constantly challenged and revised when necessary.

VALUES

Values represent the basic principles, fundamental beliefs and tenets of team members, and define what they deem important to the organization. Values state uncompromised principles that are timeless and do not change with the ever-changing climate of business operations. Some organizations use the terminology *guiding principles* to refer to values. Values guide beliefs, attitudes, and behaviors, and provide the foundation for operating the business. Key business decisions should be measured against the values of the organization so the organization never loses site of its purpose.

GOALS

Goals are more specific than the mission and vision. Nevertheless, goals are broad statements that provide direction for team members and link the mission to actions necessary to reach the desired future state of the organization—the vision. Goals that focus on activities unrelated to the organization's critical success factors have the potential of diverting leadership attention and team member energy. The number of goals should be limited for the same reasons. Goals should be stated in easily understood terms so that team members can readily link what they need to do with the mission and vision for the organization. Examples include:

- Expand Women's Services to encompass all key aspects of the business.
- Position Nurse's Heaven Medical Center as a strong community hospital with a focus on primary care.
- Develop a comprehensive health care system including primary care, radiation therapy, skilled nursing facility, home health, and durable medical equipment.

In order for the desired outcome to be achieved, objectives are designed to make each goal operational.

OBJECTIVES

Objectives describe the results to be achieved, when and by whom, and are measurable. Examples of objectives for the above goals are:

- The Director of Women's Health will direct the completion of renovations of the existing unit by December 31, 2004,
- The Chief Executive Officer will recruit six hospitalists by August 31, 2004, and
- The Chief Nursing Officer will recruit/hire 20 team members for the skilled nursing unit by November 30, 2004.

Mission, vision, values, goals, objectives, and the external and internal environment present a picture of the situation and provide a basis for strategy formulation.

Adaptive Strategies

While directional strategies provide general guidance, *adaptive strategies* are more specific and describe the process for carrying out the directional strategies. Directional strategies are the *ends*, while adaptive strategies are the *means*. Adaptive strategies describe how the organization will expand, contract, or maintain their scope of services (Ginter, et al., 2002). These are the strategies most visible to those outside the organization.

EXPANSION STRATEGIES

Expansion strategies include: diversification, vertical integration, market development, product development, or penetration (Ginter, et al., 2002). *Diversification* occurs at the corporate level when markets outside the organization's core business offer potential for significant growth. Because the organization is venturing outside the core business, diversification is generally considered a risky venture. Diversification is most often seen in health care when there are opportunities in less-regulated markets such as specialty hospitals, long-term care, or managed care.

There are two types of diversification, related and unrelated. In health care organizations, *related diversification (concentric)* includes related products and services such as home health, hospice, or radiation treatment. *Unrelated diversification (conglomerate)* includes businesses in the general environment such as a laundry, restaurant, or office buildings, and those within the health care industry such as pharmaceuticals, medical supplies, or insurance. Selecting markets and products that complement one another can reduce risk. Nevertheless, unrelated diversification has been found to be generally unsuccessful in generating revenue for health care organizations.

Vertical integration is the second corporate level expansion of adaptive strategies. The purpose of vertical integration in health care is to enhance the continuity of care while simultaneously managing the channel of demand for health care services. Health care organizations that employ vertical integration grow the business along the channel of distribution of core process (Ginter, et al., 2002) (refer to Chapter 4 for more information about core values). Vertical integration can reduce supply costs and enhance integration. A successful example would be the inclusion of technical education programs for team members in critically short supply such as nursing assistant and technicians. Vertical integration was the fundamental adaptive strategy of the 1990s. This rapid change was realized as hospitals joined networks or systems in an effort to secure resources, increase capabilities, and gain greater bargaining power with purchasers and health care plans (Ginter, et al., 2002).

Market development occurs at the division or strategic service unit level and focuses on entering new markets with existing products or services. The purpose of this strategy is to add volume through geographic expansion of the service area, or by expansion into new market segments within the present geographic area (Ginter, et al., 2002). *Horizontal integration* is a type of market development that grows the business by acquiring or affiliating with competitors. Horizontal growth of health care systems in the 1980s and early 1990s created multi-hospital systems. Many of the expected benefits such as reduction of duplication of services, economics of scale, improved productivity, and operating efficiencies did not materialize, and horizontal integration strategies slowed in the late 1990s (Ginter, et al., 2002).

Product development also occurs at the division or strategic service unit level and involves the introduction of new products or services to existing markets. Whereas related diversification is the introduction of a *new* product, product development refines, complements, or extends existing products or services such as women's health or cancer treatment. Product development may be used when customer requirements are changing, technology is changing, or when there is a need to create differentiation advantage.

Penetration strategies, like market and product development, focus on increasing volumes and market share. Market penetration is an aggressive marketing strategy centered on extending existing services. This strategy is used when the present market is growing and expected revenues are high.

CONTRACTION STRATEGIES

When the organization needs to decrease the size or scope of operations at either the corporate or divisional level, four *contraction* strategies are considered. Divestiture and liquidation occur at the corporate level, and harvesting and retrenchment occur at the divisional level (Ginter, et al., 2002).

When a service unit is viable, yet a decision to leave the market and sell an operating unit is made, *divestiture* occurs. Generally, the divested business unit has value and will continue to be operated by the purchasing organization (Ginter, et al., 2002). This strategy has become common over the past decade as health care organizations carve out non-core business. Examples of non-core health care business that may be divested include: pharmacy, laboratory, and radiology. Business units may be divested for several reasons including industry decline, the need for cash to fund priority operations, or the divested unit may have been a marginal performer. Services too far from the core business may be divested in an effort to focus on business at hand, or management expertise for the particular service may not be available within the leadership group.

Liquidation is the selling of assets of an organization that can no longer operate. In contrast to divestiture, liquidation assumes that the operating unit cannot be sold as a viable operation (Ginter, et al., 2002). Some assets, of course, may still have value, such as buildings and equipment. Reasons for liquidation include: bankruptcy, the need to dispose of nonproductive assets, the need to reduce assets, or the emergence of expensive new technology that will make the current technology obsolete.

Harvesting occurs when the market has entered long-term decline or there is a need for short-term cash (Ginter, et al., 2002). For example, despite a strong market position, revenues are expected to decline industry-wide over the next years. The unit will be allowed to generate as much revenue as possible; however, no new resources will be invested in the business. This allows for an orderly exit from the market by planned downsizing. Harvesting has occurred with many small rural hospitals that could not maintain or improve their financial positions due to the lack of physician and community support, an aging population, and the migration of the young to urban areas.

Retrenchment occurs when the market has become too diverse, and there is a decline in profitability due to increasing costs (Ginter, et al., 2002). While the market is still viewed as viable, costs are too high. Retrenchment involves redefinition of the market if it is too geographically spread out. Costs such as personnel or facility assets that are marginal or nonproductive are reduced.

MAINTENANCE OF SCOPE STRATEGIES

When current strategies are appropriate and few changes are needed, the organization may elect to *maintain* the existing strategies. This does not mean that the organization does nothing, but rather pursues either enhancement or status quo strategies (Ginter, et al., 2002).

When the organization is progressing toward its vision, yet nevertheless improvements are needed, *enhancement strategy* may be used. This may entail quality improvement efforts directed toward improving organizational processes or reducing costs. This is a time for innovation and redesign of timeworn systems. The focus should be on those identified as most important to key customers such as patients and families.

Status quo is based on the assumption of a mature market when growth has ceased. The goal is to maintain the market share. When using the status quo strategy, organizations may attempt penetration or market/product development (Ginter, et al., 2002).

Market Entry Strategies

The three major strategies to enter a market include: purchase, cooperation, and development. Market entry strategies are not ends of themselves, but rather the adaptive strategies may be used to bring market strategies to fruition (Ginter, et al., 2002).

PURCHASE STRATEGIES

There are three *purchase market-entry strategies*: acquisition, licensing, and venture capital investment. Purchase market-entry strategies allow a health care organization to quickly enter the market. Each strategy places different demands on the organization (Ginter, et al., 2002).

When health care organizations purchase an existing organization, organizational unit, or a product or service, *acquisition entry strategy* is used. Acquisition takes place at the corporate or divisional level. The acquisition may be integrated into existing operations, or it may operate as a separate unit. Acquisitions often flounder because it is difficult to integrate existing culture and operations. Often, it takes several years post acquisition to combine two organizational cultures. Despite the difficulties of integrating cultures, the synergy realized by the creation of a comprehensive health care system has demonstrated that acquisition is an effective purchase strategy.

Licensing avoids the time and market risks of technology or product development (Ginter, et al., 2002). When licensure is used as a strategy, proprietary technology is usually not purchased and therefore the organization is dependent on the licensor for support and upgrade. Health care organizations frequently use licensing strategies for implementation of clinical documentation systems. This strategy lowers the financial and market risk of technologies outside the core business.

Venture capital investment is a low-risk option whereby health care organizations purchase minority investment in a developing enterprise. This provides an opportunity to "try out," and possibly later enter into, new technology. Examples include: life science portals for bio-informatics, home-based health care services for the elderly, and cardiology arrhythmia management companies (Ginter, et al., 2002).

COOPERATION STRATEGIES

According to Ginter et al. (2002) mergers, alliances, and joint ventures—*cooperation strategies*—were the most popular strategies of the 1990s. Cooperation strategies allow organizations to carry out adaptive strategies.

Although similar to acquisitions, in a *merger* two organizations combine through a mutual agreement to form a single new organization (recall that in an acquisition a health care organization purchases an existing organization, organizational unit, or a product or service). Merger strategies are used to accomplish horizontal integration by combining two similar organizations, or vertical integration, by creating an integrated delivery system. Reasons for mergers include: to improve efficiency and effectiveness (combine resource and exploit cost reduction strategies), enhance access (broader services), enhance financial position (gain market share), and overcome concerns of survival (endure in an aggressive market). As with acquisitions, the major hurdle is the integration of two separate organizational cultures. Because a new organization is formed, mergers are often more difficult to navigate than acquisitions. In a merger, a totally new organizational culture must be developed. If mergers are to be successful, work groups must be formed to reformulate the mission, vision, and core values of the new organization. Merger of two organizational cultures into one takes years to complete (Ginter, et al., 2002).

Alliance strategies entail arrangements among existing organizations to achieve a strategic purpose not possible by any single organization. Alliances include: federations, consortiums, networks, and systems. Alliances attempt to strengthen competitive position while the organizations maintain their independence. Health care organizations often form an alliance to achieve economies of scale in purchasing. Examples include the Premier and Voluntary Hospitals of America (Ginter, et al., 2002). Although not a merger or acquisition, alliances have many of the same issues with conflicting cultures.

Joint ventures are used when risks are too high, or the project is too large or too expensive to be done by a single organization. In a joint venture, two or more organizations combine resources to accomplish a designated task. The most common health care joint ventures are:

- Contractual agreements,
- Subsidiary corporations,
- Partnerships, and
- Not-for-profit title-holding corporations.

In a contractual agreement, two or more organizations contract to work together toward specific objectives. Subsidiary corporations form a new corporation, usually to operate non-health care activities. A *partnership* is a formal or informal arrangement between two or more parties for mutual benefit of the organizations involved. Not-for-Profit Title-Holding Corporations form tax-exempt title-holding corporations to provide benefits to health care organizations engaged in real estate ventures. The dynamic health care environment mandates that organizations engage in joint ventures to lower costs (Ginter, et al., 2002).

Development Strategies

Organizations may enter new markets through internal resources. There are two types of *development entry strategies*: internal development and internal ventures.

INTERNAL DEVELOPMENT

Organizations use *internal development* for products or services closely related to existing products or services. The organization maintains a high level of control through the use of existing resources, competencies, and capabilities. While internal development presents an image of a growing organization, there is time lag to break even, and obtaining significant market share against strong competitors is difficult (Ginter, et al., 2002).

INTERNAL VENTURES

In contrast to internal development, *internal ventures* are most appropriate for products or services that are unrelated to the current products or services. Internal ventures set up separate, relatively independent entities within the organization. An example of an internal venture is a hospital that develops home health care through an internal venture (Ginter, et al., 2002). Success of this strategy is mixed, as the organization's internal climate is often unsuitable for the venture.

In the final stage of strategic formation, a *gap analysis* examines the difference in the current state and the desired state, or vision for the future. Gap analysis is the process of examining how large a leap must be taken to meet the vision and what must be done to make the leap. If organizational leaders set their vision too narrow, they will find their current state meets the vision, but lacks incentive to aspire for higher and greater things. Their task is accomplished, and the planning process ends. With this in mind, leaders must communicate the vision in a somewhat revolutionary manner. The vision should inspire team members to perform their best—there is no room for mediocrity in health care vision. The desired outcome of the gap analysis is a strategic plan that has a reasonable probability of success. To accomplish this, priorities must be established and resources allocated to narrow the gap between the current state and the desired state. This process establishes the groundwork for the strategies necessary to assure the desired outcome (Drenkard, 2001).

Planning encompasses stewardship of the organization and its resources. Care must be taken to articulate the core assumptions about the nature of the market, the competitions, and the organization; otherwise a gap will exist between the aspirations of the organization and the way the organization actually behaves. When what we do day-to-day is in contrast to what we say we do and hope to be, a paradox exists that leads to team member frustration. What does the organization value—creativity or discipline? Is the focus on short-term or long-term goals? Quality or the bottom line? While conflicts occur in every organization, successful organizations meet the challenge and reconcile aspirations and actions as part of the strategic planning process (Solovy, 2002). Decisions regarding resources must be made with the core value—what does the patient need or value and what is best/safe for the patient—as focal points of the organization. The financial bottom line is a secondary priority to safe care. When the financial bottom line is the priority, money is wasted.

An additional gap can also exist between management's view of the organization and the team members' view. Since team members are closer to the core business (patient care), input from team members must be sought as part of the planning process. A planned process whereby each business unit can share information and seek guidance and clarification will facilitate "buy-in" and avoid duplication of efforts. The alternative, top-down, directive approach may result in a high quality strategic plan, but team members who have input into planning will more readily accept the expected outcomes and so become more vested in work processes. Thus, the process includes a system of notification for team members as to the status of their suggestions—how they were evaluated, or if their ideas were not used, feedback is given to team members as to the rationale.

It is imperative that health care leaders understand and focus on their core business. Focusing on the core business provides a clear strategic vision—the big picture—in contrast to scattered plans that steal time and energy with little to show except charts and graphs. Successful organizations focus their strategy on their core rather than on the industry's competitive factors. One method of assessing the health of the organization's strategic planning process is to consider the time spent focusing on the competition. If more time is spent analyzing competitors than focusing on the core business, the process is off task. What must the organization do well to remain in business? What does the organization do particularly well? Health care dollars are scarce. Across-the-board investing often signals that competitors are setting the organization's agenda. Conversely, when an organization's strategy is formed reactively as it tries to keep up with the competition, it loses its uniqueness (Kim and Mauborgne, 2002).

Strategy Deployment

Zuckerman (1998) states that *failure to implement the strategic plan* is the most common flaw in the planning process. He emphasizes that staff may be overwhelmed with managing the day-to-day crises, leaving little time to implement strategic objectives. In addition, if the objectives are not specific, the staff may lack the direction needed to meet the established goals. Communication of the strategic plan must be coordinated throughout the entire organization—vertically and horizontally. To provide direction at the work level, goals and objectives must be established for each business unit, and must link to the overall plan for the organization. This linkage provides guidance and consistency in decision making, and allows managers and team members to understand the present and plan for the future. All team members must be able to articulate how "what they do" fits into the overall plan for the organization.

For each goal and objective, at least one person should be assigned as the primary individual responsible for planning, implementing, and monitoring progress. This is often a member of senior leadership. Specific target dates are assigned to provide a timeline for expected progress. If realization of goals involves intradepartmental work processes, performance improvement teams may be assigned. Senior leadership should establish specific dates to review progress toward each goal. Accountability is accomplished (and rewarded, or otherwise) through linkage between the goals and objectives of the strategic plan and individual team member evaluation criteria. **Exhibit 15–5** provides an excerpt from a Strategic Planning Matrix.

Exhibit 15–5 Sample of Strategic Planning Matrix

Nurse's Heaven Medical Center   Strategic Plan 2004

Goal	Objective	Actions	Measure/ Benchmark	Target Date	Responsible Party
Expand Women's Services to encompass all key aspects of the business	Complete renovations of the existing unit by 12/31/04	1) Monitor progress daily 2) Facilitate weekly construction progress meeting 3) Facilitate monthly medical staff meetings 4) Facilitate biweekly team member meetings	1) Phase I complete by 08/31/04 2) Phase II complete by 10/31/04 3) Complete Phase III by 12/31/04 Benchmark: There Medical Center, Anywhere, USA	12/31/2004	Director of Women's Health

Culture

The *culture* of the organization includes the shared assumptions, values, and behavioral norms of the group. These assumptions and values remain constant over time, even when the membership of the organization changes, and are the basis for an informal consciousness (Ginter, et al., 2002). This is significant in the current climate of mergers, acquisitions, and buy-outs. The shared values of team members may not reflect the values of the organization. When this occurs, the customary way of doing things (behavioral norms,) may sabotage the strategic plan. To assure congruency, shared assumptions (mission—who we are) must support the organizational vision and goals (what we want to accomplish). If the plan is in conflict with the culture, deployment will be a challenge. Unfortunately, if the culture is in significant conflict with the strategic plan and a strong subculture exists, change will be difficult because team members may prefer to "do things the way we have always done them."

To be cognizant of the assumptions, values, and behavioral norms of the work group, successful leaders are involved in the day-to-day operations of the organization. Healthcare leaders must schedule regular visits to each business unit. In addition, regular visits to all stakeholders are imperative. It is not acceptable to attempt to lead from the office, or through computer technology. E-mail, voice mail, and other technologies do not take the place of face-to-face contact, nor do they reflect a complete picture of the culture of the organization. Insights gleaned from involvement with stakeholders and the day-to-day operations of the organization provide vital insight during the situation analysis. Leaders must assess whether the directional strategies are still appropriate and reflect the culture of the organization. Considering the organizational culture is perhaps the most crucial aspect in the deployment of the strategic plan.

What can be done to develop a culture that is adaptive to change? Involving stakeholders in the strategic planning process cultivates an environment of trust and respect. "Buy-in" from those involved in the processes and outcomes of care is worth the extra time necessary to glean these insights. This input is especially pertinent during the shaping of directional strategies—mission, vision, values, and goals. Cultural assessment during the situation analysis may determine that additional implementation strategies are necessary to maintain or change the organizational culture. As previously mentioned, the roles of nurse leaders position them to be acutely aware of the "pulse" of the organization. Nurse leaders must feel comfortable to express views different from those in senior leadership. An atmosphere of trust encourages risk taking, and is necessary for innovation to occur. If trust is absent, personal safety and security become the priority, and the status quo will be maintained despite an elaborate strategic plan. In addition, time and money may be wasted on endeavors that do not reflect current customer needs.

Maintaining a climate of trust and respect, one that encourages risk taking and innovation, is hard work. Leaders must "walk the talk." Saying one thing, while doing another (or even more critical, rewarding another) creates confusion. The directional strategies, mission, vision, values, and goals, must be communicated often, both verbally and in writing. Prominent posting in both common areas as well as each business unit is essential. Additional successful strategies include having the mission appear on all meeting agendas and minutes, on stationery, and on laminated cards for team members. The key strategy for maintenance of an organizational culture that is adaptive to change is "live it"—as reflected in the daily business of the organization.

Structure

Ginter et al., 2002, describes three basic organizational structures: functional structure, divisional structure, and matrix structure. Similar to organizational culture, structure must not impede the overall strategy.

Functional organizational structures organize activities around mission-critical functions or processes. This is the most prevalent organizational structure for organizations with a relatively narrow focus such as health care. Departments are organized according to their function, such as clinical services, finance, marketing, or information systems. Organizations that are structured around mission-critical functions may consider clinical services as the center of the functional structure with other sections of the organization organized around clinical processes such as registration, radiology, laboratory, and so forth (Ginter, et al., 2002).

Health care is highly specialized and expertise within the specialty is highly valued. Functional structures can foster efficiency; however, this type of structure can also result in silo thinking. Functional structure can slow decision making, makes coordination of work difficult, and inhibits communication as each department "looks after their own interest" without the realization of how their processes affect others.

Divisional structures are common in health care organizations that have grown through diversification, vertical integration, or market or product development (Ginter, et al., 1998). Divisional organizations attempt to break down larger, diverse organizations into more manageable and focused sections. This division is especially important when structures of the organization are in different geographic locals, thus with a different environment and with unique customers. Divisional structures have difficulty in maintaining a consistent image and purpose. Divisional structures may additionally require multiple layers of management and duplication of services, thus increasing costs. Organizations that choose divisional structures must carefully coordinate strategic business unit activities.

Matrix structures organize activities around problems to be solved rather than functions, products, or geography (Ginter, et al., 1998). The nurse manager may have a dual reporting structure, to the Vice President (VP) of Women's Health (product) as well as the VP of Nursing Services (functional). Thus, the nurse manager would be responsible to the VP of Nursing for nursing care and to the VP of Women's Health when working on the women's health product line. In some matrix structures, the reporting relationships follow a project or program, and the relationship ends when the project is complete. Matrix structures foster creativity and innovation, nevertheless they are difficult to manage as priorities can become confused. Thus, matrix structures require expert coordination and communication.

Resources

Deploying the selected strategies uses four key resources: financial, human, information systems, and technology (Ginter, et al., 1998). Analysis of *financial resources* was a key factor in the internal environmental analysis. In addition, finance provided key input for strategy formation. Once strategies have been decided, finance is the vehicle to implement them. Leaders should require that major purchase requests be submitted with documented links to the strategic plan. Major projects require capital investment, which generally must be approved by the governing body.

Human resources must be considered prior to deployment of the strategic plan. Questions to consider include: Will additional training be required? Are additional team members needed? Will there be a need for team members with different skills and experiences? This is a critical time to complete an organizational learning needs assessment with all team members. This provides a bridge between the strategic plan, education plan, and performance improvement plan. Multiple plans should be consolidated into one master strategic plan. This is less confusing for team members and assists with unified communication of the organization's plan for improvement.

While *information resources* are crucial to develop the internal and external environmental analysis, they are equally important in the deployment of the strategic plan. As previously mentioned, clinicians can no longer be expected to complete laborious paper documentation. Likewise, leaders must be able to extract data entered into clinical documentation systems with relative ease, thereby negating the need for manual data extraction. A shared drive on the organization's computer system assists in ease of review of the strategic plan. Key business drivers selected as part of the organization's balanced scorecard should also be available on a shared computer system (balanced scorecards are discussed in more detail in the next section of this chapter and in Chapter 4, Organizational Strategies.) Large binders containing the organization's plans, placed on the highest shelf and never used, are dinosaurs.

The strategies selected will drive the needed technologies. *Strategic technology* is concerned with the type of organization, the sophistication of the equipment, and management of the technology employed with the organization (Ginter, et al., 1998). Health care organizations are high technology organizations. Equipment becomes obsolete as quickly as it is installed. This is an area of increasing concern for health care leaders as it represents major expenditures for the organization.

Strategic Management

Goals and Objectives

Exhibit 15–5 (shown previously) demonstrated a sample strategic planning matrix. Senior leaders assure that team members remain focused by assigning specific dates/times for review of the status of each goal and objective. Someone once said, "People respect what you inspect." While this may not be an example of transformational leadership, the adage is unfortunately true. Assessment of efforts toward meeting established goals and objectives not only keeps leaders aware of the status of planning efforts, it also provides team members the opportunity to "show off" their hard work. This personal time and attention by senior leaders demonstrates that the strategic plan is more than a "dusty binder on the shelf," but is rather a working document that ebbs and flows with the organization.

Follow-up reviews can be assigned by target date, or minimally twice per year. Typically, quarterly reports are assigned in order to assess if the work is proceeding as planned, or whether adjustments need to be made based on current reality. Assigning quarterly due dates for status reports on alternate months assists in time and agenda management for senior leaders as well as busy team members. Responsible parties should be forwarded a reminder of the date, time, and place of the meeting as well as the report expectations, i.e., verbal, written, visuals, and so forth. Presenters should be instructed on the amount of time allotted for their presentation. To assist team members to prepare for the meeting, it is helpful if a general format is established. Beware, however, as being too prescriptive can stifle creativity. **Exhibit 15–6** demonstrates a quarterly report matrix for follow-up of progress toward established goals and objects.

Measurement/Balanced Scorecard

Robert S. Kaplan and David P. Norton (1996) of the Harvard Business School developed scorecards (also known as dashboards, instrument panels, and data display devices) in 1991. The utility of the balanced scorecard remains unchanged—the provision of a strategic management and performance management tool. Measurement of key financial, quality, market, and operational indicators provide management with an understanding of

Exhibit 15–6 Sample Goals and Objectives Quarterly Report Matrix

Nurse's Heaven Medical Center
Strategic Plan 2004
Goals and Objectives Report Matrix

Goal	Jan	Feb	Mar	Apr	May	Jun	Jul	Aug	Sept	Oct	Nov	Dec
A	X			X			X			X		
B		X			X			X			X	
C			X			X			X			X

performance in relation to established strategic goals, and graphically displays a snapshot of the institution's overall health (Health Care Advisory Board, "Balanced Scorecards," 1999). In "Poor Performance Measurement Can Drive Financial Crisis," the Health Care Advisory Board (2002) noted that in their study of hospital downturns that "inadequate performance measurement" ranked fifth as the root cause of financial flashpoints.

Successful implementations have been documented utilizing the following process:

- The implementation for a health care facility is a 25–26 month process. Commitment from senior leadership and education for this group regarding the process and outcomes prior to initiation prevents ambiguity.
- In months one and two, a strategic planning retreat is conducted involving the entire organization (those who are unable to attend provide input and are given feedback). This retreat is critical, as consensus is sought regarding the organization's vision, strategic goals and objectives.
- During months three and four, a strategic planning committee is selected to identify objectives for each perspective in the balanced scorecard.
- In the next two months, the strategic planning committee communicates and seeks commitment from the staff for the selected scorecard.
- In the following month, the scorecard is revised based on staff input.
- In months eight and nine, the revised scorecard is deployed to employees. Each unit/department and employee is required to develop a scorecard that supports the strategies identified on the facility scorecard.
- For the next two months, the strategic planning committee reviews individual and department balanced scorecards and suggests revisions.
- At the one-year point, senior leadership formulates a five-year plan based on the finalized scorecard.
- During months 13–24, departmental and organizational progress is reviewed quarterly to identify opportunities to improve.
- At months 25–26, the hospital evaluation committee assesses staff performance based on the individual balanced scorecards. Based on the results, retention, promotion, salary increases and other rewards are realized. The strategic planning committee revises the balanced scorecard and five-year plan based on the results of the metrics

(and after scanning the environment for needed adjustments) (Health Care Advisory Board, "Balanced Scorecards," 1999).
* The cycle continues in the following years.

Theurer (as cited in Health Care Advisory Board, "Balanced Scorecards," 1999) recognized that the following pitfalls should be avoided when creating indicators for a balanced scorecard: 1) lack of context—measures should tie to strategic goals and drive organizational strategy and resource allocation, and 2) lack of benchmark data—seeing how the organization ranks against a peer group.

Leadership must empower employees and provide sufficient resources to develop unit level performance measures. Without sufficient resources, the staff will simply recycle existing measures. Bureaucratic uniformity will squelch the individualized nature of each unit and should be avoided so that each unit can be measured based on its unique attributes. Indicators must be used as tools for continuous improvement, not as tools to punish poor performance. Leadership should provide positive reinforcement for improvements realized. The Health Care Advisory Board noted in "#2 'Metric Austerity' Ensures Big Picture Awareness" that dashboards should be limited to 15 to 30 standards of measurement. Drill down data should be reserved for situations when a more comprehensive assessment is warranted.

Evaluation

Current levels and trends of balanced scorecard results are analyzed against standards of care and/or clinical practice guidelines. This analysis extracts a larger meaning from the data and supports evaluation, decision making, and organizational improvements. The frequency of evaluation depends on the volume and type of data; an adequate sample should exist before evaluating results. When opportunities to improve are recognized, actions must be taken to improve performance, and the effectiveness of these actions must also be analyzed. In addition, results are compared with local competitors, system affiliates, and regional and nationwide benchmarks. Those facilities identified as having best practice provide stretch goals for the organization. Site visits to the facilities can reap significant rewards—both personal and financial—for team members as well as for the organization. Nevertheless, it is important to consider the organization's vision, mission, values, goals and objectives when evaluating metrics.

Performance Improvement

Performance improvement (PI) is a systematic, organization-wide approach to improving the processes and outcomes of the health care system. Performance improvement shifts the focus from individual performance to the performance of the organization's systems and processes. Although individual performance must be maintained, only those team members who are unwilling or unable to change (a very small percentage of the work force) are penalized. There are four basic tenets of PI: customer focus, continuous improvement of processes, team member involvement, and use of data and team knowledge to improve decision making. To be successful, PI effects must be embraced by senior leaders and involve all departments/team members in clinical as well as non-clinical areas. Performance improvement efforts are a part of the strategic planning process, not a separate function (to comply with regulatory standards).

Tools and Techniques

Quantitative Methods

COLLECTING DATA

The *process* for measurement, assessment, and performance improvement is designed to assist the organization to effectively use resources in the provision of quality patient care. Performance improvement activities focus on interrelated factors: governance, managerial, support, and clinical processes, which affect patient outcomes and the financial viability of the facility. Clinical measurement, assessment, and improvement activities should focus on the flow of patient care and assess how well the processes in which individuals participate are performed, coordinated, integrated, and improved. When a problem or opportunity to improve care is identified, action is taken, and the effectiveness of the action is assessed. Results of performance improvement activities are used primarily to improve patient care processes. When the results of performance improvement activities are relevant to the performance of an individual, the results are used as a component in the evaluation of the individual's capabilities.

> **Priority for Data Collection**
> 1. **High Risk**
> 2. **High Volume**
> 3. **Problem Prone**
> 4. **High Cost**
> 5. **Top Money Loser**

Priority for data collection is given to those aspects of care evaluating the following areas: 1) *High Risk*—patients who are at risk of serious consequences or are deprived of substantial benefit if the care is not provided correctly (including providing care that is not indicated, or failing to provide care that is indicated). 2) *High Volume*—the aspect of care occurs frequently or affects large numbers of patients. 3) *Problem Prone*—the aspect of care has tended in the past to produce problems for staff or patients. 4) *High Cost*—the aspect of care is resource intensive. 5) *Top Money Loser*—the care provided has been documented to lose money for the facility.

Measures are used to capture performance improvement data. A measure is a variable relating to the structure, process, or outcome of care. Measures are selected based on the organization's key business drivers (what do we need to do well to remain in the business): identifiers of key quality characteristics and customer satisfaction, strategic management goals and objectives, assessment of performance relevant to functions, the design and assessment of new processes, measurement of the level of performance, and stability of important existing processes. An *operational definition* of each measure must be well defined for ease and reliability of data collection. *Measures of process* are often standards of care or practice. Measures of process include objective criteria based on authoritative sources and supported by the best available clinical and performance improvement literature. Quality control measures are also documented as required by regulatory agencies.

To be useful, data must be transcribed to information through data display, interpretation, and analysis. Tools for analyzing data over time include line graphs, run charts, or control charts. These tools allow the nurse manager to look for trends or patterns in the data (Joint Commission on Accreditation of Healthcare Organizations, 2003).

> ### Definition
>
> A *measure* is a variable relating to the structure, process, or outcome of care.

LINE GRAPHS

Line graphs aid in assessment of trends or changes in performance. These simple graphs indicate whether a process is working and may reveal areas in need of improvement. The data is plotted as the events occur over time. The horizontal axis (X) is used to plot time, for example, days of the week, months of the year, and so forth. The vertical axis (Y) is used to plot the observed level of performance. Once the data points are plotted on the graph, lines are drawn connecting from point to point allowing visualization of trends. Line graphs are used when data collection is still in the early stages prior to having sufficient data to complete a control chart (usually 24–30 data points). Nevertheless, at least 10–12 data points are needed to have a meaningful graph. If it is discovered that a problem occurs at identified times, an in-depth analysis as to the cause and resolution may be undertaken (JCAHO, 2003).

The Line Graph in **Exhibit 15–7** demonstrates data collected for an identified compliance issue for the months of October 2001 through February 2002. Five data points connected by a line provide visualization of the compliance rate that ranges from 24 percent to 43 percent. At this early stage of data collection, visualization for a beginning analysis is possible; however, additional data points are required prior to construction of more sophisticated graphs.

> ### Definition
>
> *Line graphs* aid in assessment of trends or changes in performance. These simple graphs indicate whether a process is working and may reveal areas in need of improvement. The data is plotted as the events occur over time.

Run charts are used when the nurse manager requires a more sensitive analysis of data over time than available via a line chart. While run charts are more sophisticated than line charts, they do not have the benefit of assessment of statistical process control (SPC). Typically, run charts are used until sufficient data points are available for assessment of statistical process control (SPC). In addition to the data point connections, an arithmetic mean is calculated and plotted on the graph. The following guidelines are used to determine priority for in depth analysis: 1) A run of a single data point or a series of consecutive data points on the same side of the mean (center line)

Exhibit 15–7 Line Graph

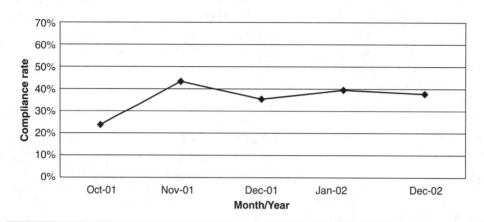

Month/Year

Definition

Run charts are used when the nurse manager requires a more sensitive analysis of data over time than available via a line chart. While run charts are more sophisticated than line charts, they do not have the benefit of assessment of statistical process control (SPC). Typically, run charts are used until sufficient data points are available for assessement of statistical process control (SPC).

and 2) a trend of a series of increases or decreases in the data points. Key to the analysis of the run chart is whether the variation is due to common cause (inherent in the design of the process) or special cause (unique events) and if there is sufficient data to plan intervention, or whether a control chart should be used (JCAHO, 2003).

The Run Chart in **Exhibit 15–8** provides a visual cue of an error rate plotted for twelve months from April 2003 through March 2004. The mean is documented to be 0.42. Two data points are worthy of analysis, May and June 2003. What is the root of these two data points, both on the upper side of the mean with successive increase—special cause or common cause? While this Run Chart provides more information than a Line Chart, a Control Chart is constructed to assess for statistical process control (SPC).

Statistical process control is a method for monitoring the "control" or extent of variation in a process or outcome. The goal is to reduce variation, thus increasing the desired result.

Control charts[1] are specialized run charts that also allow visualization of data over time. Control charts are used when the nurse manager wishes to discover how much variability in a process is due to random variation (process design), and how much is due to special cause variation (unique actions/events), in order to determine whether a process is in statistical process control (SPC). Control charts are borrowed from manufacturing where predictable results are required. In healthcare, as in manufacturing, there should not be a high degree of variation in the product. In health care, the primary product is patient care. Since these are typically called *Control* charts in manufacturing, we use this term here.

---

[1] In Chapter 3 we recommend finding other words to better express the evaluation process, rather than using the word *control*.

Exhibit 15–8 Run Chart

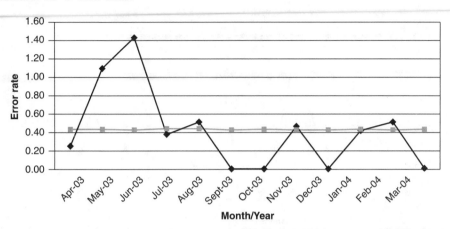

A *mean* (arithmetic average) is established for each data set/chart. Health care organizations typically calculate the upper and lower control limits at three standard deviations above and below the mean. Data points outside of the established control limits are due to *special cause*. These data points represent deviations from the way the process normally operates (Goal/QPC, 1988). A fluctuation in the data within the established control limits results from variation in the process resulting from common causes within the system (design, choice).

Criteria for interpreting control charts are as follows:

> **Definition**
>
> *Control charts* are specialized run charts that also allow visualization of data over time. Control charts are used when the nurse manager wishes to discover how much variability in a process is due to random variation (process design), and how much is due to special cause variation (unique actions/events), in order to determine whether a process is in statistical process control (SPC).

1. *Outside of the control limits*—a data point that falls outside the control limits on the chart, either above the upper control limit or below the lower control limit.
2. *Shift*—eight or more consecutive points either all above or all below the mean. Values on the mean are skipped and the nurse continues to count. Values on the mean do not make or break a trend.
3. *Trend*—six points all going up or all going down. If the value of two or more successive points are the same, the point is ignored when counting; like values do not make or break a trend.
4. *Two out of three*—two out of three consecutive points in the outer third of the chart (greater than two standard deviations). The two out of three consecutive points could be on the same side or on either side of the mean.

The control chart in **Exhibit 15–9** demonstrates a medication error rate for August 2001 through March 2004. The mean is 0.90 with an upper control limit (three standard devia-

Exhibit 15–9 Control Chart

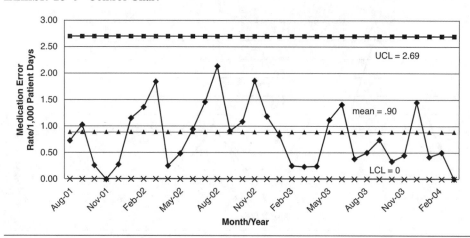

tions above the mean) of 2.69 and a lower control limit of zero (a negative error rate is not possible). All data points are within the control limits. No shifts (eight or more consecutive points all above or below the mean), or trends (six points all going up or all going down) are identified. The *"two out of three"* criteria (two out of three consecutive points in the outer third of the chart) is not demonstrated.

MATRIX

A *matrix* is used to show combinations of data. Examples include unit statistics such as: admissions, nursing hours per patient day, percent of occupancy, medication error rate, and overall rate of patient satisfaction for an obstetrical unit over a period of months. In **Exhibit 15–10** the months are documented in the matrix heading with the measures listed down the left side. This chart provides the data but it is not as easy to spot anomalies or trends using this method.

A matrix is used to show combinations of data.

Exhibit 15–10 Matrix Chart

OB Unit	Jan	Feb	Mar	Apr	May	Jun	Jul	Aug	Sep	Oct	Nov	Dec
Admissions	650	653	640	600	590	575	555	602	643	670	675	700
Nursing Hours/ Patient Day	5.9	6.0	6.1	6.3	6.6	6.8	7.0	6.7	5.8	5.9	5.7	5.5
Percent Occupancy	.75	.76	.74	.68	.67	.65	.63	.68	.74	.78	.79	.81
Medication Error Rate	1.5	1.0	.75	.54	.45	.16	.05	.50	1.45	1.3	1.7	.10
Overall Patient Satisfaction	.85	.88	.89	.90	.96	.97	.98	.95	.86	.81	.80	.78

The data in **Exhibit 15–10** could be used to assess relationships between data sets, for example, overall patient satisfaction, and nursing hours per patient day. Does patient satisfaction decrease as nursing hours per patient day decrease? Yes, in this example. Do medication errors increase when nursing hours per patient day decrease? Yes, in this example. Each data set is compared to a different data set for identification of applicable relationships. Relationships are sometimes difficult to discern using a matrix for comparison. A multiple line graph demonstrates a better visual of relationships between data sets.

MULTIPLE LINE GRAPH

Relationships of the data captured in a matrix may be better visualized in a *multiple line graph*. What does the data show happens with the rate of overall patient satisfaction when nursing hours per patient day decrease? Does patient satisfaction increase as nursing hours per patient day increase? Are data relationships more readily apparent during certain months of the year? Spreadsheet software can be used to easily convert matrix data to a multiple line graph. Caution should be exercised to not display too many indicators on the same graph, thus making it difficult to interpret. Color coding the lines to correlate with data elements assists in analysis of data relationship used (JCAHO, 2003).

The Multiple Line Graph in **Exhibit 15–11** allows for easy visualization of the relationship between a decrease in nursing hours per patient day and subsequent increase in medication error (September and October). Each applicable data set from the matrix may be plotted on a multiple line graph to discern relationships.

> *Relationships of the data captured in a matrix may be better visualized in a multiple line graph.*

COST-BENEFIT ANALYSIS

Comparison of the benefits and costs of a proposed endeavor is completed through cost-benefit analysis. *Cost-benefit analysis* (cost-benefit and break-even analysis are further explained in Chapter 10, Budgeting) is a budgeting technique used primarily by the gov-

Exhibit 15–11 Multiple Line Graph

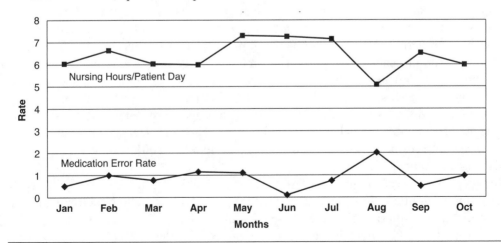

ernment. However, it is becoming increasingly popular as organizations realize the impact their business has on society and the community they serve. Cost-benefit analysis is an analytical technique that compares the social costs and benefits of a proposed program against the costs of the venture under consideration. If the benefits outweigh the costs, a positive cost-benefit is expected, and it makes senses to spend the money; otherwise it does not. Criteria for evaluation in a cost-benefit analysis include: project goals, benefits and costs, discounting cost and benefit flows at an appropriate rate, and completing a decision analysis (Finkler, 2001).

The first step in cost-benefit analysis is to determine the goals of the project—what does the organization hope the project will accomplish? What would the community gain if the project comes to fruition? Identifying goals and objectives clarifies the expected benefit for those we serve. Examples include less travel time for patients in need of cancer treatment, or local education resources for high-risk mothers.

Once project goals and objectives have been determined, project benefits must be determined. All losses and gains expected to be experienced by society are included, expressed in dollar terms. Losses incurred to some sections of society would be subtracted from the gains that accrue to others. The benefits include only those things that are a direct or indirect result of the project. Alternative strategies are considered so as to choose the option with the greatest net benefit, or ratio of benefit to cost (Finkler, 2001). Leaders would not include benefits that are a reality whether or not the project is realized. For example, while cancer treatment may be available at a tertiary medical center 100 miles away, the dollar costs related to the benefit of not having to travel such a long distance would be included in the analysis, but not the benefits of cancer treatment because it is already available.

Costs must be estimated as part of the cost-benefit analysis. All costs must be considered including opportunity costs, because when a decision is made to do something, other alternatives are sacrificed. For example, an increase in inventory requires extra cash. The cash used will not be available for use somewhere else in the organization (another opportunity). This is a critical consideration in cost-benefit analysis (Finkler, 2001). In our cancer treatment example, the facility may have to forego a transplant program in order to finance the cancer treatment program. This opportunity cost should be estimated. These calculations include the time value of money.

Project costs and benefits often occur over a period of years. Money has different value over time. If a project has a $2 million start up cost that will be paid back through revenue over a five year period, the $2 million is worth more today than over the next five years. This comparison of benefits and costs over time is referred to as *discounting cash flow*. Discounting cash flow uses an interest rate (discount rate) to convert all cost and benefits to their value at the present time (Finkler, 2001). The methodology for the discounting method is beyond the scope of this chapter. Nurse managers requiring in-depth information related to long-term financing are referred to *Financial Management for Public, Health, and Not-for-profit Organizations* by S. A. Finkler, 2001, Chapter 5, "Capital Budgeting and Long-Term Financing."

To complete the decision analysis, estimated costs and benefits are compared to each other in the form of a ratio—benefits divided by costs. If the resulting metric is greater than one, then the benefits exceed the costs, and the project is desirable. The greater the benefit-to-cost ratio, the more advantageous the project (Finkler, 2001).

BREAK-EVEN ANALYSIS

Increasingly, health care organizations must search for projects or ventures in an effort to improve financial stability, or to subsidize services for which the organization loses money, but still provides based on community need. *Break-even analysis* determines the minimum volume of services that a program or service must provide to be financially self-sufficient. This tool is useful for determining whether a new venture will be profitable. It is used in situations in which there is a specific price associated with the service such as a specific charge, or a system of cost reimbursement (Finkler, 2001). A break-even analysis is an essential part of a business Proforma.

This seems like a simple endeavor—if the reimbursement per unit of service is greater than the cost, the new endeavor would be expected to make a profit. On the other hand, if the expected reimbursement is less than the cost, the new endeavor will lose money. However, cost per unit depends on volume. When volume is low, the cost per unit will be higher. As volumes increase, the venture may become profitable. Thus, it is imperative that the organization understand at what point revenues (money expected to be received) will be equal to expenses (cost to provide the service). This is the break-even point.

In order to grasp the steps in calculating the break even-point equation, key terminology must be understood.

- *Total revenue* is the average price multiplied by the number of units.
- Total expenses include fixed and variable costs (both fixed and variable costs are further explained in Chapter 10, Budgeting).
- *Fixed costs* (FC) are costs that do not change as volume changes within the relevant range (range of activity that would be reasonably expected to occur in the budget period).
- *Variable costs* vary in direct proportion with volume. When calculating expenses, variable cost (VC) is expressed in variable cost per unit.

Finkler (2001, p. 107) describes the following calculation, included in the text boxes, to find that break-even point. In this example, 1,000 cesarean deliveries at a total cost of $2,500 per cesarean delivery, generate $2,500,000 in total revenue. The break-even point (at cost of $2,500 per case) is 450 cesarean deliveries—the point at which total revenue equals total expenses. **Exhibit 15–12** provides a visual example of the break-even point for cesarean deliveries.

Recall that the break-even point occurs when the total revenues equal the total expenses, thus the break-even point is calculated:

> *Total revenue = P (price) x Q (volume)*
>
> *Total expenses = V (Variable costs [VC] x Volume [Q]) + Fixed Costs (FC)*

> *P x Q = (VC x Q) + FC*
>
> *$1,125,000 x 450 cases = $625,000/450 (recall that variable cost is per case)*
>
> *x 450 cases + $500,000*
>
> *($1,125,000 = 450 cases at $2,500/case)*
>
> *($625,000, the variable cost = $1,125,000 total cost - $500,000 fixed cost).*

The next step is to subtract (VC x Q) from both sides of the equation:

> **(P x Q) – (VC x Q) = FC**
> *$1,125,000 x 450 cases – ($625,000/450 x 450 cases) = $500,000.*

Next, factor out the Q from the left side of the equation:

> **Q x (P – VC) = FC**
> *450 cases x ($1,125,000 - $625,000/450 cases) = $500,000.*

The resulting formula:

> **Q = FC divided by P – VC is the quantity (Q) needed to break-even**
> *450 cases = $500,000/$1,125,000 - $625,000/450 cases*
> *Q = 450 cases*

Exhibit 15–12 Break-Even Point

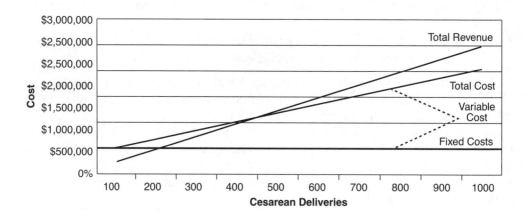

REGRESSION ANALYSIS

Understanding regression analysis is imperative for successful budgeting and strategic planning. Nurse managers must understand how to effectively predict a variable, for example, cost, based on an independent variable, for example, patient days. Without this knowledge, nurse managers are merely "guessing" as to whether their nursing unit can remain financially viable. *Regression analysis* is a statistical technique available via computer software used to forecast the relationship between two variables. The independent variable is typically plotted on the X-axis of a scatter graph and the dependent variable is plotted on the Y-axis. The computer software will require the user to enter the data for the X values and the Y values. After entering this data, little more than a command to compute the regression is required. It is important that nurse managers not be intimidated by this technique, but rather become familiar with its use in the planning process. Guessing is not suitable for professionals charged with meeting the needs of suffering society.

Regression measures the linear association between a dependent (criterion) and an independent variable (predictor). Regression assumes that the dependent variable is predictively linked to the independent variable. Regression analysis is particularly valuable for forecasting as it attempts to predict the values of a continuous, interval-scaled dependent variable from the independent variable. For example, the number of full-time equivalent (FTE) team members (the dependent variable) might be predicted on the basis of patient days (the independent variable). Forecasting in this manner is crucial to anticipate staffing needs as volumes fluctuate.

Bivariate linear regression investigates a straight-line relationship. This is not as commonly used as multivariate regression. The formula is:

$$Y = \alpha + \beta X.$$

In this example, Y is the dependent variable, X is the independent variable, and α and ß are constants to be estimated. The symbol for the Y intercept (the point at which the regression line intercepts the Y-axis) is α and ß is the slope (the inclination of a regression line as compared to the base line) coefficient. Slope can best be considered as the increase in the number of units on the Y-axis divided by the run in units along the X-axis (Zikmund, 2003). While the nurse manager may attempt to simply draw a line through the data points on a scatter graph, this method is not valid and fluctuates based on human error. Finance can assist if bivariate analysis is needed.

MULTIPLE REGRESSION

Multiple regression analysis allows for the simultaneous investigation of the effect of two or more independent variables on a single interval-scaled or ratio-scaled dependent variable. As outlined by Zikmund (2003), the formula is as follows:

$$Y = a + \beta_1 X_1 + \beta_2 X_2 + \beta_3 X_3 + \dots + \beta_n X_n$$

This method is especially useful when several factors are likely to affect the dependent variable. Nurse managers may seek input from the finance department related to multiple regression analysis.

Qualitative Methods

BRAINSTORMING

A brainstorming session is convened to understand an issue, the impact the issue may have on the organization, or to generate ideas for strategic alternatives. Members of the group present ideas with brief explanations; however, dialogue and evaluation of the ideas are not undertaken at this juncture (Ginter, et al., 2002). The ideas are usually recorded on flip charts. Team members are encouraged to verbalize ideas no matter how impossible they may seem at first. According to Brassard and Ritter (1994) there are two methods for brainstorming: structured (each team member gives ideas in turn) and unstructured (team members give ideas as they come to mind). Structured and unstructured brainstorming can be done silently or aloud. Brainstorming enhances communication, generates new ideas and alternatives, sparks creativity, and stimulates innovation.

FOCUS GROUPS

Similar to brainstorming, *focus groups* are convened to reach conclusions regarding environmental issues. Focus groups were discussed earlier in this chapter as a mechanism for generating information during the internal environmental analysis. Experts in the areas related to the identified issue provide leadership and the opportunity to discuss important issues. In addition, focus groups provide a venue to gain new insight and fresh alternatives (Ginter, et al., 2002). This insight empowers and equips them with ideas for alternative actions if necessary.

NOMINAL GROUP TECHNIQUE

Another problem identification and solving method for groups is called *nominal group technique* (NGT). In nominal group technique, team members independently generate a written list of ideas regarding the issue. After members have been given sufficient time to generate their list, each member takes turns reporting one idea at a time to the entire group. As new ideas are generated, all members record these on a flip chart for consideration. Members are encouraged to build on the ideas of fellow team members. When all ideas have been exhausted, the team discusses the ideas, and then team members privately vote by ranking the ideas in order of preference. After the ideas are ranked, the group discusses the vote, and voting continues until consensus is reached. The advantage of nominal group technique is that everyone has equal status and power, ensuring representation of the group. In addition, nominal group technique eliminates the biases of those in a leadership position (Ginter, et al., 2002).

According to Brassard and Ritter (1994), nominal group technique allows a team to quickly come to consensus regarding the importance of issues, problems, or solutions by individual rankings into a team's final priorities. Since all team members participate equally, commitment is built to the team's choice. It is especially useful for reserved team members as it places them on equal footing with more dominant team members.

DELPHI TECHNIQUE

The *Delphi technique* uses a structured group decision making technique based on repeated use of rating scales to obtain opinions about a decision. Computer software is available that summarizes the results, making the process easier and faster. Members of the group first explore the issue individually and then design a questionnaire for a larger group. The results are tabulated and given back to the group for discussion. The process continues with progressively focused questionnaires. The process is repeated until members of the group reach consensus regarding the issues and a decision is reached.

Alternately, the process may begin in a more free-flowing style with team members initially identifying important issues. This individual brainstorming technique is particularly valuable when team members are unable to meet in a group setting. Key themes are then put into a questionnaire for ranking by team members. After team members rank issues, the questionnaire is sent out again to all members for further input. This process continues as many times as necessary to reach consensus on key issues.

The Delphi technique is particularly valuable for obtaining input from team members during the strategic planning process when face-to-face conversation is not possible, but input is valued. An advantage of the Delphi technique is the protection of anonymity, making the technique particularly useful for issues where there is significant disagreement. The technique is particularly useful for groups that have historically failed to communicate effectively. The Delphi procedures offer a systematic method that ensures team member opinions are considered (Gordon, 2002).

SCENARIO DEVELOPMENT—TREE DIAGRAM

To implement an identified strategy, tasks must be mapped for implementation. *Tree diagrams* are used to break broad goals, graphically, into increasing levels of detailed actions so a stated goal can be accomplished (Brassard and Ritter, 1994). This tool encourages team members to expand their thinking while simultaneously linking the team's overall goals. Tree diagrams assist team members to move theory to reality.

The first task is to choose the goal statement. Alternately, the team may have been assigned a goal on which to work. If the team selects the goal, care must be taken to create, via consensus, a clear, action-oriented statement. Team members must have intimate knowledge of the goal topic.

Next, major tree headings, or subgoals are selected. These subgoals may be established through brainstorming, and then using the nominal group technique. These subgoals are the major means of achieving the goal statement. The first level of detail must remain broad so it does not jump to the lowest level of task. After working from the goal statement and first-level detail, the team proceeds through the three levels of detail. Some subgoals are simple, while others require more breakdown. At each level, the facilitator queries the group as to whether or not something obvious has been forgotten. An additional important question for the team is whether these actions result in accomplishment of the given goal or subgoal. Post-it™ notes may be used to create the levels of detail since they can easily be moved around. Lines are drawn when the Tree is finished. The Tree can be oriented from left to right or top to bottom.

The Tree Diagram is an effective communication tool. This technique allows for input from direct caregivers. The team's final task is to revise, add, or delete goals or subgoals as deemed appropriate (Brassard and Ritter, 1994). **Exhibit 15–13** is an example of a Tree Diagram for a health care organization.

Exhibit 15–13 Tree Diagram

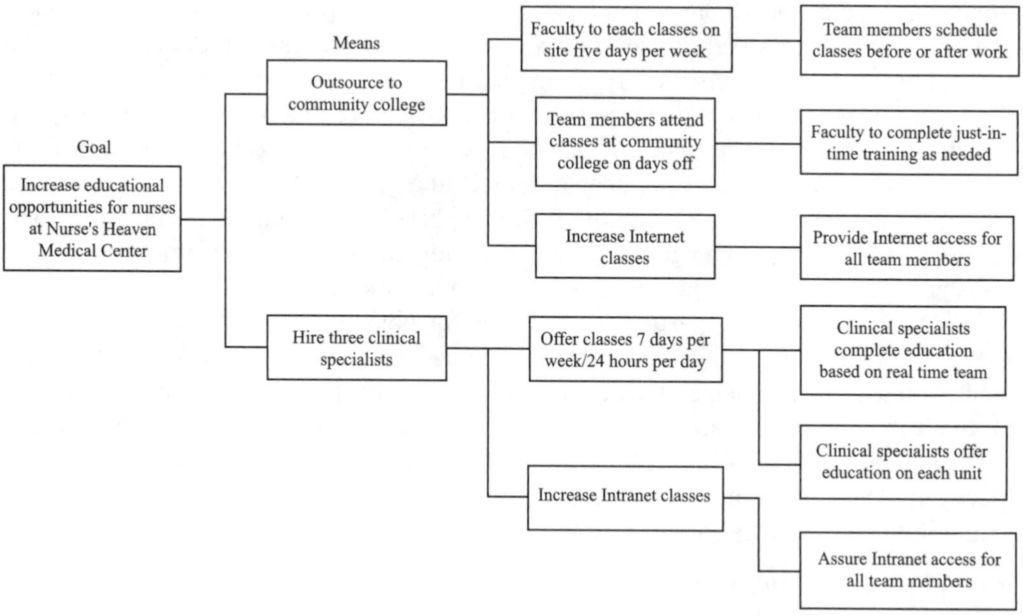

GANTT CHARTS

Project management is critical as new ventures or programs are pursued. Complex projects require that successive activities be completed in a timely fashion. Several commercial computer software programs are available; however, a simple Gantt chart can be constructed with materials at hand. A Gantt chart displays activities or goals in a matrix format. The time frame is displayed on the horizontal axis and the activities to be completed for the project are documented on the vertical axis. If dates are especially important (i.e., when one phase of the project must be completed on a specific date in order for the next phase to begin) project leaders may designate specific dates on the chart. **Exhibit 15–14** shows a sample Gantt chart for a performance improvement team. Gantt charts are also useful as a planning tool for new managers. It is easy for "time to get away" and before a new manager may realize it, evaluations are past due, reports are due the next day without adequate time to prepare, etc. Managers may also use a Gantt chart in order to "pace" themselves so they do not get overwhelmed—everything cannot be done in a week's time. Planning activities throughout the year will decrease stress and the need to "fight fires" on a daily basis. Gantt charts are especially helpful for nursing leaders who are visual learners—you can see what needs to be done, and when.

Role of the Nurse Manager

Nurse managers are situated in a unique position to recognize the need for change in the organization. Sandwiched between the front line staff and senior leaders, nurse managers

Exhibit 15–14 Sample Gantt Chart for a Performance Improvement Team

Activities	Jan	Feb	Mar	Apr	May	Jun	Jul	Aug	Sept	Oct	Nov	Dec
Select process	X											
Charter team	X											
Collect baseline data	7											
Analyze baseline data		15										
Select improvement		28										
Plan the improvement			5									
Do the improvement			10									
Check the results			31									
Act to maintain the improvement				X								

may be the first to recognize the need for changes in strategy. Nurse managers stimulate their team members by cultivating a positive culture of performance excellence and a corresponding reward system. Their challenge is to define the parameters within which team members can experiment and be innovative. Nurse managers uphold the organization's value system, and maintain systems that focus on the core business of patient care. Managers assure that strategies are in tune with the current needs of customers and are balanced so that one strategy does not suffer at the expense of another. They are sensitive to important changes all the time, and inquire of all their customers—are your needs being met? Of key importance, nurse managers maintain the system by assuring issues get picked up quickly and senior leaders are made aware. They do not just herald problems, but offer solutions as well. Nurse managers bind the organization together within the internal environment so that team members are galvanized into action. Managing a nursing unit is not an easy task and is certainly not for the faint of heart.

In his article "Future Sense: Creating the Future," H. B. Gelatt (1993) defines the skills needed to continually adapt, innovate, and change. "This 'flexpert' is open-minded, comfortable with uncertainty, delighted with change, and capable of unfreezing and refreezing beliefs, knowledge, and attitudes." (pp. 11–12) 'Flexperts' understand that the inability to shift paradigms not only restricts flexibility, but causes the individual to become out-of-date, inaccurate, and in need of revision. Culture, communities, experiences, and health care organizations change constantly and make old paradigms dysfunctional.

As nurse managers spiral toward the future, strategic planning fosters a sense of positive uncertainty that will assist team members in the acceptance of change, ambiguity, uncertainly, and inconsistency. As Erie Chapman states in *Radical Loving Care*, "Our Vision statements need to be engraved in our hearts, not just on plaques" (p. 110). Committed leadership begins with those who make up the majority of caregivers in health care—nurses.

References

Bennis, W., & Nanus, B. (1985). *Leaders: The strategies for taking charge.* New York: Harper & Row.

BrainyQuote, Aristotle Onassis. Retrieved April 10, 2004 from http://www.brainyquote.com/quotes/authors/a/aristotle_onassis.html.

Brassard, M., & Ritter, D. (1994). *The memory jogger™ II: A pocket guide to tools for continuous improvement & effective planning.* Salem, NH: Goal/QPC.

Chapman, E. (2003). *Radical loving care.* Nashville, TN: Vaughn.

Creative Quotations. (2004). Artemus Ward. Retrieved April 1, 2003 from http://www.creativequotations.com/one/1839.htm.

Drenkard, K. N. (2001). Creating a future worth experiencing: Nursing strategic planning in an integrated healthcare delivery system. *Journal of Nursing Administration, 31*(7–8), 364–375.

Finkler, S. A. (2001). *Financial management for public, health, and not-for-profit organizations.* Upper Saddle River, NJ: Prentice Hall.

Gelatt, H. B. (1993). Future sense: Creating the future. *The Futurist,* (9–10), 9–13.

Ginter, P., Swayne, L., & Duncan, W. (2002). *Strategic management of health care organizations.* Malden, MA: Blackwell.

Goal/QPC. (1988). *The memory jogger: A pocket guide of tolls for continuous improvement.* 2nd ed. Methuen, MA: Goal/QPC.

Gordon, J. R. (2002). *Organizational behavior: A diagnostic approach.* 7th ed. Upper Saddle Ridge, NJ: Prentice Hall.

Health Care Advisory Board. (1999 August). Balanced scorecards. Retrieved November 9, 2002 from http://www.advisory.com.

Health Care Advisory Board. (2002). #2 'Metric austerity' ensures big picture awareness. Retrieved November 9, 2002 from http://www.advisory.com.

Health Care Advisory Board. (2002). Poor performance measurement can drive financial crisis. Retrieved November 9, 2002 from http://www.advisory.com.

Joint Commission on Accreditation of Healthcare Organizations. (2004). *Comprehensive accreditation manual for hospitals: The official handbook.* Oakbrook Terrace, IL: Joint Commission Resources.

Joint Commission on Accreditation of Healthcare Organizations. (2003). *Staffing effectiveness in hospitals.* Oakbrook Terrace, IL: Joint Commission Resources.

Kaplan, R. S., & Norton, D. P. (1996). *Translating strategy into action: The balanced scorecard*. Boston: Harvard Business School.

Kim, W. C., & Mauborgne, R. (2002). Charting your company's future. *Harvard Business Review, 80*(6), 76–83.

Krueger, R. (1988). *Focus groups: A practical guide for applied research*. Newbury Park: Sage.

Mintzberg, H., & Markides, C. (2000). Commentary on the Henry Mintzberg interview. *Academy of Management Executive*, 39–42.

Morgan, D. (1993). *Successful focus groups: Advancing the state of the art*. Newbury Park: Sage.

National Institute of Standards and Technology. (2004). *2004 Baldrige national quality program: Health care criteria for performance excellence*. Gaithersburg, MD: National Institute of Standards and Technology.

The Quotations Page. (2004). Yogi Berra. Retrieved April 1, 2004, from http://www.quotationspage.com.wotd.html.

The Quotations Page. (2004). Marcel Proust. Retrieved April 10, 2004 from http://www.quotationspage.com/search.php3?homesearch=proust&x=31&y=5.

Solovy, A. (2002). The paradox of planning. *Healthcare & Healthcare Network, 76*(9), 32.

The Tennessee Center for Performance Excellence. (2004). *2004 Criteria for performance excellence*. Nashville, TN: The Tennessee Center for Performance Excellence.

Zikmund, W. G. (2003). *Business research methods*. 7th ed. Mason, OH: South-Western.

Zuckerman, A. M. (1998). *Healthcare strategic planning: Approaches for the 21st century*. Chicago: Health Administration.

CHAPTER 16

An Overview of Case Management

Patricia A. Hayes, PhD, RN

Introduction

Case management, a health care delivery strategy, has experienced a renaissance with the rise of managed care during the last decade. Building upon a rich history in public health nursing and social work, case management has evolved since the turn of the century from community service coordination to approaches that coordinate and deliver health care services across the care continuum. These settings include acute and subacute care, home care, and long-term care. This evolution has led to the development of new models and standards for case management practice. The models are diverse, growing in number and changing as health care systems continue to transform.

Within this context of evolving models, the definitions of case management often lack consensus. However, two major definitions have emerged, one specific to the discipline of nursing, and the other interdisciplinary.

According to the American Nurses Association Credentialing Center (ANCC):

> Case management is a dynamic and systematic collaborative approach to providing and coordinating healthcare services to a defined population. It is a participative process to identify and facilitate options and services for meeting individuals' health needs, while decreasing fragmentation and duplication of care and enhancing quality, cost-effective clinical outcomes (p. 3).

This definition is grounded in the nursing process and focuses on collaboration and client populations as important elements for nursing case management.

The interdisciplinary definition, developed by the Case Management Society of America (CMSA, 1995), describes case management as a "collaborative process which assesses, plans, implements, coordinates, monitors and evaluates options and services to meet an individual's health needs through communication and available resources to promote quality, cost-effective outcomes" (p. 8). The major difference between the two definitions is ANCC's focus on the health needs of populations, while CMSA targets the health needs of individuals.

From these two definitions have come common goals for case management models including:

- quality of care demonstrated by therapeutic and beneficial patient outcomes;
- length of stay focused on cost control through rapid movement of inpatient's through the system;
- resource utilization achieved through protocols or critical pathways derived from research and evaluation of patient outcomes;
- continuity of care achieved through the integration of services across the illness episode by a familiar case manager (Flarey, 1996; Taylor, 1999).

How organizations operationalize these goals depends upon the case management model they select to guide their particular case management delivery system.

Models of Case Management in Nursing: Past and Present

In the last decade many models of case management have appeared in the literature. A number of them have come and gone, primarily because they have lacked sound theoretical underpinnings, or failed to generate research findings that supported the core concepts within the models. Readers who are interested in the progression of nursing case management knowledge can find excellent descriptions and synthesis of key case management models in such textbooks as Cohen and Cesta (2005), and Flarey and Blancett (1996).

These textbooks, and other nursing literature, commonly categorize case management models into *within-the-walls* (hospital-based) and *beyond-the-walls* (community-based) classifications. Fitting into these classifications are two models introduced in the 1980s. They have withstood the test of time and have been studied extensively, adopted and/or adapted by health care organizations across the country. They are: The New England Medical Center Hospitals (NEMCH) *within-the-walls model*; and the Carondelet St. Mary's Hospital (CSMH) *beyond-the-walls model*—often referred to as the *Arizona model*. Both models have a strong theoretical basis, and research data has shown the models to be effective in controlling institutional costs by achieving decreased hospital lengths of stay, and decreased readmissions, while maintaining quality patient care (Ethridge and Lamb, 1989; Ethridge, 1997; Zander, 1988).

The New England Medical Center Hospitals (NEMCH) model was developed by Zander and her associates in 1985 (Zander, 1988a, 1988b), and was the first initiation of with-in-the-walls case management. According to Zander, the model structures care of clients experiencing acute illness episodes. The focus of this conceptual model is on outcomes; it is a synthesis of primary nursing care and nursing process, and introduces critical pathways and case management plans as essential concepts in structuring the episode of care. Unit-based primary care was selected as a core concept because it was known to facilitate nursing accountability, continuity, and satisfaction for patients. The nursing process, an applied scientific method, was included in the model because this process solves problems and leads to outcome definition (Zander, 1996). Case management adopts a critical pathway linked with a case management plan that creates methods for structuring, coordinating, and assessing the patients' progress. Critical pathways have proven to be one of the most innovative concepts of the model and, fifteen years later, they have been widely adapted (Renholm, et al., 2002) and have become a symbol of case management. Zander and associates define a critical pathway[1] as:

> A tool that helps practitioners manage an episode of care for a patient
> population or condition by providing a timeline of the expected course
> of care with expected patient outcomes. The critical pathway is designed
> to improve quality of patient care and promote efficient utilization of
> resources (Zander, 1988, p. 28).

In this model, the case management plan is conceptualized as a comprehensive document. The document is designed to function as a tool that integrates the nursing process and the critical pathway, as well as dealing with variance analysis (deviations from the pathway). In addition, the document is used to record the care giver relationship of care giver interventions with patient outcomes along a time line. This plan enables primary nurse case managers to coordinate a patient's entire episode of care across hospital units.

When a patient enters a hospital unit at the New England Medical Center, a primary nurse formulates a case management plan and becomes the patient's primary caregiver. If the patient transfers to another hospital unit, a new primary nurse is assigned to deliver direct care and the initial primary nurse continues to administer the patient's case management plan. Care coordination is facilitated through team meetings, case consultation, and interdisciplinary communication, focused by critical pathways. Because the model is grounded in primary nursing and nursing process it has been applied easily to a variety of with-in-the-wall settings.

Zander (1996) described the episode of illness as *finite* and the continuum of care as *infinite*. According to Zander, the infinite continuum, which links within-the-wall and beyond-the-wall models, will, in the future, focus on wellness/prevention services promoting higher levels of care. She believes the concepts contained within her hospital-based case management model will flourish in this expanded continuum of health care. This model will culminate in a need for more primary nurse case managers skilled in developing and using critical pathways, now called careMaps, across the continuum of health care, and in applying them to direct care for populations of clients (Zander, 2002). This present view of case management more closely reflects the Professional Nurse Case Management (PNCM) model developed at Carondelet St. Mary's Hospital in Tuscon, Arizona.

In 1985, Carondelet St. Mary's Hospital (CSMH) developed the first beyond-the-walls case management model (Ethridge, 1987). Changing reimbursement patterns, due to Medicare cost-containment measures and the growing number of clients enrolled in managed care, resulted in patients being discharged while still in early stages of recovery. Thus,

---

[1] An example of a critical pathway is given in Dunham-Taylor and Pinzcuk (2006) *Health Care Financial Management for Nurse Managers: Financial Applications in Hospitals, Long-Term Care, and Ambulatory Care.*

a need to provide care after discharge emerged. Rising to the challenge, nurse administrators at St. Mary's sought to meet this need by creating the Professional Nurse Case Management Model (PNCM). It was designed to offer case-managed nursing services to chronically ill and high-risk clients across hospital and community settings, moving care beyond the episode of illness into the continuum of care. One of the dominant values of the CSMH model is the belief that a continuum of care encompasses all of life and death experiences (Doerge and Hagenow, 1995). The goals of the model are to offer case managed services that improve and promote a person's health or peaceful death, and assist individuals to learn new ways of managing their illness situations.

Three qualitative studies exploring Carondelet's Professional Nurse Case Management Model (PNCM) theory-practice link have been reported in the literature (Forbes, 1999; Lamb and Stemple, 1994; Newman, Lamb, and Michaels, 1991). Findings identify the nurse case manager-client relationship as the concept in the model most integral to achieving quality and cost outcomes. Outcomes include "improved self-care skills, fewer hospitalizations and enhanced quality of life" (Lamb and Stemple, p. 12). Evidence from the studies suggests that the emphasis placed on building caring therapeutic nurse-client relationships motivates clients to engage in self-care strategies, and thereby improves functional performance.

St. Mary's used this outcome data to negotiate managed care contracts, and as a result, launched the first nursing HMO. Contracts were negotiated using a capitated reimbursement system that extended community case management services to approximately 22,000 HMO members who were experiencing chronic illnesses, disease complications, and reoccurring institutionalizations. Preliminary findings showed that nursing case management reduced hospitalizations and home health visits to below the national average, increased knowledge of health-promoting behaviors over time, and motivated more than 50 percent of the HMO enrollees to attend annual health screening programs, which contributed to decreased health risks (Ethridge, 1997). In this integrated delivery model, one professional nurse case manager may work for several months (or years) with a chronically ill individual, caring for him or her in the hospital, in the long-term care facility, in the home, or in wellness centers located within retirement complexes. Professional nurse case managers procure needed resources, provide screening, counsel, make referrals to physicians, and engage in wellness education. This broader approach to nursing practice acknowledges the interconnectedness of life and illness situations, and recognizes the individual without losing sight of the evolving whole.

Both The New England Medical Center Hospitals and Carondelet St. Mary's Hospital models are prototypes for with-in and beyond-the-walls case management models, represent pioneering efforts credited with refocusing the spotlight on case management, and have demonstrated its effectiveness on lowering use and cost of services. These innovative professional practice models are restructuring case management and the case manager role; they are proven successful in affecting continuity of care and health maintenance; they have ensured accountable resource use; they have achieved cost containment goals; and have more effectively bridged transitions among hospital-based units and integrated health care networks.

Practicing Case Management: Role and Functions of a Case Manager

A common response when one speaks of case management and the case manager role as new strategies for health care delivery is that nurses have been case managing clients for years. However, this response fails to recognize the unique body of knowledge and skills emerging over the last decade that underpins the functional role of case management. Case managers see the big picture of client care. That is, they fully integrate the total spectrum of acute to chronic phases of care within clients' lived experience, rather than simply possessing knowledge and skills limited to direct care delivery in one setting.

Practicing from this perspective requires nurses to have expert knowledge and skills in the following domains:

1. Providing direct care.
2. Procuring community resources.
3. Coordinating care across hospital units and health care delivery networks.
4. Evaluating health care services for cost effectiveness.
5. Building therapeutic nurse–client long-term relationships.

Four of these five domains of case management knowledge have been identified from a national study by the National Case Management Task Force, (as cited in Bower, 2000) which surveyed certified case managers about key areas of knowledge they used to perform their case management functions. The fifth domain, building therapeutic nurse-client long-term relationships, emerged from studies that examined the processes of nursing case management (Lamb and Stemple, 1994; Newman, Lamb, and Michaels, 1991).

In the first domain, *providing direct care*, the case manager's knowledge and skills include assessment and planning. Because knowledge development in clinical nursing is grounded in holistic assessment and care planning, nurses are well prepared to assess the interrelationships among medical, psychological, social, and behavioral components of clients' illness situations. These assessment findings are used to plan, intervene, and reassess how the components impact the client.

While assessment and planning are already core functions of nursing, from a case management perspective assessment is an ongoing, continual process that seeks to understand the patients' illness situation within the context of their total health care experiences. This expanded view of assessment provides consistency between planning and delivering care, because care of case-managed clients often occurs at multiple points of service.

Thus, nurses practicing as case managers must shift their thinking and knowing from a focus on delivering and managing episodes of illness events within one service setting to providing and managing care within a broader service context, one that includes the community. Thinking and knowing from a community perspective requires a nurse case manager to develop new levels of community consciousness and a new level of community connection to provide direct care more effectively.

Community awareness and connection also enable a case manager to procure and manage resources, the second domain. Knowing what resources are available in the community for case management clients, as well as building relationships with referral agencies that provide these resources, are essential functions of a case manager (Berg-Weger and Tebb, 1998; Mick and Ackerman, 2002). One reason it is important to have knowledge of community agencies and resources is to fill gaps in care left by family support systems and insurance. Resource identification and service planning may involve skills in linking clients to needed services. This can include such things as: transportation to medical appointments, assistive devices, home health care, meal delivery, skilled nursing services, personal emergency response systems, and restorative therapies (Schraeder, 2001). Wise allocation of resources, a goal of case management, requires a case manager to make sound clinical judgements about client needs and use of resources. To be successful in these functions, the case manager must possess a variety of skills including the ability to assess the client's present and future needs, plan creatively, solve problems, collaborate with multiple professionals, understand benefit structures, and coordinate services (Taylor, 1999).

Coordinating care and services across health care units and health care delivery networks, the third domain, is a key role of the case manager. Here the case manager must design tools that define case management responsibilities and interventions. A case manager often uses tools like critical pathways, case management plans, and protocols, to support clinical reasoning, goal, and outcome development and coordinate care across provider settings. Coordinating care by using case management tools entails tracking a client's progress, monitoring for early signs of problems, gathering and analyzing data, and communicating the results to health care organizations, providers, and consumers (Lagoe, 1998). Professional case managers who demonstrate skills in continual assessment, administration of case management tools, interpretation of data, and communication, are stewards of health care resources and dollars, and add to client satisfaction by reducing the frustration that comes from negotiating care at multiple service sites (Berg-Weger and Tebb, 1998; Kegel, 1996; Lagoe, 1998; Lamb and Stemple, 1994; Salazar, 2000).

Successful performance depends on excellent communication with other disciplines, especially physicians. Efforts to improve communication and collaboration between physicians and case managers were the focus of a summit convened in 2003 by the Case Management Society of America. Physicians and case managers from across the country attended. Barriers and solutions to effective communication were identified and used to establish a framework for successful collaboration between the two groups. This framework and other summit outcomes were reported in a consensus paper entitled, *Exploring Best Practices in Physician & Case Management Collaboration to Improve Patient Care*, which is available online at www.cmsa.org/Professional/Collaboration.

Coordinating a multidisciplinary plan that moves clients across the continuum of care, whether between hospital units or into other service settings, is the most important function of the nurse case manager (Novak, 1998). Lack of coordination within and among health care settings contributes to increased hospital readmission rates and costs of care (Burns, Lamb, and Wholey, 1996). To overcome ineffective coordination requires strong skills to negotiate with payers and providers to ensure smooth transitions and to sustain continuity of care for clients. By making communication and collaboration between physicians and case managers a priority, the CMSA summit has potentially made the coordination role of the case manager an easier function.

The fourth knowledge domain is *managing financial matters*. There are two aspects to this role: the first is to understand the payer systems, and the second is to develop and apply methods for evaluating quality service and cost-effective care. Understanding common payer systems such as health maintenance organizations (HMOs), preferred provider organizations (PPOs), point of service plans (POS), and Medicare and Medicaid, is essential. By being aware of the advantages and disadvantages of the numerous reimbursement methods within payer delivery systems, the case manager is able to bridge the gap between provider and payer, allowing them to effectively coordinate care and secure services for clients. Case managers working with specific populations learn the criteria for eligibility, benefits, and the specific process for accessing services from payer sources commonly used in these populations. Maneuvering through the provider and payer system requires the case manager to assess the client's existing health care coverage and determine if it is adequate, or determine if other sources of funding for services are available. Knowing how the process works helps when communicating with individuals in charge of referral authorization, and prevents unnecessary or excessive charges.

The second aspect of this knowledge domain is concerned with the case manager's responsibility to build his/her knowledge about the financial performance of the case management program(s) and to build support for case management services. To accomplish these functions, a case manager needs to design outcomes and use cost analysis methods to evaluate the cost effectiveness of case management services. A case manager must understand financial and budgeting methods and be able to apply outcome measures that result in a valid, reliable, and thorough assessment (Kleinpell-Nowell, 1999). In her article titled, *Measuring Advanced Practice Nursing Outcomes*, Kleinpell-Nowell compiles a helpful list of commonly used outcome measures and sources of research-based outcome instruments appropriate for evaluating case management effectiveness.

In a cost-analysis evaluation, consider factors such as external performance referents, including benchmarking, or comparing the assessment results with those of another organization(s), to add validity to evaluation findings (Ketchen, 2001). In the view of Ketchen, it is only when compared with a point of reference that cost-benefit analysis findings have meaning. This method may also reveal additional insights about the strategy used, or additional strategies to use, to facilitate cost containment. Using performance referents external to the organization can affect the future viability of a particular health care delivery strategy such as case management. For example, integrated hospital delivery systems that case manage high-risk populations of patients with chronic conditions could compare their cost-benefit analysis performance with licensed external Disease Management Organizations specializing in case managing similar populations of patients.

It is challenging to have the knowledge and skills necessary to practice in a cost-effective manner, and to have expertise in choosing appropriate outcome performance measures and tools that assess the financial performance of case management. When successfully managed, the role of case manager can be sustained, and case management will remain a vehicle for the delivery of quality cost-effective care in a managed care financing system.

The focus of the final knowledge domain of case management is *building meaningful nurse–client relationships*. Although nurse theorists' works have long touted the importance of building meaningful client-nurse relationships, there has been a current research refocus which examines client relationships in the nursing case management process. The result has been that nurse case managers have become more concerned, or need to be more concerned, with the importance and benefits of forming relationships with clients.

For example, McWilliam and colleagues (1996) explored the experiences of individuals living with chronic illness. The researchers discovered that clients wished to be involved in *mutual knowing* (mutal relationships) between client and nurse, and felt that *being known* enhanced their personal knowledge, and in turn their ability to follow through with self care. The authors concluded that more attention needed to be placed on continuity of the *caregiver* rather than on the continuity of the *care plan*.

Lamb and Stemple (1994) discovered that clients who felt they were in partnerships felt empowered to assume an active role in their health care, thus resulting in renewed efforts to become involved in health maintenance and promotion strategies. These authors grounded their research in Newman's theory of Expanding Consciousness, which describes a nurse as one who "enters into a partnership with the client with the mutual goal of participating in an authentic relationship, trusting that in the process of its evolving, both will grow and become healthier in the sense of higher levels of consciousness" (Newman, p. 68).

Practicing case management from this perspective enables clients to become partners with case managers and meets one of the goals of case management—to optimize the client's self-care ability (Taylor, 1999). Creating an atmosphere that builds respectful relationships requires a case manager to develop and use the skills of active listening and presencing; these skills enable clients to become their own "insider-experts in self-care" (Lamb and Stemple, p. 12).

On the whole, the five knowledge domains of the case manager role outlined above describe the new knowledge and skills needed to perform the role of case manager, contrasted with the basic practice of nurses. As nursing case management has evolved, there have been increased opportunities for nurses to move from basic nursing practice into this expanded role, which provides more autonomy, and possibly more job enrichment (Goode, 1995; Reimanis, et al., 2001).

Case Management Certification

The Case Management certification process ensures a common baseline of knowledge, and gives the professional and public assurance of a certain degree of competence and higher quality of case management services. There are numerous licensure, certification, and certificate programs available for case managers working in various fields of health care. Listing each is beyond the scope of this article; rather three key certifications will be described.

The Commission for Case Manager Certification (CCMC) is an independent credentialing agency that sponsors and oversees one of the major case management certifications. The CCMC, nationally accredited by the National Commission for Certifying Agencies, is the only national accreditation body for private certification organizations in all disciplines. Since the CCMC began certifying case managers in 1993, more than 20,000 case managers have earned the Certified Case Manager (CCM) credential. This credential is designed as an adjunct to other professional credentials in health and human resources.

To earn the designation of certified Case Manager (CCM), applicants must:

- Possess a good moral character.
- Meet acceptable standards of practice.
- Accomplish specific educational requirements, including a post-secondary degree program in a field that promotes the psychosocial or vocational well being of consumers.
- Provide a job description for each case management position held.
- Meet the Continuum of Care requirement.
- Hold a license that is based upon the applicant having taken an examination in the area of educational specialization.
- Insure that the license grants the ability to practice without the supervision of another licensed professional.
- Perform the six essential activities of case management:
  - assessment,
  - coordination,
  - planning,
  - monitoring,
  - implementation, and
  - evaluation in multiple environments over a minimum of five of the six core components:
    - process and relationships;
    - health care mangement;
    - community resources and support;
    - service delivery;
    - psychosocial intervention;
    - rehabilitation case management.
- Satisfy the necessary employment experience.
- Demonstrate that they possess acceptable minimum knowledge by achieving a passing score on the CCM examination. (www.ccmcertification.org/pages/121body.html)

The CCM examination is research based and covers competencies and job functions in six major domains of knowledge as listed in the above quote. It administered semi-annually in June and December; testing sites are usually located within each state.

The American Nurses Credentialing Center (ANCC) offers a second method of certification (www.nursingworld.org/ancc). The ANCC is the credentialing arm of the American Nurses Association. In 1997, the center began certifying nursing case managers and providing them with the (RN, cm) credential. Candidates for the exam must have an RN license and a baccalaureate or higher degree. A core specialty is also desired, however, individuals without a core specialty are eligible, but need 4,000 hours of registered nurse experience as opposed to the 2,000 hours of case management experience needed by those individuals who already hold a core nursing specialty certification. The framework for Nursing Case Management used by ANCC consists of the following five components: assessment, planning, implementation, evaluation, and interaction.

Both the CCM and ANCC require ongoing continuing education for recertification, which is required every five years. Each of the credentialing agencies provides written resource materials for case managers. The CCMC study guide is available through the Case Management Society of America (CMSA). They can be contacted at www.ccmcertification.org. The AANC recently published a book titled *The Case Management Review and Resource Manual: The Essence of Case Management* (Llewellyn, 2001) which the author describes as a book for individuals who are entering into case management practice, or for experienced case managers who may have practiced in only one setting. Each chapter in the book includes review questions and answers, as well as rationale, to assist with preparation for the national examination.

Certification for case management administrators (CMAC) is sponsored by the Center for Case Management (CCM) and can be obtained from the Credentialing Advisory Board (CAB). Eligibility for the certification exam occurs by meeting one of three broad categories: a baccalaureate or higher degree with experience as a case manager; a certification in a core specialty; and/or a faculty in an academic setting teaching graduate level courses or content in case management. The exam covers content about high-risk populations, assessment, strategy development, leadership, strategic planning, human resource management, and outcome management. For more information about this certification contact the Center for Case Management at www.cfcm.com/certification.html.

Trends and Issues in Case Management

The dynamic nature of health care has set the stage for the many new trends and issues now emerging in case management. After a decade of movement into fully integrated delivery systems, health care organizations have created interdependent interactive structures designed to coordinate care across the continuum, with the goal of containing cost and maintaining or increasing quality. By default, if not by design, case management has emerged as the primary strategy to coordinate services, to provide care, and to communicate across these multi-organizational systems. This trend provides an unprecedented opportunity for nurses to showcase their leadership and their accomplishments in using nursing case management as a model to both promote quality and achieve cost reductions in health care.

The recent implementation of an evaluative study of coordinated care programs, sponsored by the Centers for Medicare and Medicaid Services (CMS), was implemented by the Mathematica Policy Research organization. This study has the potential to generate measurable data that confirms nursing case management's successful impact on cost and quality. Fifteen integrated health care delivery systems from across the country were selected in January 2004 to participate. Two-thirds of these systems use case managers to coordinate care. They design and initiate interventions with physicians, and a mix of other health care professionals, for chronically ill Medicare-recipient clients.

The participating institutions have designed some very innovative programs that require new, advanced skills for practice. For instance, many of the programs are using telemedicine, in-home monitoring devices, and the Internet for counseling and interactive communication with clients. The electronic links allow important client data to be sent to the case manager for evaluation and action, or shared with the primary physician for redesign of medical care. Further, tracking client data may help to transition clients more efficiently across organizations' multiple service settings. The organizations and case managers participating in this study hope that coordinating services across the continuum and using new technologies will produce outcomes that reflect a decrease in fragmented care; an increase in client knowledge and self care; improved client satisfaction; and, of course, reduce Medicare expenditures for chronically ill individuals. The CMS demonstration projects are funded for four years and will be evaluated every two years.

A recent trend within government programs has included using the case management strategy in the management of Medicaid beneficiaries. It is a central feature of Florida's, North Carolina's, and Oklahoma's approach to health care delivery for this population (Silberman, et al., 2003). These programs are raising professional and public awareness of case management and creating increased employment opportunities for nurses who desire to function in this specialty role.

The programs, however, also cause concern for many members of the profession (Daiski, 2000), because they often adopt disease management models as guides for nursing case management practice. These models focus on medical diagnosis, illness and treatment; whereas nursing models focus on health—wellness and prevention, and illness, within the context of the patients' experience and cultural background.

After reviewing the literature on nursing case management models, my impression is that a substantial number of case management models guided by nursing theories exist that are useful for practice in all health care settings. As more government programs adopt case management as their strategy for health care, and there is every indication that they will, it is imperative that nurse case managers advocate the use of case management models that move beyond functions of medical necessity to models with nursing functions that reflect the values of health embedded within the discipline of nursing's theories. Only in this way can we hope to shape health care policy. Thus we advocate that case management models emphasize the values of nursing, and are guided by nursing theories.

The inclusion of monitoring devices, electronic links, and the Internet as sources of information reflects a trend throughout health care systems, both public and private. From a case management perspective, Internet connectivity has the power to link case managers to client's insurance plans, pharmacies, and physician offices as well as to track previous medical and nursing information about clients from the multiple service sites within the integrated system (Robinson, 2001).

The advent of Internet technology has also propelled consumers toward a greater use of technology (Adams, 2000). Recently, the consulting firm of Cyber Dialogue reported survey results that estimate that 40 million United States adults use the Internet to access health information and that by 2005, this number will increase to 88 million (Oermann, Lesley, and Kuefler, 2002). These figures suggest the consumer is seeking information beyond that provided by his or her health care givers.

Nursing case managers could develop and share a diary of reliable Internet sites with their client populations to answer questions about their health care situations, or to connect them to others who are experiencing similar illness situations. Adams (2000) believes that case managers could deliver care as an integrated package of personal services, combined with education and knowledge tailored to the patient, via the Internet. Discussions of the many revolutionary new ways e-health, and other technologies, can be used to improve health care delivery in general, and case management in particular, can be found in a number of recent publications.[2]

The phenomenal growth of Internet technology has fostered a new culture of health care, one which empowers health care providers and consumers to track clinical decisions, and access and compare information (Meadows, 2001). It will eventually move all health care professionals to embrace these tools in order to gain greater access to information, obtain better clinical outcomes (Carver, 2001), and meet the expectations of their clients.

These trends—fully integrated health systems delivering coordinated care, using multiple information technologies as mechanisms to both facilitate and measure the effectiveness of this care—produce serious issues. First, with the wide spread use of Internet technology in health care organizations, protecting data confidentiality has become a major issue. This public consumer concern prompted legislators to enact the Health Insurance Portability and Accountability Act (HIPAA) of 1996, an effort designed to achieve better electronic security of personal health information (Waldo, 2000).

The HIPAA legislation includes standards and regulations for information transmitted or exchanged electronically, and impacts any organization, provider, or payer that handles individually identifiable health information. Under these HIPAA rules the case manager may need to obtain written authorization from the individual before requesting or transmitting information from providers or payers, and most definitely needs to identify which transactions do or do not meet the HIPAA guidelines. Whether this will create barriers to the continuum model of case management, such as delaying the coordination of care and resource access, and delaying or preventing electronic information exchange, is still unclear.

Second, the trend toward providing coordinated care across the continuum and over the life span of clients is congruent with the client's expectations and satisfaction with health care (Lamb and Stemple, 1994; Dunn, Sohl-Kreiger, and Marx, 2001). How the case manager, and the organization, transitions the client from one site to another has the potential to become an issue for both providers and clients.

The literature suggests that clients prefer one provider across all settings and that this approach is the best method for clinical integration and coordination of all aspects of care (Lamb and Stemple, 1994; McWilliams and colleagues, 1996). At this time, however, case managers and organizations rarely follow this approach; rather, it is more common to link

---

[2] Some excellent resources include: Adams, J. (2000), Applying e-health to case management. *Lippincott's Case Management*, 5(4) 168–171 and Meadows, G. (2001), The internet promise: A new look at e-health opportunities. *Nursing Economic$*, 19(6), 294–295.

acute care case managers with community-based case managers. Within this type of system, case managers need to be adept at sharing information about the clients' past and current illness situations to ensure both continuity and satisfaction with care as clients transition from the illness episode to the continuum of care. The shared information needs to include clients' preferences, and successful strategies for promoting a relationship that fosters client goal attainment and produces client satisfaction outcomes.

Third, the preparation of nurses to practice case management using both continuum delivery models and effective technology has become an issue. It is generally agreed among nurse researchers and educators that there is a need for formal educational preparation of the nurse case manager, including appropriate computer skills for the role. Presently, there are inadequacies in the academic approach (Cicatiello, 2000; Halstead, 2000; Sowell and Young, 1997). Agreement ends and disagreement begins, however, when these nurse scholars discuss curricula content and debate which educational level, undergraduate or graduate, is required to prepare case managers for entry into practice.

The reality is that all nurses need content and clinical practice experiences in case management, and need to acquire skills in accessing information and managing databases via the Internet (Halstead, 2000). Often, both staff nurses and advanced practice nurses are expected to become members of interdisciplinary case management teams, and to make client care decisions based on case management concepts and electronic client data.

Sowell and Young (1997) believe that to meet the changing job expectations the baccalaureate graduate should have the expertise to be an effective case management team member, with knowledge of both databased clinical paths, and of the quality/financial issues that influence care coordination. The advanced practice nurse graduate, on the other hand, must obtain the expertise needed to perform the case manager role for a caseload of clients within a specialized target population. This view of case management education reflects the current trend in Schools of Nursing (Haw, 1996).

According to Haw's national survey of case management education in universities, ninety-five percent of nursing schools are beginning to prepare the undergraduate in basic case management concepts and processes including community resource referral, health team collaboration, client progress monitoring, and technology health services (Halstead, 2000). Haw's survey also indicates that the emphasis in graduate case management education is on role performance behaviors, and therefore the graduate curriculum incorporates many more clinical practicum experiences than offered in undergraduate education. Findings and conclusions by Haw suggest that nurse educators view the case manager role as an advanced practice role even though employers usually list the undergraduate degree as a requirement for hire. In the end, whether case management education is included at the undergraduate level or graduate level, there is an overall trend towards more formal case management preparation in nursing academia (Haw, 1996).

Finally, the emerging era of coordinating care across continuums creates issues for both integrated health system providers and case managers alike. It has been established that case managers need skills in accessing and managing patient care data across many different settings. Accurate tracking of patient visits, patient outcomes, and costs are necessary to plan for the delivery of services and the allocation of resources across the continuum. As case managers acquire these skills, there is mounting pressure for integrated health care delivery systems to provide this data. However, information systems that accurately track this data are costly (Noone and McKillip, 1996), and purchasing these new technologies requires sufficient profit margins. Unfortunately, integrated health care systems that are coordinating much of their services in community rather than acute care settings are discovering that capitated reimbursement practices by commercial and federal payers are plummeting their profit margins (Lamb and Zazworsky, 2000). Unless financial incentives are aligned with service coordination initiatives, the trend towards coordinating care across the continuum by case managers can not be sustained.

However, the ongoing research initiatives by the federal government are encouraging. The studies suggest that coordinating care across the continuum for Medicare patients does successfully reduce health care costs; thus future capitated reimbursement structures may increasingly cover these services, and be sufficient to support the cost of developing and maintaining data systems.

Anticipating the Future of Case Management

The rapid and ongoing transformation of health care systems has made anticipating the future of case management as unpredictable as the ever-changing patterns of a kaleidoscope where the crystals rearrange to form new and exciting patterns. However, this change also creates an environment where nursing case management can flourish. As health care systems pursue their goals of promoting client satisfaction, fostering client loyalty, and becoming indispensable to the community, case management is becoming the dominant strategy selected by these systems to meet their goals. In the future, it is easy to imagine that integrated health care delivery systems will link case managers to one another across their multiple service sites, and make arrangements for the same person to manage the client's care, creating client trust and confidence in both the health care system and in the case management approach.

Further twisting of the kaleidoscope creates a future in which all clients will be health managed, and the role of the health manager will expand to include an emphasis on prevention and reducing recidivism. The overall trend of managed care toward expanded benefits, which include complementary alternative medicine, prevention, and long-term care support this vision.

Consumers today are beginning to demand that health care manage their health as well as their disease, and satisfy their individual preferences over the life cycle. These expanded benefits for consumers will support and subsidize the future development of wellness models of case management.

Health managers will be expected to provide care in a variety of settings, and provide various levels of care; the goal will be to manage health risks in the community rather than in acute care settings. In the near future, case managers will be challenged to provide ways to offset the depersonalization and threat to client-nurse relationships caused by the greater use of technology for assessment and lack of communication with clients.

In the end, the shape that case management takes will depend on the diligence of both integrated delivery systems and case managers to search for new possibilities, reflect, question, and create images of care that capture the client's perspective. This reflection and partnership between the system and case manager will create new kaleidoscope colors and patterns, creating health management models that illuminate a bright future for both the care providers and the client.

References

Adams, J. (2000). Applying e-health to case management. *Lippincott's Case Management, 5*(4), 168–171.

American Nurses Credentialing Center (ANCC). (1998). *Nursing case management catalogue.* Washington, DC: ANCC.

Berg-Weger, M., & Tebb, S. (1998). Caregiver well-being: A strengths-based case management approach. *Journal of Case Management, 7*(2), 67–73.

Bower, S. (2000). *Case management: A practical guide to success in managed care.* 2nd ed. New York: Lippincott.

Brandt, M. (2002 February). "Need to know" access: Meeting HIPAA's minimum necessary requirements. *In Confidence, American Health Information Management Association,* 1–2.

Burns, L., Lamb, G., & Wholey, D. (1996). Impact of integrated community nursing services on hospital utilization and costs in a Medicare risk plan. *Inquiry, 33,* 30–41.

Case Management Society of America (CMSA). (1995). *Standards of practice for case management.* Little Rock, Arkansas: CMSA.

Carver, T. (2001). Continuum-based care coordination via the web. *Care Management, 17*(2), 14–20.

Centers for Medicare and Medicaid Services (CMS) Medicare Coordinated Care Demonstration. Retrieved February 19, 2004, from www.cms.hhs.gov/researchers/demos/coorcare.asp.

Cicatiello, J. (2000). A perspective of health care in the past—Insights and challenges for a health care system in the new millennium. *Nursing Administration Quarterly, 25*(1), 18–29.

Cohen, E., & Cesta, T. (2005). Nursing case management. 4th ed. St. Louis: Elsevier Mosby.

Daiski, I. (2000). The road to professionalism in nursing: Case management or practice based in nursing theory? *Nursing Science Quarterly, 13*(1), 74–79.

Doerge, J., & Hagenow, N. (1995). Management restructuring. *Nursing Management, 26*(12), 32–37.

Dunham-Taylor, J., & Pinczuk, J. (2006). *Health care financial management for nurse managers: Applications from hospitals, long-term care, home care, and ambulatory care.* Sudbury, MA: Jones and Bartlett.

Dunn, S., Sohl-Kreiger, R., & Marx, S. (2001). Geriatric case management in an integrated care system. *Journal of Nursing Administration, 31*(2), 60–62.

Ethridge, P. (1987). Nurse accountability program improves satisfaction, turnover. *Health Progress, 68,* 44–49.

Ethridge, P., & Lamb, G. (1989). Professional nursing case management improves quality, access and costs. *Nursing Management, 20*(3), 30–35.

Ethridge, P. (1997). The Carondelet experience. *Nursing Management, 28*(3), 26–28.

Flary, D., & Blancett, S. (Eds.). *Handbook of nursing case management.* Gaithersburg, MD: Aspen.

Flarey, D. (1996). Case management: Delivering care in the age of managed care. In D. L. Flarey & S. S. Blancett (Eds.), *Handbook of nursing case management.* Gaithersburg, Maryland: Aspen.

Forbes, M. (1999). The practice of professional nurse case management. *Nursing Case Management, 4*(1), 28–33.

Goode, C. (1995). Impact of a careMap and case management on patient satisfaction and staff satisfaction, collaboration, and autonomy. *Nursing Economic$, 13*(6), 337–348.

Halstead, J. (2000). Implementing web-based instruction in a school of nursing: Implications for faculty and students. *Journal of Professional Nursing, 16*(5), 273–281.

Haw, M. (1996). Case management education in universities: A national survey. *The Journal of Care Management, 2*(6), 10–23.

Kegel, L. (1996). Case management, critical pathways, and myocardial infarction. *Critical Care Nurse, 16*(2), 97–114.

Ketchen, D., Palmer, T., & Gamm, L. (2001). The role of performance referents in health services organizations. *Heath Care Management Review, 26*(4), 19–26.

Kleinpell-Nowell, R. (1999). Measuring advanced practice nursing outcomes. *AACN Clinical Issues, 10*(3), 356–368.

Lagoe, R. (1998). Basic statistics for clinical pathway evaluation. *Nursing Economic$, 16*(3), 125–131.

Lamb, G., & Stemple, J. (1994). Nurse case management from the client's view: Growing as insider-expert. *Nursing Outlook, 42*(1), 7–14.

Lamb, G., & Zazworsky, D. (2000). The Carondelet case management program. In E. Cohen & T. Cesta (Eds.), *Nursing case management*. 3rd ed. St. Louis: Mosby.

Llewellyn, A. (2001). *The case management review and resource manual: The essence of case management*. Washington, DC: ANA.

McWilliam, C., Stewart, M., Brown, J., Desai, K., & Coderre, P. (1996). Creating health with chronic illness. *Advances in Nursing Science, 18*(3), 1–15.

Meadows, G. (2001). The internet promise: A new look at e-health opportunities. *Nursing Economic$, 19*(6), 294–295.

Mick, D., & Ackerman, M. (2002). New perspectives on advanced practice nursing case management for aging patients. *Critical Care Nursing Clinics of North America, 14*, 281–291.

Newman, M. (1986). *Health as expanding consciousness*. St. Louis: Mosby.

Newman, M., Lamb, G., & Michaels, C. (1991). Nurse case management: The coming together of theory and practice. *Nursing & Health Care, 12*(8), 404–408.

Noone, C., & McKillip, C. (1996). Data management through information systems. In D. L. Flarey & S. S. Blancett (Eds.), *Handbook of nursing case management*. Gaithersburg, MD: Aspen.

Novak, D. (1998). Nurse case managers' opinions of their role. *Nursing Case Management, 3*(6), 231–237.

Oermann, M., Lesley, M., & Kuefler, S. (2002). Using the Internet to teach consumers about quality care. *Journal of Quality Improvement, 28*(2), 83–89.

Reimanis, C., Cohen, E., & Redman, R. (2001). Nurse case manager role attributes: Fifteen years of evidence-based literature. *Lippincott's Case Management, 6*(6), 230–242.

Renholm, M., Leino-Kilpi, H., & Suominen, T. (2002). Critical pathways. *Journal of Nursing Administration, 32*(4), 196–201.

Robinson, J. (2001). The end of managed care. *The Journal of the American Medical Association, 285*(20), 2622–2632.

Salazar, M. (2000). Maximizing the effectiveness of case management service delivery. *The Case Manager, 11*(3), 58–63.

Schraeder, C. (2001). Discharge planning. *Hospital Case Management, 9*(10), 155–156.

Sowell, R., & Young, S. (1997). Case management in the nursing curriculum. *Nursing Case Management, 2*(4), 173–176.

Taylor, P. (1999). Comprehensive nursing case management: An advanced practice model. *Nursing Case Management, 4*(1), 2–10.

Waldo, B. (2000). HIPPA: The next frontier. *Information Systems and Technology, 18*(1), 49–50.

Zander, K. (1988). Nursing group practice: The Cadillac in continuity. *Definition, 3*(2), 1–2.

Zander, K. (1988a). Managed care within acute care settings: Design and implementation via nursing case management. *Health Care Supervisor, 6*(2), 24–43.

Zander, K. (1988b). Nursing care management: Strategic management of cost and quality outcomes. *Journal of Nursing Administration, 18*(5), 23–30.

Zander, K. (1996). The early years: The evolution of nursing case management. In D. L. Flarey & S. S. Blancett (Eds.), *Handbook of nursing case management.* Gaithersburg, MD: Aspen.

Zander, K. (2002). Nursing case management in the 21st century: Intervening where margin meets mission. *Nursing Administration Quarterly, 24*(5), 58–68.

PART SIX

Finance/Accounting Issues

Although a nurse manager may never need to learn accounting and finance basics, we have included some beginning information about them in this book. We hope this helps the nurse administrator to have a greater appreciation for the finance side of the organization. We thought it would be helpful for a nurse manager to be able to read a financial statement for a health care organization, explained in Chapter 17 on Accounting, as well as to learn more about certain financial ratios commonly used in health care organizations, found in Chapter 18 on Assessing Financial Performance. If you would like more detailed background in these topics, we would suggest that you take additional accounting or financial courses.

Accounting for Health Care Entities

Paul Bayes, D.B.A. Accounting, M.S. Economics,
B.S. Accounting

Introduction

Accounting has been called the language of business because accounting information provides direction for action. Health care organizations can be classified as either for-profit or not-for-profit but much of the information is the same and requires similar decision making. Each organization has assets and liabilities. The difference occurs in the area defined as either stockholders' equity (for-profit) or unrestricted, temporarily restricted, and permanently restricted funds (not-for-profit).

The financial synopsis of management's actions is contained in the financial statements (see appendices to chapter for examples of a profit-oriented and not-for-profit entity). Excerpts from these statements will be used as examples throughout this chapter. Years ago, it was uncommon for health care entities to have financial problems. However, changing economic conditions and revenue limiting measures by third party providers (insurance companies/government) require a more proactive look at the financial condition of a business. The failure to do so may result in what has happened to many "dot-com," as well as established, companies in recent years.

Financial statements are required every year and publicly-traded health care entities must also issue quarterly financial statements. These financial statements consist of the statement of financial

> *Health care organizations can be classified as either for-profit or not-for-profit.*

Definition

Quarterly financial statements—the statement of financial position (balance sheet), the income statement (also called statement of activities-income and expenses or statement of earnings), and statement of cash flows.

position (balance sheet), the income statement (also called statement of activities—income and expenses or statement of earnings), and statement of cash flows. In recent years more attention has focused on the statement of cash flows because cash is the lifeblood of a business. To be an informed decision maker you must understand how to use financial statements, but you do not necessarily have to know how to prepare these financial statements. Thus the focus of this chapter is on the understanding and use of financial information.

Accounting Framework

$$Assets = Liabilities + Equity$$
$$A=L+E$$

One of the basic frameworks of for-profit accounting is the *accounting equation*: Assets = Liabilities + Equity. *Assets* are those items that provide future cash flow or have future economic benefit. If you were to prepare a personal financial statement for a bank loan you would list those items that have value (*assets*) and can be sold in case of default on the loan. For business organizations, assets are used to generate revenue for the firm. *Liabilities* are claims on the assets of an organization. The claims are those of creditors who have provided resources such as buildings and equipment but have not been fully paid. Using the example of a personal loan, liabilities include credit card, car or home mortgage balances. The difference between the assets and liabilities of an organization is the *equity*, or in the personal loan application example, *net worth*. Examples of these items follow. All amounts are in millions except for earnings per share.

In not-for-profit organizations the result of subtracting liabilities from assets is called *net assets* or *fund balances*. Not-for-profit entities return the excess amount to the sponsoring organization if they cease to continue stated purposes. The accounting framework for a not-for-profit organization would be Assets = Liabilities + Net Assets or Fund Balances. Examples of these differences are illustrated as follows.

Statement of Financial Position (Balance Sheet)

Assets

The balance sheet—consisting of the assets, liabilities and equity—is a "snapshot" of the health care entity and is dated for a one-day period of time. The assets, liabilities, and equity or fund balances reflect only the amounts as of a certain date. Traditional examples use December 31 as the ending day but firms have other ending time periods. The asset portion of Hospital Anywhere USA, which is dated as of December 31, appears in **Exhibit 17–1**. Complete financial statements are found in the Appendices.

Exhibit 17–1 Asset Section of Balance Sheet

(Dollars in millions)

Assets	2004	2003
Current Assets:		
Cash and cash equivalents	$314	$190
Accounts receivable, less allowance for doubtful accounts of $1,583 and $1,567	2,211	1,873
Inventories	396	383
Income taxes receivable	197	178
Other	1,335	973
Total Current Assets	**4,453**	**3,597**
Property and equipment at cost:		
Land	793	813
Buildings	6,021	6,108
Equipment	7,045	6,721
Construction in progress	431	442
Total Property and Equipment	**14,290**	**14,084**
Accumulated depreciation	(5,810)	(5,594)
	8,480	8,490
Investments of insurance subsidiary	1,371	1,457
Investments in and advances to affiliates	779	654
Intangible assets, net of accumulated amortization of $785 and $644	2,155	2,319
Other	330	368
Total Assets	**$17,568**	**$16,885**

Assets may be classified as current versus long-term, or more specifically *current assets*, *property and equipment (tangible)*, *investments*, and *intangible assets* such as patents. *Current assets* are those items that will be used to generate revenue in either one year or the operating period, whichever is longer (most often this is one year).

Generally the first item listed on the statement of financial position is cash, although many times it is combined with temporary investments which are considered *cash equivalents*. Temporary investments are *cash equivalents* because they can be sold quickly with little or no loss in value. In the Hospital Anywhere USA example, the cash equivalents have a maturity of three months or less. This is the reserve needed to meet the operational needs of the organization such as salaries, and to meet other obligations as they arise.

An important source of future cash is generically identified as *accounts (patients) receivable*. These may be represented by amounts owed by either patients to which the organization has provided services or by claims filed with third party providers such as insurance companies. These will provide future cash flows and therefore it is imperative that these insurance claims be filed quickly and accurately. Reducing the collection period provides cash more quickly for operations. This amount is often reported as a "net" number reflecting amounts that will not be collected or reductions from third party providers.

Other current assets of the organization consist of *inventory* items such as drugs in the pharmacy, surgical supplies, items maintained at nursing stations, and drinks and/or food in the cafeteria. The alternative inventory cost measures will not be discussed in this text. The income taxes receivable account is the equivalent of receiving a tax refund but waiting for the check.

PROPERTY AND EQUIPMENT

The largest item on a for-profit health care entity's balance sheet is probably buildings and equipment. This may also be defined as *tangible assets*. *Land* on which a health care facility is located is one item included in this section. Land is not written off, unless there is something that impairs value such as pollution of the land site. Other tangible assets, such as buildings and equipment, have skyrocketing costs because of the complexity of equipment and more rigorous building codes and regulations. *Buildings* are the physical facilities in which patient services are provided. *Equipment* may be items such as X-ray, Cat Scan machines, or less complex items such as patient beds. The increased costs require either the availability of large amounts of funds for purchases (cash) or credit granting sources. *Construction in progress* is an account indicating buildings that have not been completed but are being built. The account indicates progress toward completion. *Depreciation* is an accounting charge wherein the balance of the equipment and buildings is systematically written off over a period of time. *Accumulated depreciation*, which is the sum of the annual depreciation charges, is then subtracted from the plant and equipment balance providing a net figure. This number does not relate to current market value but rather is book value only, which is the original cost minus accumulated depreciation.

INVESTMENTS

Investments are classified as long-term in nature in that they are held for income purposes. These may be a result of using excess cash to either invest in items such as other organizations, joint ventures, purchase stocks, or bonds of other organizations, or donations received from external parties. As in the case of Hospital Anywhere USA, they are investments in other organizations (affiliates of Hospital Anywhere USA) or loans made to affiliate organizations.

INTANGIBLE ASSETS

Intangible assets generally are those items that have no physical presence but do have value in the form of legal rights to use or sell an asset. One example would be patents that have been developed by employees of the organization. Use of a patent may provide a strategic advantage over competing facilities or may reduce your firm's costs below that of competitors. One item that is harder to define as an intangible asset is *goodwill*. Goodwill occurs when an entity purchases another organization and there is an excess amount paid for the net assets of the purchased entity that exceeds market value. This excess amount is goodwill.

Most intangible assets are also systematically written off over a period of time like that of depreciation but the process is called *amortization*. Goodwill must be evaluated each year and a determination must be made for impairment of value. If value declines, goodwill must be reduced ("written down") by this amount.

Liabilities

To begin our discussion of liabilities, please refer to **Exhibit 17–2**.

CURRENT LIABILITIES

Accounts payables are claims on assets. These are short term in nature and are generally expected to be paid in 30–120 days based on the type of claim, but can be unpaid up to one year. The purchase of operating supplies such as surgical staples and food items are examples.

Accrued liabilities (i.e., salaries) are those that have been incurred in the course of business but have not yet been paid. For example, if employees are paid on the fifth of the month for effort in the previous month then it is an accrued expense. Employers owe employees for services provided but have not yet made payment. Accounting recognizes expenses when incurred, not necessarily when paid. Other accrued expenses could include interest incurred on debt but not paid, or taxes owed to government entities.

In the Hospital Anywhere USA example, the hospital entered into a plea agreement with various agencies to settle claims such as errors in DRG codes for calendar years 1995-1999, outpatient laboratory billings, and others. This is the government settlement accrual, which the hospital corporation owes but has not yet paid.

Exhibit 17–2 Liabilities Section of Balance Sheet

(Dollars in millions, except for per share amount)

Liabilities	2004	2003
Current Liabilities:		
Accounts payable	693	657
Accrued Salaries	352	403
Other accrued expenses	1,135	897
Government settlement accrual	840	
Long-term debt due within one year	1,121	1,160
Total Current Liabilities	**4,141**	**3,117**
Long-term debt	5,631	5,284
Professional liability risks, deferred taxes and other liabilities	2,050	2,104
Minority interests in equity of consolidated entities	572	763
Forward purchase contracts and put options	769	
Total Liabilities	**13,163**	**11,268**

Most organizations finance equipment or a building which requires a large outlay of resources over a long period of time, with some financing arrangements are up to forty years. Each year as that portion of the debt becomes due in the current year, it is considered a current liability.

LONG-TERM LIABILITIES (DEBT)

Long-term debt examples include such items as mortgages and bonds issued to borrow money. This debt will not be paid in the current year or operating period.

Other items identified as long-term debt could include professional liability risks such as unsettled lawsuits resulting from malpractice claims and employee work-related injuries. *Deferred taxes* are the differences between income reported in financial statements and that paid to the U.S. Treasury.

Minority interests in equity of consolidated subsidiaries reflect amounts, less than 50 percent, owned by others in certain organizations where Hospital Anywhere USA has majority control. *Forward purchase contracts* and *put options* are obligations that Hospital Anywhere USA has initiated to repurchase shares of its common stock to provide employees with stock purchase plans. A *forward purchase contract* is where one party agrees to buy a commodity at a specific price on a specific date and the other party agrees to make the sale. A *put option* provides the right to sell a stock at a specified price in the future. Hospital Anywhere USA entered into a contract with a third party to purchase the stock at the contract price. This creates a liability for Hospital Anywhere USA.

Stockholder's Equity

For-profit corporate firms raise funds by issuing either *preferred* or *common stock*. **Exhibit 17–3** provides an example. These stocks represent ownership shares in an organization. Both stocks generally have a par value and sell for more than this base amount (*capital in excess of par value*). The *par value* is arbitrarily established as a low amount and is used for accounting records. For example, one of Macy's stock had a par value of 0.25 (Hospital Anywhere USA is 0.01). The reason for this par value is based on legal rights or tax issues, which is beyond the scope of this chapter. The market price may be considerably more than the par value.

Preferred stock is not used as extensively as common stock but is one possible source of funds. The stock gets its name from the preference over common stock in either payments of dividends or distribution of liquidation proceeds in case of the firm ceasing business. As of 2004, Hospital Anywhere USA does not use preferred stock to raise funds for the organization. *Common stock* is the most widely used stock. Shares are described as the number authorized, issued, and outstanding. This terminology provides information concerning the legal maximum number of shares that can be sold (*authorized*), the number that have been sold (*issued*), and those that are held outside the organization (*outstanding*). For Hospital Anywhere USA the number of shares issued and outstanding are the same.

Three additional financial items are found in the stockholders' equity section of Hospital Anywhere USA. The first two are classified as "other" and "accumulated comprehensive" income, which is more substantial. *Comprehensive income* is that source of

Exhibit 17–3 Stockholder's Equity Section of Balance Sheet

(dollars in millions)

Stockholder's equity:		
Common stock $.01 par; authorized 1,600,000,000 voting shares 50,000,000 nonvoting shares; outstanding 521,991,700 voting shares and 21,000,000 shares and 21,000,000 nonvoting voting shares–2004 and 543,272,900 voting shares and 21,000,000 nonvoting shares–2003	5	6
Capital in excess of par value		951
Other	9	8
Accumulated other comprehensive income	52	53
Retained earnings	4,339	4,599
Total Stockholder's Equity	4,405	5,617
Total Liabilities and Stockholders Equity	**$17,568**	**$16,885**

income resulting from other than the typical operations of the health care entity. This data item includes unrealized (not sold) gains on available-for-sale securities (one form of investments) and gains reclassified into earnings from other comprehensive income. Also Hospital Anywhere USA had a currency translation adjustment which results from transactions in another currency. If the exchange rate changes between the time that a transaction occurs and settlement takes place, then a gain or loss occurs on the transaction.

The final item found on the statement of financial position is *retained earnings*. The name is misleading because there is no actual money in this account. Retained earnings is an account used by the accounting function to balance the books at the end of the year. The amount carried to retained earnings is the difference between all revenue sources, and expenses and costs, and dividends paid. The reason for the lack of funds can be determined conceptually. What happens to the revenue collected for providing patient services? After collection it is used to pay suppliers for services provided or employees' salaries and wages including benefits such as employer contributions to the FICA (Social Security).

The equivalent section of the stockholders' equity of a not-for-profit is called *fund balances*. These balances are either unrestricted, which can be used at the discretion of management, or temporarily and permanently restricted fund balances that are used for specific purposes. The illustration in **Exhibit 17–4** is that of the Children's Hospital.

The restricted fund balances may be for building projects or other equipment needs. When the project is completed remaining funds return to general use. Other restricted funds may be more long term in nature and would remain restricted. These could consist of either donations or fund raising activities to provide housing allowances for families visiting or staying with children requiring long-term care.

Exhibit 17–4 Not-For-Profit Fund Balance Section

	2003	2002
Unrestricted Fund Balance	213,986,611	207,562,498
Temporarily Restricted Fund Balance	53,859,722	49,333,233

Income Statement

The *income statement* is a financial statement that captures information about revenue sources, expenses, and costs of doing business during a period of time. For example, a yearly income statement would be labeled for the year ended. Hospital Anywhere USA is years ended December 31, 2004, 2003 and 2002. See **Exhibit 17–5**.

The majority of revenue sources come from providing patient services and the coding of these services via the DRG codes (hospitals) and RUGS (nursing homes). The problem with these sources is that the amount billed is not the amount received. For example, using the prospective payment system established in the early 1990s many of the major insurance companies only pay between 50 and 60 percent of the amount billed. For Medicare and state health plans, such as Medicaid, this amount is even lower—it could be as low as 25 percent. This has led to major changes in the accounting of health care providers, such as more accuracy in billing. If a claim is filed with a third party provider, payment must be received as soon as possible. Many health care providers found that claims collection

Exhibit 17–5 Income Statement

(Dollars in millions)			
	2004	2003	2002
Revenues	**$16,670**	**$16,657**	**$18,681**
Salaries and Benefits	6,639	6,694	7,766
Supplies	2,640	2,645	2,901
Other operating Expenses	3,085	3,251	3,816
Provision for doubtful accounts	1,255	1,269	1,442
Depreciation and amortization	1,033	1,094	1,247
Interest expense	559	471	561
Equity in Earnings of affiliates	(126)	(90)	(112)
Settlement with Federal government	840	0	0
Gains on sales of facilities	(34)	(297)	(744)
Impairment of long-lived assets	117	220	542
Restructuring of operations and investigation related costs	62	116	111
Total Expenses	**16,070**	**15,373**	**17,530**

was taking as many as 90 days. This means services were provided, resulting in expenditures, but the health care provider has only a piece of paper representing a claim. Many providers have improved their claims collection through improved accuracy of coding as well as by using electronic filing. The sooner the payment is received, the sooner the health care entity can use the funds to pay its own claims for services provided by creditors, and purchase new equipment or replacement equipment for improved diagnosis.

> *For example, using the prospective payment system established in the early 1990s, many of the insurance companies only pay between 50 and 60 percent of the amount billed. For Medicare and state health plans such as Medicaid, this amount is even lower—it could be as low as 25 percent.*

However, patient services may not be the only sources of revenue. Additional revenue may take the form of providing services for other health care facilities, or through the investment of funds. One example of additional services is that of a health care facility, such as Healthy Hospital (HH), doing laundry service for other hospitals. Evaluation of the laundry facility of HH found that it was only being used at 30 percent of capacity for its own use. They then contracted with other hospitals to do their laundry, earning additional revenue for HH. One section of Hospital Anywhere USA asset section illustrated the category called investments. Revenues from invested funds in the form of interest or dividends can also supplement basic operations. On the other hand, health care entities may invest in other health care organizations and receive a portion of their net income in the form of revenue.

Reductions in payments by third party providers, including government entities, have forced many health care facilities to establish an active foundation so additional funds are directed to the foundation. These additional sources of funds can be used to either cover shortfalls in revenues, or can be invested to provide interest or other forms of additional revenue.

Grants from either government agencies or firms interested in health care research can provide another source of revenue. Because most grants are available on a competitive basis, these are not guaranteed sources of revenue.

COSTS AND EXPENSES

Deductions from the revenue sources take the form of either *costs* or *expenses*. Costs and expenses, in the income statement, are those items used up or incurred in the generation of revenues. For Hospital Anywhere USA, the largest of these expenses is generally salaries and benefits paid to employees. The question for health entities is how to provide services at the lowest cost without reducing the quality of services. Can services be provided with alternative personnel, or is there a better way to utilize our facility? These are some of the major issues in health care today.

The second largest category of expenses is supplies and services as shown in **Exhibit 17–5**. Each patient for whom services are rendered will require some use of supplies, i.e., forms for patient information, swabs for testing, testing supplies, or food and beverages provided through food services.

The third largest item is the provision for doubtful accounts (*bad debt expense/provision for bad debts*) which is the adjustment for patient services that are expected not to be collected. Bad debt expense is the charge for not being able to collect patient accounts. Charges filed with third party payors are reduced according to payment schedules established by these firms. This reduces the amount of revenue from the gross (full) amount billed to the net amount. The amount over that paid by the third party payors is expected to be collected from the patient to whom services were provided. This refers to *deductibles*, and *co-payments*, which are amounts the patient pays over the reasonable and customary charges, further discussed in Chapter 6, which provides a health care economic overview. However, with Medicare and Medicaid patients, it is illegal to go back and bill the patients for whatever Medicare and Medicaid doesn't pay. In some cases, the patient will not be able to make payments. These must be taken as further charges in the form of bad debts.

Depreciation is a deduction allowed by the IRS. This is a paper and pencil amount (accounting) and is not an actual use of cash sources. Once a building or piece of equipment is acquired it may be "written off" over a designated period of time. The cost of the equipment is allocated to a specific time period and is used to reduce the net revenue and thus reduce taxes. For example, if a piece of diagnostic equipment having a 10-year life is purchased for five million dollars, using one of the many methods allowed for the calculation of depreciation (straight-line), the depreciation amount per year would be $500,000. ($5,000,000 ÷ 10 years = $500,000 depreciation per year.) As stated previously this reduces income and will lead to fewer taxes being paid.

Other forms of deductions may be interest, equity in earnings of affiliates, settlement with the federal government, and impairment of long-lived assets. If a health care facility is building, or purchases expensive equipment, it may have to borrow funds to pay for the project. The balance of the unpaid funds each year will be charged *interest. Equity in the earnings of affiliates* is your share of the firm in which you do not have the majority interest. The balance will increase if the firm in which you have invested has net income or will be reduced if the firm incurs a loss. Continuing to examine **Exhibit 17–5**, in 2004 there was a negative amount indicating losses by these affiliates. *The settlement with the federal government* is the payment that Hospital Anywhere USA has agreed to make to avoid further court actions. *Impairment of long-lived assets* is the result of an asset being reduced in value due to some market change. This could be a facility located in a part of town that has deteriorated, causing the value of the facility to decline. This is an accounting item only since you do not suffer a "real loss" in terms of cash flow until the facility is sold.

Depending on the size of the health care facility, additional costs may be incurred as a result of discontinuing an operation or selling used equipment or buildings at less than the amount recorded on the books. If a health care facility decides to sell a hospital in a neighboring town, a loss or gain can occur. Let's say five years after you purchased a five million dollar piece of equipment, you decide to sell. On the firm's books the cost was recorded at $5 M (M = million), and depreciation was taken at the rate of $500,000 per year. This is the original cost divided by the life of the asset, which was 10 years. Thus the amount shown in the financial records is $5M–$2.5M in accumulated depreciation. The book amount is $2.5M and if the asset is sold for $2M, a *loss* of $500,000 is incurred. A *gain* may also be realized by selling the equipment for an amount greater than the book value.

After payment of taxes the resulting amount is the Income or Loss from operations. If the net revenue sources exceed the expenses then a firm earns a net income. If the expenses exceed the net revenue sources then a loss occurs. Other items on the income statement are beyond the scope of this chapter.

One additional important item found on the income statement is *earnings per share* (*EPS*). This is the net income divided by the number of shares of common stock owned by stockholders outside the firm (outstanding). EPS provides a common comparison between firms having different income levels and number of shares of stock. The basic earning per share amount is presented as the net income from continuing operations, discontinued operations, and net income divided by shares of stock issued. This is the outstanding shares plus stock options, etc. divided into *income* amounts.

Cash Flow

As stated previously, cash is the lifeblood of a business. The *cash flow statement* shows one part of the financial stability of a firm. If all transactions were cash based then this statement would be easy to prepare and interpret. For-profit entities are required by Generally Accepted Accounting Principles (GAAP) to report on an *accrual basis*. This means that revenue must be reported when earned, not necessarily when payment is received, and expenses are recognized when incurred not paid. This requires several estimates during the reporting period. For example, if a service has been provided and a health care entity has a reasonable expectation of collection and can identify the amount to be collected, then it must be reported as revenue. Cash for the service may not be received until the next period.

> *For-profit entities are required by Generally Accepted Accounting Principles (GAAP) to report on an accrual basis. This means that revenue must be reported when earned, not necessarily when payment is received, and expenses are recognized when incurred, not paid.*

If employees are paid every Friday and the reporting period ends on Thursday then salaries must be accrued. For simplicity let us assume those salaries are $100,000 per week and no one works on the weekends. Each week the health care entity makes cash payments of $100,000 until the final week of the year. Since the reporting period ends on Thursday, the firm owes the employees $80,000 (4 days of pay) for services rendered. This amount must be recorded as an expense in the current period but does not require cash expenditure until the next reporting period.

The *bad debt expense* must likewise be estimated at the end of the year. The total amount of bad debts will not be known until all efforts to collect an account have been exhausted. This requires recognition of the bad debt expense for the reporting period (quarterly or yearly). The estimate is based on past experience in collection of accounts receivable, necessitated by adjustments for economic conditions. If two percent of the accounts receivable have been identified as bad in previous years and there was a major plant closing in the current reporting period, it could be expected that the amount collected would decrease and the bad debt expense would increase.

Preparation of the cash flow statement requires a thorough knowledge of the financial statements. Taking the cash balance at the beginning of the period and subtracting the ending cash balance provides the change in cash. The cash flow statement provides information explaining why cash changed. Financial statement items causing changes in cash are identified as operating, investing and financing activities.

OPERATING ACTIVITIES

Operating activities focus on the current portion of financial statements. They are the most important part of the cash flow analysis. Operating activities focus on the cash inflows and outflows from events that occur in the current operating period (see **Exhibit 17–6**). Financing and investing activities can provide funds but are limited to the extent of the time to which they can provide cash flow. There are upper limits on the amount of debt that can be issued (borrowed) on stock that can be sold. Likewise there is a limited amount of investments that can be sold to provide cash inflow. There is also a limit on the number of long-term assets that can be sold and, much like personal debt, there is a limit to the amount of money that can be borrowed.

Cash flow can be calculated in two ways but the one preferred by most entities starts with the net income or loss from the income statement. To this figure items are added or

Exhibit 17–6 Cash Flow Operating Activities Section

(Dollars in millions)			
Cash Flows From Continuing Activities:	**2004**	**2003**	**2002**
Net Income	$219	$657	$379
Adjustments to reconcile net income to net cash provided by continuing operating activities:			
Provision for doubtful accounts	1,255	1,269	1,442
Depreciation and amortization	1,033	1,094	1,247
Income taxes	(219)	(66)	351
Settlement with Federal government	840	0	0
Gains on sales of facilities	(34)	(297)	(744)
Impairment of long-lived assets	117	220	542
Loss from discontinued operating assets	0	0	153
Increase (decrease) in cash from operating assets and liabilities:			
Accounts receivable	(1,678)	(1,463)	(1,229)
Inventories and other assets	90	(119)	(39)
Accounts payable and accrued expenses	(147)	(110)	(177)
Other	71	38	(9)
Net case provided by continuing operating activities	**$1,547**	**$1,223**	**$1,916**

subtracted, indicating an increase or decrease in cash. Non-cash expenditures such as depreciation and amortization are an exception. Depreciation and amortization were deducted from net income as an expense on the income statement. This deduction reduced net income, but there was not a cash outflow. By adding this number back to the net income you are adjusting for a deduction that does not affect cash. Other items that may either be added back or deducted include the provision for doubtful accounts, gains on sale of long-term assets, settlement with the federal government, income taxes, and impairment of long-lived assets. Each of these is a non-cash expense. If a gain in the sale of long-lived assets had occurred this would be deducted from net income in the cash flow statement.

All current assets and liabilities from the balance sheet must be analyzed to determine the impact on cash flow. If accounts receivable increases, how is cash impacted? Cash would decrease. If the amount of current assets represented by accounts receivable increases you now have more paper and less cash coming in. From the perspective of the income statement, when services were provided you recorded the item as income. Net income is therefore higher than the cash generated from revenue leading to the adjustment in net income on the cash flow statement. The same is true for all other current assets. There is an inverse relationship between the change in current assets and the impact on cash flow. If current assets increase, they will be deducted from net income. Or vice versa, if current assets decrease they will be added back to net income.

Current liabilities have the opposite effect. If any current liability increases, this adds to the cash balance. What is the impact on cash if current liabilities increase? The firm has acquired either goods or services without having a cash outflow. The cash balance is improved by acquisition of assets without having a cash outflow. All current liabilities have a direct relationship with the impact on cash flow. Increases are added to net income, and decreases are subtracted from net income. The result of adding or deducting changes in current assets and liabilities to net income provides cash flow from operating activities.

FINANCING ACTIVITIES

The second portion of the cash flow statement is the *financing activities*, which focuses on long-term liabilities (those having a due date of longer than one year) or equity in the form of common or preferred stock (see **Exhibit 17–7**). If long-term liabilities increase during the year, it provides cash inflow. The firm is borrowing money to use in the business. If long-term liabilities decrease, then this implies that the liabilities are being paid off leading to a decrease in cash. Stock operates in the same manner. If either the common or preferred stock accounts increase, then the implication is that stock is used to finance firm activities. If they decrease, then stock is being repurchased and cash is leaving the firm. Likewise the payment of dividends on stock decreases cash outflow.

INVESTING ACTIVITIES

The last part of the cash flow statement concerns the *investing activities* of an organization as shown in **Exhibit 17–8**. This focuses mainly on the long-term assets of a business. If these assets are sold, cash inflows occur. On the other hand, if long-term assets are acquired then cash is presumed to decrease. An increase in investments is shown as having a decrease in cash.

Exhibit 17–7 Cash Flow Financing Activities Section

(Dollars in millons)

Cash flows from financing activities:	2004	2003	2002
Issuance of long-term debt	$2,980	$1,037	$3
Net change in bank borrowing	(500)	200	(2,514)
Repayment of long-term debt	(2,058)	(1,572)	(147)
Issuance (repurchase) of common stock, net	(677)	(1,884)	8
Payment of cash dividends	(44)	(44)	(52)
Other	(37)	8	3
Net Cash used in financing activities	**($336)**	**($2,255)**	**($2,699)**

A summary of these activities is presented in **Exhibit 17–8** to indicate the change in cash and cash equivalents.

Exhibit 17–8 Cash Flow Investing Activities Section

(Dollars in millions)

Cash flows from investing activities:	2004	2003	2002
Purchase of property and equipment	($1,155)	($1,287)	($1,255)
Acquisitions of hospitals and health care entities	(350)	0	(215)
Spin-off of facilities to stockholders	0	886	0
Disposal of hospitals and health care entities	327	805	2,060
Change in investments	106	565	(294)
Investment in discontinued operations, net	0	0	677
Other	(15)	(44)	(3)
Net cash provided by (used in) investing activities	**($1,087)**	**$925**	**$970**

Adding each category, continuing operating, financing and investing provides the change in cash and cash equivalents. Added to, or subtracted from, (if cash flow is negative as in 2003) cash and cash equivalents at the beginning of the period provide the amounts found on the balance sheet. The cash and cash equivalents account increased in both 2004 and 2002 and decreased in 2003, as shown in **Exhibit 17–9**, which provides a summary of all activites.

Exhibit 17-9 Summary of Cash Flows and Changes in Cash and Cash Equivalents

(Dollars in millions)			
	2004	2003	2002
Net case provided by continuing operating activities	$1,547	$1,223	$1,916
Net cash provided by (used in) investing activities	($1,087)	$925	$970
Net Cash used in financing activities	($336)	($2,255)	($2,699)
Change in cash and cash equivalents	124	(107)	187
Cash and cash equivalents at beginning of period	190	297	110
Cash and cash equivalents at end of period	$314	$190	$297

Schedule of Changes in Equity

The *Schedule of Changes in Equity* is required for all publicly reporting companies (governed by stock markets such as those sold on the New York Stock Exchange) and presents information for the reader to evaluate all changes in the owner's portion of the balance sheet. For each of the categories, retained earnings, and stock accounts, you start with the beginning balance and then either add or subtract items that add to, or subtract from, the firm equity during the year. For example, you would add net income, or subtract losses from the beginning retained earnings balance. Cash dividends would be subtracted from the beginning balance.

If there were no changes in the amount of stock sold or repurchased then the beginning and ending balances would be the same. However, if the firm sells additional shares of stock to finance buildings and equipment then these amounts would be added to the par values and capital in excess of par value accounts. If stocks were repurchased then the beginning balances would be reduced. Two additional items that might affect the stock accounts would occur when health care entities exercise strategies to retain employees. These stock accounts include stock options and employee benefit plan issuances that were exercised.

Stock options allow employees to purchase shares of stock at or below a future market price. This can result in non-taxable earnings for employees. For example, if an option were provided and the current stock price was $20 per share, the employee may be able to purchase the stock at some future point in time at $30 per share. Let's assume one year later the price of the stock had risen to $35 per share and the employee chooses to exercise their option. The employee would purchase the share(s) at $30 per share, adding to the par value and capital in excess of par value accounts, providing a valuable cash source. The employee now has $5 in untaxed income. It only becomes taxed if the stock sold.

Employee benefit plan issuances operate in much the same way. These are available to most employees of an organization and can be purchased at a predetermined amount. The amounts received from employees purchasing stock provide cash inflows.

Internal Accounting Information

Cost/Managerial Accounting

While public-reporting, for-profit health care entities must issue financial statements to external users, not-for-profit entities are not required to report to the general public. Accounting information used for internal or management decisions is not available to the general public but is used by management and others working within an organization. This information may be as specific as the pay rate for individual employees, or the costs to operate a function of the firm such as laboratories. For many health care workers, this is the area where management asks for employee input. This information is also used to evaluate the current operations of the organization and to solicit employee input to improve future operations. As previously mentioned, the amount of payments from third party payors has declined in recent years. Health care facilities used to receive reimbursements based on costs of operation. However, with the advent of prospective payment systems, these amounts have generally been reduced. Thus input from employees is needed to reduce costs and to improve customer services. As one nurse stated to the author, "I know the technical part of my job but I am being asked to serve on committees that are looking at changing and improving business operations." Thus the nurse needs to understand accounting information and how it can be used to support these changes.

Costs

Costs to be considered in making management decisions include differentiating between fixed and variable, direct and indirect, and marginal costs. Included in the discussion of costs is the term relevant range. To most, *relevant range* refers to the likely operating activity level expected to be incurred by a health care entity. For example, current staff can handle between 100 and 150 patients per day, which is the average use of our facilities. If the number of patients is either above or below these numbers, costs must be reconsidered, i.e., reduce or add employees to provide services.

From a revenue perspective, previous discussion centered on correct coding and use of DRGs and RUGs. Discussion also centered on the collection of these revenue items and the impact on financial statements. When health care facilities were forced to more carefully evaluate their operations they found many services offered were losing money. Since revenues were capped, cost containment became the issue.

Fixed versus Variable Costs

Evaluating operations begins with the evaluation of the costs involved. First is the distinction between fixed and variable costs. *Fixed costs* do not change with levels of services. If you are dealing with a facility that has one hundred beds, building costs such as depreciation will be the same regardless of if there is one patient or 100 patients occupying the bed(s). *Variable costs* do change with the increase of facility use. As more patients occupy the facility, costs such as food, medicines, and staff increases. These costs are variable because they change as the volume (number of patients or procedures) changes. Fixed and variable costs were previously discussed in Chapter 10, Budgeting.

Direct versus Indirect Costs

The second cost distinction is indirect versus direct costs. For an example, let's use the costs of laboratory services. The cost of the lab assistant that draws blood for analysis is a *direct cost*. Likewise, the use of needles and other supplies are direct costs. The staff person who manages the facility, handles the paperwork for the patient upon arrival, or files the claim is an *indirect cost*.

Marginal costs are those costs that are related to providing additional services. Again using the laboratory example, assume that the lab can handle 20 patients a day. If the lab is currently offering services to 15 patients, how much will it cost to provide additional services to one more patient? There will be no additional costs for the person drawing the blood sample; thus there is no marginal cost associated with this service. There will be additional costs associated with the use of needles, bandages, and testing supplies. These are marginal costs. As long as revenue for these services increases more than the costs, services should be expanded.

Average costs are those costs divided by the total number of services provided. Let us assume that it costs $500 per day to maintain the lab. If the lab performs only one test on this day then the average cost will be $500. However, if the lab performs five tests today the average cost will be $100 per test. You can operate up to a certain point without expanding facilities, personnel or equipment. As the number of tests increase the average cost decreases (this is the relevant range). Let us assume that the facility expands these services to reach 40 tests per day but can only process 20 per day with the current number of employees. The relevant range would be up to 20 tests. Over 20 tests would require the addition of personnel or equipment. Direct, indirect, and marginal costs were previously discussed in Chapter 10, Budgeting.

Activity-Based Costing

Once the types of costs are identified, they need to be allocated to the specific services performed. With the limitations on cost recovery (revenue) imposed by third party payors, health care entities must be aware of the costs to provide these services. Why should a facility pay $1.5M for an MRI machine and incur the other costs to maintain and staff the center when the revenues will not cover the costs? Recently one area of thought in accounting has been introduced to

Definition

Activity Based Costing (ABC) requires that you identify the cost drivers behind an activity. It requires that you break all services into specific functions and identify the costs associated with each activity.

help users of accounting information to focus on the specific costs of providing services. This is called *Activity Based Costing* (ABC).

Activity Based Costing (ABC) requires that you identify the cost drivers behind an activity. It requires that you break all services into specific functions and identify the costs associated with each activity. Assume you work in a physician's office and you need to determine the costs of a patient visit for a general exam. What activities are associated with the cost of providing these services? Let us assume the following, which is not a comprehensive example, for purposes of illustration:

- A general practitioner is paid $80,000 per year and spends on the average 15 minutes with each patient, seeing 24 patients per day. The physician works 45 weeks per year.
- A nurse is paid $35,000 per year and also spends 15 minutes with the patient.
- The receptionist is paid $24,000 and spends 5 minutes per patient in taking appointment calls and answering patient questions in the reception area.
- The cashier is paid $24,000 and spends 5 minutes per patient recording doctor information and verifying information for billing.
- All claims are entered electronically and it takes a data recorder 10 minutes to fill out the electronic filing version. This person is paid $20,000.
- A bookkeeper is paid $25,000 per year to capture accounting information for the facility. The bookkeeper spends 10 minutes per patient on the average collecting and reporting data for management of the facility.
- A stethoscope costs $100 and lasts two years.
- Each tongue depressor costs $.01.
- Each pair of latex gloves costs $.01.
- Each of the above mentioned individuals in the physician's office has a computer that costs $2,000 and is used for two years.
- Utility service per patient is $1.00.
- The cost per patient for building (facility) in the form of depreciation is $1.50.

Based on the previous information the following provides an analysis of the cost of providing patient services for a general physical examination. In the example shown in **Exhibit 17–10**, the patient is the cost driver.

The DRG code for medium intervention activity is billed at $50.00. A third party payor remits, on the average, 56 percent of billed amount yielding a payment of $35.60. Additional amounts may be collected from the patient but is not assumed in this case. (As mentioned earlier, this is true for coinsurance, deductibles and what is above the reasonable and customary costs with regular insurance. However, with Medicaid and with Medicare, other than billing the deductible and coinsurance, it is illegal to bill the patient for the amount of reimbursement not paid by the government.) Given the cost of the service at $41.21 there is a loss of $5.61 for each patient seen by the physician. This is where decision making using accounting data can improve the profitability of services, whether they are a single physician, nursing home, or hospital. What would you suggest to reduce the costs of the above, or improve the revenue? The physician and nurse spend 15 minutes per patient, but the others spend less time. Could the time the physician spends with each patient be reduced in order to increase the number of patients examined per year? Could

Exhibit 17–10 Activity Based Costing Example

(Dollars in millions)

Cost Driver	Cost	Cost Per Patient	Comments
Physician	$80,000	$14.81	15 minutes per patient/24 patients per day/45 weeks
Nurse	$35,000	$6.48	15 minutes per patient/24 patients per day/45 weeks
Receptionist	$24,000	$4.44	5 minutes per patient/24 patients per day/45 weeks
Cashier	$24,000	$4.44	5 minutes per patient/24 patients per day/45 weeks
Data Recorder	$20,000	$3.70	10 minutes per patient/24 patients per day/45 weeks
Bookkeeper	$25,000	$4.62	10 minutes per patient/24 patients per day/45 weeks
Utility Services		$1.00	
Computers	$12,000	$.19	6 computers/$2,000 per computer cost/life of 2 years
Gloves		.01	
Tongue Depressor		.01	
Building depreciation		$1.50	
Stethoscope	$100	.01	$100/lasts 2 years
Total		**$41.21**	

there be additional physicians or nurse practitioners employed to increase the workload of others such as the receptionist, bookkeeper, thus reducing the costs of others such as the receptionist and cashier? If the number of patients seen increase, the building and computer cost per patient would be decreased. Another alternative is to either expand the nurse's responsibilities or to hire additional nurses to reduce the MD's time with patients.

One solution would be to evaluate the use of each part of the cost structure. In the previous example, the physician was limited to seeing 5,400 patients per year. This is also the limitation for each of the other members of the physician's organization and is the cost driver. If the time spent with patients can be reduced to ten minutes per patient then the number of patients the physician can examine will be increased to 36 patients per day, or 8,100 per year. This causes a decrease in the physician cost per patient to $9.88, and receptionist cost per patient to $2.96. The overall effect causes cost to be reduced to a level below the third party payment which now exceeds cost.

Previously, different types of costs were defined. Using the previous example, we will now illustrate the costs. Fixed costs are those that do not change in total as volume (number of patients) increase. All of the costs except utilities, gloves, and tongue depressors are fixed. These costs are variable in that they change as the number of patients' increase. As seen in the revenue and cost comparison, the physician's salary is fixed and as the number of patients increased, the physician's cost per patient decreased (average cost decreases). As with any fixed costs you want to maximize the use and lower the costs to the lowest level.

Direct costs are those related to the generation of revenues. In this case, the physician and nurse are considered direct costs of providing services, as are the gloves and tongue depressors. The other costs are considered indirect because they are not directly related to production of revenue. Why is this distinction needed? If you are trying to determine whether or not to expand services you might want to look at the direct costs. Can you cover the direct costs of providing services? If so, then each patient or procedure will add to the profitability of the health care entity. For example, in the original illustration, if you can cover the direct costs (physician, nurse, gloves, and tongue depressor—$21.30), then additional amounts received can be applied to the indirect costs. The fixed costs will remain if a facility operates or closes for the weekend or vacations. If you can cover the direct cost, then any excess amount would be used to help cover fixed costs.

Marginal costs are those that increase as additional services are provided. Which costs in the illustration change as additional patients are added? Only the costs of the gloves and tongue depressor are marginal costs. What will it cost to provide service for one additional patient? When evaluating whether or not to accept additional patients you need to consider the impact on the organization. If no new costs are added for providing additional services, as long as the additional revenue exceeds the additional cost, then the service should be provided. To clarify this point, assume that a third party insurer approaches your organization offering a new client base consisting of local county employees. However, the insurer will pay a lower amount than that provided by other insurers. If you can determine the marginal costs of the services to be provided, the marginal costs may be less than the revenue received, increasing the contribution to firm profitability. This would benefit the organization.

Conclusion

Employees of health care facilities are being asked to improve patient services by generating additional revenue and becoming a valuable member of the management team. Correctly identifying services before filing claims with third parties can improve revenue collection. Additionally, making recommendations for more efficient use of services to minimize costs of these services is important for continuing organizational success. Can the health care entity substitute services for those currently being offered? Can someone in an organization provide the same quality services as others? For example, can I use an LPN for a RN? (This decision would only be best if the work performed by the person was appropriate at the LPN level.) This is one of the major issues affecting health care today.

APPENDIX

(All amounts are dollars in millions, except per share amounts.)

Hospital Anywhere USA Consolidated Balance Sheets, December 31, 2004 and 2004

Assets	2004	2003
Current Assets:		
Cash and cash equivalents	$314	$190
Accounts receivable, less allowance for doubtful accounts of $1,583 and $1,567	2,211	1,873
Inventories	396	383
Income taxes receivable	197	178
Other	1,335	973
Total Current Assets	**4,453**	**3,597**
Property and equipment at cost:		
Land	793	813
Buildings	6,021	6,108
Equipment	7,045	6,721
Construction in progress	431	442
Total Property and Equipment	**14,290**	**14,084**
Accumulated depreciation	(5,810)	(5,594)
	8,480	8,490
Investments of insurance subsidiary	1,371	1,457
Investments in and advances to affiliates	779	654
Intangible assets, net of accumulated amortization of $785 and $644	2,155	2,319
Other	330	368
Total Assets	**$17,568**	**$16,885**

Liabilities	2004	2003
Current Liabilities:		
Accounts payable	693	657
Accrued Salaries	352	403
Other accrued expenses	1,135	897
Government settlement accrual	840	
Long-term debt due within one year	1,121	1,160
Total Current Liabilities	**4,141**	**3,117**
Long-term debt	5,631	5,284
Professional liability risks, deferred taxes and other liabilities	2,050	2,104
Minority interests in equity of consolidated entities	572	763
Forward purchase contracts and put options	769	
Total Liabilities	**13,163**	**11,268**
Stockholders equity:		
Common stock $.01 par; authorized 1,600,000,000 voting shares 50,000,000		
50,000,000 nonvoting shares; outstanding 521,991,700 voting shares and		
shares and 21,000,000 nonvoting shares—2004 and 543,272,900 voting shares		
and 21,000,000 nonvoting shares—2003	5	6
Capital in excess of par value		951
Other	9	8
Accumulated other comprehensive income	52	53
Retained earnings	4,339	4,599
Total Stockholder's Equity	**4,405**	**5,617**
Total Liabilities and Stockholders Equity	**$17,568**	**$16,885**

Hospital Anywhere USA Consolidated Statement of Cash Flow for the Years Ended December 31, 2004, 2003, and 2002

Cash Flows From Continuing Activities:	2004	2003	2002
Net Income	$219	$657	$379
Adjustments to reconcile net income to net cash provided by continuing operating activities:			
Provision for doubtful accounts	1,255	1,269	1,442
Depreciation and amortization	1,033	1,094	1,247
Income taxes	(219)	(66)	351
Settlement with Federal government	840	0	0
Gains on sales of facilities	(34)	(297)	(744)
Impairment of long-lived assets	117	220	542
Loss from discontinued operating assets	0	0	153
Increase (decrease) in cash from operating assets and liabilities:			
Accounts receivable	(1,678)	(1,463)	(1,229)
Inventories and other assets	90	(119)	(39)
Accounts payable and accrued expenses	(147)	(110)	(177)
Other	71	38	(9)
Net case provided by continuing operating activities	$1,547	$1,223	$1,916
Cash flows from financing activities:	2004	2003	2002
Issuance of long-term debt	$2,980	$1,037	$3
Net change in bank borrowing	(500)	200	(2,514)
Repayment of long-term debt	(2,058)	(1,572)	(147)
Issuance (repurchase) of common stock, net	(677)	(1,884)	8
Payment of cash dividends	(44)	(44)	(52)
Other	(37)	8	3
Net Cash used in financing activities	($336)	($2,255)	($2,699)
Cash flows from investing activities:	2004	2003	2002
Purchase of property and equipment	($1,155)	($1,287)	($1,255)
Acquisitions of hospitals and health care entities	(350)	0	(215)
Spin-off of facilities to stockholders	0	886	0
Disposal of hospitals and health care entities	327	805	2,060
Change in investments	106	565	(294)
Investment in discontinued operations, net	0	0	677
Other	(15)	(44)	(3)
Net cash provided by (used in) investing activities	($1,087)	$925	$970

	2004	2003	2002
Net cash provided by continuing operating activities	1,547	1,223	1,916
Net cash provide by (used in) investing activities	(1,087)	925	970
Net Cash used in financing activities	(336)	(2,255)	(2,699)
Change in cash and cash equivalents	124	(107)	187
Cash and cash equivalents at beginning of period	190	297	110
Cash and cash equivalents at end of period	$314	$190	$297
Interest payments	$489	$475	$566
Income tax payments, net of refunds	$516	$634	($139)

Hospital Anywhere USA Consolidated Income Statements for the Years Ended December 31, 2004, 2003, and 2002

	2004	2003	2002
Revenues	$ 16,670	$ 16,657	$ 18,681
Salaries and Benefits	6,639	6,694	7,766
Supplies	2,640	2,645	2,901
Other operating Expenses	3,085	3,251	3,816
Provision for doubtful accounts	1,255	1,269	1,442
Depreciation and amortization	1,033	1,094	1,247
Interest expense	559	471	561
Equity in Earnings of affiliates	(126)	(90)	(112)
Settlement with Federal government	840	0	0
Gains on sales of facilities	(34)	(297)	(744)
Impairment of long-lived assets	117	220	542
Restructuring of operations and investigation related costs	62	116	111
Total Expenses	**16,070**	**15,373**	**17,530**
Income from continuing operations before minority interests and income taxes	66	1,284	1,151
Minority interests in earnings of consolidated entities	84	57	70
Income from continuing operations before income taxes	516	1,227	1,081
Provision for income taxes	297	570	549
Income from continuing operations	219	657	532
Discontinued operations:			
Loss from operations of discontinued businesses, net of income tax benefit of $26			(80)
Loss of disposals of discontinued businesses			(73)
Net Income	$219	$657	$379
Basic earnings per share:			
Income from continuing operations	$0.39	$1.12	$0.82
Discontinued operations:			
Loss from operations of discontinued businesses			(.12)
Loss on disposals of discontinued businesses			(.11)
Net income	**$0.39**	**$1.12**	**$0.59**
Diluted earnings per share:			
Income from continuing operations	$0.39	$1.12	$0.82
Discontinued operations:			
Loss from operations of discontinued businesses			(.12)
Loss on disposals of discontinued businesses			(.11)
Net income	**$0.39**	**$1.12**	**$0.59**

CHAPTER 18

Financial Analysis: Improving Your Decision-Making

Paul Bayes, D.B.A. Accounting,
M.S. Economics, B.S. Accounting

Numbers by themselves are data, not information. To be an informed and effective decision maker you must be able to convert raw data (numbers) into information. Putting financial data in a format that allows comparisons whether within your organization or between firms makes the information meaningful.

Benchmarking is a process that provides comparisons with the best practices of other organizations. These firms do not have to be within the same industry but traditionally comparisons are based within specific industries. This is a limiting factor in identifying best practices but simplifies the comparisons.

The purpose of this chapter is to introduce you to financial analysis and to improve your understanding of the accounting information presented earlier. An improved understanding of financial information leads to better future policies and strategic plans. Analysis may be either qualitative (non-financial) or quantitative (financial). Most of this chapter focuses on quantitative analysis because this information is more readily available. Qualitative analysis examples are provided within the text of quantitative examples. All examples use the financial statements of Hospital Anywhere USA, a for-profit entity, which were provided in Chapter 17. Selected information from Children's Hospital, a not-for-profit entity, are provided as a contrast to that of Hospital Anywhere USA. The financial statements of Retirement Homes, Inc. facility, a not-for-profit firm, are also provided as an example of a different type of not-for-profit facility. Differences in operating not-for-profit entities versus for-profit are noted.

> *Numbers by themselves are data, not information.*

> ### Definition
>
> *Benchmarking* is a process that provides comparisons with the best practices of other organizations.

Qualitative analysis requires a search of not only information in financial statements but also information from external sources. Stockholders' reports, along with financial statements, provide information. For example, the section on Management Discussion and Analysis provides information not found elsewhere in the financial statements, including strategic impetus, and changes in the market structure. Other parts of the annual reports yield information as to accounting practices (footnotes), segment information, and risk. If an organization has subsidiaries (parts of the firm either partially or wholly owned by the parent company) information on segment information reveals reliance on operations of certain products, services, or geographic areas. The Securities and Exchange Commission (SEC) for publicly traded stock companies requires supplementary information. Additional information at the SEC Edgar Database can be found at: http://www.sec.gov/edgarhp.htm. Information in Form 10-K and Form 10-Q reports is more comprehensive than the annual reports. In 10-Q (quarterly) reports, you can find information reported for each quarter of a firm. Rather than waiting until annual reports are issued analysts can better track a firm's progress using these quarterly reports. While the financial statements are the main focus of annual reports, they only make up a small portion. To illustrate, the annual report of Hospital Anywhere USA totals 51 pages of which the basic financial statements including summaries equal seven pages.

Common Size Balance Sheets

Most of the focus in this chapter is quantitative and will be based on financial statements and the standard ratio's found in both accounting and finance literature. One example of financial analysis is the use of *common size financial statements*. In the balance sheet and income statement analysts select one number and then divide into all other numbers in the statements. Total assets (balance sheets) are used as the baseline figure in balance sheets. Either gross revenue (sales) or net revenue (sales) (income statement) is used as the basis for income statements. Gross revenue is the total sales made by a firm. The difference with the net figure is deductions such as discounts and returns have been removed. Dividing all items in this set of financial statements and comparing several years provides a quick method to evaluate trends (changes). The caveat is that a two-year time frame may not be long enough to fully evaluate changes in operations. See **Exhibit 18–1**.

> *Common Size Financial Statements: In the balance sheet and income statement, one number is selected and then divided into all other numbers in the statements.*

The preceding balance sheet illustrates some minor changes in the assets, liabilities, and stockholders' equity from 2003 to 2004. The cash and cash equivalents increased from 1.13 percent in 2003 to 1.79 percent in 2004. This trend indicates that Hospital Anywhere USA had more cash and cash equivalents as a percent of total assets in 2004 than they had in 2003. This increase may be due to management anticipation of a need for more cash, or there could have been a better job of collecting patient accounts. Management may have

Exhibit 18–1

Hospital Anywhere USA Consolidated Balance Sheets, December 31, 2004 and 2003 Dollars in Millions				
Assets	2004		2003	
Current Assets				
Cash and cash equivalents	$314	1.79%	$190	1.13%
Accounts receivable, less allowance for doubtful accounts of $1,583 and $1,567	2,211	12.59%	1,873	11.09%
Inventories	396	2.25%	383	2.27%
Income taxes receivable	197	1.12%	178	1.05%
Other	1,335	7.6%	973	5.76%
Total Current Assets	**4,453**	**25.35%**	**3,597**	**21.30%**
Property and equipment at cost:				
Land	793	4.51%	813	4.81%
Buildings	6,021	34.27%	6,108	36.17%
Equipment	7,045	40.10%	6,721	39.80%
Construction in progress	431	2.45%	442	2.62%
Total Property and Equipment	**14,290**	**81.34%**	**14,084**	**83.41%**
Accumulated depreciation	-5,810	-33.07%	-5,594	-33.13%
	8,480	48.27%	8,490	50.28%
Investments of insurance subsidiary	1,371	7.8%	1,457	8.63%
Investments in and advances to affiliates	779	4.43%	654	3.87%
Intangible assets, net of accumulated amortization of $785 and $644	2,155	12.27%	2,319	13.73%
Other	330	1.88%	368	2.18%
Total Assets	**$17,568**	**100%**	**$16,885**	**100%**
Liabilities				
Current Liabilities				
Accounts payable	693	3.94%	657	3.89%
Accrued Salaries	352	2.00%	403	2.39%
Other accrued expenses	1,135	6.46%	897	5.31%
Government settlement accrual	840	4.78%		
Long-term debt due within one year	1,121	6.38%	1,160	6.87%
Total Current Liabilities	**4,141**	**23.57%**	**3,117**	**18.46%**
Long-term debt	5,631	32.05%	5,284	31.29%
Professional liability risks, deferred taxes and other liabilities	2,050	11.67%	2,104	12.46%
Minority interests in equity of consolidated entities	572	3.26%	763	4.92%
Forward purchase contracts and put options	769	4.38%		0%
Total Liabilities	**13,163**	**74.93%**	**11,268**	**66.73%**
Stockholders equity				
Common stock $.01 par; authorized 1,600,000,000 voting shares; 50,000,000 nonvoting shares; outstanding 521,991,700 voting shares and 21,000,000 nonvoting shares—2004 and 543,272,900 voting shares and 21,000,000 nonvoting shares –2003	5	.03%	6	.04%
Capital in excess of par value			951	5.63%
Other	9	0%	8	0%
Accumulated other comprehensive income	52	.30%	53	.31%
Retained earnings	4,339	24.07%	4,599	27.24%
Total Stockholder's Equity	4,405	25.07%	5,617	33.27%
Total Liabilities and Stockholders Equity	**$17,568**	**100%**	**$16,885**	**100%**

also reduced expenses, thus improving cash flow. However, the accounts receivable percentages increased from 11.09 to 12.59 percent indicating that there was an increase in the amount of "paper" held and collection slowed. This point illustrates that the person doing financial analysis may have to perform further evaluations rather than look at one piece of information. Total current assets also increased as a percent of total assets indicating that Hospital Anywhere USA was holding more *liquid assets* (ones that can be converted into cash quickly) in 2004 than in 2003.

Three changes occurred in the items defined as long-term assets. First, the buildings account decreased from 36.17 to 34.27 percent of total assets, which indicates that Hospital Anywhere USA may have sold off some of its buildings. As this account illustrates, the dollar value of buildings in fact declined from $6,108 to $6,021. Footnotes accompanying the financial statements state that three properties were sold. The second change indicates construction in progress decreased slightly, which might provide evidence of some building projects either being completed or abandoned. The third change in these assets occurred in intangible assets, which showed a decrease of 1.46 percent from the previous year. This could be due to:

- The selling off of parts of the organization thereby reducing goodwill,
- Some patents that Hospital Anywhere USA owned could have been sold,
- Patent rights could have expired, or
- A more aggressive manner used to write off existing patents or other intangible assets.

One item that appears in conjunction with this account is that the amortization, systematic writing off of intangible assets, increased from $644 to $785. This explains, at least in part, the decrease in intangible assets but does not provide evidence as to the reason for the increase in write-offs. This would come with additional research in the schedules and notes accompanying the statements.

Current liabilities show one item changing drastically. The government settlement accrual went from zero in 2003 to $840 in 2004. This indicates the settlement with the government over billing charges that cost the firm $840. The percentage change was from zero to 4.78 percent. Long-term debt, forward purchase contracts, and put options also went from zero to $769, making a percentage change from zero to 4.38 percent. A *forward purchase contract* is where one party agrees to buy a commodity at a specific price on a specific future date and the other party agrees to make the sale. In this case the agreement was for the repurchase of a limited number of common shares of Hospital Anywhere USA. A *put option* provides the right to sell stock at a specified price in the future. This again was related to the repurchase of the stock from a third party. In both instances a third party purchased shares of Hospital Anywhere USA stock in the market,

> **Definition**
>
> *Forward Purchase Contract*–where one party agrees to buy a commodity at a specific price on a specific future date and the other party agrees to make the sale.

> *A Put Option provides the right to sell stock at a specified price in the future.*

the hospital entered into a contract to purchase a set number of shares at a specified price from this third party entity. Total liabilities also increased from 66.73 percent to 74.93 percent indicating that a larger proportion of the business was financed using debt.

Analysis of *stockholders equity* indicates that the capital in excess of par values declined from $951 to zero going from 5.63 to zero percent. Although no information is directly available, one of the schedules that accompanies the financial statements provides information concerning this issue. Hospital Anywhere USA repurchased 21,281,200 shares of stock. Part of that repurchase plan would eliminate this account. A second item that negatively impacted the capital in excess of par value account was the reclassification of forward purchase contracts and put options to temporary equity. This was a result of action taken by the Financial Accounting Standards Board, which regulates reporting practices. Retained earnings declined from 27.24 to 24.70 percent as a result, partially, of the aforementioned reclassification.

Common Size Income Statements

Information in income statements is calculated in the same manner. The baseline number for analysis is either the gross revenue or net revenue. All items in the income statement are divided by this base figure which converts the information into a common basis to detect trends (changes) in operations. See **Exhibit 18–2**.

Salaries and benefits decreased slightly, which indicates that Hospital Anywhere USA may have undertaken some cost control or containment measures during the 2004 reporting period. Other operating expenses also decreased from 19.52 to 18.51 percent. These would include items such as utilities, property taxes, professional fees (legal and accounting), maintenance, rent, and lease expenses. Interest expense and settlement with the federal government increased during this time period. With the aforementioned increase in debt financing, from the balance sheet analysis, there may be an increase in interest expenses. Unless a firm can negotiate a lower rate than that used in previous financing arrangements, the increased use of debt raises the risk to creditors, which causes the interest rate to increase. A simple explanation is that as more debt is issued, even at the same rate, there will be an increase in interest cost. The settlement with the federal government went from zero to 5.04 percent. This had a major impact on the profitability of the firm. The only remaining item that had a major change, other than summative categories, such as income from continuing operations before taxes and income from continuing operations, was provision for income taxes. This amount decreased from 3.42 to 1.78 percent. This may be a result of lower income or having either tax credits or deferred taxes that can be used to reduce the current year's taxable income. *Tax credits* are provided in the tax laws and allow firms to carry losses incurred in any year back for two years and forward for twenty years. *Deferred taxes* are a result of differences between financial reporting tax requirements and those used for reporting taxes to local, state, and federal government units. In some cases alternative inventory and depreciation may be used for reporting thus creating a difference in the amounts owed and the payments may be deferred (postponed).

Exhibit 18–2

Hospital Anywhere USA Consolidated Income Statements for the Years Ended December 31, 2004, and 2003 Dollars in Millions				
	2004		2003	
Revenues	$16,670	100.00%	$16,657	100.00%
Salaries and Benefits	6,639	39.83%	6,694	40.19%
Supplies	2,640	15.84%	2,645	15.88%
Other operating Expenses	3,085	18.51%	3,251	19.52%
Provision for doubtful accounts	1,255	7.53%	1,269	7.62%
Depreciation and amortization	1,033	6.20%	1,094	6.57%
Interest expense	559	3.35%	471	2.83%
Equity in Earnings of affiliates	-126	-0.76%	-90	-0.54%
Settlement with Federal government	840	5.04%	0	0.00%
Gains on sales of facilities	-34	-0.20%	-297	-1.78%
Impairment of long-lived assets	117	0.70%	220	1.32%
Restructuring of operations and investigation related costs	62	0.37%	116	0.70%
Total Expenses	**16,070**	**96.40%**	**15,373**	**92.29%**
Income from continuing operations before minority interests and income taxes	66	0.40%	1,284	7.71%
Minority interests in earnings of consolidated entities	84	0.50%	57	0.34%
Income from continuing operations before income taxes	516	3.10%	1,227	7.37%
Provision for income taxes	297	1.78%	570	3.42%
Income from continuing operations	219	1.31%	657	3.94%
Discontinued operations:				
Loss from operations of discontinued businesses, net of income tax benefit of $26				
Loss of disposals of discontinued businesses		0.00%		
Net Income	$219	1.31%	$657	3.94%
Basic earnings per share:				
Income from continuing operations	$0.39	0.00%	$1.12	0.01%
Discontinued operations:				
Loss from operations of discontinued businesses				
Loss on disposals of discontinued businesses				
Net income	**$0.39**	**0.00%**	**$1.12**	**0.01%**
Diluted earnings per share:				
Income from continuing operations	$0.39	0.00%	$1.12	0.01%
Discontinued operations:				
Loss from operations of discontinued businesses				
Loss on disposals of discontinued businesses				
Net income	**$0.39**	**0.00%**	**$1.12**	**0.01%**

Financial Ratio Analysis

Key financial ratios can be classified into five categories. These may be called among others:
1. Liquidity Ratios,
2. Activity Ratios,
3. Leverage Ratios,
4. Profitability Ratios, and
5. Net Trade Cycle.

Each category provides an analysis of different aspects of the organization and indicates how well the firm is managed. The following ratios are limited in number and use varies by type of organization. The ones presented here are considered the more standard ratios for most businesses. Industry specific ratios would be used to provide additional information. The names used are the standard ones and those used by different firms and professional organizations may be different. To provide a more complete analysis the calculated ratios should be compared with industry averages. There are several services that provide this information on a for-fee basis. When making the comparisons you must evaluate each firm by both size and type. For hospitals, the data is provided by size and geographic regions. The information can be obtained from sources for other types of not-for-profit organizations.

Liquidity Ratios

Liquidity ratios are concerned with short-term (current items). The two most frequently used liquidity ratios are the current ratio and quick or acid-test ratio. The *current ratio* divides the current assets by current liabilities. This provides one measure of a firm's ability to pay short-term obligations, which arise in the course of operations or within one operating cycle (usually one year). For example, if the calculated ratio is two, this is interpreted to mean that you have two dollars in current assets for every one dollar in current liabilities. The limitation is that this ratio does not measure the true ability to pay obligations. A skewed example might be useful for improved understanding of this limitation. If current assets are $2M and current liabilities are $1M then there are twice as many dollars in assets as there are in liabilities. However, let us assume that the current assets consist of $1 in cash and inventories make up the remainder. All current liabilities are due tomorrow. The original answer shows that obligations can be met but, as the skewed example shows, the current debt can not be met.

> **Liquidity Ratios are concerned with short-term (current items).**

Now let's figure the actual liquidity ratio in the text box.

Ratio	How Calculated	2004	2003
Current Ratio	Current Assets/ Current Liabilities	$4,453/$4,141 = 1.08	$3,597/$3,117 = 1.15
Quick Ratio	Current Assets— Inventories/Current Liabilities	$4,057/$4,141 = .98	$3,214/$3,117 = 1.03

The current ratio declined from 1.15 to 1.08 in the above results. This would indicate that the ability to pay short-term obligations has weakened since 2003. Either current liabilities grew faster than current assets or current assets declined more rapidly than current liabilities. The common size balance sheet shows that current liabilities increased faster than current assets.

The *quick* or *acid-test ratio* provides additional information to evaluate the ability to meet short-term obligations. To compute this ratio, inventory must be subtracted from current assets. Sometimes items defined as "prepaid" may also be subtracted. The reason for the elimination of inventory from the numerator is that these items can not be converted into cash quickly without a loss in value.

In the previous example the current and quick ratio both decreased. However, most current assets of Hospital Anywhere USA can be defined as quick assets (91.1 and 89.3 percent respectively for 2004 and 2003) so the current assets are highly liquid. If items other than cash and cash equivalents plus accounts receivable are eliminated the quick ratio becomes .61 and .67 respectively for 2004 and 2003. Two years is not enough time to make a completely informed judgment about the trends but the trend is showing a decline. This is one indication that there is a decline in the ability of the hospital to meet its current obligations.

Activity Ratios

Activity ratios measure the liquidity and efficiency of asset management. The *accounts receivable collection* period measures the average time it takes a firm to collect its accounts (patient/insurance) receivable. The quicker a firm can convert the receivables to cash, the quicker they can pay their obligations or have cash for opportunities that may arise. This ratio is calculated by dividing the accounts receivable by the average daily revenue. Average daily revenue is calculated by dividing the revenue from the income statement by 365. This measures on the average how many times the organization has converted the receivables into cash.

> **Definition**
>
> *Activity Ratios* measure the liquidity and efficiency of asset management.

Inventory turnover is found by dividing the cost of goods sold by inventory (accounting) or revenue by inventory (finance). This measures how quickly inventory is sold and is important for firms with products that deteriorate or have a short shelf life (drugs, surgical supplies).

Ratio	How Calculated	2004	2003
Accounts Receivable Collection Period	Accounts Receivable/ [(Revenue)/365]	$2,211/[($16,670)/ 365] = 45.67 Days	$1,873/[($16,657)/ 365] = 45.63 Days
Inventory Turnover	Cost of Goods Sold/ Inventory or Revenue/ Inventory	$16,670/$396 =42.09	$16,657/$383 = 43.49

The above ratios for Hospital Anywhere USA indicate that the collection of accounts receivable takes an average of approximately 45 days. Once a patient leaves a facility after receiving medical services, the hospital is waiting for money from either the patient or a third party payor 45 days before the claim is settled. Inventory turnover, from an accounting perspective, can not be calculated for this hospital because cost of goods sold is not separately reported and can not be calculated. This ratio is usually provided as supplemental information to the financial statements. If they had a subsidiary that sold medical items or the information was provided in the income statements then the accounting ratio could be calculated. This is a standard ratio in all accounting literature. Finance literature supports a different calculation. As indicated previously, revenue is divided by the inventory. The turnover has increased slightly. For similar firms to Hospital Anywhere USA this number would be quite high compared to standard manufacturing organizations.

Management's effectiveness in using assets to generate revenues can be measured by using two ratios. First, *fixed asset turnover* measures how well management is using the long-term assets of the organization to generate revenue. As the balance sheet shows in Chapter 17, this asset consists primarily of buildings and equipment used for providing patient services. For a health care organization this is important in that supplying beds, and using equipment creates billable revenue. Fixed asset turnover is found by dividing net revenues by net property, plant, and equipment (cost of property, plant, and equipment minus accumulated depreciation). *Total asset turnover* measures how management is using all assets of the organization to generate revenue. The measure is found by dividing net revenues by all assets.

Ratio	How Calculated	2004	2003
Fixed Asset Turnover	Net Revenue/ Net Property, Plant and Equipment	$16,670/$8,480 = 1.966	$16,657/$8,490 = 1.96
Total Asset Turnover	Net Revenue/ Total Assets	$16,670/$17,568 = .949	$16,657/$16,885 = .986

Evaluation of the above indicates a minor change in the use of assets to generate revenue. Fixed asset turnover was relatively stable while total asset turnover has declined slightly but this may be due to the increase in current assets as previously discussed.

Leverage Ratios

Leverage ratios, also called *capital structure ratios*, are one measure of how an organization is financed. For-profit firms can either borrow funds using a debt instrument (notes payable or bonds) or sell shares of stock (equity financing). Creditors look at this important ratio to determine if they will provide more funds to an organization or if the cost of funds (interest) will be changed. Remember from the previous chapter that $A = L + K$. If an organization fails to con-

> *Leverage Ratios, also called capital structure ratios, are one measure of how an organization is financed.*

tinue in business due to financial setbacks (bankruptcy), the assets of the organization will be sold and distributed first to the creditors. If there is a remainder, the owners (those holding shares of stock) receive this amount. Thus, the more debt that you have the more risk you take on. This risk limits the amount of debt that creditors are willing to extend or finance projects cost more due to the higher risk.

However, on the positive side, debt can be used to improve the investment of stockholders (owners) of an organization. For instance, if you can borrow funds at 6 percent and invest at 10 percent then the stockholders receive the differential. Profits will be increased and these will be reinvested in the firm. For Hospital Anywhere USA the following three ratios provide an analysis of how much debt is used to finance the organization and the amount of debt compared to equity used to fund the operations and long-term projects of the firm:

Ratio	How Calculated	2004	2003
Debt Ratio	Total liabilities/ Total assets	$13,163/$17,568 = .749	$11,268/$16,885 = .667
Long-Term Debt to Total Capitalization	Long-term debt/ (Long-term debt + Stockholder's equity)	$9,022/($9,022 + $4,405) = .672	$8,151/($8,151 + $5,617) = .592
Debt to Equity	Total liabilities/ Stockholder's equity	$13,163/$4,405 = 2.988	$11,268/$5,617 = 2.006

The *debt ratio* measures how much of the total assets have been financed using debt (obligations to pay a future amount of funds). The trend from 2003 to 2004, up from 66.7 to 74.9 percent, shows an increase, which indicates that more of the operations were financed using debt and a future outflow of funds either in interest costs or repayment of debt will be required. This debt may also increase the interest rate charged on these funds based on the increased risk. Remember that analysis of the common size income statement revealed that interest costs were higher in 2004 then in 2003. The other ratios confirm this trend in that debt has increased in relation to total funding (L + K) and compared to the use of equity financing (stocks).

Long-term debt to total capitalization (long-term debt divided by long-term debt plus stockholders equity) shows that more long-term debt is being used for financing (67.2 up from 59.2 percent). This number ($9,022 for 2004) is found by subtracting total current liabilities from total liabilities and dividing by long-term debt ($9,022) plus $4,405.

Debt to equity also indicates a larger use of debt financing in the business. This ratio indicates that debt was used approximately twice as often as equity in 2003 and almost three times as much in 2004. Firms with stable revenues can borrow more (increase their debt) than others with revenues that fluctuate. However, there is generally a limitation on the amount of funds that will be provided for operations.

Profitability Ratios

Profitability ratios measure how well a firm is doing in its basic operations. These ratios measure the percent that revenues minus certain costs exceed the revenues. They also determine how well the assets of the organization and owner's investment are being used. These ratios are the gross profit margin, operating profit margin, net profit margin, return on total assets, and return on equity.

Since Hospital Anywhere USA does not engage in selling physical assets, such as beds and drugs, and these items are not reported separately, the gross profit margin is not applicable. The *gross profit* amount is determined by subtracting from revenues the cost of goods sold. However, there is no cost of goods sold for this hospital—thus this amount cannot be calculated.

> **Profitability Ratios measure how well a firm is doing in its operations.**

The *operating profit margin* is found by looking at the net revenues from the normal course of business, providing health care services, and subtracting all expenses of operations necessary to generate these revenues. This measure, sometimes called *EBIT* (earnings before interest and taxes), indicates if the firm is covering their costs of operations. This amount is then divided by net revenues. Both 2004 and 2003 indicate a reasonable operating profit margin. For 2004 this means that Hospital Anywhere USA is covering operating costs and has approximately 12 cents on the dollar left to cover all other costs including interest paid on debt and income taxes. The government settlement negatively impacted the earnings but because of cost reduction measures in 2004 other costs such as salaries were reduced helping to alleviate impact of earnings.

The remaining three measures indicate that expenses were covered but there was little, percentage wise, left over to reinvest in the firm. Without knowing how others in the industry are doing it becomes difficult to make a conclusion about the effectiveness of operations. The results presented indicate a decline in profitability of operations.

Ratio	How Calculated	2004	2003
Gross Profit Margin	Gross profit/ Net revenue	NA	NA
Operating Profit Margin	Operating profit/ Net revenue	\$2,018/\$16,670 = 12.1%	\$1,704/\$16,657 = 10.2%
Net Profit Margin	Net earnings/ Net revenue	\$219/\$16,670 = 1.31%	\$657/\$16,657 = 4.18%
Return on Total Assets or Return on Investment	Net earnings/ Total assets	\$219/\$17,568 = 1.24%	\$657/\$16,885 = 3.89%
Return on Equity	Net earnings/ Stockholder's equity	\$219/\$4,405 = 4.97%	\$657/\$5,617 = 11.69%

Trade or Cash Conversion Cycle Ratio

The final group of standard ratios used to analyze a firm's operations evaluates the *trade or cash conversion cycle*. These measure, on the average, how long it takes to collect from either the patient or third party providers or how long we are taking to pay our short-term obligations. The number of days in revenue is calculated as accounts receivable turnover previously discussed:

Ratio	How Calculated	2004	2003
Number of Days Revenue	Accounts receivable/ (Revenue/365)	$2,211/($16,670/365) = 48.14	$1,873/($16,670/365) = 41.04
Number of Days Payable	Accounts payable/ (Revenue/365)	$693/($16,670/365) = 15.17	$657/($16,657/365) = 14.40

Trade or Cash Conversion Cycle Ratio–These measure, on the average, how long it takes to collect from either the patient or third party providers or how long we are taking to pay our short-term obligations.

If creditors provide 30 days in which to pay an obligation and your organization takes 40 days, a cash flow problem may exist. For Hospital Anywhere USA the *number of days in payables*, accounts payable divided by average daily revenues, increased from 14.40 to 15.17, which indicates that the hospital took longer to pay current obligations. This is a minor change and anyone doing an evaluation would have to know the terms for payment that the hospital has with its creditors. This does however increase cash flow in that you retain cash longer by postponing the payment (cash outflow). A variation of this ratio is current liabilities divided by operating expenses minus depreciation divided by 365.

Not-for-Profit Comparisons

Not-for-profit entities have some differences that make comparisons more difficult than that of for-profit entities. Since profitability is not a mission of not-for-profit organizations, profitability ratios may not be calculated in the same manner. Health care organizations must provide an alternative performance indicator. This is normally in a footnote but must be clearly distinguished from other notes. It may take the form of either revenue over expenses, revenues and gains over expenses and losses, earned income, or performance income.

As the financial statements in **Exhibit 18–3** illustrate, there are differences between hospitals—especially between for-profit and not-for-profit firms. First, the dates of the statements are for June rather than December. The selection of a date is arbitrary. Second, other sources of revenue consist of government research grants and support provided to cover operating expenses. The latter is probably a result of donations by outside persons or organizations. The remaining accounts on the income statements are standard and would be expected to be found on both for-profit and not-for-profit organizations.

The balance sheet has one major difference with that of a for-profit entity. Instead of having stockholders (owners) of the firm, the accounts become unrestricted and temporarily restricted fund balances. *Unrestricted fund balances* are provided by others to support the mission of the hospital. Temporarily *restricted fund balances* are used for projects having a specific purpose and then returned to use for unrestricted purposes. Refer to **Exhibit 18–4.**

Exhibit 18–3

Children's Hospital Operating Revenues and Expenses
June 30, 2004 and 2003

	2004	2003
Net Patient Services and Revenue	$238,736,833	$228,094,450
Other Sources of Revenue		
Government Research Grants	45,160,159	36,757,430
Support Provided to Cover Operating Expenses	100,137,765	82,342,438
Total Operating Revenues	**$384,034.757**	**$347,194,318**
Operating Expenses		
Salaries and Benefits	$195,621,776	$172,757,651
Services, Supplies, Other	146,371,984	131,094,528
Depreciation	28,116,508	24,262,840
Interest	5,899,845	5,492,360
Bad Debt Expense	3,048,592	6,182,778
Total Operating Expenses	**$383,268,634**	**$339,790,157**
Income (Loss) from Operations	**$769,123**	**$7,404,161**

Exhibit 18–4

Condensed Balance Sheets as of June 30, 2004 and 2003

	2004	2003
Assets		
Cash and Temporary Investments	$6,084,671	$3,767,117
Patient Accounts Receivable, Net of Allowances for Uncollectible Accounts	55,084,671	49,121,350
Other Current Assets	36,059,481	27,737,663
Current Assets	$97,388,219	$80,626,130
Plant and Equipment, Net of Accumulated Depreciation	$261,633,535	$223,695,756
Funds Held in Trust	82,118,866	42,568,303
Long-Term in Trust	110,292,993	101,245,215
Total Assets	**$551,433,613**	**$448,135,404**
Liabilities and Fund Balance		
Accounts Payable and Accrued Expenses	$44,489,716	$43,222,493
Current Portion of Long-Term Debt	4,884,203	4,540,418
Current Liabilities	**$49,373,919**	**$47,762,911**
Long-Term Debt	$212,548,645	$119,007,882
Other Long-Term Liabilities	21,664,716	24,468,880
Unrestricted Fund Balance	213,986,611	207,562,498
Temporarily restricted Fund Balance	53,859,722	49,333,233
Total Liabilities and Fund Balances	**$551,433,613**	**$448,135,404**

The four ratios presented in the following table are variations of those used in the analysis of Hospital Anywhere USA, but applied to that of Children's Hospital.

Ratio	How Calculated	2004	2005
Long-Term Debt to Total Capitalization	Long-term debt/ (Long-term debt + Fund balances)	$234,213,357/ $502,059,690 = .4665	$143,476,762/ $400,372,493 = .3584
Debt to Fund Balances	Total liabilities/ Fund balances	$283,587,276/ $267,846,333 = 1.058	$191,239,673/ $256,895,731 = .744
Reported Income Index	Net Income/ Changes in Fund Balance	$786,123/ $10,950,602 = .072	NA
Long-Term Debt to Fund Balances	Long-term debt/ Fund balance	$234,213,357/ $267,846,333 = .874	$143,476,763/ $256,895,731 = .558

All three previously used ratios are smaller than those of Hospital Anywhere USA and declined in this time period. This indicates this hospital does not use as much debt to finance operations as Hospital Anywhere USA. The reported income index was not directly applicable to Hospital Anywhere USA but is somewhat equivalent to profitability ratios that used net earnings computed for Hospital Anywhere USA. Again, a direct comparison should not be made with Hospital Anywhere USA, but could be compared to other not-for-profit hospitals.

A further problem in comparing not-for-profit entities is the lack of standardized terminology or presentation formats. Some of these same problems exist with for-profit entities, but the differences are not as glaring as that of not-for-profits. The last consideration in analyzing different not-for-profit firms is that information is not as readily available as that for publicly reporting firms.

The consolidated balance sheets and statement of activities (equivalent to for-profit income statements) of Retirement Homes, Inc., are introduced in **Exhibits 18–5** and **18–6**. Selected financial ratios follow the financial statements.

Retirement Homes, Inc., shows several differences between the previously reported organizations. In addition to being a smaller entity, they have permanently restricted funds; Children's Hospital does not. They also have gift fees and long-term obligations from advance payments from persons entering their facility. Patients may pay in advance, but until the retirement facility provides the services the income is not earned. The income statement format for Retirement Homes, Inc. also includes fund balance changes which were not included in previously presented income statements.

Exhibit 18–5

Retirement Homes, Inc. Consolidated Balance Sheet		
	2000	1999
Assets		
Current Assets		
Cash and equivalents	$1,343,467	$557,494
Investments held by bond trustee	50,653	254,572
Accounts receivable, net of allowance for doubtful accounts of $166,200 and $45,200 in 2000 and 1999	444,396	371,746
Contributions and grants receivable	88,127	
Inventories	56,705	54,597
Prepaid expenses and other	62,133	90,567
Total current Assets	**2,045,481**	**1,328,976**
Investments		
Held by bond trustee, net of amount requires to meet current obligations	4,845,585	4,562,685
Board designated funds	869,603	823,758
Foundation	1,832,579	1,637,170
	7,547,767	7,023,613
Property and equipment		
Land and improvements	2,630,999	2,537,686
Buildings and improvements	34,046,631	33,359,106
Equipment	1,679,668	1,513,251
Furniture and equipment	1,440,448	1,385,729
	39,797,746	38,795,772
Less accumulated depreciation	12,289,748	11,173,504
	27,507,998	27,622,268
Construction in progress	593,335	521,608
	28,101,333	28,143,876
Beneficial interest in charitable remainder trusts	72,250	
Net deferred charges:		
Marketing and consulting costs	1,568,833	1,758,238
Financing costs	2,437,811	2,774,112
Prepayment in lieu of taxes	210,000	280,000
	4,216,644	4,812,350
Other assets	21,500	21,500
Total assets	**$42,004,975**	**$41,330,315**
Current liabilities		
Accounts payable	$308,493	$399,480
Salaries, wages and related liabilities	164,551	130,589
Accrued compensated absences	130,843	120,501
Accrued interest	81,580	83,561
Current portion of long-term debt	904,031	854,212
Other current liabilities	12,012	49,860
Total current liabilities	1,601,510	1,638,203
Other liabilities:		
Long-term obligations	33,247,449	34,163,586
Entrance fees received in advance and deposits	308,124	202,288
Gift annuities payable	377,079	254,184
Deferred entry fee revenue	23,022,153	22,865,940
	56,954,805	57,485,998
Net assets (deficit):		
Unrestricted	(18,014,253)	(19,176,458)
Temporarily restricted	1,415,676	1,382,572
Permanently restricted	47,237	
Total net assets (deficit)	(16,551,340)	(17,793,886)
Total liabilities and net deficit	**$42,004,975**	**$41,330,315**

Exhibit 18–6

Retirement Homes, Inc. Consolidated Statements of Activities Year Ended December 31		
	2000	1999
Revenue and other support		
Resident services:		
Monthly service fees	$8,340,317	$8,111,191
Amortization of deferred revenues	3,345,893	3,075,632
Patient revenue from nonresidents	2,217,990	1,629,027
Interest income	258,845	322,954
Medicare and other	804,211	615,273
Net assets released from restriction	132,171	
Total revenue and other support	**15,099,427**	**13,754,077**
Expenses		
Salaries and wages	5,059,124	4,728,354
Employee benefits	733,960	691,892
Total employment expenses	5,793,084	5,420,246
Purchased services	1,534,747	1,082,729
Supplies	1,247,315	1,286,860
Provision for Bad debts	123,404	5,000
Utilities	637,598	624,457
Rent	4,815	4,515
Insurance	204,503	42,417
Interest	2,410,079	2,426,461
Program expenses-foundation	116,924	
Foundation operating expenses	66,282	
Miscellaneous	369,046	
Depreciation and amortization Total expenses	1,672,950	1,765,252
Total expenses	**14,180,747**	**13,073,233**
Excess of revenue over expenses	918,680	680,844
Net asset reclassification	172,018	
Net assets released from restriction for capital	78,896	
Net unrealized holding losses on investments	(7,389)	1,817
Increase in unrestricted assets	1,162,205	682,661
Temporarily restricted net assets:		
Net asset reclassification	(187,018)	
Contributions	308,263	127,066
Net unrealized holding losses on investments	(168,582)	(54,993)
Investment income	291,508	244,550
Net assets released from restrictions	(211,067)	(50,443)
Increase in temporarily restricted net assets	33,104	266,180
Permanently restricted net assets:		
Net Asset Reclassification	15,000	
Contributions	32,237	
Increase in permanently restricted net assets	47,237	
Increase in net assets	1,242,546	948,841
Net deficit, beginning of year	**(17,793,886)**	**(18,742,727)**
Net deficit, end of year	**$(16,551,340)**	**$(17,793,886)**

Current Ratios

Retirement Homes, Inc. shows an improvement in its ability to meet current obligations. In 2003 both ratios were below 1, while both improved to above 1 in 2004. How does this compare to the ratios presented for Hospital Anywhere USA? The ratios for Hospital Anywhere USA deteriorated while those of Retirement Homes, Inc. improved. The trends can be compared but you cannot make a direct comparison because the firms are in two different industries and operate as two different types of organizations (for-profit versus not-for-profit).

Ratio	How Calculated	2004	2003
Current Ratio	Current Assets/ Current Liabilities	$2,045,481/ $1,601,510 = 1.28	$1,328,976/ $1,638,203 = .81
Quick Ratio	Current Assets- Inventories/Current Liabilities	$1,926,643/ $1,601,510 = 1.20	$1,183,812/ $1,638,203 = .72

Activity Ratios

Notice in the following table that the number of days in the accounts receivable collection period increased, as did the inventory turnover. This indicates that the firm has slowed the time to make collections while inventory was being used faster. Again a direct comparison cannot be made with Hospital Anywhere USA data. However, you can purchase industry comparison data (benchmarking) from either national services or associations and determine how well you are doing compared to others.

Ratio	How Calculated	2004	2003
Accounts Receivable Collection Period	Accounts Receivable/ [(Revenue)/365]	$444,396/ [($15,099,427)/365] = 10.7 Days	$371,746/ [($13,754,077)/365] = 9.86 Days
Inventory Turnover	Cost of Goods Sold/ Inventory or Revenue/Inventory	$15,099,427/ $56,705 = 266.3	$13,754,077/ $54,597 = 251.9

Notice again that both ratios improved but assets are not used as well to generate revenue for Retirement Homes, Inc. as they were for Hospital Anywhere USA. You are cautioned again not to make direct comparisons.

Ratio	How Calculated	2004	2003
Fixed Asset Turnover	Net Revenue/ Net Property, Plant and Equipment	$15,099,427/ $28,101,333 = .587	$13,754,077/ $28,143,876 = .488
Total Asset Turnover	Net Revenue/ Total Assets	$15,099,427/ $42,004,975 = .359	$13,754,077/ $41,330,315= .382

Leverage Ratios

In each case the amount of debt, long-term and total, is greater than total assets and long-term debt plus net assets. Net assets, equivalent to for-profits stockholders equity, are negative. This negative figure is probably a result of losses in previous years of operation. As a result of this negative figure the calculation is not applicable.

Ratio	How Calculated	2004	2003
Debt Ratio	Total liabilities/ Total assets	$56,954,805/ $42,004,975 = 1.356	$57,485,998/ $41,330,315 = .1.39
Long-Term Debt to Total Capitalization	Long-term debt/ (Long-term debt + Net assets)	$55,353,295/ $38,801,955= 1.43	$55,847,795/ $38,053,909= 1.47
Debt to Equity	Total liabilities/ Net assets	$56,954,805/ $(16,551,340) = NA	$57,485,999/ ($17,793,886)= NA

Profitability Ratios

Two of the following ratios cannot be calculated either due to lack of available data or because one part of the equation has a negative (deficit) balance. Two of the ratios (indicated with *) are variations of those presented previously for Hospital Anywhere USA. These ratios use the increase in net assets because a not-for-profit does not report profits but rather looks at increases or decreases in assets. All three ratios that were calculated improved in year 2004 over that of 2003.

Ratio	How Calculated	2004	2003
Gross Profit Margin	Gross profit/ Net revenue	NA	NA
Operating Profit Margin*	Excess of revenue over expenses/ Net revenue	$918,680/ $15,099,427= 6%	$680,844/ $13,754,077 = 4.95%
Net Profit Margin*	Increase in net assets/Net revenue	$1,242,546/ $15,099,427 = 8.2%	$948,841/ $13,754,077= 6.89%
Return on Total Assets or Return on Investment	Increase in net assets/Total assets	$1,242,546/ $15,099,427 = 8.22%	$948,841/ $13,754,077 = 6.89%
Return on Equity	Increase in net assets/Total net assets	$1,242,546/ ($16,551,340) = NA	$948,841/ (17,793,881)$ = NA

Additional Financial Ratios

One ratio that can be applied to both not-for-profit and for-profit entities is the *number of day's cash on hand*. This is the amount of cash necessary to meet actual daily cash operating expenses. This measure excludes both bad debt and depreciation expenses from operating expenses. Remember these are estimates and are a "paper and pencil" item only. They do not cause cash outflows. The calculation for this ratio follows.

$$Days \ of \ Cash \ on \ Hand = \frac{Cash + Marketable \ Securities}{(Operating \ Expenses\text{-}Bad \ Debts\text{-}Depreciation)/365}$$

One health care organization maintains 200 day's cash on hand. However, this amount is probably high for most firms. The more cash on hand, the less a firm has to invest in assets that have higher returns. A variation of the above ratio is the *cash flow coverage*. This measures how well you are able to cover required payments such as interest, rent, and debt payments. Information for calculation of this ratio would be found in the cash flow statements. Calculation of this ratio follows.

$$Cash \ Flow \ Coverage = \frac{Cash \ from \ Operations + Interest + Rent}{Interest + Rent + Debt \ Payments}$$

If the previous ratio is less than one it indicates that you are only able to make that percent of required payments. For example, if the above ratio was 0.8, you are only able to make 80 percent of required payments.

A ratio unique to not-for-profit organizations and one that only recently has been calculated is the *program service ratio*. This ratio is designed to determine what proportion of a firm's expenditures go directly into its program services (core business). This ratio is calculated by dividing program service expenses by total expenses. A firm should be spending a large proportion of its cash inflows on its mission.

$$Program \ Service \ Ratio = \frac{Program \ Services \ Expenses}{Total \ Expenses}$$

Other financial ratios that might be computed for either for-profit or not-for-profit entities are:

- Revenue per Employee–Net Revenue/Number of Employees
- Net Income per Employee–Net Income/Number of Employees
- Price Earnings Ratio–Market Price of Stock/Earning Per Common Share
- Growth Rate of Revenue–Percentage Change in Revenue from Previous Time Period

Ratios that are more applicable to not-for-profit and health care entities are:

- Percent of Deductibles–Deductibles/Gross Patient Service Revenue
- Reported Income Index–Net Income/Changes in Fund Balance
- Long-Term Debt to Fund Balance–Long-Term Debt/Fund Balance

In any of the previously calculated ratios where stockholders equity numbers were used, the not-for-profit sector would use the fund balance as a replacement number for calculations. Unique to the health care industry is the deductibles. As discussed in Chapter 13, the industry is impacted negatively by third-party payment systems. Once a claim is filed, deductions based on contracted rates are removed from the expected payment. The actual amount received will vary from amounts as low as 25 cents on the dollar to a high of around 60 cents on the dollar.

Conclusion

As with any comparisons that use ratios or common size financial statements, caution must be used. Comparisons must be made for a longer period than two years. Past results may not be indicative of future performance. Differences in management, risk aversive or risk takers, for one can affect how a firm is managed. Competition, geographic differences and others can impact operations. Nonetheless, ratios and common size comparisons can provide indications of action that needs to be undertaken. Benchmarking allows a firm to judge how well it is doing in relation to other organizations in both the same industry and in other industries. Recall that benchmarking is looking at best practices not just firms in your industry but in all firms.

PART SEVEN

Determining and Evaluating Staffing

Workload management is an integral component of hospital operations. Relying on experience, intuition, and historical usage to manage workloads is not viable in an age of plentiful information and customer expectations for value-based services. Systematic, replicable systems to track and monitor caregiver skill mix and hours of care are an expectation for effective leadership. In Chapter 19, an overview of patient classification system principles, and techniques, are presented along with the challenges of sustaining credible systems. Patient classification helps to achieve better workload management, with scheduling, recruitment, and retention. In addition the patient classification system/information can be integrated with the budgeting process/information.

Our most valuable and precious resource in health care is the staff. Chapter 20 deals with staffing effectiveness as shaped by administrative leadership, regulatory requirements, competency, and staffing/scheduling policies. Effective staffing is an ongoing process as it can always be improved. We have moved out of autocratic systems into a time when it is important that we are all in this together. Autocratic systems enhance turnover; while involving staff and encouraging self scheduling aids retention. The various care delivery models will be covered along with a discussion of nursing staff resources and ways that we can enhance those resources. Organizational, retention, recruitment, and monetary issues will also be discussed.

If we are staffing appropriately, we enhance productivity, as presented in Chapter 21. Effective productivity is a process of getting more out of what you put in. It is doing better with what you have. This chapter covers various types of productivity, and examines both organizational and individual perspectives. Efficiency and effectiveness, when used together, will enhance employee productivity. The productivity evaluation process involves four steps: to analyze environmental factors, staff factors, current staff productivity, and productivity standards, to make sure that we are achieving as much as we possibly can for patients.

CHAPTER 19

Patient Classification Systems[1]

Kathy Malloch, PhD, MBA, RN

Janelle Krueger, BS, RN

Introduction

Workload management is an integral component of hospital operations. Because nursing constitutes the majority of the work force in a hospital, nurse leaders in particular, are faced with the ever-increasing demand to assure efficient and effective service delivery. For years nurse leaders have relied on their experience, intuition, judgment, and traditions to create and justify their caregiver staffing plans. However, given the amount of clinical and financial data that is now available, the focus has necessarily shifted to managing the data to guide effective decision making, specifically evidence-based staffing. The challenge for nursing continues to escalate as the health care industry struggles with patient safety, demands for staffing ratio legislation, and increased collective bargaining units. Unfortunately, many leaders may eliminate this tool in their organizations based on the inadequacies (including lack of money) of many current systems—a choice that may have negative long-term consequences for nurse staffing. Indeed, many current patient classification systems are not valid or reliable, but nurse leaders may also be expecting more than is possible from a patient classification system—it is only one component of an effective workload management system. Before the nurse leader *trashes* a current system, it is incumbent on good leadership to review what is not working, what is needed for effective workload management, and how to get there. There is no substitute for information in an age of voluminous data.

The need for leaders to develop and sustain valid and reliable workload management tools has never been greater. Understanding of the role of the patient classification system as it relates to comprehensive workload management is an important step in this process. Relying on experience, intuition, and historical usage to manage workloads is not viable in an age of plentiful information and customer expectations for value-based services. Systematic, replicable systems to track and monitor caregiver skill mix and hours of care

---

[1] We recommend that nurse administrators share this chapter with their Chief Financial Officer and with their Chief Executive Officer–J. Dunham-Taylor and J. Pinczuk.

are an expectation for effective leadership. In this chapter, an overview of patient classification system principles, techniques, and the challenges of sustaining credible systems are discussed within the context of workload management scheduling, recruitment and retention, and budgeting processes.

Measuring Workload

Work measurement systems consist of several distinct techniques that quantify the time associated with tasks performed by workers. There are at least 25 techniques that assist in the study and measurement of work (Myers and Stewart, 2002). These techniques are used to understand the nature and true cost of work processes, and to address the ongoing challenge to reduce costs, reduce effort, and improve the working environment. Often times there is confusion between motion and time techniques in measuring work. An overview of the differing types of techniques and those with specific application in health care are presented in **Exhibit 19–1**.

Exhibit 19–1 Time and Motion Study Technique / Definitions

Time Study Techniques		Motion Study Techniques
	Health Care Applications	
Predetermined Time Standards System (PTSS) *All work is reduced to basic motions (bend, reach, walk, etc.) and each motion is reduced to a specific time value.*		Process charts
Stopwatch Time Study *Use of stopwatch to determine time required by a skilled, well trained operator working at a normal pace doing a specific task.*	Army Workload Management System for Nursing (WMSN)	Flow diagrams
Work Sampling *Randomly observing people working to determine how they spend their time and then drawing broad conclusions based on laws of probability.*	Logging Factor	Multi-activity charts
Standard Data Formula Time Standards *Catalog of standards developed from a database collected over years of study.*	DRG ICD-9 HPPD RVU RUG Prototype	Operation charts
Expert Opinion *A person with a great experience base estimates time to perform a specific job within his/her area of expertise.*	CUS (Comprehensive Unit of Service)	

The above five techniques often used in health care—motion and time study, work sampling, self reporting, standard data setting, and expert opinion—will be discussed briefly.

- *Motion and time studies* involve continuous timed observations of a single person during a typical time period or shift of work (Burke, et al., 2000). Primary tasks performed are measured by an observer for occurrences and duration of the specific activity. Motion study is for cost reduction; time study is for cost control. Motion studies focus on design, while time studies focus on measurement. Both studies create a cost consciousness that is desired by the industry. Many of the common measures, such as the NASA Task Load Index, were developed for use in aviation, particularly studies of aircrew workload, although they have also been applied elsewhere, such as the nuclear and other safety-critical industries.

  - A *motion study* is designed to determine the best way to complete a repetitive job. Examples of techniques to study motion include process charts, flow diagrams, multi-activity charts, operation charts, work station design, motion economy, and predetermined time standards system (PTSS). Workload measurement via motion and time studies has been applied to a number of military and industrial problems. Interestingly, these are not often used in health care to help identify time standards. Rather, these techniques are more often used in the process improvement area.

  - A *time study* measures how long it takes an average worker to complete a task at a normal pace. Examples of time study techniques include predetermined time standards system (PTSS), stopwatch time study, standard data formula time standards, work sampling time standards, expert opinion, and historical data time standards. In health care, using worked hours per patient day or procedures per year to budget or staff for the next year would be consistent with the standard data set approach.

- *Work sampling* is a time study technique that samples work activities at systematic or random intervals. It is the process of randomly observing people working to determine how they spend their time. The type and percentage of observations is assumed to represent the typical workload at any given point in time. It does not, however, determine the duration of a particular activity.

In health care, work sampling forms the foundation for some computerized patient classification systems. In work sampling, the caregiver's work is examined for the entire shift or event of care for a selected number of times to achieve a representative range of services. Once representative data is collected, the percentage of time spent on specific activities such as taking and recording vital signs, performing assessments, administering medications, or managing intravenous fluid therapy and discharge planning, is determined. These amounts then form the time standards for determining patient acuity on a daily basis (see **Exhibit 19–2**).

- *Self reporting* is another technique that is used to determine time associated with employee activities. Generally, the employee is asked to log the work performed using a data collection tool where start and stop times of each activity are recorded along

Exhibit 19–2 Example Patient Care Activity Groups: 8-Hour Shift

Activity / Time	Level 1	Level 2	Level 3	Average Total Minutes / Shift	% Time Spent / Shift
Vital Signs	5.0	9.5	5.0	19.5	5%
Assessments	10.0	19.0	10.0	39.0	10%
Treatments	20.0	38.0	20.0	78.0	20%
ADL's	20.0	38.0	20.0	78.0	20%
Documentation	20.0	38.0	20.0	78.0	20%
Medication Administration	15.0	28.5	15.0	58.5	15%
Teaching	5.0	9.5	5.0	19.5	5%
Other	5.0	9.5	5.0	19.5	5%
Total	100	190	100	390	100%

with a brief description of the activity. Self reporting may be subjective, but it has been shown to have high face validity (Burke, et al.).

- *Standard data setting* is a technique in which time standards are developed from past experiences. It is a common term given to any collection of time values and is defined as a catalog of elemental time standards developed from a database collected over years of motion and time study. From the factory perspective, machine names or numbers and job descriptions organize the catalog of time standards. When a new part is designed and the fabrication steps have been identified, the time study person looks up the machine in the catalogue, identifies the source of variance and area in which new measurements are needed. These time standards are specific to the environment and not readily transferable to another environment. Standard data time standards are typically the most accurate and least costly to determine.

- *Expert opinion* or *expert panel* is another technique for setting time standards. A panel of experts, individuals with a great deal of experience and ability to estimate time in their area of expertise, identifies the time requirements. The consensus approach uses professional judgment to assess staff required and provides a flexible approach that focuses on a critical review of nursing practice, staffing, and the use of both supply and demand information (Dunn, et al., 1995). Service work and one-of-a-kind jobs make setting time standards with the more traditional techniques cost prohibitive. Some workers never do the same thing twice, but goals are needed. An expert is needed to estimate every job and to maintain a log of estimates. The *best estimation* technique is a low cost, fast, and initially acceptable way of quantifying information using estimation and self-reporting techniques. The *expert opinion* technique attempts to remedy the criticism of the inability of the work sampling technique to capture professional judgment required in health care (Dunn, et al.). Because it can easily become biased and not always reflect current conditions, the expert opinion is only reliable if the results obtained approximate those results generated by experts, and the estimates are valid and reliable.

In health care, the expert panel approach has been used to create a *Comprehensive Unit of Service* as the foundational workload unit of measure (Malloch and Conovolaf, 1999). Experienced nurses create workload standards from a comprehensive perspective of the work performed; expert nurses compile the nurse interventions, provided to a patient for an entire shift or event, and identify the time required to provide this care as a unit rather than as summation of tasks. This approach integrates the multi-tasking processes of nurses and avoids the risk of double counting tasks. Typically, the expert panel consists of nurses who practice in clinical, educational, research, and administrative roles such as experienced staff nurses, clinical nurse specialists, nurse managers, and associate nurse executives. The panel of nurses collaborates to estimate the amount of time and level of caregiver (skill mix) required to provide the total care in the comprehensive unit of service.

- *The flaw of averages.* All of these techniques are difficult to use in health care where *both the worker and the work to be done are highly variable.* Health care is much different than the factory model in which the work is assembly-line mechanical and the majority of variation is within the activities of the worker. Accurate and credible motion and time standards specific to the health care worker provide an average time standard specific to a procedure. The flaw of this averaging process for health care is that the average situation may *never* occur. According to Savage (2002), the averaging process distorts accounts, undermines forecasts, and dooms apparently well thought-out projects to disappointing results. In health care staffing, average caregiver needs are often used to create monthly schedules. While this process is efficient, it may create more challenges in the long run. Consider the situation in which the average number of staff per shift is five and the range for each day of the week is three to nine on the basis of patient activity. No shift requires five staff persons; yet every day is staffed with five persons! **Exhibit 19–3** illustrates the flaw of averages.

Exhibit 19–3 The Flaw of Averages: Daily and Weekly Caregiver Staffing Requirements

S	M	T	W	T	F	S	Weekly Average
3	6	6	7	7	4	3	5.1 Caregivers

Using a range of relevant numbers, a distribution, rather than single values is more appropriate to the patient classification process. The wide range of time required for similar—but different—patient situations is often significant. The time required to determine specific time standards for the range of patient care profiles and combinations of needs in health care would be overwhelming and cost prohibitive to determine using motion, time, and standard data techniques. Given the range of capabilities of the techniques, a comparison of the advantages and disadvantages is presented in **Exhibit 19–4**.

Exhibit 19–4 Advantages and Disadvantages of Workload Measurement Techniques

Workload Measurement	Advantages	Disadvantages
Workload Measurement	Advantages	Disadvantages
Time and Motion	• Considered the gold standard in time estimation in the industrial environment. • Accuracy of time standards for selected tasks.	• High cost of one-on-one observations over extended periods. • Potential for observer-induced bias (changing participants' behavior when being observed). • Variable task difficulty / complexity of clinical testing and procedures not considered. • Multi-tasking events not considered. • Complex interactions of physical, social, ethical, emotional, and financial dimensions of patient care not incorporated.
Self-Reporting /Logging	• Simple and inexpensive. • High face validity. • Low cost. • Minimal training required.	• Inherent bias. • Participants have significant burden of reporting every activity performed in a time period.
Factor Evaluation / Subjective	• High face validity and hence acceptance by operators. • Most operators find it fairly easy to assign ratings.	• Operators can rate changing demands of a given task, but find it difficult to compare workload on qualitatively different types of tasks. • No unanimous agreement on the nature of the components of workload, and hence the set of scales that should be used. • Ability to capture the nursing process is questioned.
Work Sampling	• Experts are hired to validate time standards making validity level high. • Useful when new procedures and techniques are introduced.	• Large numbers of observations are required to obtain reasonable precision in time estimates. • Does not determine the duration of a work activity.

Standard Data	• Quick, easy to use. • Consistent and fair. • Economical.	• Data is unique to a specific company, and companies cannot normally use another's standard data.
Expert Panel	• Easy, efficient. • Can be reliable if results approximate those obtained by experts. • Low cost. • Considers uniqueness of situations.	• Easily biased. • Doesn't always reflect current conditions.
Comprehensive Unit of Service	• Incorporates impact of multi-tasking. • Relies on standardized nursing taxonomy for high validity. • Includes the dynamic complexity of human phenomenon including physical, psychological, and contextual realities.	• Requires use of expert or experienced nurses to develop comprehensive units of service of specific patient population. • Data is unique to the setting and cannot quickly be generalized to other settings. • Nurses are sometimes reluctant to give up task model for fear of not identifying work that is done.

Patient Classification Systems in Health Care

Simply stated, classification is the ordering of entities into groups or classes on the basis of their similarity, minimizing within-group variance and maximizing between-group variance (Gordon, 1998). *Patient classification* is a process of grouping patients into homogeneous, mutually exclusive groups to determine their dependency on caregivers or to determine patient acuity (Dunn, et al, 1995; Finkler, 2001). *Acuity* is defined as the level of need or dependency of an individual patient. The process of classifying patients is an element of workload management, the comprehensive system that includes patient classification, scheduling, staffing, and budgeting systems. **Exhibit 19–5** provides an overview.

Workload management system principles have their origins in scientific management, and began over 100 years ago. Much credit is given to Frederick W. Taylor, who in 1881 at the Midvale Steel Company, was determined to change the management system "so that the interests of the workmen and management should become the same, instead of antagonistic" (Barnes, 1980). Taylor argued "the greatest obstacle to harmonious cooperation between the workman and the management lay in the ignorance of management as to what really constitutes a proper day's work for a workman" (Barnes, p. 59).

Exhibit 19–5 Health Care Workload Management System Elements

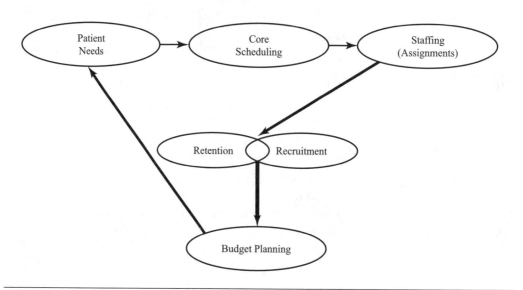

Professionals were concerned about effective workload management and focused on questions such as, "Which is the best way to do this job?" and "What should constitute a day's work?" Taylor set out to define the proper method of doing a piece of work, teaching the worker just how to perform the work that way, while maintaining stability in all conditions surrounding the work so that the worker was supported in accomplishing the tasks expected.

Not surprising, this issue exists today in most work environments. Decades later the health care industry still struggles to determine the best way to identify and to measure effective staffing resource utilization. Health care costs continue to be a persistent and growing problem for both the public and private health care funding sources. In 2001, national health expenditures increased to 14.1 percent of the GDP ($5,035 per individual) the highest ever spent on health care (Shi and Singh, 2004). Before 1965, private health insurance was the only widely available source of payment of health care, and was available primarily to middle-class working families. In 1965, Congress passed amendments to the Social Security Act creating Medicare and Medicaid programs, assuming a direct responsibility for the government to pay for some of the health care costs of two vulnerable populations: the elderly and the poor. Until October 1982, Medicare employed a retrospective cost-based reimbursement approach whereby hospitals could recover from Medicare most of what they spent for Medicare beneficiaries. Consequently, hospitals had little incentive to control costs. Medicare policy failed to constrain spending.

The behavior of health care leaders had nothing to do with any intention to diminish fiscal concern or accountability for cost issues in the provision of services; there was simply no demand for real or sustainable fiscal responsibility (Malloch, 1997). Hospitals were encouraged to acquire and to use more technology and to expand their capacity to produce a wider scope of more complex services. Caregivers were expected to give all patients the "best" of everything, to provide "rich" patient care rather than value-based care (Malloch and Porter-O'Grady, 1999). The search for a better payment system gave way to a prospective payment system in which the hospital was paid a specific amount for each patient treated, regardless of the number or types of services provided. Thus, the hospital was rewarded for reducing the cost of treating a patient over the entire course of the hospital stay. Per-case payment removed the incentive to provide more technologies and encouraged the hospital and its physicians to consider explicitly the benefits of additional services against their added costs.

This per-case payment created new challenges for the industry and did not survive due to the lack of flexibility to adjust for differences in the kinds of patients that hospitals treated. Hospitals were paid the same amount for each admission regardless of patient's clinical characteristics. Eventually, providers focused on treating patients who were less ill and avoided patients that required more resources. The challenges of health care financing reinforced the need for the industry to more clearly understand not only the types of services needed by patients, but also which caregivers could provide those services, what value or functionality would be achieved from the service, and finally what the country was willing to pay to receive these services.

These challenges have been slowly addressed beginning with the creation of classification systems to better understand patient care needs. The DRG and ICD-9 systems are examples of two classification systems, each with its advantages and disadvantages. Several other classification systems, such as the Ambulatory Payment Classification (APC), Resource Utilization Groups (RUG) and Home Health Resource Groups (HHRG), have emerged in recent years to address the need for classification of patient care needs (Shi and Singh, 2004).

The International Classification of Diseases (ICD) system is used to code and classify mortality data from death certificates. The International Classification of Diseases, Clinical Modification (ICD-9-CM) is used to code and classify morbidity data from the inpatient and outpatient records, physician offices, and most National Center for Health Statistics (NCHS) surveys. NCHS serves as the World Health Organization (WHO) Collaborating Center for the Family of International Classifications for North America and in this capacity is responsible for coordination of all official disease classification activities in the United States relating to the ICD and its use, interpretation, and periodic revision (www.cdc.gov).

Another patient classification is the Diagnosis Related Groups (DRG), which categorizes the types of patients a hospital treats (its case mix). DRGs were developed by a group of researchers at Yale University in the late 1960s as a tool to help clinicians and hospitals monitor quality of care and utilization of services. They proved to be so useful that in 1983 they became the system used by Medicare in the United States to pay hospitals. Briefly, the DRGs work by taking more than 10,000 ICD-9-CM codes and grouping them into a more manageable number of meaningful patient categories (close to 500 now). Patients within each category are similar clinically and in terms of resource usage. The groupings are based on diagnoses, procedures, age, sex, and the presence of complications or comorbidities.

Neither the DRG nor the ICD classification systems have included the fundamental work of nursing—namely the coordination of care, patient assessment, education, development of the plan of care, provision of a safe environment, and delegation and supervision of selected personnel. The challenge remains to identify the work of nursing, quantify it into health care's economic equation, and create workload management systems that assure buyers that they are getting value for their commitment of resources. Buyers want to be assured that there is some common frame of reference for clinical decisions made throughout the health system. They want to know whether there are some normative standards of clinical practice, including price, to which all providers comply; standards that can continually be validated and replicated. Further, every provider is now under the same obligation to assure that there is a connection between what one does and what is achieved; there is now a requirement that a clinical decision also be the most cost-effective choice that can be made. It is from these mandates that the continuing need for valid and reliable patient classification systems remains relevant.

Patient Classification Systems in Nursing

Historically, nursing has integrated concepts from the DRG and ICD-9 medical and disease related classifications into its own interventions and resource utilization. Because nursing lacked a common language it has been difficult to organize and include nursing terminology, work, and practice. The limitation with the DRG and ICD-9 systems is based on their ability to capture only patient diagnoses or procedures performed. These indicate only care provided and intensity/severity of illness, however, the essential work of planning, coordination, and evaluating services is not included or coded in these systems.

As knowledge development progressed and nursing diagnostic categories were identified, interest in organizing knowledge for practice, education, and research also increased. Nurses reflected on the work of Harmer (Gordon, 1998) and her efforts to classify the work of nurses. This early reference to building knowledge in nursing that supports classification is found in Bertha Harmer's *Methods and Principles of Teaching and Principles and Practice of Nursing* published in 1926 (Gordon, 1998). Harmer challenged nursing to respond to the following issues:

1. Could the organized content of nursing knowledge be identified and integrated into current systems?
2. Should nurses prescribe nursing care for each patient as doctors prescribe medical care?
3. Can the term *social diagnosis*, a term borrowed from social work, be applied to nursing?

The next significant work related to classification was when nursing theories and nursing process problem solving were introduced in the mid-20th century. Concepts of practice were emphasized and included procedures, tasks, and functions. It was in the practice milieu that Abdellah (1959) reported a classification of nursing problems based on a survey of 40 schools of nursing. Consistent with the times, the 21 problems were therapeutic problems that described the goals of the nurse, rather than health problems of the patient or family. The classification of these goals of nursing served to organize curricula and practice for many years (Gordon, 1998).

Another classification of basic, functional needs was developed by Henderson (Gordon, 1998). The components describe problem areas. Thus it is a conceptual classification into which empirical entities may be sorted. At the time no entities, such as nursing diagnoses, existed. These early classification systems and the developing theories or philosophies of nursing were influential in setting the stage for the next phase of knowledge development: diagnostic, intervention, and outcome concepts (Gordon, 1998).

In 1973, the American Nurses Association published *Standards of Nursing Practice*; the standards were followed in 1980 by *Nursing: A Social Policy Statement*, which defined nursing as the diagnosis and treatment of human responses to actual or potential health problems. In 1984 the North American Nursing Diagnosis Association (NANDA) established the conceptual framework for a nursing diagnostic classification system. This definition and taxonomy helped to establish consistent terminology, making oral and written communication easier and more efficient. In addition, definitive nursing functions were identified, and increased the nurse's accountability in assessing the patient, determining the diagnosis, and providing the treatment called for by the diagnosis.

Bulechek and McCloskey believed that the nursing process was a form of logical clinical inquiry and that the nurse made decisions about particular clinical phenomena (ANA, 1989). The nursing interventions identified and developed by the research team from the University of Iowa have become a highly regarded taxonomy for the work of nursing. Nursing intervention classifications (NIC) now represent an accepted and systemic approach to naming classes of nursing interventions, facilitating understanding, and communicating patient treatment plans. Nursing Interventions Classification (NIC) is a comprehensive, standardized language that describes treatments that nurses perform in all settings and in all specialties. NIC interventions include seven foundational domains: physiological (e.g., acid-base management), psychosocial (e.g., anxiety reduction), illness treatment (e.g., hyperglycemia management), illness prevention (e.g., fall prevention), health promotion (e.g., exercise promotion), interventions for individuals or for families (e.g., family integrity promotion), indirect care interventions (e.g., emergency cart checking), and interventions for communities (e.g., environmental management).

A standardized language for nursing provides the industry with tools to recognize the contributions and accomplishments of nursing. Using a standardized language is important in demonstrating contributions, influencing practice, and facilitating critical thinking. Nurses now have the necessary knowledge and instruments to clearly articulate the effects of their interventions on patient outcomes.

Rationale for Patient Classification Systems

Determination of manpower is dependent upon a system for assessing requirements of patients and fitting these requirements to the appropriate level of staff expertise. Nursing leaders are required to provide quantitative reports on workload allocations as well as justification on reasons for the staffing levels required. Reporting expectations of nurse leaders also includes the expectation that resources expended did indeed produce value to the patient; evidence that there is a relationship between the nursing care provided and the functionality or improvement in the patient's clinical condition.

The rationale for valid and reliable patient classification is well documented. The first of four reasons includes the need to understand the relationship between patient care needs, nursing intervention, desired outcomes, and the skill level of nurses. This prerequisite determines the appropriate type and number of caregivers and support staff needed to provide safe and effective patient care (Behner, et al, 1990; Mark and Burelson, 1995). Providing services that do not impact the outcome of patient functionality is no longer appropriate or affordable.

Second, information is needed to correlate the work of nursing and the outcomes of care. When registered nurse levels are low, nurses may not have time to provide essential education or prevention oversight of patients, or to supervise non-licensed staff. Further, there are documented relationships between registered nurse staffing and levels of medication errors, patient falls, new pressure ulcers, nosocomial pneumonia, urinary tract infections, length of stay, and unplanned readmissions (Aiken, et al., 2003; Cho, 2003; Needleman, 2002; Potter, 2003; Sasichay-Akkadech, 2003; Seago, 2001; Unruh, 2003). Given the significant costs resulting from avoidable adverse outcomes such as nosocomial pneumonia ($1,800 per infection) or pressure ulcers (up to $40,000 per pressure ulcer), the significance of valid and reliable workload management systems is not debatable (HHS Study, 2001; Kovner and Gergen, 1998; Mark and Burelson, 1995; Oerman and Huber, 1999).

Third, fixed staffing numbers (ratios) cannot be considered as remedies to improve quality patient care (Bolton, et al., 2001). Patient-to-nurse ratios identify the minimum staffing levels, while patient classification systems define the amount of staff needed for a particular situation. Ratio-staffing levels are data derived from a valid and reliable patient classification system and from knowing the range of patient care needs. Ratio data are best used in the aggregate for budgeting and scheduling, not for day-to-day staffing.

Fourth, valid and reliable systems define and defend the work of professional nursing, increase visibility of professional nursing practice, protect patients from complications, and decrease the vulnerability of nurse staffing to budget cuts. The integration of nursing science taxonomy into practice also explicates professionalism and the ethical obligations of nursing to use resources wisely while providing skilled services.

The *ANA Staffing Principles*, developed in 1999, clearly identify and support the need for empirical data to guide decision making to identify and maintain the appropriate number and skill mix of nursing staff using valid and reliable systems. The nine principles identified by an expert panel for nurse staffing include: (a) appropriate staffing levels for a patient care unit reflect analysis of individual and aggregate patient needs, (b) either retire or seriously question the usefulness of the concept of nursing hours per patient day (NHPPD), (c) unit functions necessary to support delivery of quality patient care must also be considered in determining staffing levels, (d) the specific needs of various patient populations should determine the appropriate clinical competencies required of the nurse practicing in that area, (e) registered nurses must have nursing management support and representation at both the operational level and the executive level, (f) clinical support from experienced registered nurses should be readily available to those registered nurses with less proficiency, (g) organizational policy should reflect an organizational climate that values registered nurses and other employers as strategic assets and exhibit a true commitment to filling budgeted positions in a timely manner, (h) all institutions should have documented competencies for nursing staff, including agency or supplemental traveling registered nurses, for those activities that they have been authorized to perform, and (i) organizational policies should recognize the myriad needs of both patients and nursing staff (ANA, 1999). In essence, the ANA has identified four critical factors essential in the creation of nurse staffing systems: patient characteristics, intensity of unit activity, context of care, and the expertise of caregivers.

Factor, Prototype, Relative Value Unit, and Comprehensive Unit of Service

Several techniques have been used in health care patient classification systems in an attempt to quantify the work of nursing. Most commonly, motion and time, work sampling, and standard data techniques have been used. Not surprising, varying levels of success have resulted from these endeavors. When first introduced in the 1930s, patient classification systems were based on an industrial engineering model of nurse's time and nursing tasks. Engineers believed that patient activities could be quantified by identifying the time it took nurses to complete a task related to patient care. The identified timed tasks could then be summed to identify the number of staff needed.

Over the past 60 years, system users have identified that significant variables were omitted from these historic design structures, ones necessary to accurately determine either the patient acuity or the staffing requirements (Van Slyck, 2000). To address these shortcomings, health care leaders have also integrated factor, prototype, relative values, and comprehensive unit of service concepts into traditional systems to increase validity.

- The *factor* evaluation method identifies selected elements of care, critical indicators, or tasks with associated times that are most likely predictors of nursing care needs. Individual patients are then assessed for the presence or absence of these critical indicators and based on this assessment, assigned to a category. Nursing is viewed as a series of tasks performed in a sequence. This method attempts to elicit a measure of overall workload. The factor evaluation system rates a number of indicators of care separately and then sums the ratings to designate the patient's acuity (Hasman, et al., 1993). Examples of patient conditions or nursing interventions identified as critical indicators are activities of daily living, medications, monitoring, safety needs, and complex equipment. Some factor evaluation systems include as many as 400 items for the nurse to review prior to selecting the category that most accurately matches the patient. **Exhibit 19–6** is an example of the indicators in a factor patient classification system.
- The *prototype* approach identifies the characteristics of patients in each category. Individual patients are then assigned to the category that most closely reflects their nursing care requirements. This method generally offers profiles or descriptions of patients typical of those requiring a particular type and amount of nursing care. The system, developed by Walts and Kapadi (1996) to support their staffing algorithm, is a prototype system—it classifies patients into eight categories based on required nursing

---

Exhibit 19–6 Example of Factor Patient Classification System

Circle all that apply:

Self care	Restraints	4-6 IV Medications	Neuro check q shift
Partial care	Isolation	> 6 IV Medications	Neuro check q 2 hrs
Complete bath	Wound care-simple	Telemetry monitor	Medicate for pain x3
Ambulate with assistance x2	Wound care–complex	Suction q 2 hrs.	Medicate for pain >3 times
Ambulate with two person assist x1	1 peripheral IV line	Suction > q 2 hrs	Insert foley catheter
Assistance with meals	2 peripheral IV lines	I & O q 8 hrs	Enema
Total Feed	> 2 IV lines	I & O q 1 hr	Accucheck q 4 hrs
Skin care	Oral medications	Educate patient re: diabetes	Give 1 unit of blood
Heel care	1-3 IV medications	Educate patient re: surgery	Give > 1 unit of blood

---

time. Examples of prototype profiles or descriptions include: simple or average, above average, and high or complex patient care needs. Each profile is assigned a designated number of hours for care. Typically, no skill mix differentiation is determined in the prototype method. **Exhibit 19–7** is an example of a prototype patient classification system. Unfortunately, as patients seldom fall into all of the categories in one level this approach does not allow for partial selection which often leads to inconsistent and inaccurate classification of patients.

- *Relative value unit.* In addition to grouping patients into similar categories based on nursing care needs, a patient classification system can also quantify the workload within the categories by assigning a *relative value* to each category. A relative weight is assigned to each patient category; one category is assigned arbitrarily the value of 1.0 and all other categories are assigned values in relation to it. The relative value scale is then used to describe the workload for a given unit or organization.

- The *Comprehensive Unit of Service* (CUS), developed by Malloch and Conovaloff (1999), is based on the standard data and the expert panel method. The comprehensive unit of service consists of the total care provided by nursing during a shift or event of care and integrates a multi-tasking factor to account for the overlap of care in identified patient situations. This model is designed to address the lack of sensitivity to the unique holistic nature of patients and fluctuations in economies of scale or the impact of nurses doing more than one task or process at a time. Clinical experts identify groups of interactions, activities, and tasks required by the patient on the basis of care provided. The expert nurse creates a comprehensive unit of service for the patient care situations that represent the range of patient intensity within the clinical specialty requiring a specified amount of time. Multiple comprehensive units of service are created to extrapolate time standards and skill mix for the ratings. The

Exhibit 19–7 Example of Prototype Patient Classification System: Level 1-3

	Level 1–Average Needs	Level 2–Above Average Needs	Level 3–High Needs
ADL's	Minimal Assistance	Partial Bath; Assistance with feeding	Total Care
Medications	3-8 Oral Medications	9 or more oral medications 1-3 IV medications	More than 4 IV medications
Monitoring	Routine vital signs	Telemetry monitoring	Multiple monitors; telemetry, swan and / or ICP
IV Lines / Tubes	Less than 2 lines or tubes	3-6 lines and / or tubes	More than 6 lines and tubes

expert assigns hours of care and required skill mix to each comprehensive unit of service. Patient data is then reported in hours of care and skill mix required for the patient care services rather than by levels of care or acuity category.

Note: Skill mix is defined as the percentages of each type of caregiver providing care for a particular group of patients.

For example, the skill mix for a medical unit might be 60 percent registered nurse, 25 percent licensed practical nurse, and 15 percent non-licensed caregiver. **Exhibit 19–8** is an example of a comprehensive unit of service. The clinical profile of the patient determines caregiver time and skill mix required to manage that patient.

Exhibit 19–8 Comprehensive Unit of Service Example

	Category	Caregiver Intervention	Rating
1.	Cognitive needs	1-step commands; reorient every 2 hours	2
2.	Self-Care needs	Transfer with 2 staff members; 1:1 feed; Complete bath	1
3.	Emotional/Social/ Spiritual needs	Set limits 1:1; therapeutic communication > 45 minutes; reassure every hour	2
4.	Comfort/Pain management needs	Assess /Monitor q shift; medicate x1 / shift	4
5.	Family support needs	Update family x1/shift	5
6.	Treatments	Wound care dressing change x2 / shift; 8 oral medications; 2 IV medications	3
7.	Interdisciplinary coordination needs	Coordinate 4 providers; Delegate and supervise 2 caregivers	4
8.	Transitions needs	Assess x1 / shift	5
	Time required: 3.0 hours	RN: 1.0; LPN: 1.0; NA: 1.0	

Hours as shown in **Exhibit 19–9** are aggregated to then determine the hours needed to care for all the patients on that unit.

Once the standards are established, nurses rate patients in eight categories, which represent the essence of patient care during or at the end of each shift. The hours and skill mix are generated for each patient and then summarized to identify the total unit staffing needs. Staffing hours and skill mix needed are then compared with available staff to determine adequacy of staffing or if adjustments are needed.

Exhibit 19–9 Patient Classification System: Patient Care Staffing Needs

	Patient	Clinical Profile (CUS)	Total Estimated Hours*	RN Hours	LPN/ LVN Hours	Nurse Assistant Hours
1.	Smith	3225 4335	3.50	0.5	1.00	2.00
2.	Wilson	3334 3345	2.75	0.5	0.75	1.50
3.	Murray	5434 4444	1.75	1.0	0.25	0.50
4.	Jones	3143 4434	4.50	1.0	1.50	2.00
5.	Watson	5154 3224	4.50	1.5	1.50	1.50
6.	Fox	4232 4444	2.25	0.5	0.50	1.25
7.	Michaels	4334 3345	2.75	0.5	0.75	1.50
8.	Green	3344 3345	2.75	0.5	0.75	1.50
	ENEPCS		**24.75**	**6.0**	**7.00**	**11.75**

*Total Estimated Hours and skill mix are calculated in the software and are based on the times identified by the individual organization in the Comprehensive Units of Service.

Other Units of Service/Systems

Patient care providers in areas other than the acute inpatient setting have also identified the need for systems that identify and measure staffing needs. Clinic visits, surgical procedures, deliveries, skilled nursing facilities, home health, and other procedures have been identified as service units. Specific service disciplines have identified case mix index, resource utilization groups (RUG), and home health resource groups (HHRG) as indicators for measurement. The Medicare program has adopted a case-mix method to reimburse skilled nursing facilities. This method provides a per diem prospective rate based on the acuity level of patients. The case-mix index uses the relative value unit technique and refers to the overall intensity of conditions that require medical and nursing interventions. The patient's condition is assessed and an estimate of the actual amount of resources that the patient will need is determined. The case-mix for skilled nursing facilities is driven by the minimum data set (MDS), which consists of a core set of screening elements used to assess the clinical, functional, and psychosocial needs of each resident. Using the data gained from the MDS assessment, the classification system resource utilization groups (RUG) was created to differentiate residents by their use of resources. Variables include diagnosis, functional limitations, negative health conditions, skin problems, and special treatments and procedures needed. RUG-III classifies patients into 44 categories according to their health care needs.

A relatively new classification system, home health resource groups (HHRG) uses 80 distinct groups to indicate the severity of the patient's condition. Reimbursement for episodes of home health services are bundled under one payment and adjusted based on the patient's HHRG.

Each of these models attempts to identify the qualitative aspects of clinical care and translate the care into mathematical formulations.

Essential Characteristics for a Valid and Reliable Patient Classification System

Criteria that should be considered in selecting a patient classification system to identify patient care needs for nursing include the following:

- Adequate representation of the current work of nursing,
- Use of industry standardized language,
- Inclusion of the facility geography,
- Ability to determine skill mix and staff hours required for each patient,
- Level of computerization and interface capability,
- Historical validity and reliability,
- Ability to be used with all patient care delivery models,
- Ability to identify unique patient populations of the organization,
- Ability to incorporate the caregiver's knowledge and experience, and
- Consistency with the organization's mission and vision.

Validity, Reliability, and Sensitivity of Patient Classification Systems

To be useful, the patient classification system must be credible both to nursing staff and to those outside nursing, including administrators, financial officers, and directors of health care plans. Both the validity and reliability of the system must therefore be clearly established and sustained. A valid and reliable patient classification system that defines patient care needs is the foundation of an effective workload management system.

VALIDITY

A system to determine staffing needs, typically a patient classification system, is said to have a high degree of validity when it accurately represents the work of the caregivers, correctly distributes patients among distinct classes, and defines the category of caregiver required for the care (Hernandez and O'Brien-Pallas, 1996a, b, and c). Nursing workload data must be accurate to make appropriate staffing and scheduling decisions as well as to make wise budget allocations. Accurate data cannot be obtained unless the patient classification system, the foundation of the workload management system, is both valid and reliable.

Validity of the patient classification can be described as *the degree to which it actually measures what it intends to measure*. The patient classification system is intended to measure the work of nursing. The work of nursing includes at a minimum the general categories of physiological care, behavioral support, safety measures, family education and support, coordination of care, documentation, and community integration (McCloskey and Bulechek, 2000). Validity is a matter of degree, not an all-or-none property, and the process of validation is unending (Hernandez and O'Brien-Pallas). Validity should be monitored annually and the method of assessing validity will vary with the type of classification system (Hernandez and O'Brien). Several types of validity are considered in a patient classification system, including face, content, construct, internal, and external validity. A brief description of each will be discussed.

Face validity is high when nurses believe that the system accurately reflects and represents the work that they do or the dependency of the patients for whom they provide care. Face validity is lost when the nurses do not fully understand the system or the assumptions that underlie it. If the nurse does not understand the philosophy of the system (i.e., task or process) and does not believe that the system captures all of the workload, face validity is lost and the instrument is no longer credible or usable.

Content validity is the extent to which the tool includes all of the major elements relative to the construct being measured. The evidence is typically obtained from three sources: literature, representatives from relative populations, and content experts (Burns and Grove, 2001). Most existing tools capture the procedural work of nursing but only minimally include the coordination, monitoring, and evaluation role of the professional nurse, thus resulting in a tool with less than acceptable validity.

Construct Validity is the fit between the conceptual definitions and operational definitions of variables. *Conceptual definitions* provide the basis for the definition of operational definition of variables. The measure should provide a valid inference of the construct. Does the tool measure what it claims to measure? Does the category system explain the complexity of responsibility areas and total care required (Verran, 1986)? An example is a patient assessment. The construct is the assessment and the operational definition would include those elements that comprise a nursing assessment such as body systems, psychosocial status, safety needs, family support needs, and discharge planning. Thus the tool would necessarily include items or indicators specific to the operational definition of a nursing assessment to create construct validity.

Internal validity, or the extent to which the measures used in the tool are a true reflection of reality (and not the result of extraneous variables) is another key characteristic of the patient classification tool. Internal validity of a patient classification system considers the credibility of the tool or system within the organization. Inclusion of scheduling and staffing requirements into a patient classification system diminishes the internal validity because the variables of staff competence levels, indirect support time, and /or regulatory requirements cloud the specific patient care requirement. Incorporating system requirements into the patient classification system decreases the internal validity.

External validity, or the extent to which the findings can be generalized beyond the sample used, is a critical issue for patient classification systems. While the industry is desperately seeking a measurement tool that can be used in all organizations with all patient populations and with high external validity, the achievement of this goal remains a challenge. There are some commonalities in the categories of nursing care interventions from organ-

ization to organization; there can also be significant variations in the operational definitions and processes of care for the same interventions. While the comparisons appear
appropriate, validity is uncertain until the definitions and associated time requirements are
examined. This is not to imply that some degree of external validity cannot be obtained,
but rather to note that when external comparisons of data from setting to setting are made,
the limitations to generalizations of comparability must be noted.

RELIABILITY

The *reliability* of the patient classification system tool addresses the consistency of rating. Different observers assessing the same patient at the same time should generate the
same rating. According to Finkler (2001), prototype tools are more subjective, making this
degree of reliability more difficult to achieve. Factor evaluation tools are more objective,
but their reliability depends on clear definition and consistent interpretation of the critical
indicators. Ongoing measurement of reliability is necessary and generally involves two or
more raters independently (inter-rater reliability) assessing a defined percentage of classified patients at a specified interval. Reliability scores of 100 percent (no discrepancies in
ratings) are always the target. There is disagreement about the necessary frequency for
inter-rater reliability and the number of patients to classify when doing reliability checks.
Recommended frequencies span from annually to monthly. To obtain the highest degree of
system reliability, annual review of 100 percent of system users is recommended. However,
authors agree that more frequent reliability monitoring is required if a high degree of inter-
rater reliability is not maintained (Hernandez and O'Brien, 1996a).

With prototype tools, reliability only addresses agreement of type. With the factor evaluation tools, reliability ideally is demonstrated by agreement on both patient type and individual critical indicators. Inter-rater reliability scores of less than 85 percent seriously
compromise the credibility of the system.

SENSITIVITY

Sensitivity typically refers to physiological measures and is related to the amount of
change of a parameter that can be measured precisely (Gift and Soeken, 1988). If changes
are expected to be very small, the tool must be able to detect the changes. For example,
infant scales that differentiate ounces are appropriate in the nursery. Truck scales that
measure hundreds of pounds would not be sensitive enough for the nursery. Patient classification sensitivity is about detecting those changes that determine time and type of caregiver and is a balance between estimation of time and precise time amounts. At best, the
time for patient care can only be an estimation of requirements within certain ranges
because patient events are unpredictable and patient responses to care vary. Estimates
within 15 minutes of actual time required for patient care are adequate for the complex
phenomena of patient care.

VARIANCE MANAGEMENT

Once a valid and reliable patient classification system has been created, the next process
in workload management is to compare patient classification needs for care with the actual
hours and skill mix of staff available. This essential step is often overlooked or minimized
in importance. *When this analysis is not done, the entire work of patient classification is,*

in fact, negated or at best ignored. The reality of the routine mismatch between patient care needs and available staff is an issue for the organization as a collective rather than the individual caregiver. Expecting the caregiver to *do one's best* in an impossible situation continues to fuel the flames of caregiver dissatisfaction and he or she will ultimately exit from the workforce.

Variance data for each day should be examined to determine significance and appropriate interventions. Typically, a variance is significant when the difference between required staff and available staff is greater than one-half of the length of a shift; four hours for an eight-hour shift and six hours for a twelve-hour shift. A variance is also significant if the classified hours and available staff are adequate but the skill mix available is not consistent with the classified skill mix. Existing staff can usually manage variances below one-half of a shift. When the variance exceeds one-half of a shift, the team should identify actions to manage the variance, then document and address them. Examples of variance actions include postponing or rerouting admissions, calling in additional staff, floating existing staff, reevaluating the patient acuity ratings, postponing non-emergent care, and overtime. **Exhibit 19–10** is an example of a variance management form.

Trend data for variances identifies patterns and frequency of occurrences for each patient care area as well as defines acceptable levels of variance from suggested staffing. These data are important in knowing where and when staffing problems occur and thus allowing managers to focus on fixing only problem areas rather than developing whole system changes. Analysis of aggregate variance data should be done at least quarterly and more often if significant variances are occurring. Variances specific to day of week (e.g., Mondays and Fridays may require additional labor hours due to increased admission, discharge, and transfers; or Tuesdays and Thursdays may be higher procedure days), by season (e.g., winter vs. summer), by skill mix (e.g., additional unlicensed hours needed rather than licensed hours), and by shift (e.g., additional nurse aides (NAs) needed on day shift vs. night shift) become readily apparent in this analysis.

Exhibit 19–10 Calculating the Variance: Comparison of Patient Classification and Actual Staff Hours

	Patient Classfication Hours	Actual Staffing Hours	Variance
RN Hours	28.0	36.0	+ 8.0
LP/VN Hours	30.0	24.0	- 6.0
NA Hours	35.0	24.0	- 11.0
Total	93.0	84.0	-9.0

Variance Management Actions:

_____ Control of work flow by re-routing admissions

_____ Call in additional help

_____ Staff overtime

_____ Utilize Resource Nurse

_____ Reassess patient classifications for possible over-estimation of staff needs

_____ Re-define the workload and eliminate or postpone non-essential tasks

_____ Other

Even with the best retention efforts in place, there are continuing global nursing short-ages that must be considered. Nursing is aging at twice the rate of other professions with the average hospital nurse aged 45, and by 2010, 40 percent of RNs will be over 50 years of age (Spratley, et al., 2000). While the enrollment in entry level baccalaureate programs in nursing has increased over the last three years according to the American Association of Colleges of Nursing (2002), concern still exists about the sufficiency of these increases as well as the continuing stress in the work setting. Nurses continue to describe their envi-ronment as stressful due to new technology, increased patient demands, and increased workload and overtime.

Managing the daily variances between patient care needs and available staff is but one strategy to address the shortage of nursing and will not rectify all of the challenges of staffing. Indeed, other essential long-term strategies are needed including building better communication systems between leaders and staff, new staffing patterns, flexible schedul-ing, flexible benefits, technology, new partnerships with nursing schools, and involvement in policy issues that impact patient safety and nurse staffing. These strategies are essential to address this long-standing challenge.

Putting It All Together

Using the data from a valid and reliable patient classification system is the essential data point for evidence-based staffing and scheduling. In **Exhibit 19–11**, seven steps are pre-sented to describe both the flow of data and the analysis of data as patient care needs change.

Step 1 provides summative data from a valid and reliable patient classification system and shows the associated labor costs for direct care for registered nurses, licensed practi-cal nurses, and nursing assistants. Indirect costs are factored in once direct care needs have been determined. The range of patient care needs is noteworthy because these ranges serve to guide the core scheduling process for allocation of resources on a daily basis. Step 2 dis-plays data using the projected volume and associated patient care need categories. Total salary dollars, average cost of care per patient day, total projected hours, total projected FTEs, and the average hours per patient day (HPPD) are identified in this step. In Step 3, changing patient care needs are identified and the budget is modified to reflect the changes. Step 4, includes recalculated salary dollars, average cost of care per patient day, total projected hours, total projected FTEs, and the average HPPD. Steps 5–7 present analyses of the changes in costs of care, FTEs, skill mix, and average HPPD. Prior to final-ized changes based on these data, the impact on patient care outcomes must be examined to assure optimal patient safety and desired clinical outcomes.

Exhibit 19–11 Putting It All Together: Translating Patient Classification System Data to the Annual Budget

Step 1. Patient Classification System Summary Data: Unit A 2003

	Hours			Total Hours	Cost / Job Role			Total Cost	Notes
	RN	LPN	NA		RN ($25.00/hr)	LPN ($15.00)	NA ($8.00)		
Patient Type A	1.00	1.00	1.00	2.50	$25.00	$7.50	$8.00	$40.50	Individual patient care staffing needs form the foundation for the unit budget. The patient types A–E are used to reflect common patient care needs for calculation purposes only and do not reflect the myriad patient care needs profiles that exist on patient care units. Knowing the skill mix for each patient, the range of needs as defined by hours and skill mix are essential elements for a realistic budget. In this example, hours of care range from 2.5 to 11.0 hours per patient. The average cost per patient ranges from $40.50 to $211.00 per patient.
Patient Type B	1.50	1.00	1.50	4.00	$37.50	$15.00	$12.00	$64.50	
Patient Type C	2.00	2.00	1.50	5.50	$50.00	$30.00	$12.00	$92.00	
Patient Type D	4.00	2.50	1.50	8.00	$100.00	$37.50	$12.00	$149.50	
Patient Type E	6.00	3.00	2.00	11.00	$150.00	$45.00	$16.00	$211.00	
Range of Hours / Job Role	1.0 - 6.0	0.5 - 3.0	1.0 - 2.0	2.5 - 11.0					

Step 2. Calculating the 2004 Budget: Unit A: Dollars and FTE's

	Unit Volume	Cost/ Patient	Total Cost / Patient Type	Hours	Total Hours	FTE's	Notes
Patient Type A	3,300	40.50	$133,650.00	2.50	8,250	3.97	The budget for 2004 is created based on actual patient care needs and skill mix experienced in the prior year. Calculations for total hours and dollars estimates for the 2004 budget year are based on the estimated volume of patient days (10,000) and percentages of patient care types expected by categories A through E. The range of hours (2.5 to 11.0 hours) used by skill category provides information from which to create the daily staffing plan. The total budget for RN/LPN/NA salaries for direct patient care for this unit are $782,300. The average cost of care for each patient day is $78.23. Total annual hours of care are 45,600 hours. Total FTE's are 21.92. Average HPPD are 4.56 hours. Indirect hours (e.g. unit support, employee education) are added to the core patient care needs labor budget. Typically, indirect hours range from 8-15% of the total dollars budgeted.
Patient Type B	3,500	64.50	$225,750.00	4.00	14,000	6.73	
Patient Type C	1,500	92.00	$138,000.00	5.50	8,250	3.97	
Patient Type D	1,200	149.50	$179,400.00	8.00	9,600	4.62	
Patient Type E	500	211.00	$105,500.00	11.00	5,500	2.64	
Projected Patient Days	10,000						
Total Projected Labor Cost			$782,300.00				
Average Cost / Patient Day				$78.23			
Total Projected Hours					45,600		
Total Projected FTEs						21.92	
Average HPPD						4.56	

Step 3. Patient Classification System Summary Data (Actual): Unit A 2004

	Hours			Total Hours	Cost / Job Role			Total Cost	Notes
	RN	LPN	NA		RN ($25.00/hr)	LPN ($15.00)	NA ($8.00)		
Patient Type A	1.50	0.50	1.00	3.00	$37.50	$7.50	$8.00	$53.00	The actual hours and skill mix used during the current year 2004 are then compared to the 2004 budgeted hours and skill mix.
Patient Type B	2.00	1.00	2.00	5.00	$50.00	$15.00	$16.00	$81.00	From 2003 to 2004 the range of hours of care increased from 2.50 to 11.0 to a range of 3.0 to 13.00.
Patient Type C	2.50	1.00	1.50	5.00	$62.50	$15.00	$12.00	$89.50	The range of direct salary cost per patient day increased from $40.50-$211.00 (as shown in Step 1) to $53.00-$247.50.
Patient Type D	4.50	2.00	2.00	8.50	$112.50	$30.00	$16.00	$158.50	
Patient Type E	7.00	3.50	2.50	13.00	$175.00	$52.50	$20.00	$247.50	
Range of Hours / Job Role	1.5 - 7.0	0.5 - 3.5	1.0 - 2.5	3.0 - 13.0					
Range of Cost / Job Role					$37.50 - $175.00	$7.50 - $52.50	$8.00 - $20.00		

Exhibit 19–11 Putting It All Together: Translating Patient Classification System Data to the Annual Budget (continued)

Step 4: Revising the Budget for 2005: Unit A: Dollars and FTE's

	Unit Volume	Cost/ Patient	Total Cost / Patient Type	Hours	Total Hours	FTE's	Notes
Patient Type A	3,300	37.50	$123,750.00	3.00	9,900	4.76	The 2005 hours, skill mix and dollars budget is revised to reflect the increase in patient care needs and skill mix changes.
Patient Type B	3,500	81.00	$283,500.00	5.00	17,500	8.41	The number of patient days remains the same at 10,000.
Patient Type C	1,500	104.50	$156,750.00	5.00	7,500	3.61	The budget increased 17% from $768,300.00 to $895,950. The average cost per patient day increased 17% from $76.83 to $89.60.
Patient Type D	1,200	173.50	$208,200.00	8.50	10,200	4.90	The projected hours increased 26% from 45,600 to 51,600 hours.
Patient Type E	500	247.50	$123,750.00	13.00	6,500	3.13	The total FTE's increased 24% from 21.92 to 24.81. The average HPPD increased 13% from 4.56 to 5.16.
Projected Patient Days	10,000						
Total Projected Labor Cost			$895,950.00				
Average Cost / Patient Day				$89.60			
Total Projected Hours					51,600		
Total Projected FTEs						24.81	
Average HPPD							5.16

Step 5: Analysis of Annual Hours, Dollars and Skill Mix Changes

	2003	2004	Percentage Change	Notes
Labor Cost	$768,300	$895,950	17%	From this analysis, it is concluded that both the cost and hours increased during 2004 but at differing rates. Labor cost increased 17% while total hours increased 13%. The RN % increased 27%, the LPN % decreased 15% and the NA % increased 19%.
Average Cost / Patient Day	$76.83	$89.60	17%	
Total Projected Hours	45,600	51,600	13%	
Total Projected FTEs	21.92	24.81	13%	
Average HPPD	4.56	5.16	13%	
RN hours	19,350	24,600	27%	
LPN hours	12,650	10,800	-15%	
NA hours	13,600	16,200	19%	

Exhibit 19–11 Putting It All Together: Translating Patient Classification System Data to the Annual Budget (continued)

Step 6. Skill Mix Analysis 2003

Patients	Hours					Total Hours / Skill Mix			
	RN	LPN	NA	Total		RN	LPN	NA	
3,300	1.00	0.50	1.00	2.50		3,300	1,650	3,300	8,250
3,500	1.50	1.00	1.50	4.00		5,250	3,500	5,250	14,000
1,500	2.00	2.00	1.50	5.50		3,000	3,000	2,250	8,250
1,200	4.00	2.50	1.50	8.00		4,800	3,000	1,800	9,600
500	6.00	3.00	2.00	11.00		3,000	1,500	1,000	5,500
10,000						19,350	12,650	13,600	45,600
						42.4%	27.7%	29.8%	100.0%

Notes
The skill mix is 42.4% Registered Nurse, 27.7% Licensed Practical Nurse and 29.8% Nursing Assistant.

Step 7. Skill Mix: Unit 2004

Patients	Hours					Total Hours / Skill Mix			
	RN	LPN	NA	Total		RN	LPN	NA	
3,300	1.50	0.50	1.00	3.00		4,950	1,650	3,300	9,900
3,500	2.00	1.00	2.00	5.00		7,000	3,500	7,000	17,500
1,500	2.50	1.00	1.50	5.00		3,750	1,500	2,250	7,500
1,200	4.50	2.00	2.00	8.50		5,400	2,400	2,400	10,200
500	7.00	3.50	2.50	13.00		3,500	1,750	1,250	6,500
10,000						24,600	10,800	16,200	51,600
						47.7%	20.9%	31.4%	100.0%

Notes
The skill mix for 2004 is 47.7% Registered Nurse, increased from 42.4%; 20.9% Licensed Practical Nurse, decreased from 27.7% and 31.4% Nursing Assistant, increased from 29.8%.

Threats to Valid Patient Classification Systems

Often patient classification systems lose credibility over time for reasons not readily evident. Several threats or explanations for lower validity are consistent with those identified in experimental study design (Burns and Grove, 2001). Examples include history or outdated measures in the tool, maturation or "over-familiarity" with the tool, and instrument complexity. An outdated classification system, or one that has not been reviewed in over a year, can be lower in validity if new procedures or equipment have been added to the practice area and are not included in the tool. If nurses automatically classify patients without consideration to the tool, opportunities for inaccurate ratings exist. Annual review and validation of the appropriate use of the tool is essential to assure meaningful data results. Finally, if the classification tool is too complex and requires extensive time, system users tend to misuse or to not use the tool at all, thus negating the validity of the data.

History of Misuse and Mistrust

Skepticism about patient classification systems has existed since they were introduced. With the variety of patient classification systems available and the years of trialing new and innovative ways of capturing time estimation, the nursing profession still struggles with the creation of credible workload management systems. Several sources of the patient classification system mistrust exist: low validity, misuse, failure to use the data generated, and lack of tool simplicity.

LOW VALIDITY

Task-based acuity systems do not always account for professional nursing care practices, such as patient education, interdisciplinary collaboration, family support, and delegation and supervision of other caregivers. As a result, while the system appropriately captures increasing patient severity, the assumptions used to structure staffing models are flawed (Shaha, 1995). Because much of nursing is mind-work rather than hand-work, it is not surprising that the task-based methods of some systems only capture a part of nursing work. Additionally, the effects of multi-tasking are not captured.

Patient classification systems are often developed based on mathematical assumptions of linearity and constancy. This lack of variability—with standard times allotted for each patient acuity level—assumes that the patient care needs within the category or level are constant, regardless of unit activity, staff skill mix, physical layout, or support services (DeGroot, 1994). The number of patients in each category is multiplied by the standard times to project staffing needs. The mathematically fixed nature of linear staffing models, the customary lack of objective work load data, and the lack of an explicit relationship to the staffing budget or skill mix make this type of system unreliable.

At present, there is no single agreed upon patient classification system that describes the commonly accepted nursing practice components of assessment, diagnosis, intervention, and outcomes. Because there is no agreed upon system, there are few, if any, empirical data sets to describe nursing practice across clinical settings, client populations, diagnosis-related groups, medical diagnoses, geographic areas, or time. The lack of consistent nursing language makes it extremely difficult to know with any degree of accuracy which type of patient classification system provides the most valid and reliable data for workload management decisions.

MISUSE OF THE TOOL

The most common problems with classification systems relate to a phenomenon called *acuity creep*. Acuity creep occurs when the reported acuity of patients increases slowly over time, while the actual care does not appear to change. In other words, acuity levels *creep* to higher and higher levels often to justify higher resource use by managers in affected areas. Creep becomes a problem because it assumes there is an ever-increasing need for patient care resources and labor in an industry where financial resources for such care are ever decreasing (Shaha, 1995).

The use of a system with low validity makes it difficult to distinguish inappropriate acuity creep from those changes in patient care that are real. Reimbursement changes and growth in alternative areas beyond the inpatient arena have not only changed the actual acuity of inpatients, but also changed the typical model of patient care delivery. Nurse aides, for example, were not factored into original acuity systems, but provide a significant portion of care in current inpatient and outpatient settings.

The lack of trust between administration and caregivers stems in part from the belief that patient classification systems are an attempt to decrease staffing levels. Caregivers believe that initiatives in redesigning nursing work have emphasized efficiency over patient safety. Poor communication practices between staff providing patient care and health care leaders have also led to mistrust. This loss of trust has serious implications for the ability of hospitals and other health care organizations to make the fundamental changes essential to providing safer patient care (Page, 2004).

PREDICTION VS. PLANNING

The general consensus of nurse leaders and staff nurses is that they want a patient classification system that prospectively determines the amount of staff and skill mix that will be sufficient for meeting the patient needs on the following shift. Yet the greatest frustration with staff nurses is that there is no system that can accurately predict the staffing needs for the next shift and when attempts to formulate estimations for the next shift are implemented, caregivers are quick to challenge the results.

While there is a core of expected care for the next shift, a minimum of 20 percent of the workload in most units is highly variable. New admissions, unplanned clinical condition changes, family crises, and provider rounding times make the prediction process difficult—if not impossible—without a crystal ball! The most that a patient classification system can tell you is *on average what the staffing should be based on history* (Seago, 2002). The severity of patient illness, need for specialized equipment and technology, intensity of nursing interventions required, and the complexity of clinical nursing judgment needed to design, implement, and evaluate the patient's nursing plan are often not predictable. Given the uncertainty of at least 20 percent of the work systems to provide real-time staffing must be planned for well in advance to assure that there are resources for both the planned (core) work and the unplanned work.

Patient classification data is best used to *plan* for the next shift, not *predict* staffing needs. Planning for the next shift requires not only information about the patient needs, but also information about the oncoming staff competencies, the previous similar shift staffing (yesterday's afternoon shift to compare with the upcoming afternoon shift), facility support for housekeeping, pharmacy, transportation, and teaching staff available. Only a human being—such as a clinical leader—can best determine the best staffing mix for the next shift.

TOTAL HOURS VS. SKILL MIX REQUIRED

Despite the name implying a measurement of severity of illness, patient acuity or patient classification is in truth more concerned with determining the *time* required for care; the patient acuity level is secondary information. There is indeed some correlation between acuity and amount of care required, but the correlation is not absolute. A chronic ventila-tor-dependent paraplegic may score high in severity of illness but not require a large number of care hours due to condition stability and established plans of care. Many systems do not differentiate between the two measurements, and make the leap from quality to quantity of nursing care a significant challenge. The patient classification system must identify not only the needs of the patient but also what level of caregiver is required to perform the work.

FAILURE TO USE THE DATA GENERATED

The patient classification system is typically managed by the nursing department and requires the input of staffing supervisors, unit directors, and unit staff that will be affected by the data. Financial officers and leaders of other clinical services are typically not involved in the initial design and management of nursing systems. Often times, the credibility of the data and the possibility of manipulating the data to the advantage of nursing is challenged, particularly if the data demonstrates increased workload and increased need for resources (Finkler, 2001). As a result, the fundamental trustworthiness of the system is questioned by non-nursing hospital leaders and the system is merely tolerated or ignored. System users are well aware and strongly believe that the data from the system is merely window dressing to meet regulatory requirements. In the highly litigious health care marketplace, leaders are also concerned about the liability of not reacting to the data and have legitimate concerns when systems generate data that is not used, but could negatively impact the organization. Given that a patient classification system identifies the need for five caregivers and only four are available, the question becomes whether the organization is at risk when it fails to provide the fifth nurse. These are pertinent and legitimate questions, and nursing must be prepared to respond by demonstrating reliability and a team approach to managing the variance between needs and resources.

LACK OF TOOL SIMPLICITY

To address the credibility gap, clinicians have worked to develop all-inclusive, objective lists of interventions to create a valid system. Unfortunately, these systems become lengthy and risk losing reliability very quickly. Some systems require the user to review and select 100 or more categories for each patient each shift; this process seldom results in good data. Classification systems that try to list every intervention possible within a unit become perceived as overwhelming, time consuming, and not worth the effort needed to assure accuracy. When the system cannot be easily integrated into the workflow, it is seen as *one more thing to do*, and becomes a lower priority—often getting completed only *after* the shift is over. Systems that are easily misused, mismanaged, or inaccurate generate inaccurate data that cannot be used by managers to defend their staffing decisions. The time it takes to complete the tool can also be a significant barrier in the collection of necessary data.

This conundrum of attempting to identify every intervention but doing so in an efficient manner sets the stage for mistrust in any patient classification system. The low validity achieved when nurses attempt to identify every intervention ultimately makes the product mistrusted by nursing staff, nursing leaders, financial managers, and administration. Many of the current models of patient classification systems continue to struggle with this challenge. Resolving conflicts that arise from the use of a patient classification system for staffing have often ended up at the bargaining table and in the regulatory arena (DeGroot, 1994).

Limitations: What Patient Classification Systems Cannot Do

While patient classification systems have become the primary professional vehicle for measuring patient needs and the caregiver interventions required to meet those needs, there are limitations. Given that understanding patient's needs is the primary or leading data element for an effective patient classification system, health care workers are challenged to complete this process *before* developing core schedules and daily staffing guidelines. Patient care needs must be the driver for staff schedules of hours and skill mix. Continuing to attempt to combine patient classification, scheduling, staffing, retention, and recruitment into one process serves only to decrease system validity and frustrate workers with additional unproductive tasks. Further, validity of the patient classification system is also compromised when daily staffing trends are used as primary data elements to determine patient needs. **Exhibit 19–5** illustrates the relationships among the six components in a workload management system and further illustrates the importance of the sequence of creating the elements in the workload management system. The first step is always to determine patient needs prior to creating a core schedule, the daily staffing plan, retention and recruitment plans, or the budget. The patient classification system is one component of a comprehensive workload management plan which also includes the core schedule, staffing (assigning patients to nurses), recruitment and retention efforts, and the budgeting process.

Patient Classification Systems Are Not Core Schedules

Core schedules represent the number and skill mix required for patient care and focus on having sufficient staff to care for the population served. Scheduling is the long-range plan that becomes the organization's template for the required number of staff. The schedule incorporates the organization's goals; available staff; state and national legislation; scope of practice defined by licensure, regulations, and accreditation requirements; and planned patient demand (Gardner and Gemme, 2003).

The scheduling plan also considers indirect caregiver role requirements such as the health unit secretary. Those roles that support the operations of the unit should be categorized in the *schedule* portion of the workload management plan. This time, traditionally labeled as indirect time, is defined and measured in a variety of ways in organizations. Regardless of how it is defined, indirect time must be measured consistently. Whenever possible, direct care or interventions specific to patient care that can be directly attributed to the patient, as well as daily planning, and documentation should be identified in the patient classification system. According to O'Brien-Pallas and colleagues (1997), health care leaders are challenged to examine the traditional concept of direct and indirect care and to define the main constructs that may influence nursing work. Patient care work should include work that is directly attributed to the patient whether it is at the bedside or in the conference room supporting the planning process. Support hours such as shift report, and counting supplies and medications, are typically a percentage of time, and are calculated for inclusion in the core schedule. Once patient needs are determined and validated, the department director can then determine the core staffing hours and skill levels needed to run the department efficiently and effectively.

Patient Classification Systems Are Not Daily Staffing Guidelines

Daily staffing is the real-time adjustment of the schedule based on current census, acuity, and the mix of available resources (Gardner and Gemme). To illustrate the differences in patient classification, scheduling, and staffing, consider the following scenario:

There are six patients in the intensive care unit. Assessment of patient care needs using a valid and reliable system indicates that the required staffing is one registered nurse, one licensed practical nurse, and one nursing assistant. In developing the core schedule, the manager considers federal regulations, community standards, and state licensure requirements. These standards call for one registered nurse for every two patients in the intensive care unit; thus the core schedule for this unit is a minimum of three registered nurses for six patients. Continuing with the same patient care needs, the daily staffing might need to be four registered nurses if one of the nurses is a new graduate. Thus, each component of the workload management process adds new information until the real time outcome is determined. Patient needs may be less than regulatory requirements and less than the available skill of the nurses.

Flexibility and continual daily adjustments are integral to an effective workload management system. Attempting to create and justify a core schedule based only on patient needs could compromise the organization's licensure, patient safety, and the ability to monitor and rescue patients in unstable conditions. Attempting to identify patient care needs based solely on the budget is expecting patients to conform to the resources available, and creates unrealistic staff expectations. This is not to infer that the financial resources are not essential elements of the system, but rather that the identification of patient needs is necessary to determine if the resources are adequate and if there is a gap. Dialogue about what care and service will be provided within the available resources can then begin between the care giver and payers (Malloch and Porter-O'Grady, 1999).

Patient Classification Systems Are Not Patient Care Delivery Systems

A patient classification system does not determine how care is delivered; rather it identifies what care is needed. A *patient care delivery system* is the method or system of organizing and delivering nursing care. It is the manner in which nursing care is organized to deliver the care necessary to meet the needs of the patients. The delivery system encompasses work delegation, resource utilization, communication methodologies, clinical decision making processes, and management structure (Manthey, 1991; Huber, 1996). Examples of patient care delivery models are: (1) functional nursing, (2) total patient care, (3) team nursing, (4) primary nursing, (5) case management, and (6) patient-focused care.

Typically, the nurse executive, in collaboration with key stakeholders, is responsible for establishing an overall staffing plan for the division or departments of nursing and needs to include levels of patient care needs identified in the patient classification system. The plan describes the professional practice model used in the hospital and indicates how that model supports the delivery of patient care and the environment in which care is delivered. Further, the staffing plan describes adherence to the American Nurses Association's Code of Ethics, Social Policy Statement, and Standards of Practice. The intended benefits of such a plan are: (1) improved quality of patient care, (2) positive impact on patient outcomes, (3) improved work environment, (4) increased staff satisfaction, retention, professional growth, and development, and (5) improved organizational outcomes. The amount of patient care staff, skill mix, and necessary support staff needed to assist in providing the care is adjusted based on patient needs (the daily staffing process). The staffing plan also describes the structure and process by which responsibilities for patient care are assigned and how the work is coordinated among caregivers. In addition, it describes the mechanism for documenting and reporting staffing concerns. This integrated set of processes, or the patient care delivery model, integrates data from a valid and reliable patient classification system. For example, the patient classification system will identify the required skill mix necessary to best manage the typical patients on any given unit. Trended data may identify a need for a change in the skill mix and staffing plan that incorporates the use of greater numbers of registered nurses, or greater numbers of LP/VNs and nursing assistants providing adjunctive care.

Patient Classification Systems Do Not Direct Nurse-Patient Assignments

The patient classification system identifies the specific hours of care and skill mix required by a specific patient. The system is not intended to complete or direct the process of matching caregivers with patients based on qualifications and competencies of the caregiver. The assignment of patients to specific caregivers is currently the duty of the nurse manager or staff nurse because there are multiple variables to be considered. This process includes giving consideration to: (1) the competency of caregivers, (2) yesterday's assignment (continuity of care), (3) preference of the caregiver, (4) previous shift staffing (RN follows LP/LVN), (5) pending admissions, discharges, and transfers and (6) geography of the unit, or proximity of patients to the central station. The ultimate goal is to match patients with a nurse who has the experience, qualifications, competencies, and interest required to provide the care that is needed and will support the best possible outcomes.

Assignment planning should also include time allotment for those indirect and administrative unit activities that support the operations of the unit, such as shift report, narcotic counts, and crash cart checks. Time devoted to the routine tasks needed to keep the department operating can be as much as 30 percent of the human resource time, whether there is related patient volume or not (Brady, 2001). In the Nursing Interventions Classification (NIC) taxonomy, indirect care interventions are described as treatments that direct care providers perform away from the patient but on behalf of a patient or group of patients. Administrative interventions, in comparison, are actions performed by a nurse administrator, nurse manager or middle manager, to enhance the performance of staff members to promote better patient outcomes (McCloskey and Bulechek, 2000). Failure to include time in the core schedule of the workload management system for indirect and administrative interventions can result in feelings of inadequate staffing due to an undocumented but very real variance.

Patient Classification Systems Do Not Direct the Budget; They Provide Information to Support the Process

The annual staffing budget is developed and incorporated into the hospital budget. The data collected from the workload management system provides the baseline for preparing the labor component of the nursing budget. The primary responsibility for this process belongs to the nurse executive, but nursing supervisors and unit managers are accountable for direct and worked productive hours. As part of the budgeting process, the nurse executive assures that the job description of the supervisor or unit manager includes bottom line accountability for operations, including labor expense. Resource allocation decisions begin with the assumption that the budget will be met and not exceeded.

Budgeting for staffing needs requires historical patient classification trend data. Historical data analysis also includes:

- Census comparison by unit,
- Average census by time of the day,
- Admissions, discharges and transfers by time of the day,
- Actual direct hours versus indirect hours per patient day,
- RN hours as a percent of the total hours worked,
- Education hours, orientation and training hours by unit,
- Overtime hours both scheduled and incidental,
- Unexpected absences,
- Days over and under hours per patient day (HPPD),
- Dollars per patient day ($PPD) targets, and
- Staff vacancies by unit.

The initial patient care hours estimate is adjusted for any changes in assumptions for the upcoming budget year, such as increases in expected patient volumes, new patient care programs, or equipment purchases that would impact staffing requirements, as well as decisions made based on the above analysis. It is evident that this phase cannot be achieved as planned without success at the previous levels. Failure to respect the order of the process often results in inaccurate forecasting and financial overruns.

The Patient Classification System Is Not a Recruitment or Retention Tool

The patient classification system is not a recruitment or retention tool, but can be either supportive or non-supportive of staff satisfaction. Nurse retention is positively impacted when staff believes their assignments are doable and equitable. Experiencing a sense of accomplishment at the end of a shift, and believing that appropriate care was given, enhances staff satisfaction and ultimately retention. Recruitment becomes the result of satisfied employees who share these perceptions with other potential employees. The environment is noted for its sensitivity to quality patient care and safe staffing.

Indeed, retention strategies are complex and are more directly related to a realistic workload management plan. Recognizing all elements of the workload management plan (patient classification system, staffing, scheduling, assignments, recruitment, retention, and budgeting) reinforces the environment for professional practice. The effective health care leader of today has a clear understanding of the procedural work of providers and possesses the skills to connect providers to the service and system infrastructure in such a way as to ensure value-based care is delivered within the limits of the available resources (Porter-O'Grady and Malloch, 2002). An effective plan reinforces the recommendations of the American Organization of Nurse Executive's retention strategies including: (1) setting flexible care priorities, (2) encouraging staff to exercise critical thinking skills for implementation of appropriate solutions to problems that may occur during their shifts, and (3) communicating expectations to nursing supervisors. Consistency, trust, and control of professional practice can help make even the worst of shifts go well while providing excellent patient care and strengthening retention efforts (AONE, 2003).

The Patient Classification System Is Not a Caregiver Competency Tool

A patient classification system is not a caregiver competency tool because it contains no information about the level of experience and competency of caregivers. Despite the fact that caregiver skills vary widely, caregivers continue to support *equal numbers of patients for all nurses*. Yet, nurses are reluctant to take on the challenge of identifying skill differences and assigning patients to nurses using competency criteria. A nurse is not a nurse! Nurses and health care leaders are challenged to revisit this notion and to develop systems to address the reality of variability in caregivers as well as variability in patients. There is a wide range of the levels and achievements of skill acquisition for caregivers. Incorporating the evolutionary roles of novice, advanced beginner, competent, proficient, and expert practitioners is essential to further increase the effectiveness of a workload management system. Examples of caregiver competency indicators are listed in **Exhibit 19–12**.

Admissions, Discharges, and Transfers Are Not a Part of a Patient Classification System

Finally, patient classification systems cannot manage the activity level of the unit, namely the number and frequency of admissions, discharges, and transfers (ADT). While the transfer activity factor is generated from patient activity, this data is a component of the sched-

---

Exhibit 19–12 Caregiver Competency Indicators

1. **Years of experience**
   a. In the organization
   b. In the profession
   c. In the specialty
   d. In related disciplines (LP/LVN, CNA)
2. **Certifications**
   a. ACLS/ BLS/PALS
   b. Specialty—Critical Care (CCRN), Rehabilitation (CRRN), Monitor Tech, Wound/Ostomy (WOCN and ET Nurse)
3. **Continuing education**
   a. Skills lab
   b. Course work (dialysis, chemotherapy)
   c. Inservices (internal)
   d. Workshops (external)
4. **Other**
   a. Critical thinking skills
   b. Ability to delegate effectively
   c. Manual dexterity
   d. Attitude
   e. Relationship building skills
   f. Organizational skills

---

uling plan. Failure to understand and manage unit activity or unit turbulence results in chaos and frustration of even the most organized and experienced nursing staff. Specific trend data include the results of historical data from admission, discharge, and transfer activity by day of the week and time of the day. A factor for each admission is incorporated into the core schedule to minimize unit chaos and to adequately provide needed patient care services.

It is interesting to note that some health care leaders still believe that the transfer activity is a non-issue. They believe that because staffing has been allocated for the patient being discharged, time for the admitted patient is available from the unused time of the discharged patient; it is essentially a *wash* as admissions replace discharged patients. The reality is that the admission process is significantly more intense than the discharge process and requires an additional 45 minutes of registered nurse time and 15 minutes of unlicensed time (Cavouras and McKinley, 1998). As the environment becomes less stable with frequent admissions and discharges, the patient classification system becomes less accurate at predicting workload. The notion of taking data from a population (annual data) and applying it to a single point in time (shift) means that you will be correct (or nearly so) on average (Seago, 2002). Given the current health care turnaround time and inpatient length of stay at 3.5 to 4.0 days, the need to trend and integrate this data into the core schedule is essential.

Legislative and Accrediting Agency Efforts

The health care industry's failure to create systems that manage cyclical nursing shortages and assure patient safety has led to both legislative and accrediting agency initiatives to control and monitor safe staffing. Both patients and the public are concerned about their ability to get quality health care as a result of insufficient staffing. As health care resources become more scarce, patients are finding it increasingly difficult to gain access to services. At the same time, patients and the public are concerned about the rising cost of health care. Legislators have responded by both studying the issues and enacting laws to prevent harm to patients and support safe staffing.

The first legislation related to safe staffing was developed in California in 1995, calling for institutions to develop valid staffing systems. Nevada regulations were adopted a few years later. New Jersey regulations require that licensed nurses shall provide at least 65 percent of the direct care hours (NJSNA Annual Survey, 1997; ANA, 2003).

The California Assembly Bill 394 was signed into law in 1999. This legislation requires specific standards for unlicensed assistive personnel (UAP), patient classification systems, and minimum nurse staffing ratios. Several phases of implementation were planned to enact this complex legislation. The first phase limited the use of UAPs, and became effective in January 2000. UAPs cannot be assigned to perform nursing functions in lieu of RNs in acute care facilities. These restricted functions include:

- Administration of medications,
- Venipuncture or intravenous therapy,
- Parenteral or tube feedings,
- Invasive procedures including inserting nasogastric tubes and urinary catheters,
- Tracheal suctioning,
- Assessment of patient condition,
- Education of patients and their families concerning the patient's health care problems, including post discharge,
- Moderate complexity laboratory tests, and
- Other functions requiring scientific knowledge and technical skills.

The second phase of the legislation included the provision for a patient classification system. The patient classification system must have patient indicators for severity of illness, need for specialized equipment and technology, complexity of clinical judgment needed to design, implement and evaluate the patient care plan, ability for self care, and licensure for personnel required for care. Specific requirements are defined in Title 22: 70053.2 and 70217 of California AB 394 (presented in **Exhibit 19–13**).

The last phase of the California staffing regulations requires the establishment of minimum, specific, and numerical licensed nurse-to-patient ratios by licensed classification and hospital unit for all acute care facilities. Initially, the regulations required that these minimum ratios be effective in 2003, but were delayed until 2004 because the task to establish a minimum ratio proved more challenging than originally expected. The initial ratios for medical-surgical units and mixed units are higher for the first 12 to 18 months after the law takes effect (as shown in **Exhibit 19–14**). These rules also include a provision that the staffing standards regulation be reviewed five years after adoption and any proposed changes must be reported to the legislature.

Exhibit 19–13 California Title 22: Patient Classification System Requirements
(www.calregs.com)

California Title 22: 70053.2 and 70217

1. Patient Classification System means a method for establishing staffing requirements by unit, patient and shift that include:

   a. A method to predict nursing care requirements of individual patients,

   b. An established method by which the amount of nursing care needed for each category of patient is validated for each unit and for each shift,

   c. An established method to discern trends and patterns of nursing care delivery by each unit, each shift, and each level of licensed and unlicensed staff,

   d. A mechanism by which the accuracy of the nursing care validation method described in (b) can be tested. This method will address the amount of nursing care needed by patient category and pattern of care, on an annual basis or more frequently, if warranted by the change in patient populations, skill mix of the staff, or patient care delivery model,

   e. A model to determine staff resource allocation based on nursing care requirements for each shift and each unit, and

   f. A method by which the hospital validates the reliability of the patient classification system for each unit and for each shift.

2. The hospital shall implement a patient classification system for determining nursing care needs of individual patients that reflects the assessment made by the registered nurse, of patient requirements and provides shift-by-shift staffing based on those requirements. The system developed by the hospital shall include but not be limited to the following elements:

   a. The individual patient care requirements,

   b. The patient care delivery system, and

   c. Generally accepted standards of nursing practice as well as elements reflective of the unique nature of the hospitals patient population.

3. A written staffing plan shall be developed by the administrator of nursing service or a designee, based on patient care needs determined by the patient classification system. The staffing plan shall be developed and implemented for staffing levels for registered nurses and other licensed and unlicensed personnel. The plan shall include the following:

   a. Staffing requirements as determined by the patient classification system for each unit on a day-to-day, shift-by-shift basis,

   b. The actual staff and mix provided, documented on a day-to-day-, shift-by-shift basis,

   c. The variance between required and actual staffing patterns, documented on a day-to-day, shift-by-shift basis, and

   d. The staffing plan shall be retained for the time period between licensing surveys, which includes the Consolidated Accreditation and Licensing Survey process.

4. The reliability of the patient classification system for validating staffing requirements shall be reviewed at least annually by a committee appointed by the nursing administrator to determine whether or not the system accurately measures patient care needs.

5. At least half of the members of the review committee shall be registered nurses who provide direct patient care.

Exhibit 19–13 California Title 22: Patient Classification System Requirements (www.calregs.com) (continued)

6. If the review reveals that adjustments are necessary in the patient classification system in order to assure accuracy in measuring patient care needs, such adjustments must be implemented within 30 days of that determination.

7. Hospitals shall develop and document a process by which all interested staff may provide input about the patient classification system, the system's revisions, and the overall staffing plan.

This ratio regulation requires that once the minimum number of licensed nurses has been allocated, additional staff be assigned in accordance with a documented patient classification system to determine nursing care requirements. Serious challenges have been presented as to the need for ratio legislation in light of existing patient classification system legislation. Many believe that if patient classification systems had been implemented as prescribed by Title 22, the need for ratio legislation would be redundant and wasteful of regulatory resources.

Exhibit 19–14 California Nurse to Patient Ratios (www.applications.dhs.ca.gov/regulations)

California Minimum Ratios	
Critical Care	1:2
Burn Units	1:2
Step-Down / Telemetry	1:4
General Medical Surgical	1:6, then 1:5
Specialty Care (Oncology)	1:5
Mixed Units	1:6, then 1:5
Pediatrics	1:4
Behavioral Health	1:6
Labor & Delivery	1:2
Postpartum	1:8 (1:4 couplets)
Well-Baby Nursery	1:8
Intermediate Nursery	1:4
Neonatal ICU	1:2
ER	1:4
ER: Critical Care	1:3
ER: Trauma	1:1
Operating Room	1:1
PACU	1:2

Nurses and policy makers across the United States who face similar nursing care crises are closely monitoring the impact and outcomes of California staffing legislation. Some believe the California ratio law could well become the model for the nation. In 2003, fourteen states are considering legislation pertaining to nurse staffing (CO, FL, HI, IA, IL, MA, MO, NV, NJ, NY, PA, RI, VT, and WA). Many of the bills also include guidelines identified in ANA's *Principles of Nurse Staffing* (1998) and require each patient care unit to have written staff plans based on essential items such as patient acuity, staff skill mix, patient outcomes, delivery systems, patient classification systems, and labor laws. These broad-based bills assign a numeric nurse-to-patient ratio for many specific patient care units such as pediatric recovery rooms, trauma, and psychiatric units. Strict enforcement is another hallmark of these bills. Violations can lead to any combination of the following: loss of hospital license, fines, termination of Medicaid reimbursement, private right of action, and civil penalties. As of May 2003, none of the staffing bills had passed (http://www.nursingworld.org/gova/state/2003/ratio.pdf).

Other related legislation was enacted in 1998 by Kentucky and Virginia to set appropriate staffing methodology. In 2001, Oregon enacted legislation that requires hospitals to develop and implement nurse staffing plans and to establish internal review processes. Random audits of hospitals for compliance are mandatory and failure to comply will result in civil penalties or revocation of licensure. In 2002, regulations adopted in Texas require hospitals, under the administrative authority of a chief nursing officer and in accordance with an advisory committee comprised of nurse members, to adopt, implement, and enforce a written staffing plan. This plan must be consistent with standards established by the Texas nurse licensing boards and be based upon the nursing profession's code of ethics. Patient outcomes related to nursing care will be evaluated to determine the adequacy of the staffing plan. Also in 2002, Florida passed legislation that specifies the establishment of minimum staffing standards and quality requirements for a sub-acute pediatric transition care center to be operated as a two-year pilot program.

According to Curtin (2003), there is some merit to legislatively mandated nurse-patient staffing ratios. More and more research indicates that nurse staffing has a definite and measurable impact on patient outcomes, medical errors, length of stay, nurse turnover, and patient mortality (Aiken, et al., 2003; Cho, et al., 2003; McCue, et al., 2003; Needleman, et al., 2002; Seago, 2001). Yet, the evidence for what the specific numerical ratio should be continues to vary widely. These study results suggest that the California hospital nurse staffing legislation represents a credible approach to increasing both patient safety and nurse retention. However, ratios must be modified based on the nurses' level of experience, the organization's characteristics, and the quality of clinical interactions between and among physicians, nurses, and administrators (Curtin, 2003).

Many believe that legislating staffing ratios is good for nursing (Mason, 2003). Leaders of the American Nurses Association have noted that if hospitals could be trusted to staff properly they would have done so. Proponents for staffing ratios do not believe that minimum legislated ratios will become the maximum, but rather that the best hospitals will exceed those standards and the worst will be forced to stop assigning eight or more patients to the medical-surgical nurse. Further, failing to set minimum standards will not be impossible due to the shortage; rather poor staffing is a cause of the shortage and will continue until staffing is fixed.

Opponents to staffing ratios have been equally strident about the ineffectiveness of this approach. Their belief is that nurse-patient ratios are counterproductive to evidence-based decision making and inappropriate as a staffing methodology for the complex phenomenon of patient care. Ratios assume that care is constant within each level of care, regardless of length of stay, skill mix, care delivery model, cost, competence, and unit geography. This assumption is clearly counterintuitive and contrary to what nurses tell us about patients—that they can all be very different, require very different interventions, and have a variety of holistic needs while residing within the same unit. When nursing units adopt standards that are not appropriate, a continuous cycle of unfulfilled expectations can result (DeGroot, 1994). Further, some leaders may actually lower current effective registered nurse staffing to the required minimum. Using the legislated minimum ratios is particularly ineffective in rural settings and trauma settings with wide ranges of patient care needs. The potential for *failure to rescue* patients in possible danger increases dramatically in these situations and results in unplanned negative patient consequences—consequences for which the nurse is often blamed, but which are really unavoidable because of the minimum staffing.

Ratios do not consider or recognize caregiver delegation ability, critical-thinking skills, experience, motivation, organizational skills, technical skills, or attitude. Even if the total number of care hours might be sufficient with a certain ratio, differentiation among the type of caregivers required to meet the patient needs is not identified. The fallacy of mandating licensed nurse-patient ratios rather than registered nurse-patient ratios assumes that all licensed nurses are equal—specifically, the registered nurses is the same as the licensed practical nurse. As the literature continues to recognize the improved outcomes with the use of registered nurses, staffing ratios may be of lesser value than intended. Assuming all patients are alike and all nurses are alike is an inappropriate and faulty assumption.

Even the proponents of staffing ratios mandates recognize that ratios do not resolve all the issues; hence the requirement to institute a patient classification system along with the minimum ratios. If hospitals had ensured the use of a valid and reliable patient classification system and relied on that system as a tool for determining nursing workload management, the lack of trust that historically has misaligned the credibility of staff, managers, and administration would not exist. Staffing would thus be based on patient needs rather than the need to comply with mandated ratios that are arbitrary and without empirical support. Despite the best of intentions in which legislated nurse-patient ratios were created, the complexity of staffing is yet to be addressed adequately. Competence, experience, and education all affect productivity and patient outcomes. These variables have not been addressed in legislated staffing ratios. The debate continues regarding the staffing ratio laws enacted. **Exhibit 19–15** is a synopsis of the advantages and disadvantages of staffing ratios.

The Joint Commission on Accreditation of Health Care Organizations (JCAHO) provides recommendations to organizations through standards. Current efforts to assure that staffing effectiveness is achieved using an evidence-based approach reinforces the need to enhance current practices. JCAHO standards require organizations to assess the number, competency, and skill mix of their staff by linking staffing effectiveness to clinical outcomes. This approach relies on the use of multiple clinical and human resource indicators

Exhibit 19–15 Staffing Ratios: Advantages and Disadvantages

Advantages	Disadvantages
Considers historical average patient acuity.	Does not consider the range of patient care acuity and fluctuations in daily care.
Incentives for nurses to return to the bedside.	Assumes nurses are available.
Simple to regulate specific numbers.	Minimum ratios could become maximum ratios; facilities can manipulate ratios by moving patients to units that have higher ratios when staff is not available.
Alleviates nurse stress (short term).	Do not reflect the differing skills of nurses.
Decrease the need to justify nurse staffing in the annual budgeting process.	Will force closure of hospital beds.
Increases nurse satisfaction.	Devalues the role of nurse critical thinking and judgment.
Improves patient safety / outcomes.	Assumes a manufacturing model is appropriate for patient care.
Marginally supported by evidence.	Removes staffing accountability from the organization to the government.
Nurses traditionally support equal numbers of patients assigned to each nurse, not taking acuity into account.	Patient care is widely varied in required hours and caregiver skill level.

rather than a single data element. Organizations collect and analyze data on multiple screening indicators, which are believed sensitive to staffing effectiveness such as overtime, vacancy rates, and adverse drug events. JCAHO standards do not rely on arbitrary ratios but rather emphasize the need for an ongoing informed review of staffing based on credible screening indicators (retrieved December 2, 2003 at http://www.jcaho.org).

Collective Bargaining Units

Another strategy to address safe staffing has been the use of collective bargaining. Recent changes in health care have subjected nurses to the effects of cost cutting, shuffled duties, reorganization, and the chronic nursing shortage. While only 17 percent of the nation's 2.2 million registered nurses belong to unions, labor groups are looking to nursing to boost their dwindling ranks. Two AFL-CIO affiliated unions actively pursuing nurses are the Service Employees International Union (SEIU) and the United Food and Commercial Workers Union (UFCW). There have been several instances of already formed collective bargaining units represented by the state nurses' association switching to AFL-CIO affiliated unions. The American Nurses Association (ANA) is reeling from the defections, including the defection of the 20,000 member California Nurses Association (CNA) from the ANA in 1995. California nurses believed CNA and ANA leadership did not do enough to combat layoffs and staff shortages (Jaklevic, 1999).

To assure safe staffing conditions for nurses and to correct inconsistent staffing, nurses have resorted to the collective bargaining process to address the issues. Unions have taken on the challenge to mandate organizations to provide not only adequate staffing but also to provide valid and reliable patient classification systems within their contracts. Nurses organize not only to protect themselves, but also to protect the patients under their care, as evidenced by the recent activity regarding staffing levels and acuity systems.

Coupled with the overwork and concern for patient safety, the health care industry is currently experiencing a critical shortage of nurses. As long as nurses continue to feel disenfranchised, unprotected, and under siege by doctors and health care administrators, interest in unions will grow stronger. The protection of collective bargaining and the belief that greater benefits can be extracted with an intermediary, provide a powerful force for health care workers. Increasing numbers of nurses believe that their voice in decision making can best be heard through a legally binding contract between the employer and a bargaining unit. The contract prevents arbitrary decisions by the employer and enforces the right to participate in determining wages, hours of work, standards of practice, pension and benefits, and all other terms of employment.

Given the complex nature of health care staffing and the strident nature of collective bargaining units, new and visionary partnerships between health care organizations and collective bargaining units are desperately needed. The mutuality of goals for safe staffing positions incite both groups to rise to the challenge to address this pressing need and make recommendations to modify the health care system processes and beliefs to achieve the desired goal in a way that is beneficial to both nurses and patients.

It is important to note that while membership in unions was historically focused on wages, benefits, and schedules, the emphasis is now on workload. This is similar to the recent challenge in California where the marathon contract dispute between Kaiser Permanente and the California Nurses Association (CNA) is legendary. Alleged bad-faith bargaining, poor quality of care, understaffing of licensed beds, and improper closures of facilities highlighted the discontent of nurses. In 1997 the union issued daily press releases alleging poor quality of care and cited daily instances in which Kaiser sacrificed patient welfare to save money. The issues included not only wages, but also the fight for the clout nurses wanted in setting and enforcing standards (Sherer, 1998). California nurses also wanted to be equal team members in reviewing and evaluating whether acuity systems and classification methods were effective.

At the same time, California Nurses Association (CNA) organized and led the process to enact legislation that mandated minimum nurse-to-patient ratios (Sherer, 1998). In August 1999, the tight health care labor market along with nurses' frustration with their hospitals allowed the California Nurses Association to make strong gains in organizing and collective bargaining (Moore, 1999). Further, the California Nurses Association won a 20 percent pay increase over three years, and the provisions on the joint staffing/patient acuity committees at four Columbia HCA hospitals in California. Research is increasingly available and supports the need for effective staffing systems. Collective bargaining units are using these data to support their positions and demands for safe staffing. Yet, the shortage of nurses often creates an impasse between employers and unions.

Most hospitals nationally are experiencing a nursing shortage despite a recent shift upward in enrollment trends. The number of students in the educational pipeline is still insufficient to meet the projected demand for a million new and replacement nurses over the next 10 years (AACN, 2002). Nurses in the United States consistently report that hospital nurse staffing levels are inadequate to provide safe and effective care. Physicians agree, citing inadequate nurse staffing as a major impediment to the provision of high quality hospital care. A 2002 report by JCAHO stated that the lack of nurses contributed to nearly a quarter of the unanticipated problems that result in death or injury to hospital patients.

The JCAHO report also found that the shortage of nurses might be linked to unrealistic workloads. A previous study by Aiken and others (2001) and found that 40 percent of hospital nurses have job burnout levels that exceed the norm for health care workers and that job dissatisfaction among hospital nurses is five times the average for all U.S. workers (Aiken, 2001).

In April, 2001, the Health Services Research Administration released a study that was subsequently reported in the New England Journal of Medicine. The study, *Nurse Staffing and Patient Outcomes in Hospitals*, was based on 1997 data from more than five million patient discharges from 799 hospitals in 11 states (Needleman, et al., 2002). This study found a strong and consistent relationship between nurse staffing and five outcomes in medical patients: urinary tract infection, pneumonia, shock, upper gastrointestinal bleeding, and length of stay. Staffing that had a higher number of registered nurses was also associated with a three-to-twelve percent reduction in the rate of adverse outcomes, while a higher staffing level for all types of nurses was associated with a decrease in adverse outcomes, ranging from 2 percent to 25 percent (Curtin, 2003).

Pronovost et al., in a 1999 study of organizational characteristics' effective outcomes in the intensive care units, found that high nurse patient ratios (1:3 or more) during the day were associated with a mean increase of 49 percent in the days patients spent in the ICU (Curtin, 2003, p. 3). Aiken and colleagues (2002) found an association between nurse patient ratios, mortality, and failure to rescue amongst 232,342 general, orthopaedic, and vascular surgery patients during and following their hospital discharge. The results of the study demonstrated that the odds of patient mortality increased by seven percent for every additional patient (over four) in the average nurse's workload. The same increase in odds was evident with respect to the failure to rescue rate. Additionally, nurses in hospitals with the highest patient-to-nurse ratios were more than twice as likely to experience job-related burnout and almost twice as likely to be dissatisfied with their jobs compared with nurses in the hospitals with the lowest ratios. These data cited can serve as the focal point for discussion to avoid the adversarial scenarios like the Kaiser conflict through the creation of meaningful partnerships between organizations and unions. Making decisions on the basis of evidence is the most appropriate approach to alleviating the historical tension and increasing the safety of the patient care environment.

The Future

When patients always receive exactly the care they need at the appropriate time, health care will have achieved its ultimate altruistic goal—the holistic, humanistic, and seamless integrated health care delivery system (Malloch, 1999). This lofty goal is often overwhelming and considered impossible by many in health care because of lack of predictability and uncertainty of future patient care needs. Yet, as information technology continues to advance, progress in meeting this goal is becoming more apparent.

Information systems now play a central role in providing efficient clinical services. Bedside computers and clinical information systems promise to revolutionize hospital nursing (Shi and Singh, 2004). The use of bar coding for supply charging and medication dispensing and administration, instant test result retrieval and analysis via computer systems, hand-held charting devices, transcription options, and telemedicine technology have all impacted care outcomes and the structure and processes of health care delivery. Using technology for real time matching of patient care needs with caregiver skill profiles from staffing and scheduling systems will be the focus of the next generation of patient classification systems.

The challenge is to integrate nursing informatics with engineering principles using a scientific inquiry aspect to create a better future (Huber, 1996). The engineering aspect applies technology to perform a function, or uses computers for very specific functional purposes. The scientific inquiry aspect determines the necessary data and information, and how this information should be captured, represented, processed, and stored so that it provides a realistic reflection of practice, adequate support of decision making, effective management of resources and knowledge, and sound hypothesis testing.

As the cost of health care continues to rise and public and private funding decreases, new and effective ways to control costs and monitor productivity are urgently needed. The patient classification system for nursing is one tool that is available but used sporadically and with little trust in the data produced. The nursing profession is again challenged to reshape the essence of the patient classification into a meaningful system and respected management tool to meet current marketplace demands.

A credible patient classification system provides objective information about the specific patient care allows for comparison to available staff and calculations of the cost of the care. These data provide the foundation for managing the variances between actual hours available and the required hours of care. Changing technology and procedures can be monitored more effectively, thus allowing for more timely and value-based responses. The responsibility to manage the variance appropriately will be seen as an essential function of the team rather than as an individual accountability. With staffing variances well articulated, nurse leaders will again be challenged to examine the work of nursing, prioritize that which is essential and valued, eliminate that which does not add value to the patient's outcome, and assure value to the community for resources expended.

Nursing must embrace the technology that is available today and use it to further evolve the validity and reliability of patient classification systems. Computerized systems can record the actual times of all direct and indirect nursing care activities. The next challenge is to interface documented caregiver interventions and their associated time standards with scheduling systems. Time computations and acuity ratings can be automatically calculated and updated in real time. If all activities of caregivers can be labeled and documented, the computer can capture actual activity performed for the patient. It can rapidly and automatically calculate data and determine patient needs, interventions required to meet those needs, and the time associated with those processes. Staffing can then be calculated while avoiding subjectivity and information delay (Huber, 1996). Indeed, such technology would render the calculation of staff hours and skill mix *transparent* in the process and *eliminate the need for caregivers to rate, score or select interventions in a separate process*. It would be the end of patient classification systems as we know them today!

Summary

Patient care executives need reliable management measurement tools for nursing practice. Although tools such as patient classification systems were initially developed decades ago, much work is still needed to make these tools useful and trusted. The updates to current tools reflect some of the changes in technology, care delivery, and patient populations being served, and unfortunately still result in varying degrees of success.

With the development of new approaches to patient care, new parameters with corresponding methodology to measure the resources required for that care will be essential to progress in the technological age. The measurement of patient care services has moved away from the specific cost accounting approaches popular ten years ago to the analysis of data from relational databases. Collaboration with management engineers and financial experts will be necessary to advance current systems. At the patient care and caregiver level, variance from predicted, expected, or best practices provides data needed by not only nurse executives, but also by financial officers, managed care plan administrators, and state and federal governments administering health benefits. At the service and system level, data that provides insight into cause, effect, and system interactions are more useful for improving care. At the organized delivery system level, data specific to the extent to which processes and management methods influence the quality of practice can provide new insights into resource utilization, prioritization of services, and patient safety.

Indeed, patients do benefit from appropriate staffing. Hospitals also improve their reputations, save money by avoiding costly errors and recidivism, benefit as stewards of resources, decrease turnover, and capitalize on providing the information that helps determine what is appropriate staffing (Curtin, 2003). Patient classification systems that consider holistic care delivery, the unique and specific needs of each patient, and identify skill mix and cost of labor on the basis of actual work rather than pre-set standards, will be most valid and ultimately most successful. Only valid and reliable systems integrated into the components of a workload management system will provide the evidence required to justify staffing needs and explain its relationship to patient outcomes.

References

Abdellah, F. (1959). Improving the teaching of nursing through research in patient care. In L. E. Heiderken (Ed.) *Improvement of nursing through research*. Washington, DC: Catholic University Press.

Aiken, L., Clarke, S. P., Sloane, D. M., Sochalski, J. A., Busse, R., Clarke, H., Giovannetti, P., Hunt, J., Rafferty, A. M., & Shamain, J. (2001). Nurses' reports on hospital care in five countries. *Health Affairs, 20*(3), 43–53.

Aiken, L. H., Clarke, S. P., Sloane, D. M., Sochalski, J., & Silber, J. H. (2002). Hospital nurse staffing and patient mortality, nurse burnout, and job dissatisfaction. *Journal of the American Medical Association, 288*(16), 1987–1993.

Aiken, L. H., Clarke, S. P., Cheung, R. B., Sloane, D. M., & Silber, J. (2003). Education levels of hospital nurses and surgical patient mortality. *Journal of the American Medical Association, 290*(12), 1617–1623.

American Association of Colleges of Nursing. (2002, December 20). Though Enrollments Rise at U.S. Nursing Colleges and Universities, Increase Is Insufficient to Meet the Demand for New Nurses. Retrieved December 1, 2003 from http://www.aacn.nche.edu/Media/NewsReleases/enrl02.htm.

American Nurses' Association. (1989). *Classification systems for describing nursing practice*. Kansas City, MO: Author.

American Nurses' Association. (1999). *Principles for nurse staffing with annotated bibliography*. Kansas City, MO: Author.

American Nurses' Association. (2003). *Nurse staffing plans and ratios*. Kansas City, MO: Author.

American Nurses' Association. (2003). *Workplace issues: ANA: The right choice for organized and collective bargaining*. Retrieved December 1, 2003 from http://www.nursingworld.org/dlwa/barg/.

AONE. (2003). *Talking points—Institute of Medicine Report on nurse staffing and quality of care*. November 5, 2003.

Barnes, R. M. (1980). *Motion and time study design and measurement of work*. 7th ed. Hoboken, NJ: Wiley & Sons.

Behner, K. G., Fogg, L. F., Fournier, L. C., Frankenbach, J. T., & Robertson, S. B. (1990). Nursing resource management: Analyzing the relationship between costs and quality in staffing decisions. *Health Care Management Review, 15*(4), 63–71.

Bolton, L. B., Jones, D., Aydin, C. E., Donaldson, N., Brown, D. S., Lowe, M., McFarland, P. L., & Harms, D. (2001). A response to California's mandated nursing ratios. *Journal of Nursing Scholarship, 33*(2), 179–184.

Brady & Associates. (2001). Sitting in the dark. *Organizational Effectiveness, 1*(7), 1–3.

Burke, T. A., McKee, J. R., Wilson, H. C., Donahue, R. M., Batenhorst, A. S., & Pathak, D. S. (2000). A comparison of time-and-motion and self reporting methods of work measurement. *Journal of Nursing Administration, 30*(3), 118–125.

Burns, N., & Grove, S. K. (2001). *The practice of nursing research: Conduct, critique & utilization*. 4th ed. Philadelphia: Saunders.

California Title 22: Patient Classification System Requirements. Retrieved December 20, 2003 from http://www.calregs.com.

California Nurse to Patient Ratios Retrieved December 20, 2003 from http://www.applications.dhs.ca.gov/regulations.

Cavouras, C., & McKinley, J. (1998). Annual survey of hours. *Perspectives on Staffing and Scheduling, 17*(3), 3.

Cavouras, C., & McKinley, J. (2002). Legislated nurse patient ratios: A help or hindrance to quality patient care. *Perspectives on Staffing & Scheduling, 21*(2), 3–4.

Cho, S., Ketefian, S., Barkauska, V. H., & Smith, D. H. (2003). The effects of nurse staffing on adverse events, morbidity, mortality and medical costs. *Nursing Research, 52*(2), 71–79.

Curtin, L. (2003 September). An integrated analysis of nurse staffing and related variables: Effects on patient outcomes. Online Journal of Issues in Nursing. Retrieved November 30, 2003 from http:// www.nursingworld.org/ojin/topic22/tpc22_5.htm.

DeGroot, H. A. (1994). Patient classification systems and staffing: Part 1. Problems and promise. *Journal of Nursing Administration, 24*(9), 43–51.

Dunn, M. G., Norby, R., Cournoyer, P., Hudec, S., O'Donnell, J., & Snider, M. D. (1995). Expert panel method for nurse staffing and resource management. *Journal of Nursing Administration, 25*(10), 61–67.

Finkler, S. (2001). *Budgeting concepts for nurse managers.* 3rd ed. Philadelphia: Saunders.

Gardner, A., & Gemme, E. M. (2003). Virtual scheduling: A 21st century approach to staffing. *Nursing Administration Quarterly, 27*(1), 77–82.

Gift, A. G., & Soeken, K. L. (1988). Assessment of physiologic instruments. *Heart & Lung, 17*(2), 128–133.

Gordon, M. (1998 September). Nursing nomenclature and classification system development Online Journal of Issues in Nursing. Retrieved November 19, 2003 from http://www.nursingworld.org/ ojin/tpc7/tpc7_1.htm.

Hasman, A., Wiersma, D., Halfens, R., & Algera, J. T. (1993). Evaluation of a patient classification system for community health care. *International Journal of Bio-Medical Computing, 33*, 109–118.

Hernandez, C. A., & O'Brien, P. (1996a). Validity and reliability of nursing workload measurement systems: Review of validity and reliability theory. Part 1. *Canadian Journal of Nursing Administration, 9*(3), 16–25.

Hernandez, C. A., & O'Brien, P. (1996b). Validity and reliability of nursing workload measurement systems: Review of validity and reliability theory. Part 2. *Canadian Journal of Nursing Administration, 10*(3), 16–23.

HHS. (2001). Linkages between patient outcomes and nurse staffing in hospitals. *Health Resources and Services Administration.* Rockford, MD: US Department of Health and Human Services.

Huber, D. (1996). *Leadership and nursing care management.* Philadelphia: Saunders.

Jaklevic, M. (1999). Associations join pro-union ranks: Doc, nurse organizations want to give their members a stronger voice, new services. *Modern Health Care, 29*(27), 6–14.

Joint Commission on Accreditation of Health Care Organizations. (2002). *Health Care at the Crossroads: Strategies for Addressing the Evolving Nursing Crisis.* Retrieved December 2, 2003 from www.jcaho.org.

Kirk, R. (1997). *Managing outcomes, process, and cost in a managed care environment.* Gaithersburg, MD: Aspen.

Kovner, C., & Gergen, P. (1998). Nurse staffing levels and adverse events following surgery in U.S. hospitals. *Image: The Journal of Nursing Scholarship, 30*(4), 315–321.

Malloch, K. (1997). Health care economics. In R. K. Nunnery (Ed.). *Advancing your career: Concepts of professional nursing*. Philadelphia: F.A. Davis.

Malloch, K., & Conovolof, A. J. (1999). Patient classification systems, Part 1: The third generation. *Journal of Nursing Administration, 29*(7), 49–56.

Malloch, K., & Porter-O'Grady, T. (1999). Partnership economics: Nursing's challenge in a quantum age. *Nursing Economic$, 17*(6), 299–307.

Manthey, M. (1991). Delivery systems and practice models: A dynamic balance. *Journal of Nursing Administration, 22*(11), 57–63.

Mason, D. J. (2003). How many patients are too many? Legislating staffing ratios is good for nursing. *American Journal of Nursing, 103*(11), 7.

Mark, B. A., & Burleson, D. L. (1995). Measurement of patient outcomes: Data availability and consistency across hospitals. *Journal of Nursing Administration, 25*(4), 52–59.

McCloskey, J. C., & Bulechek, G. M. (Eds.). (2000). *Nursing Interventions Classification* (NIC). 3rd ed. St. Louis: Mosby.

McCue, M. (2003). Nurse staffing, quality and financial performance. *Journal of Health Care Finance, 29*(4), 54–76.

Moore, J. (1999). Nurse union gains in California: CNA uses favorable market conditions to win pay increases, organize new units. *Modern Health Care*, Crain Communications, Inc.

Myers, F. E., & Stewart, J. R. (2002). *Motion and time study for lean manufacturing*. 3rd ed. Upper Saddle River, NJ: Prentice Hall.

New Jersey State Nursing Association (NJSNA) annual survey. (1997). *New Jersey Nurse, 27*(7), 6–7.

National Center for Health Statistics. (2003). Centers for Disease Control. Retrieved November 20, 2003 from http://www.cdc.gov/nchs/about/otheract/icd9/abticd9.htm.

Needleman, J., Buerhaus, P., Mattke, S., Stewart, M., & Zelevinsky, K. (2002). Nurse staffing levels and the quality of care in hospitals. *New England Journal of Medicine, 346*(22), 1715–1722.

O'Brien-Pallas, L., Irvine, D., Peereboom, E., & Murray, M. (1997). Measuring nursing workload: Understanding the variability. *Nursing Economic$, 15*(4), 171–182.

Oerman, M., & Huber, D. (1999). Patient outcomes–a measure of nursing's value. *American Journal of Nursing, 99*, 40–47.

Page, A. (2004). *Keeping patients safe: Transforming the work environment of nurses: Quality Chasm series*. Institute of Medicine The National Academy of Sciences. Washington, DC: National Academy Press.

Porter-O'Grady, T., & Malloch, K. (2002). *Quantum leadership: A textbook of new leadership*. Gaithersburg, MD: Aspen.

Potter, P., Barr, N., McSweeney, M., & Sledge, J. (2003). Identifying nurse staffing and patient outcome relationships: A guide for change in care delivery. *Nursing Economic$, 21*(4), 158–166.

Pronovost, P. J., Jenckes, M. W., Dorman, T., Garrett, E., Breslow, M. J., Rosenfeld, B. A., et al. (1999). Organizational characteristics of intensive care units related to outcomes of abdominal aortic surgery. *JAMA: Journal of the American Medical Association, 281*(14), 1310–1317.

Sasichay-Akkadechanunt, T., Scalzi, C. C., & Jawad, A. F. (2003). The relationships between nurse staffing and patient outcomes. *Journal of Nursing Administration, 33*(9), 478–485.

Savage, S. (2002). The flaw of averages. *Harvard Business Review, 79*(11), 20–21.

Seago, J. (2002). The California experiment: Alternatives for minimum nurse-to-patient ratios. *Journal of Nursing Administration, 32*(1), 48–58.

Seago, J. (2001). Nurse staffing, models of care delivery, and interventions. In Shojania, K. Duncan, B., McDonald, K., and Wachter, R. eds. *Making health care safer: A critical analysis of patient safety practices, evidence report/Technology assessment No. 43*. Rockville MD: AHRQ.

Shaha, S. (1995). Acuity systems and control charting. *Quality Management in Health Care, 3*(3), 22–30.

Sherer, J. (1998). Kaiser's labor pains. *Hospitals & Health Networks, 72*(8), 30–32.

Shi, L., & Singh, D. A. (2004). *Delivering health care in America: A systems approach*. 3rd ed. Sudbury, MA: Jones and Bartlett.

Spratley, E., Johnson, A., Sochalski, J., Fritz, M., & Spencer, W. (2000). *Findings from the national sample survey of registered nurses*. U.S. Department of Health and Human Services: Bureau of Health Professions Division of Nursing.

Unruh, L. (2003). The effect of LPN reductions on RN patient load. *Journal of Nursing Administration, 33*(4), 201–208.

Van Slyck, A. (2000). Patient classification systems: Not a proxy for nurse "busyness". *Nursing Administration Quarterly, 24*(4), 51–59.

Verran, J. A. (1986). Testing a classification instrument for the ambulatory care setting. *Research in Nursing and Health, 9*, 279–287.

Walts, L., & Kapadia, A. (1996). Patient classification system: An optimization approach. *Health Care Manager Review, 21*, 75–82.

CHAPTER 20

Staff—Our Most Valuable Resource

Janne Dunham-Taylor, PhD, RN

By 2010, less than half the work done in organizations will be done by full-time employees. Companies which will compete successfully for the small number of workers entering the workforce in the next 30 years will have to change the way they treat their employees. Drucker says that increasingly, employees, though paid, must be treated like volunteers. We know when dealing with volunteers:

- They must get more satisfaction from work.
- They need a challenge.
- They must know and buy into the organization's mission.
- They need continuous training.
- They have to see RESULTS (Wieck, 2000, p. 4).

Introduction

Our most valuable, precious resource in health care organizations is the staff. (The physician may be a staff member or may be a supplier, but without the staff the organization would be unable to fulfill its mission.) What a patient consistently needs in health care settings—care and treatment—is provided by the staff. The problem and richness with staffing is that people are involved. People deliver services to other people; all of whom have certain preferences, competencies, and differences. This is compounded by patient acuity and volume fluctuations; by cost or resource constraints; and by changes caused by technology developments and changing treatment protocols. The problem is that there is no "one best staffing solution." What is best in one setting or cost center may not work in another because staff have different competencies and gifts and patients' needs vary. All this presents day-to-day challenges for the nurse administrator. The nurse administrator is constantly weaving an ever-changing tapestry to achieve the best staffing outcome—*having an appropriate, safe, cost-effective, competent, committed work force present at the right times to deliver needed patient services (what the patient values) that meet quality standards.*

Staffing is such an IMPORTANT issue, yet so many times is not managed appropriately. There is nothing worse than disgruntled staff—all because the nurse manager has failed to follow certain general staffing principles as discussed in this chapter.

> ### Definition
>
> *Staffing*—Having an appropriate, safe, cost-effective, competent, committed work force present at the right times to deliver needed patient services (what the patient values) that meet quality standards.

It is easy to get involved with the day-to-day hassles of not having enough of the right staff scheduled to meet the daily patient needs. We can get so tied up with this issue that we sometimes forget our patient outcome—what the patient values delivered in a safe, cost-effective manner.

Each staff member is unique, and has certain gifts no one else possesses. In order to achieve the best staffing, each person's gifts, competencies, and work-related needs and life priorities have to be supported, nourished, and enhanced. When we do it right, all this is woven into a tapestry to produce a beautiful result. Staffing is just like quality—no matter how well it is done, there are always better ways to do it! The tapestry achieves beauty when everyone in the organization works together as a team of proactive, committed people consistently working toward this goal (Pinkerton and Rivers, 2001); and the tapestry changes as the patients and staff change. Together, all can figure out better ways to more effectively meet the patient needs.

Staff Effectiveness

> ### Definition
>
> *Staff effectiveness*—the number, competency, and skill mix of staff involved in providing effective, efficient, safe health care services that the patient's value.

This staffing definition sounds so simple. Yet implementation is very complicated, and holds many financial implications. Staffing is not simply providing a schedule for staff so they know when to show up for work. Instead, staffing must take into account staff preferences aside from the obvious—taking into account patient needs, what the patient values, and the desired patient outcomes. In fact, accrediting bodies are very concerned with staff effectiveness, defining staff effectiveness as the number, competency, and skill mix of staff involved in providing health care services, tying these factors to the patient outcomes achieved and what the patient values. The idea behind this is to aid organizations to screen for potential staffing issues and to improve patient safety. Besides this chapter, another source for evaluating staff effectiveness is in White (2000).

Staff effectiveness is further compounded by financial factors. For instance, when an *understaffing* situation occurs, it is best to choose less expensive options first. Perhaps a staff member can work the next shift and not work a scheduled shift later in the week or can work overtime. However, if staff have already been working overtime, they may be so tired that working another shift would be unsafe for the patients. Perhaps a part-time staff member could work the extra shift; or perhaps a staff member could be floated from another unit or float pool. The last resort might be to hire agency or traveler staff. It is best if there is an established staffing plan, as discussed in the next section, that specifies priorities. Otherwise, one may resort to more expensive staffing options than necessary, or, if no additional staff can be found, nurses might be forced to work short-staffed, causing staff dissatisfaction and potential safety issues.

Organizationally, it is important to ask why the understaffing situation occurred. Is it just an immediate circumstantial situation that only occasionally occurs? Or is it happening regularly? If regularly, is the staffing level inadequate? Is there a leadership problem on the unit, or within the organization? If this problem is not resolved, increased turnover will occur which spirals into more safety/legal issues, less satisfaction on the part of everyone involved, and more money being spent unnecessarily all around.

At the same time, as the patient census dips, a common practice is to give staff excused absences without pay for that shift, or to have staff float to another unit. Is there an established mechanism that clearly spells out what happens and to whom? In general, staff hate to be floated. Has cross training occurred? Do staff have a choice whether or not to float? An unpaid shift has serious implications for staff. How can one plan on a certain level of income if one might be sent home with no pay for a shift? Remember the quote at the beginning of this chapter? Is this the way we would want to be treated? Does this practice influence our loyalty to the organization?

The chaotic nature of staffing has become a huge issue for nurses. Patient acuity has been on the rise. Length of stay has decreased. "Norrish found that nurses reported patient turnover rates of 40 percent to 50 percent in a single shift. Lawrenz found similar unpredictability with the number of admissions, discharges, and transfers averaging from 25 percent to 70 percent of midnight census" (Mark, p. 240). Thus staffing might be adequate at the beginning of the shift, but insufficient later in the work day causing poorer, more expensive patient outcomes or patient safety issues.

Even today, staffing occurs on a day-to-day, or even shift-by-shift, basis with the person responsible for staffing operating from a staffing plan that exists only in his/her head based on past experience. Perceptions of staffing adequacy may therefore vary due to the varied experiences of nurses. It is also possible that the perception of what the appropriate staffing level should be on a unit may vary between those doing the staffing and the staff on a particular unit. Recent studies on perceptions of staffing adequacy (Mark, 2002) indicate several actions that nurse administrators can take to improve staff perception of staffing adequacy:

- As the unit size increases, staff are more likely to perceive staffing to be inadequate.
- As patient acuity and the number of admissions increase, it is important to increase staffing levels.
- Another source influencing staffing adequacy is that appropriate technology is available, and that staff know how to use it.

Aside from direct staffing problems, there are many contextual issues that directly impact staffing effectiveness. For instance, the Hay Group found that "when the nurse manager is viewed as an advocate, nurses perceive workloads to be more manageable. This occurs even when workload measurement is actually higher than comparable nursing units with a lower workload score" (Flannery and Grace, p. 36). Pinkerton and Rivers (2001) identified an extensive list of these issues outlined in **Exhibit 20–1**. These issues need to be considered when determining whether staffing is appropriate.

How do we know that we are staffing appropriately? Partial answers are provided in this chapter, and in other chapters such as the previous one on Patient Classification Systems. However, we need to continually assess and reevaluate staffing.

Exhibit 20–1 Understanding Contextual Variables/Factors Impacting Staffing Needs

I. Support

  A. Interdepartmental
    1. Number of support staff from other disciplines.
    2. Adequacy of support services, for example, patient transport team, volunteers.
    3. Ineffective discharge planning.
    4. Quality and/or evidence of pre-hospital patient teaching.
    5. Presence or absence of services in the hospital that support nursing care 24 hours.
    6. Increased ancillary service utilization.
    7. Quality of relationship with physician.
    8. Changes in other departments impacting nursing.
    9. Effectiveness of interdisciplinary teams.
    10. Effectiveness of communications.
    11. Accuracy and thoroughness of patient education by other disciplines.

  B. Intradepartmental
    1. Number of unit-based support staff.
    2. Number of orientees scheduled (training time).
    3. Teamwork or no teamwork/unit cohesiveness.
    4. Communication from patient to nurse (is there a person answering call light who can adequately communicate problems to nurses)?
    5. Ineffective discharge planning.
    6. Full or part-time, shift worked.
    7. Number of tasks per staff type.
    8. Health of nurse, pregnancy, work restrictions.
    9. Skill mix.
    10. Patient care modality.
    11. Consistency of patient care assignment.
    12. Staff turnover.
    13. No working preferred shift/rotating shifts.
    14. Paperwork expectation—nursing documentation.

II. Care Environment

  1. Bed turnover (combined number of admits and discharges).

  2. Environmental layout impacting efficiency.

  3. Presence of extender system (for example, tube systems, fax machines, PCs).

  4. Availability of patient safety devices (fall prevention, restraint reductions measures) or is the nurse required to have direct sight?

  5. Shift of patients from one level of care to another.

  6. Midnight census may be an outdated way of tracking work load as so many patients have early evening d/c and midnight census does not reflect work between 7 am-7 pm when most patients come and go.

  7. Medication delivery system.

  8. Having weighted factors for outpatients housed on impatient units. Most care provided in first 6 to 10 hours. If they go home at 2300 only partial credit given for intensive care.

  9. Impact of academic presence/students.

 10. Technology development: automatic blood pressure machines at bedsides, auto charting,medication dispensing, etc.

 11. User-friendly technology.

 12. Information systems: data retrieval.

 13. Information systems: order entry.

 14. Chaos factors impacting the delivery of nursing care.

III. Professional Competency.

  1. Experience level of staff, new graduates especially with diverse patient population.

  2. Organizational skills of the nurse.

  3. Delegation skills of the nurse.

  4. Level of education (degree): continuing education certifications.

  5. Charge capable (charge nurse).

  6. Philosophy and leadership style of the nursing leadership team.

  7. Participation on hospital/unit/community related activities: gets overall richer understanding of nursing.

  8. Frequency of new procedures produced (learning curve).

  9. Impact of generalist vs. specialist practice.

 10. Number of float/temporary staff.

 11. Professional attribute/professional practice model.

 12. Autonomy level of the nurse.

 13. Cultural competence/diverse composition of teams (correlate with diversity of patient population).

IV. Physician Driven

  1. Number of consultants on case (writing excessive orders and/or conflicting orders requiring confirmation re-work).

Exhibit 20–1 Cont'd

2. Number of different physician groups, with greater impact when patients are off service.
3. Variation in physician practice/medical staff rules and regulations.

V. External

1. Changes in nursing workforce.
2. Declining nurse productivity with an aging workforce.
3. Decreased commitment to suffering.
4. Aging workforce.
5. Generational differences.
6. Regulatory requirements.
7. Legal/liability for RNs.
8. Fatigue
9. Frequency and complexity of changes.

From: Pinkerton, S., and Rivers, R. (September–October, 2001). Factors influencing staffing needs. *Nursing Economic$*, 19(5), p. 237.

Regulatory Requirements

It is not uncommon for nurses to turn to the state licensing board when they have questions about "unsafe" assignments. A common response is to advise nurses to document the staffing problem with a supervisor and put their concerns in writing. From an administrative perspective, this issue should be considered with a policy and procedure to cover this eventuality. It is not appropriate to assign nurses in a situation where the administrator knows that it is unsafe because of inadequate staffing. In this case, it is necessary to make some other arrangements to cover the patients, or to divert patients to other facilities.

Regulatory issues vary depending upon the regulatory body as discussed in Chapter 2. However, there are some regulatory issues that involve nurse staffing. For instance, accrediting or licensing agencies want to see: 1) that staff are adequately credentialed and that staff are competent to do the assigned work; 2) that there are policies and procedures describing how nursing assignments are completed on a shift-by-shift basis; and 3) that the nurse staffing is adequate. As a required part of the regulatory process, the nurse administrator will need to demonstrate each of the above by using the staffing plan, plus having accurate records of actual staffing in each area for every shift.

The Patient Safety Act of 1999 (H.R. 1288/S. 966) requires Medicare providers (health care organizations) to make public information on the following:

- Number of RNs providing direct care.
- Numbers of unlicensed assistive personnel.

- Average number of patients per RN.
- Patient mortality.
- Incidence of adverse patient care incidents.
- Methods used for determining staffing levels and patient care needs (AONE Nursing Shortage, 2000).

Several states have mandated all or parts of this Act to be required for all health care organizations, even when they are not certified for Medicare.

At the state level skill mix is, or may be, governmentally mandated in the future. Some states currently require staffing ratios to be reported to the state department of health. California has implemented minimum nurse-to-patient ratios for each unit of every hospital (See Chapter 19, Patient Classification Systems). With the nursing shortage, the mandated staffing ratios have resulted in increased wages and other bonuses in order to have enough nurses to meet the requirements. The other problem is that a set staffing level does not take into account patient and staff variability and experience nor other issues that may be occurring in the environment, i.e., that rural hospitals have to traditionally have a higher level of RN staffing. Staffing ratios currently are being considered at both federal and state levels.

Competency

Part of the accreditation process for health care organizations includes validation and documentation that staff are actually credentialed (Payne, 2001), i.e., RN licenses are current, and that staff are competent to do their work. It is important to maintain records showing that nursing staff are working within the scope of practice determined by the state licensing board, meet current health requirements such as appropriate immunizations, and that staff are safe, competent practitioners.

The state licensing board sets minimum standards for nurse competency. To determine how to define competency within an organization, the American Nurses Association (ANA) suggests, "The specific needs of various patient populations should determine the appropriate clinical competencies required of the nurse practicing in that area.... All institutions should have documented competencies for nursing staff, including agency or supplemental and traveling RNs, for those activities that they have been authorized to perform" (American Nurses Association, p. 5). Other sources for establishing clinical competency are the nurses who have a great deal of experience caring for a patient population, professional nursing organizations, the literature (LaDuke, 2000; Taylor, 2000; McConnell, 2001), benchmarking, and regulatory agencies. Meretoja and Leino-Kilpi (2001) reviewed the available competency instruments and found that most measured "nurses' self-perception of competence.... It is important to have more comparative studies of nurse competence from managerial, patients,' and other health e-team members,' points of view" (p. 351). Within each organization, nurse administrators will need to determine how to measure staff competency, to document that this competency has been met, and to make appropriate educational opportunities available for staff.

Staff competency must be continually assessed and documented systematically. One system used to achieve that objective is the Performance Based Development System

(PBDS). Both reliability and validity have been reported for this system. The PBDS uses an extensive series of methods to assess employee competence, and rates the findings on a continuum that ranges from "does not meet" to "exceeds" expectations (Del Bueno, 2001).

Staffing/Scheduling Policies

As a nurse manager decides what staffing and scheduling options to use, it is helpful to have some policies. Often these are established organizational policies for such things as use of vacation time, how many staff can be on vacation at one time, how to make requests for time off, when and how to use overtime, and self-scheduling guidelines. It is important that policies enhance staffing and scheduling, as guidelines are helpful. However, too many policies can often impede creativity, and discourage someone from working for us. Instead, if we give staff more freedom to determine work time and time off, staff are more satisfied, retention greatly improves, and turnover lessens.

Resource Management System

Staffing is part of a resource management system. Ideally, a carefully planned resource management system needs to link anticipated budgetary information (discussed in Chapter 11, Budget Development and Evaluation), reliable and valid patient classification data (patient classification data is most ideal when taken directly from RN charting. Patient classification is discussed in Chapter 19) that is actually used, a staffing plan, human resource data, staff competency data, a very flexible scheduling system, actual staffing, time and attendance data, productivity data (discussed in Chapter 21, Productivity), and payroll data. There are existing computer systems that effectively accomplish this interface. For example, ANSOS [the Automated Nurse Staffing Office System] system from Per-Se Technologies—is one system. Unfortunately, there are still many organizations that do not have an integrated[1] information system in place.

The Staffing Plan

A *staffing plan* specifies how many of each category of staff are needed when the patient volume is at certain specified levels (Manthey, 2001). Ideally, if a reliable and valid patient classification system is in use, the staffing plan would be based on patient acuity. Because people within the organization do not always staff the same way, staffing plans are predetermined for better consistency. It is best if staffing plans are implemented across the organization but a plan can be developed and used on a single unit. If only used on a unit level it works best to have a closed unit. In this section we discuss the elements to consider

---

[1] In integrated information systems all the computer systems can interface with one another. It is specifically important that the nursing systems interfaces with the human resource system, with the documentation system, and with the budget system.

when establishing or evaluating a staffing plan: staff resources, skill mix, care delivery models, distribution of staff, staff recruitment and hiring practices, and cost issues.

Staffing plans are most effective when the nurse manager and nurse executive regularly evaluate the plan, particularly when significant patient or staffing issues have occurred. This evaluation process includes the effectiveness of the staffing plan, if it exists—or the need to develop a staffing plan if it does not exist. In addition, the evaluation involves other factors such as current staffing patterns; availability of staff; other staffing issues/systems such as effective scheduling; whether there is a good system in place to make sure that the right number of competent staff are there at the right time; contextual variables (Pinkerton and Rivers, 2001) that are problematic; and staff competencies with the current patient population.

> **Definition**
>
> *Staffing Plan*—a plan that specifies how many of each category of staff are needed when the patient volume is at certain specified levels.

Professional organizations provide further guidelines for this evaluation process. The American Organization of Nurse Executives' (AONE) *Perspectives on the Nursing Shortage* (2000) recommends that regular evaluation reflect the value of nursing services. "Patients, providers, payers and policymakers will demand to know that changes in health care delivery in response to the diminishing size of the nursing workforce have not adversely affected patient care" (p. 15). They stress the importance of actual quantitative data and evidence-based policies that can be used to demonstrate the quality of the care given to patients. This data "must provide a solid foundation for decisions on staffing and financing. Voluntary initiatives should incorporate:

- Collecting of nurse-sensitive indicators, especially those seeking to associate patient outcomes with care delivery models and staffing patterns.
- Collecting data on workforce supply, employment patterns and vacancy rates on an ongoing basis.
- Evaluating state practice acts to recommend policy changes that facilitate innovation in patient care.
- Working with regulatory bodies to facilitate communication between patients and health care providers within systems that cross state lines (p. 15).

The American Nurses Association (ANA), in *Principles for Nurse Staffing* (1999) drawn up by an expert panel of nurses, provides more specifics about evaluation data to be collected:

> Changes in staffing levels, including changes in the overall number and/or mix of nursing staff, should be based on analysis of standardized, nursing-sensitive indicators. The effect of these changes should be evaluated using the same criteria. Caution must be exercised in the interpretation of data related to staffing levels and patterns and patient outcomes in the absence of consistent and meaningful definitions of the variables for which data are being gathered. [Thus the following data should be used to determine staffing levels.]

- Number of patients,
- Level of intensity of the patients for whom care is being provided,
- Contextual issues including architecture and geography of the environment and available technology, and
- Level of preparation and experience of those providing care (1999, p. 5–6).

See **Exhibit 20–2**.

Exhibit 20–2 Matrix for Staffing Decision Making

Items	Elements and Definitions
Patients	Patient characteristics and number of patients for whom care is being provided
Intensity of unit and care	Individual patient intensity; across-the-unit intensity (taking into account the heterogeneity of settings); variability of care; admissions, discharges, and transfers; and volume
Context	Architecture (geographic dispersion of patients, size and layout of individual patient rooms, arrangement of entire patient care unit(s), and so forth); technology (beepers, cellular phones, computers); same unit or cluster of patients
Expertise	Learning curve for individuals and groups of nurses; staff consistency, continuity, and cohesion; cross-training; control of practice; involvement in quality improvement activities; professional expectations; preparation and experience

Reprinted by permission: American Nurses Association *Principles for Nurse Staffing with Annotated Bibliography*, 1999, p. 6.

Along with these issues ANA specifies that certain *nurse characteristics* should be taken into account when determining patient care unit staffing. These include:

- Experience with the population being served;
- Level of experience (novice to expert);
- Education and preparation, including certification;
- Language capabilities;
- Tenure on the unit;
- Level of control of practice environment;
- Degree of involvement in quality initiatives;
- Measure of immersion in activities such as nursing research that add to the body of nursing knowledge;
- Measure of involvement in interdisciplinary and collaborative activities regarding patient needs in which the nurse takes part; and

- The number and competencies of clinical and nonclinical support staff the RN must collaborate with and supervise (ANA, 1999, pp. 6–7).

In addition the following staff-related data should be analyzed:

- Work-related staff illness and injury rates (Shogren, Calkins, and Wilburn 1996);
- Turnover/vacancy rates;
- Overtime rates;
- Rate of use of supplemental staffing;
- Flexibility of human resource policies and benefit packages;
- Evidence of compliance with applicable federal, state, and local regulations; and
- Levels of nurse staff satisfaction (ANA, 1999, p. 9).

"Organizational policy should reflect a climate that values registered nurses and other employees as strategic assets, and exhibit a true commitment to filling budgeted positions in a timely manner" (Gallagher, Kany, Rowell, and Peterson, 1999, p. 50). Organizational policy needs to account for both patient and staff needs. Gallagher, et. al. suggest the following services will enable more efficient and more effective staffing:

- Effective and efficient support services (such as a laboratory, clerical support, housekeeping, and transport) to reduce time away from patient care and to decrease the need for the RN to engage in "rework;"
- Access to timely, accurate, and relevant information that links clinical, administrative, and outcome data;
- Sufficient orientation and preparation, including the availability of nurse preceptors and nurse experts to ensure RN competency;
- Preparation regarding technology used in providing patient care;
- Sufficient time to collaborate with and supervise other staff;
- Support in ethical decision making;
- Opportunity for care coordination, continuity of care arrangements, and patient and family education;
- Adequate time for coordination and supervision of unlicensed assistive personnel by RNs in order to facilitate transitions during changes in work design, mergers, and other workplace changes;
- The right of staff to report unsafe conditions or inappropriate staffing without suffering personal consequences; and
- A logical method for determining staffing levels and skill mix (p. 50).

Other aspects to take into consideration when determining who will provide appropriate, safe, and cost effective staffing include the following:

- Provide evidence-based care (see Chapters 2 and 8 for additional information);

- Have clinical specialists more involved in planning care for complicated patients;
- Be sure that staffing levels reflect all program requirements, i.e., the budget and productivity data include observation patients even though the midnight census is used to determine this data;
- Make sure that staffing accounts for specific physician practice patterns, such as extensive use of sitters for 24-hour observation of patients;
- Resolve organizational issues that impact staffing—such as no clinical pathways, never confronting physicians, or a low RN staffing ratio so patient length of stay is higher.
- Provide new technological, pharmaceutical, or genetic advancements, as well as training staff to use them;
- Ensure that ancillary nursing personnel are competent, and, when appropriate, licensed and certified;
- Have nursing personnel involved in all organizational planning and changes—as well as being aware of how patient outcomes and satisfaction are impacted by the changes;
- Effectively maximize the staff we have. This could include reevaluating: staff scheduling; the skill mix; RNs assuming professional roles; appropriate delegation; and staffing most effectively to meet the needs of the patient population; and
- Improve team work between staff members—including the physicians.

After evaluating the staffing plan, it may be necessary to change the way the staffing has been done. Various components of staffing, as well as ideas as to what might work best, are discussed in the next sections of this chapter.

Where to Find the Answers? An Ongoing Process

If a staffing plan is not already in place or needs to be evaluated, there are many approaches that nurse administrators can take to determine an effective plan. One approach, advocated by the authors, is to use an expert panel comprised of individuals who are most knowledgeable about the patient population being served (Dunn, Norby, Cournoyer, Huded, O'Donnell, and Snider, 1995). In this example, outcomes are given to the expert panel. Panel outcomes might include:

- Increase or decrease the bed capacity on each unit [or number of patients served by specific staff];
- Identify patient mix or acuity changes;
- Change staff mix;
- Shift existing resources;
- Coordinate shared resources among units;
- Obtain better support services;
- Modify the role/function of care providers;
- Explore the expanded role of volunteers;
- Decentralize or establish better utilization of float personnel; and/or

- Develop new programs or delivery systems, e.g., same-day surgery, short stay unit, primary care (pp. 65–66).

The expert panel then develops a staffing plan to meet these outcomes. The advantage of using an expert panel to develop the staffing plan is that this method involves the staff who will actually implement the plan. This panel could also annually evaluate the staffing plan.

Staff Empowerment

Staff empowerment, which is part of effective leadership (until a leader reaches Stage 4 in Hagberg's power levels, the leader is not able to empower others [see Chapter 3]), needs to occur consistently to have the best staffing outcomes. Staff need to be empowered to be creative, and must come up with solutions to the problems they face, including their schedules. After all, who knows best what needs to be done better than the staff who do it day after day? It is important that the manager encourage all to try to implement new ideas, knowing that some will succeed and some will fail. Staff may not agree on the answers, disagreements are part of this process, but if all—manager and staff—keep the patient outcome in mind, they will come up with some innovative ideas.

Brainstorm Together

Get everyone into the act! The outcome—everyone figures out ways to more creatively, and cost effectively, provide care. Have staff brainstorm together. Use some of the techniques Joyce Wycoff suggests in her book, *Mindmapping* (1991). Another excellent resource for creative ideas and ways to work with groups is *The Dance of Change* (1999), which promotes developing a learning organization. Have fun with the suggestions. Nothing is too "off the wall!" (Here's the box again. Fly through it with the suggestions!)

While brainstorming, *the only parameter is that all solutions are based on the value—what is best for the patient?* What achieves quality care yet is cost effective?

Let the ideas and solutions develop—it is an ongoing process. It involves everyone giving and receiving the care. One step at a time—a small step here, a setback, then a giant step, then another step. It often happens in uneven increments. *There is always a better way to do things!* It is like a spiral that continues to get better. (The spiral also happens with poor leadership only then things get progressively worse!)

Experiment, Experiment

After brainstorming, encourage everyone to experiment and try things. Some will work; some will bomb. Remember nothing ventured, nothing gained. We all make mistakes. But the mistakes mean that someone cared enough to try, and some of the experiments will be shining stars! As the successes occur celebrate together. What a wonderful way to establish commitment… and teamwork… and pride… and retention… and effective leadership!

What Are We Thinking?

If we are continuing here with a quantum leadership perspective, as discussed in the Leadership Chapter, we must examine our own thinking. If we think it is not possible to achieve this goal—quality services that are valued by each patient/family unit in the most cost-effective way—the first thing we need to do is to change our thinking. If we do not think something is possible, chances are it will not materialize. Instead of concentrating our thoughts on wringing our hands that there are not enough staff—after all, we don't want *that* to materialize—we need to picture that there *are* enough staff. That is a better self-fulfilling prophecy! Instead we need to think, "There is a way to do this somehow." The answer may not be forthcoming immediately, but it will come if we believe that this is possible. And the answer may come in the most unexpected way—from a chance remark from a patient or from the housekeeper!

We always need to challenge our thinking. Continually ask—and encourage all the staff to always ask—

Why do we do it this way?

Or better yet,

Is there a better way to do this?

Question everything. Why do we need an eight-hour shift or a twelve-hour shift, etc? Be creative. Get out of the box!! Isn't the bottom line that we need enough staff giving quality care in a cost-effective way?? We need to break down our own Berlin wall within our profession! Throw away set start times, shifts, positions, job descriptions, our usual ways of giving care, and even the location where we do the care. As long as the work gets done well, why let the sides of the box get in our way? We are only limited by our own minds—there are endless possibilities! Let yourself go and have some fun!

We Are All in this Together

And don't figure it all out yourself because you do not have all the answers. This book does not provide all the solutions! Heaven forbid if it did! If it did, there would be nothing new to discover!! Instead there are an infinite number of better solutions to try. Brainstorming provides the starting point. We all take it from there. And the same is true for our staffing dilemmas. With all of us working together, and with different answers emerging in different systems, we can continue to share these answers and successfully resolve our dilemmas.

And We Can Always Do It Better . . . and Better . . . and Better. . .

Whatever the reason, in times of crisis, we professionals are good with turning the situation around, drawing together, and fixing it or making it better. Now, as the nursing shortage gets worse, it is time to draw together and try new solutions to insure more effective care for our patients.

Evaluation or Development of the Staffing Plan

As the panel develops or evaluates the staffing plan, it is helpful to examine actual patient usage peaks and valleys. Ideally staff scheduling is heavier during the patient usage peaks and lighter when the valleys occur. However, if this is not occurring, the staffing plan needs to change to more accurately schedule staff when needed. For instance, perhaps the patient population has changed and the acuity and/or patient census has increased which results in a recurrent understaffing problem. This situation is discussed in more detail in the Productivity, Chapter 21. Perhaps there are not enough staff, or not enough of the right kind of staff present at the right times, to adequately staff the unit. After determining the solution, it might be necessary to develop a new budget and different staffing requirements from the average nursing hours of patient care (NHPPD–Nursing Hours Per Patient Day) needed for adequate staffing. (Chapter 11, Budget Development and Evaluation shows how to create a budget from acuity data.) A change in budget, staff mix, or better use of staff resources might result. The staffing plan specifies which staff are needed as patient volume increases and which staff do not work when patient volume decreases. Planning ahead for the peaks and valleys provides more consistency for both patients and staff.

A measurement of the patient population acuity, determined from a valid and reliable patient classification system, will provide more accurate data for the staffing plan, rather than just using census data. If patient classification system data is available, Fralic (2000) advocates creating a staffing schedule based on a slightly lower NHPPD number, (i.e., 7.3 NHPPD or 7.4 NHPPD if the actual NHPPD was 7.5) to give some flexibility to the nurse manager. Then if suddenly the average NHPPD goes above 7.5 NHPPD, a staff member could be added on a shift without going over budget. This strategy also saves money when less staffing is needed on certain shifts.

There are three problems with patient classification system data—even when valid and reliable. The first issue is that patient classification data is historical. This will improve as present documentation systems are linked with providing patient classification data so data will be available at any point in time. This capability is currently being trialed (See Chapter 19). This newer method has the advantage of not taking additional staff time.

The second problem with patient classification systems is that different systems do not agree on actual hours of care needed by the same patient. Cockerill, Pallas, Bolley, and Pink (1993) used four nursing workload measurement tools including GRASP and found "discrepancies of up to 30%… in the costs associated with caring for exactly the same patients" (Shullanberger, 2000, p. 132). Shullanberger reported 19 studies that showed discrepancies in measuring patient acuity. We still need a consistent national measurement of patient classification. However, patient classification data is the best measurement presently available.

The third problem with patient classification is that some patients require more staff time due to personality or situational issues.

If patient classification data is not available, comparative data such as benchmarking with other units serving a similar patient population can be used. Benchmarking data is available from: other health care organizations, the literature, patient classification system companies, professional organizations, or group purchasing organizations such as VHA and Premier. When benchmarking secondary data it is very important to ensure that there is data consistency (Garry, 2000; Hall, Pink, Johnson, and Scraa, 2000).[2]

Once basic staffing levels are determined, one can set up several scenarios to determine when the staffing would change as patient volume increases or decreases. When the patient volume goes below the minimum staffing level, as explained in Chapter 11 on Budget Development and Evaluation, staffing cannot be cut further and other options, such as combining services with another cost center, must be considered.

Staffing plans also need to look at a typical day. Overstaffing situations may be occurring inadvertently. For example, on an inpatient unit where everyone works 12-hour schedules with an equal number of staff on both shifts, this may not be an efficient or best use of staff FTEs. See the example in Chapter 21, Productivity.

The staffing plan must also define who is in charge during a shift. This person will provide leadership, make assignments, and deal with unusual incidents or difficult situations. This person provides the leadership on issues as they occur during a shift or for a specified length of time.

Staffing plans may need to temporarily change when new employees are hired. As the new employee is oriented, this person will not be able to take care of as many patients. If a preceptor is used, this person will need to work the same schedule as the new employee.

As a nurse administrator establishes a staffing plan it is important to have this plan reflect productive hours actually worked, as defined in Chapter 11 on Budget Development and Evaluation. It is best if the budget can reflect productive hours separately from nonproductive hours. A nurse manager can directly affect productive hours by having an effective staffing plan. It will be harder for the nurse manager to change non-productive hours as these are based on benefits given. It is generally not within the nurse manager responsibilities to change benefits. However, nurse manager leadership can affect non-productive hours. For example, when staff morale is low, staff will be more likely to take more more sick and scheduled time off. In addition, the budget should reflect appropriate non-productive hours. There are still organizations who have a budget that only covers staff productive time, so when staff are using non-productive time the unit works short!

Within the staffing plan, another important evaluation activity is to examine the nursing workload. Are there certain nursing personnel who consistently have lighter assignments? Or who seem to more easily care for the more complicated patients? The patient classification acuity data—if available—can be used to compare nursing workloads. This data can also be used for staff evaluation. If one staff member can safely care for a higher volume of patients, this staff might deserve additional merit pay. This staff member would be an excellent role model and possible mentor for other staff. Or a staff member might need to be mentored and/or counseled as to how to safely care for a higher volume of patients. Expectations or staffing standards might need to be established.

---

[2] For a staffing example using benchmark data to determine appropriate nursing workload, see Chapter 3 in Dunham-Taylor and Pinczuk (2006) *Health Care Financial Management for Nurse Managers: Applications From Hospitals, Long-Term Care, Home Care, and Ambulatory Care.*

Are nursing workloads reasonable with the right staff mix? This should be evaluated periodically as patient safety issues can result if RN workloads are too heavy.

Other factors can affect staffing plans. For instance, staff shortages could occur, or cost issues might arise, necessitating a change in the staffing plan. As these factors occur, reevaluation of the current staffing plan, of the number of patients that can be safely cared for, and of unit configurations may need to be reexamined.

Samples of staffing plans are included in *Health Care Financial Management for Nurse Managers: Financial Applications in Hospitals, Long-Term Care, Home Care, and Ambulatory Care* (Dunham-Taylor and Pinczuk, [2006]). There are several staffing plans in the literature (Strickland and Neely, 1995; Schmidt, 1999; Douglas and Mayewshy, 1996; Fralic, 2000). One is reported by Hollabaugh and Kendrick (1998) at Good Samaritan Regional Medical Center in Arizona. They developed a five-level pyramid to staff for peak times (winter) as well as low census/acuity times (summer), a hiring plan for the varying census times, and a more equitable cancellation policy. This plan achieved cost savings, more continuity and job satisfaction, fewer patient and physician complaints as well as establishing a more effective way to adequately staff despite large variations in census.

Nursing Staff Skill Mix

An important factor in determining appropriate staffing is the *nursing staff skill mix*, the various types of nursing staff by job classification necessary to care for the patient population being served. To determine the skill mix one should ask several questions: How do we deliver the care? Who is best to deliver the care? How is the care divided amongst the various caregivers? What skill mix provides the safest care? Which is cost

> **Definition**
>
> *Nursing Staff Skill Mix*—the various types of nursing staff by job classification necessary to care for the patient population being served.

effective? Unfortunately there is no ideal answer. What works best in one setting, (i.e., in a stepdown unit), may not be best in another, (i.e., a skilled unit). And the answer to any one of these questions may depend upon current circumstances such as patient acuity, turnover of patients, discharges pushed to Fridays, admissions arriving on the evening shift, staff competencies or availability, or budget deficits. So skill mix is partially determined by current circumstances and must change to meet new situations as they occur.

As a rule of thumb, areas where there are a lot of admissions, discharges, and transfers generally need a higher RN ratio to do the necessary assessment. Rural hospital staffing also has a greater number of RNs because patient needs widely differ.

One fallacy that can occur is that RNs are more expensive than unlicensed nursing staff. On the surface one might think RNs are expensive because their salaries are higher than LPNs and aides. But is this really the case? Research is beginning to refute this notion (McClung, 2000). Melberg (1997) shows that a hospital budget with a 96 percent RN staff mix is less expensive than another hospital budget with a 64 percent RN mix. In fact, the hospital with the highest costs had the lowest RN skill mix (64 percent).

> A high RN mix [96 percent] does not correlate with higher nursing costs per patient day in acute or critical care. Diluting the RN mix does not always reduce staffing costs. Although hospital A has a 96 percent RN-skill mix, the highest in the system, total nursing salary per patient day falls exactly in the middle. The highest costs occurred at hospital C where, in fact, the 64 percent RN mix is the lowest in the system. This finding is consistent in acute care, in critical care and on the orthopedic units, specialty nursing areas found in all five hospitals and therefore used for comparison. This difference is not explained by regional variations in RN salary, since RN salary at hospital A during the period of study was higher than at any hospital in the system except hospital E (p. 48).

One advantage noted with the high RN mix was that less time was needed to communicate with less skilled workers. RNs save patient care costs in other ways. RNs possess an extensive knowledge base and assessment capability that places them in a position of significance to the patient. Outcomes research so far is showing that a higher RN skill mix results in lower length of stay, and fewer complications, safety, and legal issues (ANA, 1997; ANA, 2000; Blegen and Goode, 1997; Melberg, 1997; Bliesmer, Smayling, Kane, and Shannon, 1998; Blegen, Goode, and Reed, 1998; Blegen and Vaughn, 1998; Kerr, 2000; Shullanberger, 2000; Blegen, Vaughn, and Goode, 2001; Bolton, et al., 2001; Hendrix and Foreman, 2001; Needleman, 2001; Aiken, Clarke, Sloane, Sochalski, and Silber, 2002; Aiken, Clarke, Cheung, Sloane, and Silber, 2003).

Research linking RN skill mix with patient outcomes has been an exciting ongoing process with more information becoming available each month. To date these studies are finding that higher RN ratios make a big difference in the quality of patient care. This started with ANA's *Implementing Nursing's Report Card*, followed by ANA's *Nursing Staffing and Patient Outcomes: In the Inpatient Hospital Setting* (2000). This last study used data from nine states—using all-payer data sets (9.1 million patients in almost 1,000 hospitals) for six states (Arizona, California, Florida, Massachusetts, New York, and Virginia) and just using a Medicare sample (3.8 million patients in more than 1,500 hospitals) for an additional three states (Minnesota, North Dakota, and Texas). As nurse staffing increased, the outcomes—length of stay, pneumonia, postoperative infections, pressure ulcers, and urinary tract infections—decreased. There was close congruence between data from each hospital regardless of payer mix.

Additional skill mix/outcome research has followed:

- Blegen and Goode (1997) found that when there were more RNs proportionately, medication errors decreased as did respiratory and urinary tract infections, skin breakdowns, and patient complaints. Then a year later, Blegen's two studies (Blegen, Goode, and Reed, 1998; Blegen and Vaughn, 1998) found that there "were the fewest number of patient and family complaints, patient falls, medication administration errors, and observable decubiti" when the RN to non-RN ratio was 85–87 percent (Shullanberger, p. 147). Blegen, Vaughn, and Goode (2001) further reported that "controlling for patient acuity, hours of nursing care, and staff mix, units with more experienced nurses had lower medication errors and lower patient fall rates" (p. 33).

- Needleman, Buerhaus, Mattke, Stewart, and Zelevinsky (2001) sampled 799 hospitals from 11 states and found consistent relationships between nurse staffing levels and "five patient outcomes, urinary track infections, pneumonia, length of stay, upper gastrointestinal bleeding, and shock in medical patients" and death in major surgery patients (p. ii). A weaker relationship was found for urinary track infections and pneumonia in surgery patients.
- Similarly, "Socalski and Fagin (1997) found that 'magnet hospitals,' those known for first-rate nursing care, had significantly lower mortality rates than matched (similar size and type) hospitals. They had slightly higher RN-to-patient ratios and a considerably richer skill mix than equivalent hospitals. They also enjoyed higher rates of patient satisfaction, lower nurse burnout, and a safer work environment" (Shullanberger, p. 132).
- Another variable that has an influence on patient outcomes is the organizational context in which nurses practice. Aiken and Patrician (2000) developed, and established reliability and validity, for a Revised Nursing Work Index instrument to measure the organizational context. Subscales within this instrument measure: autonomy, control over the practice setting, the nurse-physician relationship, and organizational support. Other research using these variables find that Magnet Hospitals—known for good nursing care—have a lower patient mortality rate of 9 fewer deaths per 1,000 Medicare discharges (Aiken, Smith, and Lake, 1994).
- Brewer and Frazier (1998) conducted a multivariate analysis of RN staffing in western New York and found that the type of unit, nursing model, rural location, and use of aides and unit secretaries affected RN staffing. Intensive care, pediatric, and maternity units had higher levels of RN staffing than medical/surgical/gynecologic units. Rural hospitals used more RNs than other hospital settings. Adding nurse aides increased the RN ratio while use of LPNs did not significantly change the RN ratio. A unit secretary decreased the RN ratio.
- Mark, Salyer, and Wan (2000) examined the skill mix in 67 hospitals in 11 southeastern states. They found that "high-tech services and a larger percentage of admissions in which managed care organizations were the primary payer were associated with a higher proportion of RNs on the unit. Lower RN skill mix was associated with more regular stay admissions. One nursing unit characteristic, complexity of patients' needs for nursing care, was predictive of nursing unit skill mix, with increasing complexity associated with a higher proportion of RNs" (pp. 557–558).
- In the long-term care setting, Bliesmer, Smayling, Kane, and Shannon (1998) found that greater use of licensed nurses in the first year of admission resulted in improved functional ability, increased probability of discharge home, and decreased probability of death. There was no difference found with chronic patients who had been in long-term care over a year.
- Hendrix and Foreman (2001) found that, NAs have substantially more impact than RNs on minimizing long-term care decubitus costs, but both were significant. This study shows that the average nursing home operator would need to spend approximately $380 per resident for RNs and $569.98 to $1,820.32 per resident for nurse aides to achieve this staffing ratio. Increased LPNs did not achieve fewer decubiti so

this study advocated reducing or eliminating LPNs. *When staffing was not at the minimum suggested by this study, the researchers found that the nursing homes spent $84,085,167 within the industry on decubiti—a cost that could have been eliminated with adequate staffing.*

- After eight years of research on nursing home patient care levels, Federal health officials (Pear, 2000) have found that 54 percent of all nursing homes fall below minimum nurse staffing standards and further said that patients were endangered with low staffing levels. They found that staffing levels were much higher in non-profit nursing homes compared with for-profit nursing homes. In their study results, Federal officials advocated that minimum staffing standards for all care facilities should be two hours per day per patient of nurse aide time and twelve minutes per day per patient of RN time. Outcome measures in this study included: decubiti, malnutrition, weight loss, dehydration, need for hospital admissions, and possible death. When there were low staffing ratios the staff turnover rate increased.

- Aiken, Clarke, Cheung, Sloane, and Silber (2003) found that patients had a greater chance of survival when more highly educated nurses were providing the direct patient care.

- Aiken, Clarke, Sloane, Sochalski, and Silber (2002) linked survey data from 10,184 staff nurses with 232,342 general, orthopedic, and vascular surgery patients from 168 Pennsylvania hospitals, and found that:

> Fifty percent of the hospitals had patient-to-nurse ratios that were 5:1 or lower. Each additional patient per nurse was associated with a 7%... increase in the likelihood of dying within 30 days of admission and a 7% ... increase in the odds of failure-to-rescue (deaths within 30 days of admission among patients who experienced complications—examples included aspiration pneumonia and hypotension/shock). After adjusting for nurse and hospital characteristics, each additional patient per nurse was associated with a 23%... increase in the odds of burnout and a 15% ... increase in the odds of job satisfaction (p. 1987).

- Correspond this with a telephone survey of 601 RNs reported by Peter D. Hart Research Associates, Inc. in 2003:

> Three in five hospital nurses (59 percent) say that the staffing level at their hospital is having a negative impact on the quality of care patients receive. More than half (54 percent) say that when it comes to the quality of care, understaffing at their hospitals is a very or fairly serious problem, and Med-Surg nurses with higher patient-to-nurse ratios (more than 6:1) are especially likely to agree. When it comes to nurse burnout, fully three in five (62%) nurses have considered leaving the patient-care field during the past two years, and Med-Surg nurses with higher

patient-to-nurse ratios are more likely than average to have considered leaving the patient-care field.... Med-Surg nurses report that on average they are caring for 8.0 patients per shift, with 50 percent caring for more than six patients and 82 percent caring for more than four. [When asked] how many patients they should be caring for, [they indicated] an average of 5.2 patients (pp. 1–2).

These data would indicate that part of the problem causing the nursing shortage is that hospitals are not adequately staffing units, so nurses decide to leave and work in other settings. Note that the March 2004 issue of *Research in Action* from the Agency for Healthcare Research and Quality reviews the literature on hospital staffing and quality of care (www.ahrq.gov).

Nursing Care Delivery Models

The nursing care delivery model being used is another important factor with staffing. There are several nursing care delivery models and many variations of these models in individual facilities. Historically in nursing the pendulum seems to swing back and forth between RNs being the predominant patient care giver and RN scarcity spurring more auxiliary health care workers sharing patient responsibilities.

> **Definition**
>
> *Care Delivery Models*—deciding the way the patient care is actually assigned to specific personnel categories.

Case Method

In the 1920s there were private duty nurses in the community. In inpatient settings the RN gave all the care for one shift until another RN came on duty (case method).

Functional Nursing

Then in World War II, RNs were needed for the war effort. The RN shortage from the war continued in the 1950s resulting in *functional nursing*. Much of the care was given by nurse aides. In functional nursing, specific job functions/tasks were assigned to different workers, i.e., administration of medications (RN function), giving the bed bath (nurse aide function). No one took care of the patient totally. Care could become fragmented and depersonalized—much like an assembly line. When safety issues occurred it was not always clear whose responsibility it was to have discovered, prevented or dealt with the problem. On the positive side, skills could be enhanced. For instance, one RN starting all the IVS became an expert at it.

Team Nursing

Team nursing came about as more nurses became available. In this case a group of different types of care workers (RN, LPN, and/or nurse aide) work together on a team with an RN team leader. The team could then function in different ways—functional nursing on a small scale, or the RN might care for more critically ill patients while the LPN and/or nurse aide cared for less acutely ill patients. In team nursing there was no consistency in the patients they care for from day to day. In times of understaffing this could quickly revert to functional nursing or an unorganized level of priorities. At its best, when the group is a well-functioning team, the care could be effectively completed. Marie Manthey (1988) observed that the best way to accomplish team nursing is to schedule staff teams, RN plus Assistive Person(s), to consistently work the same schedule. This increases the productivity of teams. In this arrangement team members are used to working with each other, know they can count on each other, and better care results.

Modular Nursing

Modular nursing was a spin-off of team nursing. However, in modular nursing the team consistently cares for a patient until the patient is discharged. If the patient is readmitted later, usually this same team again cares for the patient each day until discharge. Generally patients are all geographically located in close proximity on a unit.

Primary Nursing

The pendulum swung back with *primary nursing*. With primary nursing some units hired only RNs to care for patients, just like the case method. Usually though units staffed more heavily with RNs. *Total patient care* was the new buzz word. When the primary nurse went off duty, an associate nurse assumed responsibility for the patient, following the plan the primary nurse had set up and communicated.

In times of plenty primary nursing worked well. However, it was perceived to be more expensive. RN salaries cost more than other types of nursing personnel, however, as we pointed out in the Nursing Staff Skill Mix section of this chapter, higher numbers of RNs may actually be less expensive. As managed care began to take effect, the cost factor came into play. Suddenly some thought it was too expensive to have an all RN staff. All sorts of assistive staff were dreamed up and trained. A common theme was to combine functions of a couple workers within one assistive person. For example, the former nurse aide would give basic nursing care, pass trays, feed patients, transfer patients, turn patients, help with laundry, housekeeping duties, or whatever. By this time, patients' lengths of stay had shortened and patients were more acute. RNs were still needed but it cost too much to have the RN replacing the ice water at the patient's bedside, changing linens, or passing food trays. LPNs became popular again. LPN schools that had been closing during the primary nursing era were suddenly booming again.

In the managed care era, the RN became taxed when LPNs would take a patient assignment because the RN had to take care of assessing and supervising the care of the LPN's patients as well as complete a full patient assignment him/herself. Meanwhile aides often did not have enough to do.

Team Nursing and Case Management

Presently, with a nursing shortage, team nursing has become the predominant method. As the RN became more taxed, and as patients were often transferred to less expensive locations, *case management* was created to achieve more patient consistency and to coordinate services for a specific patient population throughout an illness episode with others following up on the plan of care the case manager plans. (See Chapter 16 on Case Management.)

Another case management or interdisciplinary team method is sometimes used to coordinate care. Here an interdisciplinary team meets about and/or with patients (the second is preferable), arriving at a specific plan of care for each patient. The goal is to get patients into the least expensive care as quickly as possible by anticipating all services needed at specified times including those services that would prevent certain complications from occurring.

Nursing Staff Resources

Now let us consider some specific components of nursing staff resources. Although nurse managers may be responsible for interdisciplinary staff, they are not discussed here.

Advanced Practice Nurses

The group of advanced practice nurses includes many different kinds of nurses with advanced degrees (most often master's degrees). Acute nurse practitioners and clinical specialists can plan, educate, coordinate, and provide care for the more complicated hospitalized patients, while primary care nurse practitioners and clinical specialists can see patients, prevent health care complications, teach patients, and encourage prevention of disease. Nurse anesthetists provide anesthesia under the guidance of an anesthesiologist. In some states nurse midwives can actually deliver babies; in other states they function more like a clinical specialist.

Clinical specialists are presently underused in health care organizations, yet could be a valuable resource well worth the money. They can provide clinical leadership for complex patients in a cost-effective way, as well as educate staff on ways to better care for patients. Although their salaries are higher than a staff nurse salary, they can actually save money by more effectively dealing with complex patient management issues. Even the Institute of Medicine recommends more extensive use of advanced practice nurses!

Perhaps the best new role has been developed by the American Association of Colleges of Nursing (AACN) on the Clinical Nursing Leader. This advanced practice role

> functions within (the health care delivery system) and assumes account-
> ability for health care outcomes for a specific group of clients within a
> unit or setting through the assimilation and application of research based

information to design, implement, and evaluate client plans of care (*AACN Working Paper on the Role of the Clinical Nurse Leader,* 2004).

Registered Nurses

In the United States, there are approximately 2.5 million RNs, with 2.1 million actually working in nursing. RN employment growth has been occurring at about two to four percent per year. The increase has been greater in states with low HMO enrollments. Although in 1991 72 percent of RNs worked in hospitals, by 1999 this number decreased to 63 percent. And as the acuity increased in hospitals, RN FTEs per hospital occupied bed have risen from 1.15 in 1994 to 1.22 in 1997. RN employment in nursing homes has been increasing since 1983; it has been growing in physician offices since 1991. Most RNs (77 percent) are still paid by the hour rather than being salaried.

Legally, the registered nurse scope of practice is specifically defined in each state. Although there are individual differences in this definition, there is a consistent core definition that includes the nursing process (assessment, diagnosis, planning, intervention, and evaluation), expert knowledge or professional judgment, and specialized skills needed for this independent, professional role. "The RN has the responsibility and accountability to delegate or not delegate direct patient care activities based on such factors as the complexity of the task, potential for harm, abilities of the [LPN or] UAP, and the necessary problem solving skills" (Kido, 2001, p. 28).

The RN has certain areas of expertise—assessment of the patient, discharge planning, patient teaching—that other nursing care givers do not have. It is important to "articulate the unique contributions of the registered nurse in meeting patient outcomes so that these aspects of the work of registered nurses are preserved if addressing nursing shortages involves fulfilling non-RN tasks with other licensed or certified personnel" (*AONE Nursing Shortage*, 2000, p.16). We will also need to look at what the RN is doing and facilitate this as much as possible.

The RN issue for staffing is further complicated because all nurses are not the same: 27 percent have diplomas, 32 percent have associate degrees (AD), 31 percent have BSNs, and 10 percent are prepared at the masters or doctoral levels. Presently, 59 percent of new entry-level graduates are from AD programs. There are 876 AD programs and 661 four-year colleges and universities contributing to the RN workforce. Until recently BSN enrollments have been declining. Only 16 percent of the AD graduates go on for baccalaureate degrees. One difference, for example, is that an associate degree or diploma RN may not have had the pathophysiology or pharmacology knowledge base and may be more task oriented; while a baccalaureate-prepared RN often has better assessment and critical-thinking skills. Presently, 82 percent of RNs are employed with 59 percent of RNs being employed in hospitals (General Accounting Office, July 2001).

Another factor when determining RN staffing is their availability. Presently there are critical staff shortages occurring in several professions. Here we will just discuss the RN issues.

First, the RN workforce is getting older (the average staff nurse age is early forties). Projections indicate that by 2010 the average staff nurse would be 45.4 years and that 40 percent of the RN workforce will be over 50. Staff nursing can be physically demanding

(GAO, 2001). Older nurses often physically cannot do as much. Thus any ergonomic or robotic improvements—outlets at midwall level, supplies within a few steps—that can be made available for nurses are helpful. In addition, scheduling differently can help the older nurse. Nurses may not be able to physically work an 8-hour, or 12-hour, shift because of the physical demands, but could work fewer hours.

Nursing faculty are also getting older (average age is mid-fifties), and are grossly underpaid (by $20,000 to $30,000 per year) which is presenting a very critical shortage because as more nurses are needed, there will not be enough faculty to teach those interested in entering the profession. Baby boomers were more willing to sacrifice salary to teach. Newer generations are not as willing to do this. It is anticipated that by 2010, half the present faculty will retire.

Second, not as many young people are choosing the nursing profession. "The number of working RNs under the age of 30 fell from 419,000 in 1983 to 246,000 in 1998, a 41% decline.... Of all working RNs in the United States, the percent under 30 years of age dropped from 30% of the RN workforce in 1983 to 12% in 1998" (Staiger, Auerbach, and Buerhaus, 2000, p. 231). Current RN enrollments have increased but are not enough to fill the gap.

Third, after 2010 many baby boomer RNs will begin to retire. Projections indicate that 20 percent of RN FTEs will not be able to be filled. This retirement group will also include nursing faculty, needed to train new nurses.

A fourth issue is that presently many RNs have become frustrated, stressed, and disillusioned with hospital and long-term care inpatient nursing. Studies are finding that nurses report the quality of their care is not as high as it used to be—or needs to be (*2001 ANA Staffing Survey*). Nurses are saying that the work is too hard and thankless. "Thirteen percent of the RNs who participated in the AJN Patient Care Survey stated they were likely to leave the nursing profession" (p. 39). The General Accounting Office (2001) report states that half the RNs surveyed by The Nursing Executive Center had considered leaving the patient care field. Aiken, Clarke, and Sloane (2000) found that nurses are choosing to leave these settings for better, equal—or even less—pay, better schedules, less physically demanding work, and/or a position where they can feel that they can still give good patient care and have more autonomy.

At times these RNs find work in other health care related jobs, but sometimes they leave the profession altogether. The nursing profession is not alone in this. Pharmacists can receive more pay working in a retail pharmacy and radiology technicians are choosing software-related jobs.

This dissatisfaction with nursing—caused by inadequate staffing, heavy workloads, increased use of overtime, and not enough support staff—has resulted in another disturbing outcome. The ANA survey found that 55 percent of both RNs and LPNs said they do not recommend the nursing profession to others. This could cause far reaching problems for the nursing profession. Do you see how important the RN:patient ratios are? When RN workloads are too heavy, more RNs leave the nursing profession.

It is always best to match employee's gifts with the patient assignment. For example, on a psychiatric unit one staff member works well with paranoid schizophrenic patients while another does better with bipolar patients. Nurses will be more satisfied taking care of the patients they enjoy, and patients will receive better care. Everybody wins.

This problem can be fixed in part when nursing administrators create better work environments. For instance, one frustration is that the RN is often spending time looking for something or for someone. Having things readily available, or using infared devices to find things or people may be helpful. In addition, computer systems linked with physician offices help to decrease trying to reach physicians. Instead the RN can just send a note to the physician and the physician can send an order back to the RN. Every chapter of this book contributes to creating better work environments. Creativity and change are part of this process. In addition to this goal, some organizations are offering additional personal services for RNs such as housecleaning services or having groceries delivered.

Nurses Are Professionals, Not Blue-Collar Workers

"The role of the Professional Nurse is to establish a therapeutic relationship with the patient that includes responsibility for managing the patients' care over an episode of care" (Manthey, 2001). This statement is deceptively simple yet *too often we treat RNs, and they see themselves, as blue-collar workers*. For example, we use time cards and pay salaries at an hourly rate. Forte and Forstrom's (1998) definition of this problem says it beautifully:

> What is wrong is the way the RN thinks about work—and most of this is our doing. The staff nurse sees work as:
>
> • Allocated to all caregivers, not delegated by the RN;
>
> • Task based not knowledge based;
>
> • Determined by job descriptions;
>
> • Described in policy and procedure;
>
> • Constructed to be performed by interchangeable performers.
>
> These beliefs preclude the RN from taking responsibility for professional practice.
>
> Additionally, nursing's informal norms against risk-taking and confrontation are intensely strong and often prevent the RN from commenting on practice patterns or trying new ways. There is a lack of conscious reflection on practice and a reluctance to direct the actions of others. Operating in this mode, the RN fails to:
>
> • Conceptualize a clearly defined professional role;
>
> • Recognize what is different about patients today;
>
> • Spot the interventions that have the greatest impact for the patient;
>
> • Identify "RN-only" work (nondelegable) both for everyday (based on external constraints) and for this particular day (based on clinical judgment);
>
> • Determine how other caregivers use their time (set the priorities);
>
> • Direct how assistants provide care (set the standard);

- Instruct assistants regarding what they need to know and observe today; and
- Clarify which data the assistants need to bring back to the RN (pp. 46–47).

Yet all these things are precisely what RNs need to do.

Perhaps this difference in perception comes partially from the educational preparation of the nurse; only 31 percent of RNs in the United States have BSNs. Goode, Pinkerton, McCausland, Southard, Graham, and Krsek (2001) reported a survey of 43 hospital CNOs who defined a difference between AD/diploma RNs and BSN RNs. They rank-ordered the differences by describing the BSN RN as having greater critical thinking skills, less task orientation, more professionalism, stronger leadership skills, more focus on continuity of care and outcomes, greater focus on psychosocial components, better communication skills, and greater focus on patient teaching (p. 58). In this study, only 43 percent of hospital employers paid a salary differential for educational credentials.

On the professionalism issue, there is hope. Certainly there are many AD/Diploma RNs who exhibit professionalism. Our nurse administrator group is becoming better educated—most CNOs are now master's prepared. Many RNs do not realize that they are using a blue-collar, task-oriented approach. As more nurse managers and staff nurses achieve higher levels of education this may help the professionalism issue. The first step, however, is recognizing that we are in the task-orientation mode. This is an old paradigm, and is defined in **Exhibit 20–3**. It will take a concerted effort on all our parts to change to this new paradigm.

As we implement a professional model, as outlined above, we need to examine, and change, our way of thinking in everything we do. For example, do we schedule based on the blue-collar model? In the blue-collar model, the RN does not determine the best schedule to work to give the needed patient care. Instead the RN works a specific, predetermined shift. In the professional model, the RN determines the best schedule to accomplish the work—this means the nurse may work five hours one day and ten the next. Following this model, some hospitals have designated *attending* nurses assigned to specific patients. Skeletal staff cover the open hours, so the attending nurses can set their own work times to best meet the needs of their patients. There are many other ways to achieve the professional model. Creativity is the key.

Also in the blue-collar model, an aide and LPN are assigned patients and/or tasks along with the RN. The RN has to sign for the LPN's patients. This can double the RN's workload meaning that the RN may be responsible for 12–14 patients! In the professional model, the aide and LPN *report to* the RN. Patients are assigned to the RN who then determines what the aide and LPN will do with the group of patients. The RN is the leader, the delegator, and is the one who determines the patient needs in total. The RN does not have to give all the care, but chooses to do those things that require the extra knowledge base and assessment skills the RN possesses.

We are further hampered by our Achilles heel in the nursing profession. Lamentably, for some reason, most often RNs do not view themselves as leaders unless they have an administrative title. Perhaps this is perpetuated by the fact that nurses are women; or

---

Exhibit 20–3 Paradigm Shift

Old Paradigm

Nursing assistants have their own work, predetermined by lists and job descriptions, but they are also supposed to help the nurses.

Divide the patients among available RNs and LPNs who then operate in a total-patient-care mode.

RNs are expected to cover for LPNs by doing tasks which, by policy, LPNs may not perform, but RNs would not comment on the LPNs' care or the priorities they set—this would be interfering.

RNs may ask LPNs or nursing assistants for help, but since everyone has his/her own care assignment, help may be rarely requested or offered.

Who does what is determined by lists and policies, not by individual competencies or specific patient needs.

New Paradigm

Nursing assistants are assigned to care teams and receive their patient care work from the RN as delegated work each shift.

Assign each of the patients to an RN who manages his/her required care either by doing it or by delegating it to other care-team members.

LPNs and nursing assistants work with an RN in two or three person care teams, sharing the workload, each making a maximized contribution. The RN is free (and expected) to influence all the care that is performed by the care team.

RNs determine what they will do and what they will delegate. When help is needed, care-team members can assist each other or reorganize their work plan for the shift.

Work is divided up using each care-team member's skills to the fullest extent, freeing the RN to do the work that only the RN can do.

From: Forte, P., & Forstrom, S. (January 1998). Work complexity assessment: Decision support data to address cost and culture issues. *JONA*, 28(1), 46–53.

---

maybe it is because we get doctor's orders. However, in our present paradigm *nurses need to be leaders in the delivery of care*. As more of the care is given by an RN, quality of the care is higher. However, having unlicensed personnel is also helpful—just not in huge quantities. Both the RN and the unlicensed person(s) need to be working as an effective team. The RN needs to be the leader of the care—but not have to do it all.

Changing to the professional model will require the nurse manager—or better yet one of the RNs—to do a lot of teaching about the professional model change. The expectations for LPNs and aides are for them to report to the RN. The RN will need to learn how to lead and delegate effectively, which will be a lot of work because many RNs have trouble with delegating—"It's easier to just do it myself."—and do not view themselves as leaders. As the professional model is first introduced, chaos will occur. However, with the nurse manager's support and consistency, higher job satisfaction will develop. However, if the nurse manager does not believe in the professional model, it probably will not happen!

LPNs/LVNs

LPN growth has remained relatively flat other than home health hiring more ten years ago. In fact they have been declining in hospitals while growing in physician offices. More and more, it is the LPNs who are administering medications on inpatient units. When this is done, it is important that the LPN is communicating effectively with the RN and aide caring for a patient, or critical information could be missed that would affect patient safety.

Unlicensed Assistive Personnel

Unlicensed assistive personnel, when in the right proportion to RNs, can aid the RN to more effectively carry out professional activities. Unlicensed assistive personnel are at the low end of the pay scale so other jobs can look more attractive and are not as hard physically. Yet many in this position really enjoy their relationships with patients. Another benefit for nurse aides are the health care benefits they receive when they work full time. One retention strategy for both RNs and unlicensed assistive personnel are to couple the same employees consistently together at work (Manthey, 1988).

> There is no universally accepted description of UAPs. Hospitals use these workers in a variety of roles, some that are more focused on supporting the patient care environment rather than the patients themselves.... The use of lower-cost workers in delivering nursing care is a concept that has taken on a greater importance to hospitals and other healthcare institutions grappling with real and threatened declines in reimbursement, coupled with an aging nursing force. UAPs have been used in a variety of roles [besides the traditional primary support functions at the bedside]; some perform simple housekeeping or secretarial tasks, and others perform higher-level clinical or technical tasks such as electrocardiograms and phlebotomy. Because there is no one accrediting body common to all types of UAPs, and because state laws vary regarding their use, hospitals have been relatively free to experiment with different care models under the guidance of their internal nursing leadership (McClung, 2000, p. 531).

The Omnibus Budget Reconciliation Act of 1987 (OBRA '87) required states to license nursing assistants in long-term care facilities and to define the knowledge base and competencies required for nurse assistant certification. State requirements vary (training may be less than one week to four or more weeks) but must include those requirements federally mandated. Some boards of nursing require CNAs to submit proof of additional education to the state board in order to be recertified. (So in long-term care a nursing assistant must be licensed while hospitals can hire unlicensed nursing assistants.)

The research also tells us some facts about unlicensed assistive personnel. Anthony, Standing, and Hertz (2000) found that "more negative events occurred when there was no direct observation of the unlicensed assistive personnel by the licensed nurse during the delegated activity.... There was a consistent trend in which closer, planned, and intentional supervision was more likely to be associated with positive outcomes" (p. 480). The RN professional model discussed previously achieves this goal when coupled with Manthey's strategy of coupling the same aide with the same RN consistently.

Sago (2000) found that both RNs and unlicensed assistive personnel (UAPs) "seek 'positive interpersonal relationships, are generally accepting and cooperative, need to do well, and enjoy helping and assisting others'" (p. 284). So both groups "want to help others and want to do a good job" (p. 284). This study also recommends that both staff nurses and the nurse manager "[listen] and [act] on suggestions by the UAPs, . . . [allow] the UAPs to make decisions as much as possible about their work, [and include] the UAPs in decision-making about patient care, the way the day's work is structured, and how they carry out their work" (p. 284).

In Kansas the Mennonite Manor hired local people to be a Manor Care Attendant. These people did not do hands-on care with residents but assisted aides whenever possible. For instance, they could provide wheelchair escort, "make beds, organize resident's closets, empty and clean commodes and urinals, fill water pitchers, lay out clothing and supplies, help with mechanical lifts, and visit and read to residents" (Wineland, 2003, p. 33).

Volunteers

Another strategy for RN retention and to ease an RN's job and to increase patient service, is to find volunteers that can do various services for patients and families. Volunteers are used most often by hospitals but can be used in any setting or by individual units. This is a fairly untapped resource. Specific guidelines would need to be developed as to their qualifications, training, and specific services they would provide.

Enhancing Staff Resources

There are numerous ways to enhance and to better appreciate our staff resources. For example, we know from the job satisfaction research that we need to have new challenges or changes in our work—even when we work in the same place. Thus it is conducive to support and encourage employees if they decide to change specialties to develop a new area or process at work, or to take on a special assignment, to encourage them—and give them the time—to do this. Here are a few other examples of how to enhance staff resources.

Generational Differences

Generational differences can influence how staff approach their job and their work. Five different generations are represented in our current workforce: pre-boomers or silent generation (birth in 1934 to 1945), baby boomers (birth in 1946 through 1959), cuspers (1960 to 1968), busters (1969 to 1978)—sometimes cuspers and busters are lumped together as Generation X—and, netsters or Generation Y (1979 on). See **Exhibit 20–4**. If a boomer nurse manager is supervising a buster employee, the boomer nurse manager may not understand why the buster chooses to put lifestyle first. The cusper would need help from the net-

Exhibit 20–4 Generational Differences

Pre-Boomer 1934-1945	Boomer 1946-1959	Cusper 1960-1968	Buster 1969-1978	Netsters 1979-1984+
Traditional work ethic	Money/work ethic	Money/principle	Principle/satisfaction	Principle/satisfaction
Work first	Work first	Some of both	Lifestyle first	Lifestyle first
Born to lead	Expect to lead	Lead and follow	No need to lead	Lead if necessary
Loyal to employer	Loyal to employer	Some of both	Loyal to skills	Loyal to skills
Independent but conventional	Care deeply what others think	Some of both	Don't care what others think	Care little what others think
Value working well with others	Want others to work with them	Want others to work with them	Prefer to work alone	Will tolerate small groups
Technically competent	Technically challenged	Technically challenged	Technically savvy	State-of-the-art
Believe in the mission	Lip service to mission	Care about mission	*Must* have mission	*Must* have mission
Strong chain of command	Chain of command	Some of both	Individual first	Individual first
Want to win	I win, you lose	Want to win	I win, you win	I win, you win

Older Workers: Born 1935 - 1959	Younger Workers: Born 1960-1981
"We're invincible as a team."	"I work best alone."
"I want, think, would like…"	"I need."
Softened style: "I'd love it if you…"	Blunt style: "Just do it…"
Long preambles	Abrupt speech patterns
Care deeply what others think	Care little about what others think
Like to process and talk about ideas and issues	"Just tell me what you want done and I'll do it."
Highly value participation and consensus	Do not participate, attend meetings or need to hear others' opinions
Want people to want to do something , to want to be part of the team	Want people to get the result quickly and quietly as possible; often astonished by employee feelings/discontent
Believe people can be motivated by a stirring, well-expressed idea	Believe motivation is pushing on the end of a string
Recognition means a great deal; want acceptance, popularity, group identity	Doesn't work and isn't needed. They think "I know what kind of job I'm doing. If a boss recognizes my work, that's nice but its frosting on the cake."

MOTIVATION ACROSS AGE GROUPS				
Pre-Boomer 1934-1945	Boomer 1946-1959	Cusper 1960-1968	Buster 1969-1978	Nesters 1979-1984+
• Money • Responsibility • Public recognition • Accomplishment • Desire to lead • Control • Organizational loyalty	• More money • Promotion • Public recognition • Peer recognition • Desire for subordinates • Control • Loyalty to self	• Do well by doing good • Meeting organizational goals • Recognition from boss • Bonuses • Stock options	• Time off • Mentoring • Meeting own goals • Recognition from boss • Skills training • Stock options	• Time off • Mentoring • Portable skills training • Meeting own goals • Stock options • Preparation for self-employment • Sales training

ster with computerized anything. Flexibility of work schedules will be very important to both busters and netsters. Support for on-site and off-site personal services will make a more attractive work package for this younger group. Being aware of these differences can enhance the workplace as staff of all ages bring different perspectives that will make the workplace richer (Santos and Cox, 2000; Kupperschmidt, 2001; Ulrich, 2001).

Coaching—Self Care

Savage (2001) has written a wonderful article on executive coaching. Although she writes this only for nurse executives, it is important for any care giver at any level in the organization. Nurses consistently deal with "anxiety inherent in the life and death nature of health care organizations" (p. 178) and often are taught to be self-sufficient. Yet having a coach that focuses on an individual and focuses on specific issues or concerns can actually enhance a person's ability to do the work. Productivity, job satisfaction, and job retention are the result of this process. She gives pointers on choosing a coach and setting up contacts with this person. It is so easy to not pay attention to our own needs when others needs are so great.

Preceptors serve the coaching function for less experienced nurses. The ANA advocates that *"clinical support from experienced RNs should be readily available to those RNs with less proficiency"* (1999, p. 5). Benner's work has certainly shown the importance of the "expert" nurse being helpful to the "novice" nurse. Unfortunately, on inpatient units, the novice often works the off shifts—evenings and nights—while the expert gets to work more days. Thus, a preceptor should be offered for orientation, or an internship should be available where novice nurses can learn the ropes with more experienced nurses. Expert nurses will be more efficient, more caring, and will more effectively prevent adverse patient outcomes. Providing expert nurse support can make a significant difference for the new nurse. Although these programs can be expensive in the short run, in the long run they can be cost effective as they tend to improve retention (Beeman, Jernigan, and Hensley, 1999).

Reality Shock

Kramer and Schmalenberg (1977; Schmalenberg and Kramer, 1976) identified and researched a typical dilemma a new nurse experiences and labels this "reality shock." Actually this dilemma occurs, although less pronounced, anytime a person starts a new job. As new graduates start a new job, there are generally four predictable phases that they will experience. First they usually experience the *honeymoon phase* where "everything is wonderful." There are two major issues to resolve in this phase—skill and routine mastery, and becoming socially integrated. As the new graduate tries something and is blocked either by a person or because of a lack of certain skills, the second phase begins to develop—the *shock phase*. Here one of four possible characteristics can occur with the new graduate: moral outrage (the "shoulds"—"You should care about the patient."); rejection of either the schooling or the work scene; fatigue—go home and sleep until you have to go to work again; and perceptual distortion—"Nothing is good, everything is bad." In this phase some resolution is needed. Then the third phase, the *recovery phase*, hits. Things start to look better. Humor returns. One cannot resolve everything. If balance can be achieved, the *resolution phase* will occur. In this phase the resolution can be either constructive or destructive.

> There are two specific dimensions to constructive conflict resolution. First of all, it must be growth producing and self-actualizing for the individual as a person. Secondly, it must enable the individual to contribute toward improving the health care system and/or quality of nursing care (p. 40).

There are several ways the new graduate resolves this dilemma: 1) "go native" adopting the behaviors of the work scene, throwing out the school values; 2) go back to school—a lateral arabesque; 3) become a "rutter" and just work for the money; 4) become burned out; 5) start job hopping; 6) completely withdraw from nursing; or 7) achieve "biculturalism" constructively resolving the work-school dilemma. In the 1976 study, a third of new nurse graduates left the nursing profession with another third being burned out—turning into complainers. "A scant handful" achieved biculturalism.

Kramer and Schmalenberg (1977; Schmalenberg and Kramer, 1976) suggest five ways to help more of these graduates achieve biculturalism. They expand upon these suggestions in their book, *Biculturalism*.

- First, "resocialize our socialization agents—the instructors of nursing, head nurses, and inservice personnel who are the chief socializing agents of new nurses. These agents need to maintain, or acquire, biculturalism" (Schmalenberg and Kramer, 1976, p. 42).
- Decide the skills every nurse needs and teach those skills. A preceptor or coach working alongside the new nurse can make such a significant difference for the new graduate.
- Education and "service must emphasize the productive, non-wasteful use of available time and also that there is time" for such things as patient teaching (p. 43).
- "Provide nurses with the tools of and practice in constructive resolution of conflict" (p. 43).
- "Faculty and head nurses… be supportive of students and new graduates to maintain their innovativeness" (p. 43).

Two more recent studies corroborate and add to the reality shock data (McNeese-Smith, 2000; Duchscher, 2001). "Nurses in the entry stage were primarily new on the job, and the majority of nurses who had been on the job less than 6 months considered themselves to be in the entry stage.… Some nurses began to disengage almost immediately on beginning their job" (McNeese-Smith, p. 145). The study found a correlation between organizational commitment and mastery. Disengagement was less likely to occur with these nurses. Study recommendations include: "Involve every nurse in an active goal-setting, self-evaluation process that includes annual (or biannual) examinations of the nurse's goals, level of job satisfaction, organizational commitment, and personal and professional needs in relation to the job, and opportunities for challenge" (p. 146). The coaching process, available from the start, would make a tremendous difference in this engagement process. Duchscher examined the first six months of employment, outlining the various issues that need to be resolved by the new graduate at the beginning, at two months, at five months, and at six months. She found that the nurses really needed a preceptor/mentor.

Mentors

One aspect to always think about as an administrator is that we all need to be mentoring others so they can eventually take over our work. The mentoring process gives others a boost because the mentees know that someone believes in them and in their capabilities. It also helps to enhance the mentees current work. This needs to happen at every level in the organization—from aide to president.

Clinical Ladders

Clinical ladders have been established in many settings as a way of increasing and rewarding the professionalism of staff. For example, Goode, Pinkerton, McCausland, Southard, Graham, and Krsek (2001) report that 43 percent of the hospitals in their study had such programs. Staff who possess different capabilities, and/or educational or certification requirements, are at different levels of the clinical ladder. Salaries correspond with the level achieved. There can be many criteria used for a clinical ladder such as national certification, ability to care for different kinds of patients effectively, developing new programs or different ways of accomplishing care, achieving better patient outcomes, and orienting/precepting new staff, to name a few. Clinical ladder programs provide advancement opportunities, and are a wonderful retention tool. Clinical ladders can be for RNs, LPNs, or unlicensed assistive personnel. Most often clinical ladders exist for RNs. Krugmen, Smith, and Goode (2000) describe a clinical ladder program.

Staff Learning and Development

Ultimately people need to find meaning in their work. If our staff are feeling so overworked that they are exhausted, this is not conducive to providing a helpful, replenishing environment where they can expand and grow. One constant in this world seems to be that there is so much more to learn! As we learn, we grow. This also applies to our staff. Learning can occur in so many ways—a mentor; a conference; reading; things we hear and see with patients and their families, other employees, and physicians; professional meetings; or just in the living process. Job satisfaction increases when there are new things to learn. This opportunity also tells staff that they are appreciated. As a nurse manager, please do all you can to create a learning environment for all employees.

Staff Recognition and Celebrations

Staff appreciate hearing that something they did meant a lot to a patient or family, or to a colleague. Receiving a letter, a small gift of thanks, or an award can be a very moving experience. Other forms of recognition are also appreciated at all levels. Usually an organization has several forums for staff recognition—newsletters, postings on bulletin boards, awards ceremonies, sharing at staff meetings, thank you notes, prizes and drawings, or even just asking staff, if they would you like to thank anyone.

Sources and Distribution of Staff

As life circumstances occur, staff are not always able to work when needed, so other forms of staff distribution or staff sources are necessary. Although we list the common ways to deal with this problem, if problems are consistent it probably indicates a serious underlying administrative leadership problem that will need to be fixed (see Chapters 3 and 4).

It can also be tempting to get into "quick fix" solutions like sign-on bonuses, to only give salary increases to new staff, to pay relocation expenses, and so forth. These do not deal with the basic underlying problems and, in the long run, will only make the situation worse as current employees are not rewarded. (See Chapter 4.)

Full-Time/Part-Time Staff

To schedule most effectively, it is generally best to have both full-time and part-time staff. If there are too many full-time staff, there are not enough staff available to cover weekends, vacations, and sick time. If there are too many part-time staff, continuity of care suffers. For an inpatient unit it is preferable to have approximately 60–70 percent full-time and 30–40 percent part-time to allow for some flexibility yet still have continuity. (See Chapter 11, Budget Development and Evaluation for more details.) Also, think of different options for staff. For example, a 35-year-old experienced staff RN would work when her children are in school but needs to be home during the summer. Isn't it better to have her for 9 months than not at all?

Part-time staff can be helpful, and besides working a regular schedule, may be willing to work extra shifts as long it it fits with their other life circumstances. However, if used too much the staff will begin to dread and avoid calls. When used occasionally, extra shifts for part-time employees can really help to keep staffing more evenly distributed for patients.

OVERTIME

Overtime is often used when there are not enough staff present. Standard policies regarding the use of overtime should exist as it can become abused and really burn up staff as well as budget dollars. However, overtime is useful for occasional use and less expensive than other options such as hiring an additional person for peak times or paying for agency staff. A problem arises when overtime becomes a regular event. It is most costly because staff get tired, make mistakes, will become less efficient, and can begin to resent the extra hours of work. When prolonged use of overtime becomes an issue, first examine the situation to diagnose the problem. Is the unit run well or is there a leadership problem? Is it that one cannot find a person to fill the position? Be creative, fix problems, and picture that you will fix the problem in the best way possible. Involve staff in the issue. If team work is occurring, staff will offer to help. However, as one fixes the problem, a temporary solution, rather than mandating overtime, may be necessary, (i.e., close beds or hire agency nurses even though they cost more).

As the nursing shortage has developed, mandatory overtime has become an issue. It is best not to resort to this measure—it is a "quick fix" that will backfire as patient safety issues and turnover may result. ANA advocates restrictions on mandatory overtime further specifying that "no staff member in a health care organization should be required or forced to accept work in excess of a predetermined schedule. Any employer who violates the provisions would be subject to sanctions. Nurses do not want to be forced to work overtime when they are tired or when they have other commitments" (*ANA Staffing Survey*, p. 2).

Another issue with overtime is that the federal government recently passed a law that salaried "whitecollar" workers are entitled to overtime pay. This new law ("FairPay") was passed to cover workers making $23,660/year or less. This could apply to LPNs or other health care workers who are salaried, rather than being paid on an hourly basis.

POSTING OPEN SHIFTS ON THE WEB

Thrall (2003) discusses another effective staffing strategy:

> St. Peter's Health Care Services, Albany, N.Y., posts vacant nursing shifts on the Web and lets nurses bid to work them in a process similar to that of Priceline.com.... 'It gives nurses more choice and more control, and it's convenient—they can look at the available shifts from a home computer.'... When an open shift is listed, nurses see 'most likely,' 'least likely' and 'likely' bid ranges.... Two-thirds of the 300 nurses who typically bid on jobs are existing staff. Nurses who want to work extra shifts know early what's available and hear back quickly from managers, who are paged when bids register (p. 38).

Third Seasoners

As the shortage worsens, "it is imperative that older nurses be retained, not only for their experience and expertise, but also to prevent worsening an already critical nursing shortage. . . . most administrators are aware of the aging workforce and wish to retain older nurses. Unfortunately, 94 percent of facilities have no policies in place to address the needs of older nurses" (Letvak, 2002, p. 387).

A strategy for the understaffing problem is to employ RNs who are in their third season of life—aged 55 and older—to work part-time, come back from retirement to work, or take a post-retirement option to work. It may be that physically they cannot work full time but could work two or three days a week. Most often post-retirement nurses work a part-time schedule such as working one weekend a month or working shorter shifts. First, consult the Human Resource Department about the federal and state laws concerning these workers and about guidelines for employment. For example, they might be directly employed by the organization or work as an independent contractor. They could also be hired to complete a specific project. In addition they may not need as many benefits as other personnel (Powell, 1999). Third seasoners could also help do coding for the facility.

Job Sharing

Job sharing occurs when two nurses share a full-time position so that one of the two is consistently on duty each scheduled day. This expands the part-time concept by placing the responsibility on the two nurses to figure out who covers which scheduled shift. They also share the benefits (Sherry, 1994; Gliss, 2000).

On Call

On call time has been another arrangement to attempt to have adequate staffing. This involves paying staff who work a regular schedule and then get extra pay to be "on call," meaning that they are available to come in, if needed, after hours or on weekends. This is a popular option in operating rooms and labor and delivery areas but is also used in other areas.

Floating Staff

When there is inadequate staffing on one unit, a common practice is to "float" staff from another unit. Unless part of a regular float pool, nurses hate being floated and find it to be a very stressful experience. "One study of ICU nurses showed that only death outranked floating as a source of stress" (Davidhizar, Dowd, and Brownson, 1998, p. 33). The problem is that often they have not been cross-trained, do not know staff on that unit, and, on problem units, may receive the hardest assignments. The greatest fear though is that they will violate patient safety.

Cross training is essential—although it does not always happen. Rudy and Sions (2003) have written a very thoughtful process to use with staff, as well as guidelines to make floating more tolerable to staff and safer for patients. Regulatory bodies, such as JCAHO, specify that health care organizations should document cross training and that there must be a systematic plan in effect to accomplish this. Staff being floated will be less stressed if they have had a chance to orient to the unit, get to know some of the staff, bone up on skills needed for different types of patients, and are rewarded for floating. Ideally, one criteria for a salary increase or merit pay should include the capability to float to other units, if this is expected. This option could also be included in a clinical ladder.

Staffing Pools

Sometimes an organizational staffing pool [supplemental staff pool, float pool] exists where staff work a regular schedule but float from unit to unit as needed. Regular float pool nurses love the challenge and change of working on different units with different kinds of patients. Cross training is still important with float pool staff. Staff have regular schedules and can be part-time or full-time.

Another twist with staffing pools is to hire a number of nurses that do not want to work a regular schedule but promise to work a few shift(s) each month. In this arrangement, the nurses often have more flexibility of work schedules. Then as more staff are needed, these nurses are called to see if they can work. These nurses may just want part-time work but they also may have other full-time jobs. In some cases these nurses are part of a standby pool and "are paid a per diem rate to be available to work if called on assigned days" (Sherry, 1994).

Staffing pools may be unit specific, for the entire organization, or even exist for several organizations in a region or state (Fralic, 2000; Sherer, 1994; Sherry, 1994). For instance, in Vermont twelve hospitals developed an interhospital staff-sharing network. For $30,000 annually per hospital, this network schedules staff from one hospital with low census to another with greater staffing needs. This has been less costly than using agency nurses and has an added benefit of providing nurses with a picture of how other places accomplish the work so nurses bring ideas back home.

Another variation on the staffing pool, SWAT (smiling, willing, available, and talented), is a team of two experienced nurses on each shift who are "dispersed to nursing units for 1 to 2 hours to provide care for newly admitted patients, to assist with special procedures, or to assist in emergency situations. . . . Once the care is provided and the situation is under control" the team moves on to another site (Taylor, p. 432). This can also be accomplished by having a resource nurse available at peak times to help the regular staff.

At the Mountain States Health Alliance Johnson City Medical Center (Johnson City, Tennessee), a "Code Alert" can be called to any patient care area that needs extra help. Any employee that is available goes to help the area and assist with such things as feeding patients or other basic care issues.

Agency Staffing

Of course, if all else fails one can turn to agency nurses—especially in large urban areas. These nurses are more expensive because one has to pay the agency to administer their program as well as pay for the nurse's time. In this case, continuity can be a problem and the agency nurse might not be aware of the organization's policies. For accreditation purposes, one must provide orientation information and these staff need to meet credentialing and care standards (Herringer II, 1999).

There are two kinds of agencies: a supplemental staffing agency and a registry. A supplemental staffing agency hires staff, contracts with organizations needing the staff, and provides staff as needed for those organizations. A registry does not actually employ staff, but will notify staff that an organization needs help. The staff member calls the organization directly and contracts directly with the organization to work there.

Traveling Nurses/Foreign Nurses/Internet Nurses

Sometimes it is not possible to find enough staff on a local basis. In this case the health care organization may directly advertise, contract a traveling nurse agency, or get on the internet to bring in nurses from other states or countries. This can involve licensing issues. When bringing in nurses from other countries, there may be cultural, language, competency, and regulatory difficulties (Bola, Driggers, Dunlap, and Ebersole, 2003).

Immigration visas limit the number of foreign nurses who can immigrate. And there may be limitations—on a national or state level—on positions the nurses can fill based on their educational preparation. *JONA* published a supplemental on *Choosing a Travel Nursing Agency* (March 2003) that is helpful for nurse administrators. Additionally, there is a worldwide nursing shortage so there are ethical implications with "robbing Peter to pay Paul." Plus there are not enough foreign nurses to address the United States' nursing shortage.

Sometimes traveling nurses are available for a short-term arrangement of three to six months. Here the nurse manager will interview by phone. However, traveling nurses may also be recruited for a long-term basis, if the traveling agency contract permits. Moving expenses might be involved as well as a finders fee (a couple month's salary) for the agency. This can be quite expensive.

Effective Staff Scheduling

Historically, the nurse manager would do the schedule each month with staff submitting requests. Usually, requests were honored. Staff might be required to rotate across different shifts, or occasionally a staff member could be scheduled on all three shifts—day, evening, night—in one week. However, this method was also abused, causing much staff anguish. Obviously, this is not a schedule conducive to either staff satisfaction

> **Definition**
>
> *Scheduling*—implements the staffing plan by assigning designated personnel to work specific hours and days.

or patient safety, not to mention the nurses's sleep deprivation issues. A nurse was expected to work every other weekend, or occasionally one weekend out of three. Sometimes nurses were penalized if they took the weekend days off and would have to make up the days. Unfortunately, this still occasionally happens today. Doesn't this sound like an example of the blue-collar model? It does not take into account personal issues that may arise, does not consider what patients need in terms of consistency and relationships, and satisfaction levels are not the greatest for anyone concerned.

Another issue with scheduling occurred as budgets were tightening. In this situation if the census went down, nurses were sent home and not paid for the shift; nurses could not depend upon a steady paycheck.

Scheduling will affect employee morale, productivity, work satisfaction, job tenure, and patient outcomes. There is no one best way to achieve effective scheduling. However, the authors advocate self-scheduling with established guidelines, with staff working the same shift as much as possible. This achieves more staff autonomy. Staffing becomes a real challenge when there are shortages. Since there is no ideal answer, be creative and open to new ways to schedule. If staff do not like their schedules, if schedules are used to reward or punish staff if the nurse manager/staff do not know how to effectively schedule, or if the nurse manager leadership is not effective, then staff will be unhappy, tired, and their low morale issues will get passed on to negatively affect the patients. In fact, in a study by

Strachota, Normandin, O'Brien, Clary, and Krukow (2003) they found that 50 percent of the nurses changed positions for one reason: *work hours*—they worked "every other weekend/still working majority of holidays/working nights with no possibility of days off/no flexibility" (p. 115).

To repeat an earlier theme, the important issue with scheduling is to always ask,

WHY DO WE DO IT THIS WAY?
HOW COULD WE DO IT BETTER?

There probably is a better, less costly way, to meet patient needs. For example, if a staff member would rather get a child off to school and then come to work, maybe this could work. Why does everyone need to work the same shift times? What are the peak times that staff are needed? As we discuss in Chapter 21 on Productivity, it is more expensive to have everyone work the same shift times having times when staff are not as busy and times when there are not enough staff to cover patient needs. Let's get out of the box!

Self Scheduling

In self scheduling, staff work out their own schedules within set guidelines. Guidelines might include following the staffing plan, number of days or hours worked each pay period or week, and weekend/holiday coverage expectations. Staff need to be able to negotiate with each other and resolve differences. The nurse manager intervenes if negotiations are unsuccessful but in a way that helps staff to work out the differences themselves. Mainly the nurse manager role is one of support. Is it any surprise that this works best on units lead by effective nurse managers, and usually is a disaster when there is an ineffective nurse manager? Self scheduling contributes to higher productivity and job satisfaction (Miller, 1992; Abbott, 1995; Hoffart and Willldermood, 1997; Irvin and Brown, 1999; Hung, 2002). Nurses have more control and predictability in their lives. Shullanberger, who reviewed the current staffing literature for the past 10 years, recommends "self scheduling of staff with the nurse manager's only related responsibility being the minimum number of nurses required to adequately care for patients each shift" (p. 146).

Self scheduling can have other positive benefits. Hausfeld, Gibbons, Holtmeier, Knight, Schulte, Stadtmiller, and Yeary (1994) reported that this worked on a unit with a widely fluctuating census. Overtime and sick calls decreased and there was much less floating into or out of the unit. Staff autonomy and satisfaction was higher. And staff felt that the patient care improved. A win-win situation occurred.

Using the professional model, the next step in self scheduling is to have the professional RN group schedule themselves based on their patients' needs while a skeletal staff continues to schedule using regular shifts.

Be creative. You do not have to use the "same old" shift times—in fact if you are using the same shift times, you probably need to go back and redo your work.

Permanent Shifts

Staff like being able to work a permanent shift. Generally, there is less turnover, less sick time, less tardiness, less absenteeism, and more work satisfaction, when staff are assigned a permanent shift. It promotes better teamwork between staff because they all work together consistently. Ultimately both staff and patients benefit when nurses are more satisfied. It is a win-win situation.

When staff are expected to rotate shifts, staff are more likely to get sick, be tired, be less satisfied with the job, have more accidents, and increased turnover will occur. Ineffective leadership is often the cause. Unfortunately, nurses may be expected to work different shifts within the same week. This disrupts circadian rhythms. This chaotic work schedule promotes a lose-lose situation for everyone concerned—including the patients.

When more staff are needed for a shift, an effective leader involves the staff in coming up with the best solution. It may be that one staff is willing to work a different shift for an entire week. Or staff may come up with a rotating list and take turns each doing a different shift. There are endless possibilities but it is always best to have staff decide for themselves what is best.

Flextime

Other scheduling options, such as flextime, allow staff to choose to work times that work best for them and for accomplishing their work. This is a nice option for staff. As stated above, when one treats staff as professionals, rather than blue-collar workers, the staff will know when their patients need them and be there. However, one practice with flextime is to have nurses identify shifts and units where they will be available to work and receive an hourly wage and no benefits for their work—more of a blue-collar approach (MacPhee, 2000).

Block or Cyclical Schedules

Traditionally block, or cyclical, schedules have been a popular way to do scheduling (Marchionno, 1987; Fralic, 2000). In a block schedule, a nurse consistently works the same schedule for a biweekly, or monthly, pay period. Using a block schedule allows the nurse to plan ahead and schedule personal activities for the consistent days off. Be careful using this, as the expectation that stall will work every other weekend regardless of staff personal needs can affect nurse retention. The block schedule then repeats itself and is used cyclically.[3] Schedules need to be individualized for specific units. This can be a helpful way to achieve minimum staffing while letting other staff determine work times based on patient needs.

---

[3] Gillies (1994, p. 262) gives 2 examples of patterns for cyclical scheduling.

Shift Times

Shift times are starting to change to be anything that works. Evaluate possibilities for shift times that would better serve patient needs on a regular basis. For instance, it is possible that the shift start and end times occur right when the peak patient needs occur. It makes more sense to use a skeletal staff to give coverage during open hours, and when there are heavier patient demands—like afternoons on an inpatient unit when there are a lot of admissions and discharges—having additional staff scheduled with different start and end times to cover the peak times. This saves money too.[4]

Loevinsohn (1992) advocates using "every conceivable combination and permutation of 8, 10, 12 (even 4-hour shifts for mothers with young children)... [that] may be staggered or overlapped with preceding or succeeding shifts" (p. 56). We go beyond this description to emphasize shifts of any duration. This optimizes scheduling to meet the nurses' personal needs as well as meeting the patient needs. There are limitless possibilities for other scheduling options. Shifts of any length, and of different start and end times, can be used so more staff are available to cover typical peak patient use times. Staff will prefer more flexibility in shift start times, shift length, different options for days or weekends off, consecutive days off, flexibility to change shift times or days off, flexibility to move from full-time to part-time or vice versa, flexibility to be off with children in the summer, etc.

The key is that nurses have unique preferences for schedules and these preferences tend to be quite consistent (Gray, McIntire, and Doller, 1993). Taking into account everyone's scheduling preferences and needs is important for staff satisfaction. It is the authors' philosophy that everything will work out perfectly if all this is taken into consideration!! After all, if what we think about is what will occur, better that we think about what is best!

TWELVE HOUR SHIFTS

Sometimes a mixture of 8- and 12-hour shifts are used. Twelve-hour shifts are popular because staff have more days off. One problem with twelve-hour shifts is that if the nurse is scheduled three or four days in a row, the nurse is tired and more prone to error. Many nurses hate 12-hour shifts because they find working a 12-hour shift very tiring, especially as they get older. Others love it—they tend to be the younger staff! There are several options with twelve hour shifts: 1) a nurse could work three 12-hour shifts each week and one 8-hour shift every two weeks, and receive full-time pay, 2) a person could work seven 12-hour shifts in one pay period—accruing 4 hours of overtime each pay period—a costly way to staff, 3) staff could work six 12-hour shifts in the pay period and either be paid full-time pay or only be paid for worked hours, 4) give full-time pay for working two 12-hour shifts every weekend, or 5) pay 36 hours weekly for working two 12-hour shifts on weekends. Think carefully about doing the more expensive options. Aside from being too expensive, if it is later stopped, staff will view it as something that is taken away, and lower morale will result.

---

[4] Reese (1998) discusses doing this for an ER.

One research study (Gillespie and Curzio, 1996) described nurses who worked 12-hour shifts as feeling less fatigued (20 percent) than those working 8-hour shifts (80 percent). They also found that the nurses' documentation was better on the 12-hour shifts. From the patient perspective it did not matter whether nurses worked 8- or 12-hour shifts. Working these shifts lets some nurses work full-time at one organization and then moonlight working additional shifts somewhere else.

STAFF SCHEDULING SOFTWARE SYSTEMS

Software packages are available for scheduling. It is best if these programs interface with the larger resource management system software so it can be linked with the patient classification system data, the human resource system, and the budget. The scheduling system must have the capability to use the current staffing plan and must be flexible enough to input any specified work hours. Does it reflect needed staff information, i.e., each worker classification, specified hours each staff member routinely works, staff availability, scheduling requests, staff experience, and vacation, sick or other nonproductive hours? Guidelines in choosing self-scheduling programs are provided by McConnell (2000).

Organizational Issues

Daily Staffing Communication

In more centralized situations, there may be a daily staffing meeting attended by the CNO, nurse managers, the shift supervisors, and other administrative personnel such as the nursing office staffing person. These meetings are used to identify unusual situations, to work out solutions, to find out bed availability, to share staffing concerns, to share what positions are open or filled, along with other administrative issues.

Position Control

Organizationally, position control is an important issue. This term, used by human resources, specifies actual FTEs assigned to a unit. Generally there is a position control format, computerized or paper trail, that tracks each person filling every FTE in the organization. Thus no one can fill a position that is already filled nor fill a position for more hours than the specified FTEs allocated to a cost center. Although the human resource department usually keeps track of the position control documentation, this responsibility is often shared with the nurse executive and/or nurse managers. **Exhibit 20–5** shows a typical position control document that specifies the total number of FTEs and lists all staff members, their positions, and their correct FTE designation. The authors recommend that the nurse manager be sure that records are updated, noting such things as leave of absence (LOA), vacancies, new employees, changes in FTE designations for positions, and any other issues that would effect the FTEs. Then in the future if some question arises regarding actual number of FTEs, the nurse manager has the documentation to show the accurate amount. Usually a nurse manager can decide to split the FTEs differently, the main issue would be that the total FTEs still remain the same.

Exhibit 20–5 Position Control

Position Title	FTE	Hours/Year	Hours/Week	Name
Nurse Manager	1.0	2,080	40	S. Rutherford (8/19/82)
RN	1.0	2,080	40	J. Smith (2/14/95)
RN	0.6	1,248	24	C. Jones (0.3) (4/25/01), K. Wilson (0.3) (10/7/01)
LPN	1.0	2,080	40	T. Blair (11/17/98)
Nurse Aide	1.0	2,080	40	D. Dixon (6/3/04)
Nurse Aide	0.8	1,664	32	R. Thomas (6/18/97)
Unit Secretary	1.0	2,080	40	E. Simmons (7/15/03)

Job Analysis

Sometimes job analysis can be useful. A person may have so many job responsibilities that they cannot do the job well. One example of this would be a nurse manager responsible for 150 FTEs. In this case, it becomes necessary to create another nurse manager position. In fact, the industry standard is that approximately 50 FTEs or less is the cut-off point for nurse managers. In this case, two additional nurse managers are needed. In fact, the industry standard is below 50 FTEs depending upon unit complexity, size, patient acuity, case mix, and scope of responsibilities. One study found that the best average was 36.8 FTEs per nurse manager (Altaffer, p. 37).

Job analysis is also used when an employee is expected to perform duties that were not included in the original job description. The human resource department can evaluate job responsibilities by performing a task-based job analysis, where one defines tasks, duties, knowledge, and skills; or use a competency approach, where one examines necessary competencies required for the job.

Centralization versus Decentralization

How much should be centralized into one nursing office, and how much should be handled on the unit level by the nurse manager? The authors advocate decentralizing as much as possible. With staffing issues, this means that the nurse manager or staff on a unit has the responsibility for scheduling staff, not a centralized nursing office. The budgetary accountability would also fall to the nurse manager. Decentralization also means that the nurse manager has the responsibility to interview and choose staff, orient staff, evaluate staff, and be there on a day-by-day basis to handle the many problems that occur. In some decentralized systems there are no shift supervisors. The nurse manager staffs for all open hours. When someone calls in sick, the unit secretary, or another staff member, will need to find someone to work. If no one is available, one of the staff will have to stay and work overtime. In this situation, it is best to have a designated list of employees to call in to work—that all staff have agreed upon. Then staff are more likely to support each other, and accept more responsibility for using teamwork across shifts.

Even though much is decentralized, there is still a useful place for certain centralized functions such as staff development, and nurse recruitment. In a centralized system there are often shift supervisors that attend to last minute staffing changes or unusual patient needs that occur when the nurse manager is not working. This does not always encourage staff autonomy but does help when staffing is tight.

Closed versus Open Unit Concept

Organizationally, the authors advocate a closed unit concept as being best. On a *closed unit*, when there is effective leadership, staff on that unit cover for each other. In this arrangement, teamwork is more likely to happen. If the staff do not come to work at the assigned time, the other nurses working on that unit would have to work overtime or come in on a scheduled day off. Peer pressure—along with good leadership—encourages staff to work together, support each other, and not call in sick unless really ill. Overtime usage goes down and staff cohesiveness increases. Patient and physician satisfaction improves and turnover goes down (Ruflin, Matlack, Holy, Sorbello, Nadzan, and Selden, 1999). The only problem with this arrangement is if the unit becomes drastically understaffed and occasionally needs help.

In a closed unit arrangement, there is no need for a nursing supervisor. As previously discussed, when someone calls in sick the current staff take care of it. Staff on one shift cannot leave until the next shift is properly staffed. The nurse manager—or another administrator—can be available by pager for emergencies. A few organizations do this but more often there are evening and night nursing supervisors on the premises—especially in hospitals.

In the closed unit arrangement, designated nurses are in charge so staff always know who assumes this role. The staff figure out amongst themselves how to cover absences. For instance, everyone's name may be on a list, rotating the calling so everyone has a turn.

Today however, the majority of units are *open units*, meaning that if a nurse calls in sick, a nursing supervisor will call in another nurse from that unit, find another nurse from a float pool or another division, or even call in an agency nurse to fill in for the sick nurse. The problem with open units is that this situation does not foster teamwork and self-responsibility. After all, someone else will worry about the staffing problems. In the open unit concept, ineffective leaders do not have responsibility to do anything about the problem. If anything, they are rewarded—staff are found for them—while an effective nurse manager, who did staff well on another floor, is penalized when their staff are pulled for units where there are ineffective nurse managers. *The authors recommend a closed unit!*

Sister Units

Sister units (or it probably is better to say *sibling* units) were developed so that two or more units in close proximity or that have fairly similar patients, would help each other out with staffing when needed (Wing, 2001). Cross training is important in this arrangement.

Which to Use?

As you can see, some scheduling options are more advantageous for a unit or department than others. Often several of the options are used. Good leadership is always critical for success. The main thing is to never forget the underlying outcome: *to provide quality services that each patient/family unit values in the most cost effective way.* After all, *the way we treat staff is the way they will treat patients.*

Retention

> ### Definition
>
> *Retention*—staff choose to stay for long periods within a cost center; turnover is under 10 percent annually.

> ### Definition
>
> *Turnover*—The number of staff that leave a cost center annually.

Retention begins with effective leadership, as described in Chapter 3 on Leadership. Retention is *always* important yet, unfortunately, receives more attention when there is a shortage. Think about a well-run department with committed staff. Retention is good. Chances are the manager is excellent; even if this manager has left, the staff continue with the principles established by themselves and that leader.

And think about the problem department. Staff morale will be low, causing high turnover. More overtime is needed, and so is more float staff. The first problem to be dealt with in such a department is to evaluate the leadership. Chances are, there is a leadership problem. It could be poor nurse manager leadership but may extend up to upper or top level administrators and the board.

If the leadership problem is not fixed, retention will not be realized and turnover will continue to occur. In fact, it spirals. Overall morale suffers. Overtime increases resulting in staff burnout if the problem is not fixed. There are more temporary staff being used. Costs go up. The present staff constantly have to orient new employees—and then the new employees do not stay. Productivity decreases. More safety issues or patient complications will occur. Satisfaction levels of staff, patients, physicians, and families suffer. Excellent employees leave or do not choose to work on that unit. And those who do work there begin to realize others do not want to work on their unit.

Everyone in the organization pretty much knows which departments are well run and which are not. Additionally, they know which departments to bypass or circumvent at all costs—the problem departments. As other people—including patients and their families—deal with the problem areas, the entire organization gets a bad reputation. And if the administration does not deal with the problem, the administration gives others the message that this is acceptable performance in the organization.

In well-run departments, good outcomes occur with high retention—staff, patient, and physician satisfaction; better patient outcomes; higher patient safety; fewer legal-ethical issues; and a better bottom line. In fact, "Alexander, Bloom, and Nichols (1997) in an organization-level study found that *combined voluntary and involuntary turnover of RNs was positively related to hospital operating costs per patient day*" (Anderson, Issel, and McDaniel, 1997, p. 70). Other research supports the costliness of turnover.

- Shader et al. (2001) found that higher turnover occurred when there was more job stress, lower group cohesion, lower work satisfaction, and weekend overtime. Retention was enhanced by higher work satisfaction, higher group cohesion, a more stable work schedule, and less work-related stress (p. 210).
- The Hay Group (2001) conducted research in 300 companies in 50 countries to help understand why nurses plan to stay for more than two years, or why they plan to leave in less than two years. Although they found wide disparities between what these two groups said about seven factors—use of my skills and abilities, ability of top management, company's sense of direction, advancement opportunities, opportunity to learn new skills, coaching and counseling from one's own supervisor, pay, and training—staff that planned to stay rated themselves considerably higher on each factor.
- Thompson and Brown (2002) studied RNs in skilled nursing facilities and found that "pay/benefits, work environment, and teamwork were factors in retention, while poor pay/benefits, schedule conflicts, and relocation were perceived as drivers of turnover" (p. 66).

Retention of unlicensed assistive personnel can be a big problem. For instance, it can reach 80 percent–400 percent in long-term care. Kupperschmidt (2002) advocates having realistic job previews so job expectations will be more realistic and improve retention.

Do you know why staff stay? It might be worthwhile to ask. Hill and Ingala (2002) advocate doing a *presence interview* to find out this information. Upenicks (2003) discussed a magnet hospital retention approach which includes: bonuses for longevity; 10–16 hours of continuing education per RN; 3 to 4 RNs on a unit attending a national conference each year; tuition reimbursement; premium pay when a nurse does overtime ($200 per shift); increasing staffing ratios (more RNs per patient); and both nursing and hospital-wide shared governance councils (p. 12).

The more staff are involved with the decision making at their level—from scheduling to patient care—the more likely they will be satisfied and stay. As a nurse manager, we are challenged to constantly involve staff in actually running the cost center. The core values, as discussed in the Organizational Strategy Chapter, provide the base for a well-run unit. Everyone is a contributing member. No one is more important than another. All have wonderful contributions to make. Every person has special gifts—gifts that no one else has. The leader's job is to recognize those gifts and to match an employee's gifts with the parts of the job they will do best.

Retention starts at the top—it is always helpful to have consistent, competent leadership—and needs to flow throughout the organization. That is why an organization's reputation is so important. Word gets around. Retention of competent, effective administrators—from the CEO through the nurse managers (Squires, 2001)—is as important as retention of nurses (Fralic, 2000; AONE *Nurse Recruitment and Retention Study*, 2000), and retention of unlicensed personnel (Kupperschmidt). Employees are more likely to stay and feel valued in well-run organizations.

There are many examples of well-run departments, fewer examples of well-run organizations, but they exist. It takes constant work to keep it that way.

One example of *nurse retention* was achieved at Poudre Valley Health System in Ft. Collins, Colorado. Its vacancy rate was 4.6 percent (650 nursing positions) where the board "earmarked an additional $1 million annually to bolster the nurse staffing ranks. It's a small price to pay—total payroll is $67 million—to stabilize staffing…. [They established] a low patient-to-nurse ratio—about two to three medical-surgical patients per nurse during the day—Poudre Valley minimizes its need to make sudden personnel shifts. 'The nurses have a schedule they can count on…. They are in control of their personal lives.' Also, having more nurses helps keep length of stay low" (Thrall, 2001, 18, 20). In addition Poudre Valley has achieved four other factors contributing to retention:

- CEO and board support to discourage disruptive doctor behavior.
- Extra pay for nurses who help orient new hires for three months.
- Higher pay rates for nurses who serve as clinical coordinators or patient coordinators.
- Donates $350,000 a year to a nearby nursing school for scholarships in an accelerated program in which students with a B.A. can become nurses in 18 months. In return, the system gets 10 new nurses a year (p. 18).

High Turnover—The Antithesis of Good Leadership

When turnover on a department or unit rises above 10 percent per year, that is a sign that there is a leadership problem. Serrow, Conwart, Chen, and Speake (1993) found that

> estimates of nursing staff turnover ranged from 48% to 86% in non-profit nursing homes compared to only 20% to 30% in non-profit hospitals and ranged from 72% to 118% in for-profit nursing homes compared to only 30% to 44% in for-profit hospitals…. Turnover captures managers' attention because it is related to organizational performance in areas of cost efficiency,… certification violations, and death rates (Anderson, Issel, and McDaniel, p. 69).

Note that this is an overall average for the facilities included in this study—not the turnover from individual units. This means that some units had a better turnover rate while the turnover on other units was much higher.

Benchmarking data can also provide turnover rates. Remember however, that an average for an organization is not as meaningful as one for individual units. Additionally, be sure that the benchmarking measures similar criteria. Does the criteria include both voluntary and involuntary turnover? Are the following criteria included: 1) resignations, retirements, and deaths; 2) layoffs; 3) temporary workers; 4) staff changing from full time to part time; and 5) staff transferring to other units, to the staff pool, or to temporary positions? With benchmarking we can think we are comparing like circumstances yet in reality differences exist in the data. There are also factors such as not wanting to look bad with colleagues, or not knowing the actual figure but guessing.

What causes turnover? There have been a number of studies examining issues that correlate with higher turnover (Anderson, Issel, and McDaniel; Thompson and Brown, 2002). Thompson and Brown found that size was the only factor that approached significance—the larger the facility, the higher the turnover rate. Anderson, Issel, and McDaniel, individually examined turnover in nursing homes for RNs, LVNs, and nurse aides. They found that turnover was lower for all three groups in non-profit homes, homes with higher profit margins, and higher financial investment in administrative functions and roles.

How is turnover calculated? As with other budgeting terms, there is no industry standard. For instance, if a staff member transfers to another unit within the organization, some organizations do not include this person in the turnover figures while in other organizations they are included. The usual way to calculate turnover is as follows:

It is important to *use the actual number of people working on a unit* rather than FTEs

> *Number of people leaving positions on a unit/year ÷ Number of positions for the unit*
> *x 100 = % of turnover/year*

(full-time equivalents) because it is possible that two or three part-time people fill one FTE. For example, if a nurse manager is responsible for 40 FTEs, in actuality there might be 65 people filling the available FTEs. The authors recommend counting people who transfer as well as those who actually leave the organization. This gives a more accurate representation as to whether there is a leadership problem on the unit. Turnover rates must be examined on a consistent basis.

Turnover rates can be collected in more detail as well. For instance, one could separate full-time staff and part-time staff. One could count those who left the employer, numbers of filled or unfilled positions, numbers of contracted staff used as well as numbers of those who transferred to another cost center.

The turnover rates with excellent nurse managers will range below the 10 percent turnover mark while a problematic manager experiences a higher turnover. A couple caveats are necessary here as nothing is absolute. When a new nurse manager who is an effective leader takes over a problem unit, the turnover rate may continue to be higher than the 10 percent range while the nurse manager is stabilizing the unit and establishing standards of performance. In long-term care aide turnover is often 80 percent—leadership can be improved here too!

Turnover is very expensive. Actual costs that are easy to measure include a temporary worker or overtime, advertising, interviewing, orientation; these cost $10,000 to $12,000. However this number does not account for other hidden costs such as the person who temporarily assumes the role left empty, coworker and supervisor time dealing with the temporary nurse, lower productivity of a new nurse, and preceptor time spent orienting the new nurse. These circumstances can considerably raise the cost to $40,000 or more per nurse. In addition, the productivity loss can result in poorer patient outcomes, more legal issues, and other safety, quality, or accreditation concerns.

Another cause of turnover can occur when filling positions. If all applicants for a position look marginal, it is best not to hire any of the applicants for the position. We recommend only hiring those staff who look like they will do well on the unit. It can be a trap to hire a marginal person because one is desperate. [Desperate means that one has lost hope in finding a good applicant. It is better to change the thinking to, "The right person will be there at the right time." Even if there is a shortage, *all you need is one person!*] In the end, the nurse manager spends more time dealing with a marginal employee, and probably terminates them anyway. The nurse manager's time could have been better used actually helping to take care of patients! Renew the search process and rely on other methods to achieve the needed staffing.

Realistically, there will always be some turnover. This is good; it brings new, fresh people with different ideas into the workforce. To have no turnover is undesirable because this promotes stagnation. The issue is to keep turnover below 10 percent for the year.

Absenteeism

Absenteeism is another costly problem for organizations. The National Institute of Labor Studies reported that absenteeism was 2.5 percent in 1998 (Harter, 2001). Absenteeism can have many causes. When an employee experiences an illness, it can be nice to have sick time benefits so pay is not disrupted. However, there are employees that use a sick day as soon as it is accrued. Absenteeism is something that becomes a counseling issue when it occurs too frequently. It is best to directly discuss this issue with the employee. Why is the employee gone so much? Personnel laws prohibit the manager asking about specific medical problems. However, one can ask an employee to bring in a note from their physician. In some organizations the note is to be given directly to the human resource department; the nurse manager never sees it. Sometimes the employee will volunteer information about their illness or their reason for the absence. This can then be discussed. The employee may be absent for other reasons such as child care, adult care of a relative, a divorce, or other family or personal reasons.

Another issue that can be the root of the problem is whether the employee likes the work and the work setting. If the employee's gifts are not enhanced by the work, then perhaps the employee is in the wrong job. Or perhaps employee morale on the unit is low. The workplace culture may not promote teamwork so being absent may not be seen to affect others. Dialogue between employee and supervisor are essential here. Whatever the reason, it is helpful to have a consistent policy throughout the organization with all administrators supporting this policy—consistently discussing absenteeism issues with employees and counseling when appropriate. Extensive absenteeism does affect patient care.

Many of these issues gets back to the leadership. How involved are the employees in decision making about their work? How many opportunities are available to employees so they can stretch and try new things? How are employees treated? If they are devalued—treated like a menial worker who does not have a brain or personal aspirations—they will begin to act like that. (See the pygmalian effect discussed in Chapter 3.) The unit leadership may be the underlying cause of the absenteeism.

Now that both parents generally work in our society, both child care and parent care can become a problem for the employee. Sometimes it is necessary to take time off to care for other family members who are sick. Some organizations have dealt with that problem by offering day or night care services for sick relatives. This enables the employee to work while the relative receives care. This is a win-win situation for both employee and employer.

Sometimes absenteeism requires employee counseling. If someone is continually needing to be off, the work is not getting completed in the workplace. Absences affect the entire work team. There is a fine balance between absenteeism for reasonable reasons and absenteeism that is not acceptable. This remains a judgment issue for the nurse manager. When questioning such a circumstance, it can be helpful to discuss the situation with the nurse executive and with human resource personnel. There must be consistent standards for each employee. When discussing the absenteeism issue with staff be sure to find out whether there are other workplace problems that may be contributing to the employee's absence. It may be remedied by both you and the employee working out some new approaches or resolving some conflicts, or by finding some new challenges for the employee. No one likes doing exactly the same work day after day. We all need some new and different challenges. When taking disciplinary action, we recommend the involvement of the employee as described in the Disciplinary Action section later in this chapter.

Staff Recruitment and Hiring Practices

The most important recruitment tool is word of mouth. The organization's reputation out in the community is so important, both from the potential employee and patient perspective. Perhaps the most important source for recruitment are current employees. Succession planning is important—is everyone mentoring someone, or several people—to take over their jobs? Is this activity rewarded in the organization? If we think of this at all, we tend to think of doing this for management positions (Husting and Alderman, 2001). It is best if it can happen at every organizational level.

The American Organization of Nurse Executives (AONE) conducted a *Nurse Recruitment and Retention Study* (2000), which found that there is a strong association between recruitment and retention strategies. This makes sense as knowing and providing "what nurses want" is the key. This study identified eight important strategy categories:

1. Diverse and Personal Methods of Recruitment

   - Affiliations with nursing schools and outreach to new graduate nurses with internships, residencies, and extensive orientation programs aimed to ease the transition from school to workplace (Olson, et al., 2001).

   - Highly personal approach when talking with candidates at open houses, job fairs, and on-site interviews.

   - Pairing new technologies such as the Internet and consolidated applicant databases with direct mail and advertising.

2. Competitive Compensation and Flexible Benefits

   - Competitive salaries that recognize marketplace realities while maintaining equity with incumbent staff.

- Good, flexible benefits, especially tuition reimbursement, health insurance, retirement plans, paid time off, and child-care benefits.

3. Respect and Recognition

- Respect from management and ongoing recognition of nurses' efforts.

- A positive, collegial working environment.

- Attention to patient, staff, and physician satisfaction levels, recognizing that high morale leads both to successful word-of-mouth recruiting efforts and to better retention.

4. Outstanding Communication Between Management and Staff

- Consistent and skillful listening, sharing of information, and follow-up from management.

- Mechanisms such as surveys, meetings, forums, discussion sessions, focus groups, one-on-one conversations, suggestion boxes, and newsletters to support communication and feedback.

5. Adequate and Flexible Staffing Protocols

- Flexible scheduling that offers nurses control over what shifts they will work and number of hours worked, with attractive incentives for night, weekend, and holiday coverage.

- Support in balancing personal and professional lives by flexing hours to meet family and educational needs.

- Adequate staffing that allows the ability to spend appropriate time with patients.

6. Participation in Decision Making

- Input and participation in decision making that affects nursing practice, such as a shared governance model.

7. Professional Development

- Support for continuing education and professional practice development to ensure appropriate skill levels and enhance retention.

- Policies to facilitate advancement and mobility within the organization.

8. Strategic Planning for the Future

- Strategic planning to further identify issues and develop tactics regarding the aging nurse population.

- Active promotion of the features, benefits, and rewards of the nursing profession to young people (2000, pp. vi–vii).

Mentoring New Employees

Once the new employee is hired a carefully planned orientation is critical because the more helpful and friendly everyone is, the more likely the person will be to stay. So often new nurses are assigned to the night shift with very little support. Discuss this problem with the entire staff and be creative with solutions. Having a regular mentor is so important in the beginning, especially with new graduates. New staff need helpful role models. With the nursing shortage, consider having retired or "older" expert nurses mentor and precept new staff. The mentor would work the same schedule and help the new nurse plan and implement work with assigned patients. The mentor will encourage the development of good work habits and help the new employee successfully resolve reality shock. It is important for the nurse manager to sit down regularly with the new employee as well. The same is true for unlicensed staff; have someone that does the job orient the new staff member. Then as the manager, be sure to regularly discuss how things are going with the new staff member.

Often, to save money (!), we give the new nurse little or no support and have them work the midnight shift. In the long run, this is an expensive option. Work habits are established during this time. Staff are more likely to leave due to the lack of support. Initially if more expense is incurred to give that nurse a solid foundation, a lot is saved in the future—including retention of the employee, and dollars saved that have resulted from not only employee retention and job satisfaction but patient safety.

Staff Education

Providing opportunities for staff education is always a priority in well-run organizations. According to Kinney (2001) the three most frequent learning needs in hospitals (the authors would add *any* organization) are leadership and management development, developing teams and teamwork, and learning how to use technology. He clumps other learning needs into orientation; customer service; and professional development, continuing education, and training. In well-run organizations staff education is a core value.

Some educational needs can be met within the organization, and many are achieved by going outside the organization for computer-assisted instruction or attending live educational events. Live educational events also give staff the opportunity to network and to find that other staff experience similar circumstances. Tanner (2002) examines costs and outcomes of professional staff development to help the administrator determine whether to meet these needs internally or externally. As the nursing shortage increases, chances are there will be a shortage of nurse educators within the organization, and outsourcing more education than usual may be necessary. Retired, experienced nurses and nurse educators may provide an additional source for staff education.

It is important to determine whether educational outcomes are achieved. This includes both short-term outcomes—directly learning certain knowledge, skills, or competency achievement—and the long-term outcomes—job satisfaction, retention, and patient safety.

Educational costs, outlined by Tanner, include direct costs of the person teaching or precepting the staff receiving the education, the cost of replacing the staff attending the educational event, competency assessment tools and other direct teaching expenses, and the cost of tracking the educational event; and indirect costs such as course preparation time, education department overhead, cost of staff errors that may have been prevented with more educational opportunities, staff retention and satisfaction, and the resultant patient satisfaction. Educational costs can be difficult to determine because staff, such as clinical specialists or intensivists, may provide education while actually taking care of patients.

Monetary Incentives

Individual Incentive Plans

NURSE COMPENSATION

The dilemma with staffing monetary incentives is that it seems like we are always cutting costs yet we must be competitive with the current staffing market. When there are shortages, generally everyone increases salaries for new employees to facilitate recruitment. The problem with this quick-fix solution is that long-term employees often do not get commensurate salaries raises—and they are the most valuable employees as they are already oriented, fully functional, and have been loyal to the organization. Unfortunately, research bears this out. "RNs with five or more years tenure in a setting had lower pay and benefits costs per admission than did the other categories of nurse staff" (Shullanberger, p. 128). In this situation the long-term employees feel less valued. We do not want to send this message. So let's not forget the tried and true employees with better compensation and benefits.

This issue illustrates another dilemma. As nurses stay within an organization, eventually their pay reaches the maximum amount for their personnel classification. These experienced nurses begin to feel devalued. And because they are not as likely to leave, the organization does not concentrate additional dollars to this group, or, if they do, it is a bonus that may not be renewed the following year. The salary is not permanently raised. Yet these are our most valuable employees!

Another related problem is a salary/gender issue. Women in the United States earn 74 cents for every dollar a man earns. This has improved over the last 30 years, but continues to be a problem. Although more men are going into the nursing profession, RNs are predominantly women. Unfortunately, it usually takes a shortage before RN compensation makes any gains above the rate of inflation. For instance, throughout the 1990s RN salaries never increased above the inflation rate. Now as the shortages are occurring, salaries are increasing.

Another related policy issue is that presently in many pension plans there is a maximum pay limit a retired person can receive to remain eligible. This may need to be changed if the professional shortages get serious enough that we do not have enough professionals to do all the work.

The benefit package—both traditional sick, vacation, and holiday time; a health and life insurance package; social security, unemployment, and worker's compensation; retirement plans; and other options—must be examined. Presently many organizations use a cafeteria approach to benefits, where employees choose which benefits they will have. In addition most health insurance plans charge deductibles and coinsurance. In the past, as budget cuts were made, sometimes benefits like tuition reimbursement were axed. To do this is like shooting oneself in the foot! In this time of staff shortages and increased emphasis on safety, the better educated our nurses are, the better they can safely serve the patients. In addition, education is a recruitment and retention factor for nurses. AONE (2000) recommends having tuition reimbursement, scholarships, loan assistance, and forgivable loans for nurses obtaining their BSN and MSN. In addition nurse faculty loans need to be forgiven. Another enhancement some organizations offer is paying the deductibles and coinsurance for employees' health insurance.

Additional benefits are being added with the shortages—things like child (or older adult) care; housecleaning; grocery shopping; home mortgage loans; providing massage; providing close, free parking, meals, movie tickets, shopping certificates; and other stress-releasing options at no cost.

It can be helpful to know what nurse compensation is being paid at competitive organizations. Yet it is price fixing to actually get all the organizations together and have each organization offer the same salary. While comparing, do not despair if another organization's salaries or benefit package is better than your organization. Nursing staff will consider other factors when looking for positions such as a helpful, more friendly work environment, adequate staffing, more vacation time, a more flexible schedule, a salary package that maintains equity with incumbent staff, better retirement plans, and child or adult care.

It is interesting to note that over the last twenty years, looking at health care organization costs, the overall costs have gone up more than nursing costs have increased. This is because we have added so many new services such as information systems, risk management, quality assurance, and bioengineering.

As an organization examines the salary question, the question is, how much can the organization afford yet still get qualified applicants?

DIFFERENTIATED PAY STRUCTURE/MERIT PAY/PAY FOR PERFORMANCE

When examining salaries, another important concept must be considered. Differentiated pay, merit pay, and/or bonuses, if carefully thought out, can provide a boost, or extra "thank you," to deserving staff, and can serve as a good retention tool. After all, a bird in the hand is worth two in the bush! What are the desired characteristics of various workers within the same profession? For instance, we all know that certain nurses are able to successfully give safe, effective care to more patients than other nurses. Does our merit criteria identify these high achievers? And what about things like teamwork? If a high achiever never helps anyone else, this is not desirable. What about floating? If someone can do this effectively, perhaps this person deserves higher pay. Desired characteristics can include specialty certification, a BSN or higher degree, clinical specialty, helpfulness to patients and families, ethical behavior, professionalism, or leadership. Involve staff in setting the criteria. What is valued? The idea is to pay more/reward for the desired performance.

DIFFERENTIALS AND BONUSES

Differentials and bonuses are extra money given to employees in certain circumstances. It is money that is not included in the base salary. It is a common practice to pay evening and night shift differentials—extra pay per hour worked. Sometimes this applies to weekends. On-call pay is another source of additional pay. It is easy to decide to give other differentials—or special pay or bonuses—when staff shortages occur. For instance, paying a differential to staff who work in areas experiencing shortages such as critical care; or giving sign-on bonuses paid to new employees who sign a contract to work for a certain time period.

The authors would caution starting special pay or bonuses for two reasons. First, *once given to staff it is hard to take it away*. Staff expect it. Morale is affected when taken away. Second, *it sends a message to other staff not getting the pay that their work and loyalty is not appreciated*. With specialty differentials the unintended message is that employees in one type of specialty *are more valuable than another*. For example, if a critical care differential is started because there is a shortage of critical care nurses, how do the medical nurses feel? Like they are unappreciated. Our recommendation is to

> ***think of the long-term effects before ever starting a new differential or bonus.***

Gainsharing is another bonus program where specified amounts are paid to employees if the company achieves certain profits or productivity levels. Generally certain performance levels are set and this is paid quarterly, semi-annually, or annually only when the goals are achieved. The same is true of team-based incentive plans.

Be aware that in many health care organizations, bonuses, stock options, and perks—automobile, cell phone, first-class air travel, country/health club membership, and/or low-interest loans—may be given to the president and, sometimes, to the executive or physician group. This is included as an additional incentive(s) for the executive because these are given above base pay. Sometimes bonuses and stock options are only given as incentives for achieving certain goals (i.e., having saved a specified amount of money, increased employee productivity, and/or making a specified amount of profit).

Another type of bonus is the *golden parachute*—a specified severance lump sum payment and benefit package given to executives if suddenly fired or "let go," especially if involved in mergers or acquisitions. In large corporations, over half the CEOs have a severance package. A *silver parachute* can be given to middle- and lower-level managers for the same purpose.

Group-Based Incentive Plans

EMPLOYEE STOCK OWNERSHIP PLANS (ESOPs)

Another monetary incentive program, which can be available for employees at all organizational levels, is the *employee stock ownership plan*. Here each employee has stock ownership in the organization. This employee incentive can improve productivity, although sometimes employees can feel that they are "forced" to participate in the program. It is best when employees are consulted when changing over to the plan. There are tax benefits by establishing such plans. Sometimes ESOPs have been used to avoid an unfriendly takeover.

SICK TIME/VACATION TIME/ABSENTEEISM ISSUES

In many organizations one of the benefits for employees is sick time, personal time off, or vacation time (i.e., one day per month). Usually employees do not use all their sick time and it accrues from year to year. Vacation time can also accrue from year to year. Employers may face a problem if everyone took all their time at once because it would create a large deficit for the organization. Thus many employers cap accruals for sick and vacation time.

A few people will take their sick time as soon as it is accrued. They are consistently calling in sick about once a month. Because it is not planned time, no arrangements have been made to cover for this "ill" staff member. One way that some organizations have dealt with this issue is to give all employees PTO (personal time off) days instead of sick and vacation time. The idea here is that employees plan to take time off before they take it, and the organization can plan for their replacement.

PROFIT INCENTIVES

There are other kinds of monetary profit incentives. For example, sometimes administrators—presidents and the executive team—participate in a profit-sharing plan (or other titles such as incentive plans, cash awards, bonuses, revenue-enhancing programs, incentive plans) when productivity is at a certain level, and/or costs are decreased or remain at specified levels. When financial or other goals are reached, a specified amount of profit or bonus is earned. Incentive programs are dangerous, not only for ethical reasons, but that: 1) quality may not be even mentioned, and 2) the message is that the administrator(s) solely reached the goal. In actuality it took everyone in the organization to achieve the goal(s). It would be better, if starting such a plan, to include all in the organization and to include quality and patient safety goals. A few organizations do this but it is rare. If only the executive team receives the bonus, everyone loses—even the administrator, because the administrator will need to look in the mirror in the morning.

The ethical implications of some of the productivity bonuses are another matter. It is easy to sit in an office, never see a patient, and cut costs. In this scenario the bottom line is all important. The fact that more harm is caused to the patient is not seen by such people. This is ineffective leadership. Quint Studer (2000), a former CEO, discusses the danger with this mentality and with the trappings that go along with it—the cherry furniture and the private parking space close to the building.

It is much harder to be in touch with the patients and families, with the staff, and then determine whether money is cut! When the administrator is in touch with all concerned, productivity will go up, staff will feel better about their jobs, and there will be fewer patient complications and deaths because patients and their families will receive better care. In this case, everyone wins.

DISCIPLINARY ACTION

When employee performance is not up to the desired standard, disciplinary action must be taken. If not, it becomes a large cost to the organization. If disciplinary action is not taken, we inadvertently give the message that this is acceptable behavior. It is important to use a positive disciplinary approach and involve the employee as much as possible in dealing with the change needed to fix the problem. A wonderful classic article by Campbell,

Fleming, and Grote (1985) describes this disciplinary process and outlines what to do at each step. Disciplinary actions can be punitive and belittling when done in a negative way. However, it can be a time for growth and opportunity by involving the employee more positively in solving the problem. The employee and supervisor can dialogue on the changes that need to be made to fix the problem. The positive approach uses "reminders" rather than "warnings" and in this article they even advocate for the final step, giving the employee pay to take a day, not come to work, but to have time to ponder on whether they want to work to solve the problem or lose their job. Using the positive approach, the employee still has a choice as to whether or not to change, but the employee takes responsibility for the problem and chooses to change or lose the job.

Disciplinary action is usually defined by human resource policy. Generally it involves, first, talking with the employee about the issue; second, if the issue still occurs then getting together again and writing the changes needed; third, if the issues continue use suspension—a negative way to do it versus giving the employee a day off with pay to decide whether or not they choose to change; and fourth, dismissal if the employee still chooses the same negative actions. Defining the problem, and needed changes, in an objective way is essential. It is always best to discuss the issues with the nurse executive and with human resource personnel who usually can help to identify objective ways to deal with the problem. When dealing with unionized employees, there is generally a procedure already set up defining the disciplinary process, which often involves having a union representative being present during the disciplinary interview. You may want to have another person sit in to both support you and to be a witness as to what happened. Discuss this with the nurse executive.

Immediate dismissal issues are usually also found in the human resource policies. Typical issues for immediate termination (the word "firing" is generally not used) are: falsifying the employment application; physically harming a patient intentionally; intoxication, drug use, or drinking at work (here the employee often is first referred for peer assistance); possession of weapons; theft; or fighting.

Where Do the Extra Dollars Come from?

All of these monetary incentives cost money. However, if a health care organization is well run, like Quint Studer advocates, money for employee incentives will be available from money saved from law suits and the other results of poor leadership. Some of that money could be used to provide merit pay or incentive plans to deserving employees. When there is good leadership, everything else follows—less overtime; less turnover; more employee, patient, and physician satisfaction; fewer patient complications; less costly legal issues. This is money well spent.

References

Abbott, M. (September 1995). Measuring the effects of a self-scheduling committee. *Nursing Management, 26*(9), 64G–64G.

Agency for Healthcare Research and Quality. (March 2004). *Research in Action.* (www.ahrq.gov).

Aiken, L., Clarke, S., Cheung, R., Sloane, D., & Silber, J. (September, 2003). Educational levels of hospital nurses and surgical patient mortality. *Journal of the American Medical Association, 290,* 1617–1523.

Aiken, L., Clarke, S., Sloane, D., Sochalski, J., & Silber, J. (October, 2002). Hospital nurse staffing and patient mortality, nurse burnout, and job dissatisfaction. *Journal of the American Medical Association, 288*(16), 1987–1993.

Aiken, L., Clarke, S., & Sloane, D. (October 2000). Hospital restructuring: Does it adversely affect care and outcomes? *JONA, 30*(10), 457–465.

Aiken, L., & Patrician, P. (May/June 2000). Measuring organizational traits of hospitals: The revised nursing work index. *Nursing Research, 49*(3), 146–153.

Aiken, L., Smith, H., & Lake, E. (1994). Lower medicare mortality among a set of hospitals known for good nursing care. *Medical Care, 32*(8), 771–787.

Albany Times Union. (October 29, 2001). Nursing scramble persists.

Altaffer, A. (July 1998). First-line managers: Measuring their span of control. *Nursing Management,* 36–39.

American Association of Colleges of Nursing. (June 2004). *Working paper on the role of the clinical nurse leader.*

American Nurses Association. (1997). *Implementing nursing's report card: A study of RN staffing, length of stay and patient outcomes.* Washington, DC: American Nurses Publishing.

American Nurses Association. (1999). *Principles for nurse staffing: With annotated bibliography.* Washington, DC: American Nurses Publishing.

American Nurses Association. (2000). *Nurse staffing and patient outcomes: In the inpatient hospital setting.* Washington, DC: American Nurses Publishing.

American Nurses Association. (2001). *2001 ANA staffing survey.* Washington, DC: American Nurses Publishing.

American Organization of Nurse Executives (AONE). (January 2000). *Nurse recruitment and retention study.* Chicago: AONE.

American Organization of Nurse Executives Monograph Series. (October 2000). *Perspectives on the nursing shortage: A blueprint for action.* Chicago: AONE.

Anderson, R., Issel, M., & McDaniel, R. (Spring 1997). Nursing staff turnover in nursing homes: A new look. *Public Administration Quarterly,* 69–95.

Anonymous. (May 2000). Getting & keeping the best and the brightest. An AONE executive summary. *Nursing Management,* 17.

Anonymous. (July 1999). A special report: Nursing Management's salary review exclusive nurse manager, executive. *Nursing Management,* 21–23.

Anthony, M., Casey, D., Chau, T., & Brennan, P. (November–December 2000). Congruence between registered nurses' and unlicensed assistive personnel perception of nursing practice. *Nursing Economic$, 18*(6), 285–293, 307.

Anthony, M., Standing, T., & Hertz, J. (October 2000). Factors influencing outcomes after delegation to unlicensed assistive personnel. *JONA, 30*(10), 474–481.

Barigar, D., & Sheafor, M. (January 1990). Recruiting staff nurses: A marketing approach. *Nursing Management, 21*(1): 27–29.

Bednash, G. (June 2000). The decreasing supply of registered nurses: Inevitable future or call to action? *JAMA, 283*(22), 2985–2987.

Beeman, K. L., Jernigan, A. C., & Hensley, P. D. (March–April 1999). Employing new grads: A plan for success. *Nursing Economic$, 17*(2), 91–96.

Blegan, M., & Goode, C. (Spring 1997). Nurse staffing effects on patient outcomes: Results of main/mnrs joint collaborative grant. *MAINlines*, 7, 22.

Blegen, M., Goode, C., & Reed, L. (1998). Nurse staffing and patient outcomes. *Nursing Research, 47*(1), 43–50.

Blegen, M., & Vaughn, T. (1998). A multisite study of nurse staffing and patient occurrences. *Nursing Economic$, 16*(4), 196–203.

Blegen, M., Vaughn, T., & Goode, C. (January 2001). Nurse experience and education: Effect on quality of care. *JONA, 31*(1), 33–39.

Bliesmer, M., Smayling, M., Kane, R., & Shannon, I. (August 1998). The relationship between nursing staffing levels and nursing home outcomes. *Journal of Aging & Health, 10*(3), 351–372.

Bloom, J., Alexander, J., & Nuchols, B. (1997). Nurse staffing patterns and hospital efficiency in the United States. *Social Science Medicine, 44*(2), 147–155.

Bola, T., Driggers, K., Dunlap, C., & Ebersole, M. (July 2003). Foreign-educated nurses: Strangers in a strange land? *Nursing Management, 34*(7), 39–42.

Bolton, L., Jones, D., Aydin, C., Donaldson, N., Brown, D., Lowe, M., McFarland, P., & Harms, D. (Second Quarter 2001). A response to California's mandated nursing ratios. *Journal of Nursing Scholarship, 33*(2), 179–184.

Brewer, C., & Frazier, P. (September 1998). The influence of structure, staff type, and managed-care indicators on registered nurse staffing. *JONA, 28*(9), 28–36.

Buerhaus, P., Staiger, D., & Auerbach, D. (May–June 2000). Why are shortages of hospital RNs concentrated in specialty care units? *Nursing Economic$, 18*(3), 111–116.

Buerhaus, P., Staiger, D., & Auerbach, D. (November–December 2000). Policy responses to an aging registered nurse workforce. *Nursing Economic$, 18*(6), 278–303.

Campbell, D., Fleming, R., & Grote, R. (July–August 1985). Discipline without punishment—at last. *Harvard Business Review*, 162–178.

Capuano, T., Fox, M., & Gresh, B. (1992). Staffing nurses according to episodic census variations. *Nursing Management, 23*(10), 34–37.

Cockerill, R., Pallas, L., Bolley, H., & Pink, G. (1993). Measuring nursing workload for case costing. *Nursing Economic$, 11*(6), 342–349.

Connelly, L., Yoder, L., & Miner-Williams, D. (May 2000). Hidden charges: Top competencies to develop in a charge nurse. *Nursing Management*, 27–29.

Coughlin, C. (January 2000). Incentive compensation for nurses: Is this professional practice? *Journal of Nursing Administration, 30*(1), 3–5.

Cullen, K. (May 1999). Strong leaders strengthen retention. *Nursing Management*, 27–28.

Davidhizar, R., Dowd, S. B., & Brownson, K. (April 1998). An equitable nursing assignment structure. *Nursing Management*, 33–35.

De Groot, H., Burke, L., & George, V. (May 1998). Implementing the differentiated pay structure model: Process and outcomes. *JONA, 28*(5), 28–38.

Del Bueno, D. (November–December 2001). Buyer beware: The cost of competence. *Nursing Economic$, 19*(6), 250–257.

Douglas, D., & Mayweski, J. (February 1996). Census variation staffing. *Nursing Management, 27*(2), 32–36.

Duchscher, J. (September 2001). Out in the real world: Newly graduated nurses in acute-care speak out. *JONA, 31*(9), 426–439.

Dunham-Taylor, J., & Pinczuk, J. (2006). *Health care financial management for nurse managers: Applications from hospitals, long-term care, home care, and ambulatory care.* Sudbury, MA: Jones and Bartlett.

Dunn, M., Norby, R., Cournoyer, P., Hudec, S., O'Donnell, J., & Snider, M. (October 1995). Expert panel method for nurse staffing and resource management. *JONA, 25*(10), 61–67.

Fagin, C. (2001). *When care becomes a burden: Diminishing access to adequate nursing.* New York: Milbank Memorial Fund.

Flannery, T., & Grace, J. (Summer 1999). Managing nursing assets: A primer on maximizing investment in people. *Nursing Administration Quarterly, 23*(14), 35.

Fletcher, C. (June 2001). Hospital RN's job satisfactions and dissatisfactions. *JONA, 31*(6), 324–331.

Forte, P., & Forstrom, S. (January 1998). Work complexity assessment: Decision support data to address cost and culture issues. *JONA, 28*(1), 46–53.

Forte, P., Forstrom, S., & Lindquist, L. (July/August 1998). Work complexity assessment: Notes from the field. *JONA, 28*(7/8), 39–44.

Fralic, M., Ed. (2000). *Staffing management and methods: Tools and techniques for nursing leaders.* Chicago: AHA Press.

Frase-Blunt, N. (December 2001). Peering into an interview. *HR Magazine*, 71–77.

Gallagher, R., Kany, K., Rowell, P., & Peterson, C. (April 1999). ANA's nurse staffing principles. *AJN, 99*(4), 50–53.

Garry, R. (September 2000). Benchmarking: A prescription for healthcare. *JONA, 30*(9), 397–398.

Gillespie, A., & Curzio, J. (1996). A comparison of a 12–hour and eight-hour shift system. *Nursing Times, 92*(39), 36–39. (Reported in Shullanberger article.)

Gillies, D. (1994). *Nursing management: A systems approach.* 3rd ed. Philadelphia: W.B. Saunders.

Gliss, R. (January–February 2000). Job sharing: An option for professional nurses. *Nursing Economic$, 18*(1), 40–41.

Goode, C., Pinderton, S., McCausland, M., Southard, P., Graham, R., & Krsek, C. (February 2001). Documenting chief nursing officers' preference for bsn-prepared nurses. *JONA, 31*(2), 55–59.

Gray, J., McIntire, D., & Doller, H. (May/June 1993). Preferences for specific work schedules: Foundation for an expert-system scheduling program. *Computers in Nursing, 11*(3), 115–121.

Hall, L., Pink, G., Johnson, L., & Schraa, E. (July/August 2000). Developing a nursing management practice atlas: Part 1, methodological approaches to ensure data consistency. *JONA, 30*(7/8), 364–372.

Hall, L., Pink, G., Johnson, L., & Schraa, E. (September 2000). Development of a nursing management practice atlas: Part 2, variation in use of nursing and financial resources. *JONA, 30*(9), 440–448.

Harter, T. (March–April 2001). Minimizing absenteeism in the workplace: Strategies for nurse managers. *Nursing Economic$, 19*(2), 53–55.

Hausfeld, J., Gibbons, K., Holtmeier, A., Knight, C. S., Stadtmiller, T., & Yeary, K. (1994). Self-staffing: Improving care and staff satisfaction. *Nursing Management, 25*(10), 74–80.

From "The Retention Dilemma: Why Productive Workers Leave-Seven Suggestions for Keeping Them." Copyright (c) 2001 Hay Group, Inc. (July/August 2001) *Healthcare Executive*, 17.

Hendrix, T., & Foreman, S. (July–August 2001). Optimal long-term care nurse staffing levels. *Nursing Economic$, 19*(4), 164–175.

Herringer II, J. M. (April 1999). Duties and direction for managing contract nurses. *Nursing Management,* 24.

Hill, K., & Ingala, J. (October 2002). Just ask them! *Nursing Management*, 21.

Hoffart, N., & Willdermood, S. (April 1997). Self-scheduling in five med/surg units: A comparison. *Nursing Management, 28*(4), 42–45.

Hollabaugh, S., & Kendrick, S. (February 1998). Staffing: The five-level pyramid. *Nursing Management, 29*(2), 34–36.

Hung, R. (January–February 2002). A note on nurse self-scheduling. *Nursing Economic$, 20*(1), 37–39.

Husting, P., & Alderman, M. (September 2001). Replacement ready? Succession planning tops health care administrators' priorities. *Nursing Management*, 45–50.

Irvin, S. A., & Brown, H. N. (July–August 1999). Self-scheduling with Microsoft Excel. *Nursing Economic$, 17*(4), 201–206.

JONA Supplement. (March 2003). Choosing a Travel Nursing Agency. A supplement to *JONA, 33*(Supplement 1).

Jones, C. (1990). Staff nurse turnover costs: Part II. Measurements and results. *Journal of Nursing Administration, 20*(5), 27–32.

Kalist, D. (July–August 2002). The gender earnings gap in the RN labor market. *Nursing Economic$, 20*(4), 155–162.

Kerr, P. (2000). Comparing two nursing outcomes reporting initiatives. *Outcomes Management for Nursing Practice, 4*(3), 144–149.

Kido, V. (November 2001). The uap dilemma. *Nursing Management, 32*(11), 27–29.

Kieltyka, C., Robertson, S., & Behner, K. (January 1997). A flexible staffing model for patient service associates. *JONA, 27*(1), 48–54.

Kinney, T. (2001). Highlights of the Report on Human Resource, Education, Nurse Retention Issues in Hospitals, *thomaskinney–msn.com*.

Kramer, M., & Schmalenberg, C. (1977). *Path to biculturalism*. Wakefield, MA: Contemporary Publishing.

Krugman, M., Smith, K., & Goode, C. (May 2000). A clinical advancement program: Evaluating 10 years of progressive change. *JONA, 30*(5), 215–225.

Kuhnert, K., & Lewis, P. (1987). Transactional and transformational leadership: A constructive/developmental analysis. *Academy of Management Review, 12*(4), 648–657.

Kupperschmidt, B. (November–December 2002). Unlicensed assistive personnel retention and realistic job previews. *Nursing Economic$, 20*(6), 279–283.

Kupperschmidt, B. (March 2001). UAPs: To have and to hold. *Nursing Management,* 33–34.

Kupperschmidt, B. (December 2001). Understanding net generation employees. *JONA, 31*(12), 570–574.

LaDuke, S. (April 2000). Nurses' perceptions: Is your nurse uncomfortable or incompetent? *JONA, 30*(4), 163–165.

Letvak, S. (July/August 2002). Retaining the older nurse. *JONA, 32*(7/8), 387–392.

Livingston, J. (September–October 1988). Pygmalion in management. *Harvard Business Review,* 121–130.

Loevinsohn, H. (July 1992). A new perspective on scheduling: Freedom and cost control. *Nursing Management, 23*(7), 56–61.

Luthans, F. (1988). Successful vs. effective real managers. *The Academy of Management Executive, 11*(2), 127–132.

MacPhee, M. (April 2000). Hospital networking: Comparing the work of nurses with flexible and traditional schedules. *JONA, 30*(4), 190–198.

Manthey, M. (March 1988). Primary practice partners (a nurse extender system). *Nursing Management, 19*(3), 58–59.

Manthey, M. (March 2001). Creative Health Care Management, 1701 East 79 St., Suite #1, Minneapolis, MN 55425.

Manthey, M. (September 2001). A core incremental staffing plan. *JONA, 31*(9), 424–425.

Marchiono, P. M. (October 1987). Modified cyclical scheduling: A practical approach. *Nursing Management, 18*(10), 60–64.

Mark, B. (May 2002). What explains nurses' perceptions of staffing adequacy? *JONA, 32*(5), 234–242.

Mark, B., Salyer, J., & Wan, T. (November 2000). Market, hospital, and nursing unit characteristics as predictors of nursing unit skill mix: A contextual analysis. *JONA, 30*(11), 552–560.

McClung, T. (November 2000). Assessing the reported financial benefits of unlicensed assistive personnel in nursing. *JONA, 30*(11), 530–534.

McConnell, E. (March 2000). Staffing and scheduling at your fingertips. *Nursing Management,* 3, 52–53.

McConnell, E. (May 2001). Competence vs. competency. *Nursing Management, 32*(5), 14.

McNeese, D. (March 2000). Job stages of entry, mastery, and disengagement among nurses. *JONA, 30*(3), 140–147.

Mee, C. (May 2000). What does nursing pay? *Nursing Management,* 27–28.

Melberg, S. (November 1997). Effects of changing skill mix. *Nursing Management, 28*(110), 47–48.

Meretoja, R., & Leino-Kilpi, H. (July/August 2001). Instruments for evaluating nurse competence. *JONA, 31*(7/8), 346–352.

Miller, K., Grindel, C., & Patsdaughter, C. (July 1999). Cardiac surgery's calculated risk: Use risk classification to predict clinical outcomes and staffing needs for cardiac surgery patients. *Nursing Management,* 34, 36.

Miller, N. (May 1992). Job satisfaction through self-scheduling. *Nursing Management, 23*(5), 96B–96D.

Mitty, M. (1998). *Handbook for directors of nursing in long-term care.* Albany, NY: Delmar.

Munroe, D. (December 1988). Commitment of part-time nursing personnel: A challenge. *Nursing Management,* 59–61.

Needleman, J., Buerhaus, P., Mattke, S., Stewart, M., & Zelevinsky, K. (2001). *Nursing Staffing And Patient Outcomes In Hospitals.* Final Report, US Department of Health and Human Services, Contract No. 230–99–0021.

Nursing Executive Center. (2000). *Reversing the flight of talent: Nursing retention in an era of gathering shortage.* Washington, DC: The Advisory Board Company.

Olson, R., Nelson, M., Stuart, C., Young, L., Kleinsasser, A., Schroedermeier, R., & Newstrom, P. (January 2001). Nursing student residency program: A model for a seamless transition from nursing student to RN. *JONA, 31*(1), 40–48.

Payne, D. (February 2001). Credentialing and privileging complementary care providers. *Nursing Management,* 16.

Pear, R. (July 2000). U.S. recommends strict new rules at nursing homes: Concern over staffing: Officials say patients may be endangered by shortages of both nurses and aides. *New York Times.*

Peter D. Hart Research Associates. (April 2003). *Patient-to-Nurse Staffing Ratios: Perspectives from Hospital Nurses.*

Pinkerton, S., & Rivers, R. (September–October 2001). Factors influencing staffing needs. *Nursing Economic$, 19*(5), 236–237.

Powell, D. H. (November/December 1999). Retaining third-seasoners: The time is ripe. *Healthcare Executive,* 5–10.

Prescott, P., & Bowen, S. (June 1987). Controlling nursing turnover. *Nursing Management,* 18, 60–66.

Reese, S. (July/August 1998). Emergency department productivity improvement through a management-staff partnership. *JONA, 28*(7/8), 27–31.

Rudy, S., & Sions, J. (April 2003). Floating: Managing a recruitment and retention issue. *JONA, 33*(4), 196–198.

Rufflin, P., Matlack, R., Holy, C., Sorbello, S., Nadzan, L., & Selden, T. (June 1999). Closed-unit staffing speaks volumes. *Nursing Management, 30*(6), 37–39.

Salvatore-Magalhaes, J. (May 1999). Remember where you came from: Personal interviews put nurses' motivational needs in perspective. *Nursing Management,* 29–30.

Santos, S., & Cox, K. (January–February 2000). Workplace adjustment and intergenerational differences between matures, boomers, and xers. *Nursing Economic$, 18*(1), 7–13.

Savage, C. (2001). Executive coaching: Professional self-care for nursing leaders. *Nursing Economic$, 19*(4), 178–182.

Schmalenberg, C., & Kramer, M. (1976). Dreams and realities, where do they meet? *Journal of Nursing Administration, 6*(6), 35–43.

Schmidt, D. (Summer 1999). Financial and operational skills for nurse managers. *Nursing Administration Quarterly, 23*(4), 16.

Seago, J., & Ash, M. (March 2002). Registered nurse unions and patient outcomes. *JONA, 32*(3), 143–151.

Senge, P. (1990). *The fifth discipline: The art & practice of the learning organization.* New York: Doubleday/Currency.

Senge, P., Kleiner, A., Roberts, C., Ross, R., Roth, G., & Smith, B. (1999). *Dances of change: The challenges to sustaining momentum in learning organizations.* New York: Currency.

Serrow, W., Conwart, M., Chen, Y., & Speake, D. (September–October 1993). Health care corporatization and the employment conditions of nurses. *Nursing Economic$, 11*(5), 279–291.

Shader, K., Broome, M., Broome, C., West, M., & Nash, M. (April 2001). Factors influencing satisfaction and anticipated turnover for nurses in an academic medical center. *JONA, 31*(4), 210–216.

Sherer, J. (September 1994). Personnel power: In Vermont, hospital workers pool talents to fight short-staffing. *Hospitals & Health Networks*, 60–62.

Sherry, D. (1994). Coping with staffing shortages: Strategies for survival. *Home Healthcare Nurse, 12*(1), 38–42.

Shindul-Rothschild, J., Berry, D., & Long-Middleton, E. (November 1996). Where have all the nurses gone? Final results of our patient care survey. *AJN, 96*(11), 25–39.

Shogren, E., Calkins, A., & Wilburn, S. (1996). Restructuring may be hazardous to your health. *American Journal of Nursing, 96*(1), 64–66.

Shullanberger, G. (May–June 2000). Nurse staffing decisions: An integrative review of the literature. *Nursing Economic$, 18*(3), 124–148.

Sochalski, J., Aiken, L., & Fagin, C. (1997). Hospital restructuring in the United States, Canada, and Western Europe: An outcomes research agenda. *Medical Care, 35*(10), OS13–OS25.

Squires, A. (March 2001). Sink-or-swim tactics? *Nursing Management, 33*, 35.

Staiger, D., Auerbach, D., & Buerhaus, P. (September–October 2000). Expanding career opportunities for women and the declining interest in nursing as a career. *Nursing Economic$, 18*(5), 230–236.

Strachota, E., Normandin, P., O'Brien, N., Clary, M., & Krukow, B. (February 2003). Reasons registered nurses leave or change employment status. *JONA, 33*(2), 111–117.

Strickland, B., & Neely, S. (March 1995). Using a standard staffing index to allocate nursing staff. *JONA, 25*(3), 13–21.

Studer, Q. (March 2000). *Taking your organization to the next level.* American Organization of Nurse Executives Annual Meeting. National Nursing Network Inc., 4465 Washington St., Denver, CO 80216.

Tanner, A. (February 2002). Professional staff education: Quantifying costs and outcomes. *JONA, 32*(2), 91–97.

Taylor, K. (September 2000). Tackling the issue of nurse competency. *Nursing Management*, 35–37.

Taylor, M. (November–December 1991). SWAT team: Aggressive approach to the '90s. *Nursing Economic$, 9*(6), 431–433.

Thrall, T. (September 2001). Skipping gimmicks, keeping nurses. *Hospitals and Health Networks*, 18, 20.

Thrall, R. (March 2003). Filling those shifts. *Hospitals and Health Networks*, 20, 38.

Thompson, T., & Brown, H. (March–April 2002). Turnover of licensed nurses in skilled nursing facilities. *Nursing Economic$, 20*(2), 66–69.

Ulrich, B. (September 2001). Successfully managing multigenerational workforces. *Seminars for Nurse Managers, 9*(3), 147–153.

United States General Accounting Office (GAO) Report to the Chairman, Subcommittee on Health, Committee on Ways and Means, House of Representatives. (July 2001). Nursing Workforce: Emerging Nurse Shortages Due to Multiple Factors. *GAO*, -01-944.

Upenieks, V. (January–February 2003). Recruitment and retention strategies: A magnet hospital prevention model. *Nursing Economic$, 21*(1), 7–13, 23.

Urden, L. D. (May 1999). What makes nurses stay? *Nursing Managment,* 27–30.

Van Servellen, G., & Schultz, M. (April 1999). Demystifying the influence of hospital characteristics on inpatient mortality rates. *JONA, 29*(4), 39–47.

Wieck, L. (June–July 2000). Tomorrow's nurses: Are we ready for them? *Texas Nursing,* 1–4.

Wheatley, M. (1999). *Leadership and the new science: Discovering order in a chaotic world.* San Francisco: Berrett-Koehler.

White, K. (July 2003). Effective staffing as a guardian. *Nursing Management, 34*(7), 20–25.

Wineland, J. (January 2003). We grow staff, not just wheat, in Kansas. *Nursing Homes, Long Term Care Management,* 33–34.

Whitman, G., Davidson, L., Rudy, E., & Wolf, G. (February 2001). Developing a multi-institutional nursing report card. *JONA, 31*(2), 78–84.

Wing, K. (January 2001). When flex comes to shove: Staffing and hospital census. *Nursing Management,* 43–47.

Wycoff, J. (1991). *Mindmapping: Your personal guide to exploring creativity and problem-solving.* New York: Berkley Books.

CHAPTER 21

Productivity

Janne Dunham-Taylor, PhD, RN

What Is Productivity?

The American Productivity and Quality Center defines *productivity* as "a process of getting more out of what you put in. It's doing better with what you have" (from the American Productivity Center, Health Education Associates, p. 105). From the health care perspective, we want "to achieve positive health outcomes at the lowest possible cost" (Chang, Price, and Pfoutz, p. 433). Using these definitions, to achieve better productivity, we need to examine both the *quality* and the *quantity* of the outcome, as well as scrutinize the resources and processes necessary to achieve that outcome. Enhancing productivity involves achieving more efficiencies, and must be linked with effectiveness. Productivity is one of those elusive things that is hard to measure, and where, no matter how well we accomplish it, there is still room for improvement.

Productivity has been measured nationally, organizationally, and individually. *Nationally,* when there is high productivity, higher standards of living result. When productivity increases and costs remain the same, the country benefits. However, often when productivity increases, costs can increase. Then, purchasing power can decrease and inflation can occur. When productivity decreases, labor costs often go up, and a less competitive position results.

Organizational productivity is necessary to stay competitive. It is something to consider every day as we do our work. Every chapter in this book speaks to productivity, because if

> **Productivity**
> - *"A process of getting more out of what you put in. It's doing better with what you have."*
> - *"Achieve positive health outcomes at the lowest possible cost."*
> - *Measures both the quality and the quantity of the outcome taking into account the resources and processes it took to accomplish this outcome.*
> - *Takes into account both efficiency and effectiveness.*

anything is wrong, such as poor leadership or ineffective organizational systems, more resources will be used, and thus productivity will suffer. If allowed to continue, the organization will not be able to remain competitive and could eventually close. There are many strategies people in organizations use to increase productivity, including: outsourcing services; purchasing capital equipment to support workers; replacing people with machines, (i.e., in the pharmacy with counting pills); purchasing available technology, (i.e., a computerized documentation system); and redesigning work so the work goes faster, is easier, and is more rewarding.

Individual productivity can be important in any setting, at work or at home. Three factors are important with individual productivity. First, the person needs to have the ability to do the work. This includes education and experience, competency, as well as the capability and intelligence to understand the work. But it also includes an adequate orientation to specifics that need to be accomplished; an ability to correctly prioritize activities; the quality of the work that is completed; and the ability to work cooperatively with others. The second factor with individual productivity comes from within—how much effort is the person willing to put into accomplishing the work? This can be influenced by the environment—the amount of teamwork, chemistry with the supervisor, and whether one enjoys the people one works with. But this is also influenced by whether the work is a match with a person's gifts. This willingness is exemplified by such things as promptness, good attendance, reliability, accuracy, honesty, adaptability, creativity, integrity, caring, and love, as defined in Chapter 3. A third factor involved in individual productivity is the support given to a worker, such as having a computerized documentation system, purchasing the latest equipment that makes the job easier to do, and, as nurses are get older, changing to shorter shift times and providing assistance to help with the physical part of the work. Individual productivity is affected by all three factors, increasing or decreasing accordingly.

Besides these issues, additional complications can influence productivity in health care. First, our product is not a widget being produced, but instead *our product is service*. When producing widgets, it is easier to make sure that each widget has consistent quality. Normally, as one purchases the widget, one can inspect it, and can determine whether it is something one wants to buy. However, when producing a service, no two people are alike, even when we are treating patients with similar problems. In service, *people, with all their differences, are serving people, who all have different needs.* Thus one client or patient may be quite satisfied with a service, while another person receiving a similar service may be displeased with it.

The problem with our service industry is that as one experiences it, one purchases it. One has not had the opportunity to have first inspected it. In fact, often the purchaser has no prior historical knowledge as to the quality of service given to others by a provider:

> Estimating the quality of health care services is a particularly vexing problem. In purchasing goods such as household appliances and automobiles, the consumer is usually able to judge the quality of a product by inspection or by referring to a consumer's guide for information on that product's durability and performance. If a manufacturer consistently

creates inferior goods, consumers can express their quality preferences by not purchasing those products.

> The purchase of health care services is fundamentally different. Because health care is a service, production and consumption of the service are simultaneous events. The consumer cannot return a defective product and often cannot reverse the effects of poor service. Furthermore, few consumers have access to a guide to health care services. Evaluation of quality is left to the consumer, who has neither the time nor the necessary knowledge on which to base this decision. Instead, the health care consumer must rely on the ethical obligation of the professional to exercise sound judgment about the type and quantity of health care required.
>
> . . . Measuring effectiveness is difficult because the ultimate outcome of many episodes of illness care or treatment encounters is not known for some time after the case ceases (Sullivan and Decker, p. 121).

Other issues, such as the chemistry that occurs between people, affect quality. Administratively, this becomes very complicated because staff, administrators, and physicians differ in the way they respond to situations, to each other, and to patients and their families. In fact, the same person can respond differently when part of a different work group, when the person has a different boss, or with different patients.

Second, *our service product is not well defined.* Are we providing disease care, or are we providing health? More often, we treat disease, and, as we do this, our client experiences more discomfort. Our client may achieve better health as a final outcome, *although better health may never be discussed.* In fact, the best outcome may be a peaceful death. Most often it is the insurer(s), by defining what will be reimbursed, that determines what services will be provided.

Third, unless someone likes to be sick and wants the attention, *no one wants our product, unless they need it.* Then we want to be better or cured. Think about it. We are not eagerly saving our money so that we can purchase care for a disease! In fact, everyone is complaining that the costs of health care are too high.

Fourth, *it is difficult to quantify our service output.* We can measure patient days or visits, but it is more difficult to say that we cured x number of people with pneumonia; or x number of clients with heart disease. If there is a cure, chances are it happens after the patient no longer needs our services.

Fifth, *the service we provide may not be what our customers want or value.* What do they want, or expect, from our service? Do we even ask this question? Then if the question is asked, *how do we measure if we achieved it?*

The Open Systems Model

Productivity can best be described using the open systems model. In this model, a system has inputs, throughputs, and outputs. Or, put another way,

Input + Throughput = Output

INPUTS

> **Productivity**
> *Input + Throughput = Output*

The *inputs* include all the resources—human and non-human (materials, equipment, buildings). In health care, inputs might be labor hours, number and skill mix of nursing staff, other staff needed for various services, payroll expenses, money spent on equipment, supplies used, and remodeling or building expense. However, labor hours do not capture abilities. For example, two nurses that have the same educational background and years of experience can differ considerably in their ability to achieve appropriate patient outcomes, or in their ability to care for a certain number of patients safely and effectively.

THROUGHPUTS

Throughputs are all the *processes*—the things that people do—to achieve the output, the final product, or service. Throughputs include environmental factors that affect the quality of the output. In health care throughput is the actual care that is given, and the processes used to give that care. This can include leadership issues; employee issues—satisfaction, motivation, and sense of self confidence; organizational issues—group affiliations, and job design; equipment and supply availability; and technology.

Another aspect of the throughput is an examination of the *equity of services given*.

> In other words, which population receives the services and whether the services are fairly distributed. How one defines *fairly distributed* is based on agency philosophy and policy. Horizontal equity is how the effects of production are distributed across the population as a whole, e.g., all the types of clients who are seen by the agency from the geographic areas served. Vertical equity is how a given production function affects a specific target population, e.g., among all the clients who need intravenous (IV) therapy, have all received the service, and does the agency wish to provide service to all or only a segment of the population? Determine what the agency philosophy is regarding equity (for example, service to clients with the ability to pay or quality care to all), and use that as a framework when analyzing productivity (Harris, pp. 472–473).

Throughput can be difficult to measure in any service industry because it involves many interdisciplinary staff working effectively and collaboratively together. Organizational processes can enhance or impede productivity. It is also difficult to measure because care for one patient may involve a different number of resources than care for another patient. Additionally, factors such as whether there is a computerized documentation system, whether the care givers have all the necessary supplies and equipment at their fingertips, whether the staff are oriented properly, and whether the appropriate staff member is caring for the patient, exist.

OUTPUTS

Outputs result from the application of the throughputs and inputs. The output is *the material, goods and/or services, produced.* Reimbursement occurs based on the outputs. We continue to have difficulty measuring the true outputs. For example, did the patient get better? Presently reimbursement is made regardless of the output. The patient may be better, or may be worse or may have died! Perhaps the output was a planned, peaceful death.

Presently in health care we use *time* measurements as our outputs, such as the number of discharged patients within a DRG, patient days, procedures, and/or number of visits. Unfortunately, time measurement does not identify the quality of the outcome—did the patient get the necessary care, was the patient safe, and was the best outcome achieved? Better yet, did the patient get what s/he wanted or valued? Time measurement also does not reflect the amount of throughput needed, such as one patient requiring many more resources than another.

To capture quality or what the patient values, other measurements are necessary. Some may be qualitative. These output measurements include patient outcomes and patient satisfaction. Both are often measured after the care was received. Unfortunately, this is too late to change the care that was given. It would be more advantageous to find this out as much as possible during the care process so it could be changed before the patient leaves. We need a good measurement for determining what the patient wanted or valued, and whether this was achieved. This is probably the most important output in the health care industry, yet is generally not happening. This provides room for growth in the future!

ORGANIZATIONAL VIABILITY

Effective productivity and viability go hand in hand. When productivity is not as good as it could be, the bottom line suffers. A problem at any level, if unresolved, will detract from the everyone else's productivity. All these factors are interrelated. If one problem is ignored and allowed to continue, chances are, the overall productivity needs to be improved.

PRODUCTIVITY MISCONCEPTIONS

There are some misconceptions about productivity (see **Exhibits 21–1** and **21–2**) that can lead to viability issues if they get too far out of hand. As with all concepts, at times, even though we all use the same words, we are actually operating using different definitions. These differences should be identified and clarified early. When allowed to continue over years, the effects of the misconceptions can be considerable. We will identify some common misconceptions about productivity here.

Porter-O'Grady and Malloch (2003) identify three misconceptions that involve staff productivity:

> Business still operates under questionable assumptions regarding productivity—that the more hours employees work, the more productive they are; that the faster employees work, the more they accomplish; and that the more employees are paid, the more motivated they are to be productive—leaders are challenged to better understand the reality of employee productivity (**Exhibit 21–1**). Health professionals in this

country are working more hours than ever before and getting less done. In fact, Americans have the dubious distinction of being first in the number of hours worked each year. The U.S. Department of Labor, Bureau of Labor Statistics, noted only a slight increase in productivity from 1960 to 1990, and the productivity increase in the last 10 years is attributed to technological advances, particularly the development of the Internet.

Health care employees are burning out faster than the replacements are coming in, yet they are still being pushed to become more productive. They are working 12-hour days, are commuting up to 2 hours a day, and are held by an electronic leash to the office. Their opportunity to relax is almost nonexistent.

Contrary to popular beliefs, we need to learn how to slow down our thinking at times, not speed up. Time for reflection and contemplation of ideas and issues is sorely missing in health care. The never-ending checklist is always present and demanding attention. Further, experts report that pay is *not* the chief motivator for productivity. In general, employees desire to do meaningful work most of all, next they desire opportunities for collaboration through group decision making, and then they want equitable pay (pp. 317–318).

Exhibit 21–1 Myths and Truths About Employee Productivity

Accepted Notions

- If employees work more hours, they will be more productive.
- If employees work faster, they will be more productive.
- If employees are paid more, they will be motivated to work harder and produce more.

The Reality

- Employees perform optimally for six to seven hours and may be able to work longer in a burst of energy or inspiration, but then they must rest.
- Employees need balance; they need a life outside of work.
- Slower, intuitive thinking is often more effective in solving problems than mental agility.
- Studies show that, in Germany, where individual performance is not rewarded with pay increases, productivity is often higher than the United States.
- Employees are most productive when their employers pay them *equitably* and then do everything possible to help the employees put money out of their minds.

From: Johnson, C. B. (2000). When working harder is not smarter, *Inner Edge, 3*(2), pp. 18–21.

Exhibit 21–2 Productivity Misconceptions

- Work is not meaningful for staff.
- There is no opportunity for staff to collaborate with others.
- Pay is not equitable.
- Quantitative productivity measurements are "the be all and end all."
- Productivity is synonymous with budget cuts, or with unrealistic increases in workload.
- Budget cuts always result in negative outcomes.
- When a department experiences a productivity problem, the department head is directed to fix the problem.
- Productivity issues are an employee issue, not a management issue.
- As productivity increases, quality suffers.
- Staff need to work faster.
- Productivity improvement is the only way of improving income generation.
- Only internal issues cause productivity problems.
- Contract staff or contract services result in better productivity.

This provides us with three important ways (questions to ask) that will enhance productivity (see **Exhibit 21–3**). *First, is our work meaningful? Do staff feel that way about their work?* If not, what is the problem? Are they doing work that does not match their gifts? Do others treat them like they are unimportant? *Second, do staff have opportunities for collaboration?* Does group decision making occur? *Third, is the pay equitable?* How can we, as administrators, improve these issues in our workplace?

A fourth misconception is that *quantitative measurements are "the be all and end all"* to measure productivity. In other words, quantitative measurement is assumed to be the most effective measurement. In reality, quantitative productivity measurements provide a barometer about productivity, but need to be considered with other qualitative and efficiency data. More importantly, the quantitative measurement may not include other important productivity or quality factors. It is very dangerous to think that quantitative measurements alone provide all the data about actual productivity.

A fifth issue with productivity measurement is that in some cases productivity has gotten a bad reputation with some nursing staff, as the word "productivity"—as defined by the finance department—has been used *synonymous with budget cuts, or with unrealistic*

Exhibit 21–3 Ways to Enhance Productivity

- Is our work meaningful?
- Do staff feel that way about their work?
- Do staff have opportunities for collaboration?
- Is the pay equitable?

increases in workload. The short-term result can be not having enough staff to safely deliver care; dissatisfied nurses, physicians and patients; and more patient safety and legal issues.

> Slash-and-burn cost cutting brings only a series of onetime efficiencies. In the end, there's only one encore—another round of cost cutting. And that's the catch. This approach leads to increasingly hollow companies that ultimately are unable to maintain market share in an ever-expanding global economy (Roach, p. 154).

This view of productivity by nursing staff is unfortunate because the true meaning of productivity is that, chances are, we all could be more efficient and effective. But the slash-and-burn tactics are not the way to accomplish this goal. These tactics devalue staff and do not follow what employees most want—to have meaningful work, to collaborate in decision making, and to have adequate pay. Following these three precepts, if budget cuts are needed, all need to be involved in the identification of where the cuts will occur. And maybe staff will have other ideas as to different ways to make money and offer better services that will negate the need to cut the budget!

A sixth misconception is that *budget cuts always result in negative outcomes.* This is not necessarily the case. This is related to a seventh misconception, that as *productivity increases, quality suffers.* Let's look at an example of a budget cut that actually enhanced both quality and productivity improvement.[1]

You are the nurse manager on a general surgical unit. Nurses work 12-hour shifts on this unit. Starting with the day shift, mornings are not that busy. However at 2PM there suddenly are a lot of admissions, discharges, and transfers. Beds get held up either because patients have not left them, or because the beds have not been cleaned. The emergency room, recovery room, and intensive care units get into a holding pattern because they cannot transfer patients. This chaos continues until by 7PM, the day nurses have been deluged in their workload and cannot wait to leave—yet still need to spend one and a half to two hours charting. This becomes overtime. And the chaos continues until about 8 or 9 PM. During the chaos, the new shift group comes on and needs report right when the day nurses are trying to finish their work. Between 9 PM and 1:30 AM the workload becomes more manageable. Then things really taper off from about 1:30 to 5 AM. [Note: this may not taper off on a medical unit.] Then it starts to get busy again by the time the day shift arrives.

Staffing on days is the same through the morning and through the chaotic afternoon. The night shift staffing is the same for both the busy time and the later time when things taper off. Do you see anything wrong with this scenario? How is productivity affected?

Let's examine this from a productivity standpoint. *When do the patients actually need staff services?* Staffing should increase during the busy times and decrease during the less busy times, right? And having a shift change right in the middle of the chaos does not make any sense, right? Sometimes we can get so used to "the way we have always done it," we do not try to fix it. A skeleton crew working 12-hour shifts for overall coverage would

---

[1] The authors thank Cindy Hoehn for her input with this example.

make more sense. The rest of the staff could have other shift options—like having extra staff work 1:30 PM to 9:30 PM—to cover the chaotic period. A better schedule would help staff to meet the various levels of patient volume at appropriate times. Some staff will enjoy working different hours—or not working an eight- or twelve-hour shift. And why have shift change occur during the chaotic time? Other shift times, or variable shift times, would be far more preferable. Most often, when these changes occur, it actually costs less to run the unit after the changes (less staff is needed overall), and staff are more efficient and effective because the help is there at the appropriate times. Better patient safety results. It is more productive and has saved considerable budget dollars.

When this change occurs there will probably be many difficulties with staff adjusting. They will be sure that additional staff are needed, will think that this budget cut is wrong, and will be sure that patient care will suffer. However, if staff are involved initially, and help to collect and analyze the data, and determine solutions, the transition is easier. Although some staff will insist, "We need *more* staff," some will realize that this makes sense and make helpful suggestions. Dialogue together about what would be the best way to staff. Have staff help to revise the staffing plan. Using this example, it is usually possible to cut several FTEs yet still have more staff there during peak work times. As all work through these issues, remember that *the core value is what is best for the patient*? Not the budget cut. Everything follows what the patient values (as defined in Chapter 2).

In the long run, if implemented appropriately by involving everyone concerned, this staffing solution could achieve better efficiency (or productivity), save money, and result in better staff and patient satisfaction, as well as achieve better patient safety.

Several other *organizational* issues with productivity efficiencies are raised by this scenario. If the nurses are spending all that time charting, a computerized documentation system is really needed. This can be a very large purchase. So to avoid mistakes, involve everyone in the process of choosing such a system (see Chapter 5 on choosing information systems).

Another organizational issue is that support services are a problem. Why are the beds not being cleaned promptly? Depending upon worker function, this may involve the housekeeping department, or nurse aides. But it also might come right back to the nurses and unit secretary who have not communicated ahead with those workers that a discharge is about to occur. If everyone involved can get together and discuss both their frustrations and suggestions for improvement, chances are better efficiencies can be achieved.

Another support staff issue could be the unit secretaries. Is unit secretary staffing the same regardless of patient census? It is probably best not to include a unit secretary as a fixed cost (see the Budget Development and Evaluation Chapter for more information on determining fixed staff). It may be best when the census is down or when units are small, to assign a secretary to two or more units. This can be especially helpful if the units are in close physical proximity with one another. But even when they are not, efficiencies occur splitting a secretary between two units. That allows more flexibility with staffing. If the unit is very busy between 1:30–9 PM, having a secretary there for that entire time (no change of shifts occurring for secretaries during that time) could both improve staff efficiency, and provide consistency because the secretary would know who was being discharged, who was being admitted, and could facilitate communication with other departments, including housekeeping, admitting, the OR, the ICUs, physicians, and so forth.

An eighth misconception with productivity is that *when a department experiences productivity problems, the department head is directed to fix the problem.* Here the department in question tries to either increase their productivity number, (i.e., number of visits or patient days; or spends time attacking the quality of the data) while a larger, more important problem is not being dealt with at all. It is a silo mentality to believe that *poor productivity lies within that department alone.* Chances are that although the department needs to improve, there are other organizational systems problems that need to be fixed as well.

Let us look at some examples that directly impact nursing productivity. As nursing staff are working, supplies are not available because materials management has not filled the supplies to par levels or the supplies are not coming up during the time frames that staff need them, or orders are going in late because admitting couldn't forward orders without the charts being stamped; the pharmacy closes at 5 PM; surgeons do not make rounds until 4 PM; or the patient transport waiting time is one hour. It quickly becomes obvious that more departments than nursing need to be involved in these situations.

In fact, when examining organizational systems, Brady and Associates (1999) found that an interdisciplinary department-based work team, using a structured group process for one or two days:

> will typically identify potential cost savings in the range of $250,000 to $460,000 per department, per year. Only about 10% ! or less of these are caused by factors that the department has control over or can 'fix' internally. The rest will require cooperation and coordination with others outside the department (p. 2).

In reality, systems problems actually cause a lot of productivity problems.

If systems problems are allowed to go on, the organization experiences less than optimal productivity throughout the organization, even though productivity measurements may look like certain departments are problems!

> Improving only one component of an agency will not affect overall productivity. Productivity improvement involves a systematic assessment of the entire organization rather than just a staffing review. For example, a physical therapist's job tasks may be tied to secretaries who answer the phones and screen calls, to data processing (records may not be transcribed and given back to the therapist for use during the scheduled visit), and to other disciplines. The therapist may have to wait for the home health aide to arrive to supervise the visit or to meet with an RN regarding the client. One provider group cannot improve or change productivity unless other components of the system are evaluated. Therefore, do not expect the RN staff to increase productivity unless productivity improvements occur in other components of the system in which RNs work (Harris, p. 471).

There is another misconception, that *the productivity issue is an employee issue, not a management issue.* As we have been saying throughout this book, we are all in this together. Getting into a "we-they" mentality is harmful to the organization. In fact, it may be poor leadership on the part of any administrator that is contributing to the organizational productivity problem; we need to start with ourselves. Are *our* actions causing productivity problems? Are *we* allowing productivity problems to continue?

The administrative role goes beyond personal examination. Part of our responsibility involves our looking at the system, identifying issues that need improvement, involving staff to be doing the same, and then getting everyone involved to bring about the changes necessary to fix the problems.

The staff, or the administrators, or the finance department, may hold a tenth misconception, that *productivity improvement is the only way of improving income generation in the organization.* If this were true why is it so important to change and add new services? Using this scenario we would just continue doing the same thing until we eventually went out of business from our antiquated business practices.

Eleven, *just paying attention to internal issues,* can be another misconception. It is possible, for instance, that the supply chain has malfunctioned and the organization cannot get needed supplies and equipment in a timely way, thus causing serious productivity problems. Here the problem lies with the supplier, although, chances are, staff in the organization are helping to cause the problem as well. For instance, as something becomes scarce, staff squirrel it. They hide whatever they cannot get easily, and this may actually cause the shortage to get worse! Additionally, the paperwork is so ponderous it is impossible to get needed supplies quickly. Perhaps someone is forgetting to order promptly. We are all in this together! Each of our actions can effect the outcome.

Components of Productivity Enhancement

Productivity enhancement can be achieved by becoming more efficient and more effective. Let's elaborate.

EFFICIENCY

Efficiency describes the competency of performance—how much work needed to be done, with how many resources, to achieve the maximum feasible product or service. Efficiency involves throughputs—the way we accomplish work, or the work processes; the resources used (including identification of who can best accomplish the work); and the amount of time taken to produce a product or service. It is said that work expands to meet the time allotted to it.

Efficiency, however, reflects time or resources saved, or used, more wisely. Efficiencies can be achieved by finding a better process, one that more effectively uses the resources to accomplish the work. One place to look, when examining efficiency, comes from the old adage, "what is taking 80 percent of staff time yet only getting 20 percent back in output or budget revenue." In this case, examination of the situation might show some efficiencies that need to be taken. For example, one might look into what is being provided to the patient, what the patient expects or values, and how we might change the process to involve fewer steps, and to stop doing activities the patient does not expect or need.

An efficiency issue can be caused by using *contract staff or contract services*. Contracted services such as purchasing can save costs, but can increase the amount of time needed to teach staff how to use different supplies and equipment, as the supplies and equipment change to save money. Contract staff can be expensive both monetarily and time-wise. Contract staff may not be aware of how the organization operates, of policies and procedures, of necessary paperwork that needs to occur, and so forth. Serious productivity problems can result, not to mention serious reimbursement issues and possible patient complications or legal difficulties. If registry staff is used, they need to be properly oriented, and agree to follow certain guidelines and standards.

Efficiency might also examine whether revenue could be increased, (i.e., if one could attract additional patients, this might result in better revenues if some of the current staff might be able to care for the additional patients). Better efficiency can be achieved if one devised a new procedure that was more cost effective and used fewer staff—especially if the same amount of reimbursement was paid for the new procedure.

Perhaps the most difficult part of achieving efficiency is "getting out of the box," thinking of better, or different ways to accomplish the work that will save money and resources, yet achieve the same or better patient outcomes. For example, using the Friesen design:

> A unit has no nursing station in the belief that nurses will spend more time with patients if all supplies, records, drugs, etc., are supplied by non-nurse personnel, and if nurses have no station at which to congregate. One Canadian hospital found that with the Friesen system, nursing time in patient rooms increased from 20% to 108%, staff was reduced 9% and workload increased 30% (Hoffman, p. 52).

The final outcome of efficiency is that one has achieved no waste in either employee time nor use of materials.

Although this data is from an old study, we could really make an impact on productivity by considering options that we normally would not consider. Presently the RN is spending 50–60 percent of the entire shift time on indirect activities and is not in the patient's room while doing it. This includes such things as: getting medications using Pyxis, looking up medications, doing double checks on chemotherapy, documenting care, doing miscellaneous things in utility rooms, cleaning, calling physicians, checking physician orders, shift report, checking crash carts, and so forth. On a 12-hour shift the average time the RN spends in each patient's room is 12 minutes! *The final outcome of efficiency is that one has achieved no waste in either employee time nor use of materials.*

Efficiencies may represent different time allotments for different circumstances. For instance, if one nurse is making home visits in an urban area, one might expect this nurse to make more home visits than another nurse making home visits in a rural area. In both cases, the expectation would be that whenever possible, the staff member achieves mileage efficiency by visiting homes in close proximity with one another. However, this needs to be a judgment call with staff taking into account client needs and availability.

In nursing *introducing new technologies* or *changing work processes* are most likely to improve efficiency.

> Real and sustained gains in productivity are achieved by introducing new technologies and work processes. The scale of the work activity affects potential changes in productivity. A 90 percent improvement in an activity that consumes 1 percent of the nurse's time saves 4.3 minutes, whereas a 20 percent improvement in an activity that takes 40 percent of the nurse's time saves 38.4 minutes per shift. If there are 5 nurses on the unit, the latter improvement would make 3.2 hours available for other activities. If the activity under scrutiny involves a large component of time, such as medication administration or documentation, changes in process may achieve a productivity gain.
>
> Technology may also provide a mechanism to improve productivity. In the medication administration example, it could be enhanced by purchasing PYXIS units, or having robots fill prescriptions in the pharmacy. Technology analysis must focus on currently available technology because potential technologies are not available for application (Chang, Price, and Pfoutz, p. 432).

EFFECTIVENESS—WHAT HAS VALUE?

The second component of productivity is *effectiveness—the degree to which the final result achieves the desired outcome*, the output. This means that we need to know the final result of the care. Yet, most often the outcomes are achieved later, after clients have experienced the care and are discharged. How do we find out what the outcome actually was? If the client remains in the same system receiving care at another site, it is possible to monitor outcomes. But if the patient leaves and the provider does not see the patient again, it is more difficult to find out what happened. In some cases, a staff person can call the patient to help with problems, answer questions, and find out how the patient fared. But often we simply do not know what happened.

Even though we might not know the outcome, we have examined effectiveness by asking such questions as: Was the patient safe? Were the standards of care met? Was the care adequate or excellent? Did the staff do the work correctly?

However, there is another unknown in this equation, what outcome did the patient want or value? Unless we asked, we may not know or understand the client perspective. Patient satisfaction is one component of what is valued. It implies client expectancy. But the actual value piece, what the client actually wanted as an expected outcome, may remain unknown. The other problem with value is that we presently do not have enough research to know whether present practices actually affect the client outcome. For example, what specific actions enhance or detract from healing? Why do some patients respond positively to treatment while others do not? How can we anticipate whether a particular patient will experience side effects of a medication, while another patient will not? Why do some patients, who believe they will die, actually do; while other patients, expected to die, live? So the significant question, *Were desired patient outcome(s) achieved?*, is difficult to answer at best.

A very important component of productivity effectiveness is making sure that all care givers are using *best practices* or *evidence-based practice*. Examples of this are given in Chapter 2 and in Chapter 8.

This question is compounded by the fact that we continue to treat *disease*—not the factors that will produce better *health*. Does our client value health? Is the care we are giving promoting the client's health? Does the client want to participate in his/her care? Do we encourage this? Do we even find out what the patient wants? This is a wonderful field for further research exploration.

Then there is actual productivity measurement. Presently, productivity is usually measured before we know what the patient outcomes will be. After all, if we do not find out the patient outcome until after discharge, yet we measure productivity while staff are giving the care, how do we know what productivity level is appropriate? It is possible that, if we tinker with increasing productivity, or with changing skill mix, more patient complications could result. Our current research does not provide an answer to this issue.

> The measurement of health care outcomes is gradually becoming more meaningful and reflective of patient needs. Unfortunately, indicators are often looked at in an order that fails to take into account the basic goal of health care—health improvement. For example, *productivity measures are typically examined prior to clinical outcomes.* [our emphasis] If productivity targets are exceeded, increases in productivity are mandated without consideration of their potential impact on care provision (Porter-O'Grady and Malloch, p. 316).

This question leads to another aspect of effectiveness, which has to do with staff response. How well do staff adapt to changing circumstances? This will affect the through-put and efficiency as well as the final output (effectiveness). Determining all the process variables that will affect this final output is very complicated. One would examine such things as: How well did the staff do the job? Were staff there at the right time to do the work? Did the staff work together well as a team? How effective was the equipment or the facility/home layout to produce the final product? Were appropriate supplies readily available? Did staff easily document the care given? Did staff change the care when appropriate?

> From an open systems perspective, organizational *effectiveness* means sensing a change in the environment, inputting and digesting relevant information, using that information... to make creative decisions, changing the throughput according to those decisions while managing undesired side effects, outputting new products or services in line with perceived environmental demands, and obtaining feedback on the change.... Effectiveness is measured by [the organization's] ability to survive, adapt, maintain themselves, and grow. Effectiveness is defined by how well an organization copes with its environment. Managerial philosophies must change to allow innovative, non-status quo thinking to be integrated into organizational decision making (Sullivan and Decker, p. 118).

Enhancing Productivity: Linking Efficiency with Effectiveness

The best way to enhance productivity is to link efficiency with effectiveness, always stretching to do better, even when, comparatively, we are already doing well in these areas. Productivity is like quality. Continuous improvement is important, or the product or service—or even the organization—can become obsolete.

> Sustained productivity enhancement, along with its associated improvements in living standards, is not about working longer—it's about *adding more value per unit of work time....* Unlike the manufacturing jobs of the agricultural or industrial revolutions, much of the added value of the information age takes place within the very mortal confines of the human brain. . . .Future prosperity depends on the link between new technologies and workers' skills (Roach, p. 160).

The last sentence of this quote provides us with a clue as to what we need to do to enhance productivity. How can the available technologies help us to do our work better? Have you noticed that health care is becoming less invasive? Have you noticed how evidence-based practice is changing? What we do or what is appropriate care? Do we even know what technologies are available? The first problem may be that we need to investigate what technologies are available. This is why it can be so invigorating to go to a national conference where one can see and hear about new technologies and different ways of doing work. Some of you may be thinking, "But all these technologies cost money. Where is the money coming from?" Remember the discussion in Chapter 2? If we *believe* something is possible we can do it. If we do not believe it is possible, someone else will do it and leave us behind.

Actually productivity enhancement starts with ourselves—are we productive in our work? Are we administratively doing our best? What can we improve? How are we contributing to increased productivity? Are we using available technologies successfully? Chances are, since we are all human, we could be doing better in this matter personally.

Organizationally, every person must make constant refinements. Productivity is not just an activity for the finance department to measure or to be concerned with.

> Health care teams that recognize the interconnectedness of members and acknowledge the unique contributions of each to the delivery of services are able to make substantial contributions to the achievement of organizational goals. Specifically, they are able to help improve patient care outcomes, implement strategies in a shorter time, apply new knowledge as it becomes available, use organizational resources more productively, problem solve more creatively, and manage work processes more effectively (Porter-O'Grady and Malloch, p. 207).

Productivity is most effective when every person in the organization is constantly discovering better ways to do the work, exploring new technologies that are available, finding and developing new services, letting go of old practices that are no longer effective, and having consistent interdisciplinary dialogue about improvements or enhancements. Our newest generations have a lot to offer us as they are growing up with technology and can automatically do things on a computer, for instance, that their parents cannot do as well. They have a lot to contribute that will enhance our productivity!

Another problem with productivity is getting out of the box. Have you thought about all the rituals and practices we do in the workplace? It is easy to continue doing them the same way because it is what we know. With productivity:

> Most costs are embedded in the rituals and practices of the clinical process and are simply not short-term costs. Thus, a lot of individuals must be involved and we must look at things other than hours per patient day and other narrowly defined measures.

> Instead, we should be looking at costs per discharge and costs in a unit-of-service basis. [See Chapter 13, Comparing Reimbursement with Costs of Invoices Provided, for more details.] We must engage in utilization management processes and try to change the way that healthcare resources are being consumed. For example, we can use urgent care as an alternative to an emergency room or decrease utilization of critical care units. These obviously can decrease labor costs in clinical areas; but in reality, many of the labor costs we can control are outside the bedside location.

> I would like to talk about the integration of financial and clinical processes. This is one of the greatest opportunities for cost reduction and improving productivity within our organizations. A very simple example of that is pulling medical records, admitting and authorization, and all those processes into the patient care environment, where they can be fully integrated. Our nurses look at cost per discharge, not our length of stay. We are looking at total costs for a patient over an episode of care, not necessarily what we did on an inpatient basis. We see cost reduction as a critical skill for our nurse in terms of looking at how providers can more effectively manage the patient care environment and ensure that patients are receiving value for care.

> Finally, there is the concern of quality issues that are nurse sensitive. In looking at outcomes and productivity, we have discovered that many of the things we tend to wrap our arms around, in fact, are not nurse sensitive, meaning that nursing hours or the level of registered nurse staffing do not truly impact some aspects of outcome and productivity. We would like to think they do, but, in fact, they do not. This allows us to look more creatively at how we use resources in our organizations. Nurse leaders and patient care leaders in our provider organizations can be responsible financial managers of resources. We can position our provider organizations so that they can be competitive in a contracting[2] environment (Van Slyck, pp. 51–52).

There are many factors that can enhance or decrease productivity. As previously noted, every chapter in this book not only has financial implications, but affects productivity.

---

[2] Remember that the environment is only contracting if we think it is!

Poor leadership, poor management, poor performance, all result in productivity ineffectiveness. And vice versa. Productivity is enhanced when positive things are happening. Productivity and quality go hand in hand. Productivity and leadership go hand in hand. Productivity and the bottom line go hand in hand.

For example, productivity is affected by such things as *staff issues*: their level of experience, amount of staff scheduled, not being oriented properly, not having been taught how to do something, or not having enough information about something they are expected to do. Tardiness and absenteeism, sick and vacation time, conference time, overtime, and use of agency staff can all effect productivity. Staff mix could be inappropriate for the work that needs to be done—either overqualified personnel are doing a task; or staff are underqualified to do the required work.

Sometimes lower productivity has *environmental causes*, such as not having enough supplies, equipment, or technology to properly do the work; there are problems with the physical layout; or there are long distances for staff to travel in home care.

Sometimes low productivity may be happening overall, even when productivity seems high. For example, if not enough staff are available to work, staff may be doing as much as possible for patients, yet know that more needs to be done. As staff frustration mounts, it is easy to start missing important things that should happen. In this case efficiency looks wonderful but effectiveness suffers. Putting all productivity measurements together, the result is actually low productivity.

Low productivity may occur due to *inter-organizational issues*. For instance, perhaps an insurer has not paid for the care a patient received in a timely manner. Perhaps the diagnosis was not put on the insurance claim by the physician, or a coder put the wrong CPT code on the claim, or the patient did not give the correct address as to where the payment should be sent. In such instances, this problem will take more of the patient's time, more of the insurer's time, more of the provider's time, and even after all this, the outcome—payment—may not occur, even after several people, and organizations, were involved in trying to resolve the issue.

Another question is to ask, *what is necessary*?

> Look for the best outcomes and the best practices in all areas—clinical and administrative—and seek to replicate those practices throughout the organization.... And stop doing and stop paying for things that do not contribute to quality.... Basically, what the cost of quality boils down to is the cost that is involved that would be eliminated in your organization if there were absolutely no quality problems. Studies of administrative and service industries dealing specifically with healthcare show that 20 percent to 50 percent of the activities are nonreal work. What is nonreal work? It does not mean that you and your staff are not busy; you are busier than ever. But the tasks that many are doing do not necessarily contribute to quality care. A few examples:
>
> • System delays such as laboratory tests that come back late and delay discharges, which can increase patient days and staffing;
>
> • Variations in physician practices, which generate medically unnecessary patient days and test procedures;

- Drug doses that are discarded because they are mislabeled or put on the wrong cart;

- Skill mix problems—not just in the context of nurse versus unlicensed staff; nurses have taken over a lot of the tasks that a few years ago were done only by physicians; and

- Excess inventory, such as hoarding supplies on the floor because you cannot quite count on your ordering delivery system to get you the product you need when you need it.

All these things cost. Every time you have staff turnover, patient falls, infections, litigation, in short, any time that you are doing any reprocessing or rework activities, that is a cost of quality. . . .

Look for ways to cross departmental boundaries to achieve your strategic goals. When you get your staff working together, they can be a gold mine of information. They know exactly where the rework and reprocessing occurs because they do it everyday, day in and day out (Van Slyck, p. 53).

Productivity Monitoring System

As we try to get a handle on productivity and determine if productivity has improved, a productivity monitoring system can really help. Then we can look at the measures we have taken, and compare data to see if the measures had any effect on productivity. However, our current productivity measurements are inadequate. We are able to capture part of the picture in our monitoring system but part of the picture is unaccounted for and missing.

> A productivity monitoring system is most effective when it can capture the plan of what one wants to achieve as well as the report of what actually happened. The system's design should make pertinent patient data available, on time, to unit management and staff (VanSlyck, p. 18).

Productivity measurement should define a *reasonable expectancy*, a standard for determining people power needed to accomplish the work. This reasonable expectancy is used to build a budget and set an expected allocation of resources. Productivity measurement is most effective when it includes both *quantitative* and *qualitative* data. Our present models tend to avoid the "squishy" quality and value factors that are, as yet, more difficult to measure. For instance, Leah Curtin says that efficacy is a factor that needs to be included in the productivity data. This would include measurements of "years of formal education, levels of academic achievement, evidence of continuing education and skill development, and years of experience" (Swansburg, p. 97). Also, there are many variables that might impact productivity that are not included in the measurement at all, (i.e., new staff who are getting oriented who are not as efficient, unnecessary patient days occurring, or unopened supplies being discarded because they were lying in the patient room). Additionally, finding out what the patient wants is rarely measured. However, even though we are in the toddler stage with productivity measurement, it helps to understand what is currently available and being used.

Historically, our first attempts were to *only* quantify productivity. Many organizations still do this. Although this measurement provides useful data, it is only a *partial* measurement. As we have already said, both efficiency and effectiveness are part of productivity, so quality must be added to the measurement. Presently, quality measurements include patient outcomes and patient satisfaction. That is a good start, but we have a long way to go.

As with budgets, when encountering various productivity measurements, one will need to *always get a definition of how these figures are determined*, then evaluate how effectively these figures capture actual productivity. Thus various examples of productivity measurement are presented in this chapter, even though there are definite problems with each of them and they should not be used alone.

PRODUCTIVITY MEASUREMENTS

Industrial Model

Historically, the first form of productivity measurement was a quantitative one called the *industrial model*. Olson (1983) defined this as "the relationship between the use of resources and the results of that use" (p. 46). It was called the industrial model because it was first used on the production line. As certain resources—supplies and people (the input)—worked to produce something (the output), one could measure productivity. For example, Henry Ford's company produced a certain number of cars in one day. As he worked out more efficient ways to produce cars, (i.e., by using an assembly line), he increased productivity, he increased the number of cars produced without needing to increase the work force. By calculating productivity in this way, one could try to improve productivity by increasing the output without increasing the input, or by increasing the output more than the input was increased.[3]

So the first productivity measurements could examine the ratio of outputs to inputs. In health care, examples of industrial model ratios are staff hours per patient day, per test, per visit, per treatment, per procedure; FTE-to-bed ratios sometimes written as FTE per adjusted occupied bed (AOB); nursing salary costs per patient day, visit, and so forth; or cost per unit of service, i.e., the cost per home visit, the cost per DRG, or the number of patients per overall facility budget amount, within a specific time period. When measured at regular intervals over time, this data can provide an idea as to whether the productivity level has improved. If productivity was improved, more outputs (patient days or bed ratios) were able to be produced using fewer resources (inputs–staff hours or FTEs). If productivity worsened, more resources (inputs–staff hours or FTEs) were used without significantly increasing the outputs.

---

[3] Note that the quality of the cars was also important but is not reflected in this equation. (After all, producing more cars in one day will not be helpful if the cars do not work properly.)

Using the home visit as the output, Harris (1997) discusses inputs:

> In home care the use of resources may include everything necessary to complete the home visit, known as the product. This can include the caregiver's time, supplies, agency management time, and other indirect expenses. Historically, the results or output of using these resources have been defined as the number of visits per discipline per time period. The time period may be 1 day, 1 week, or 1 month. Visits may be separated by type—maternal-child, pediatrics, or hospice—and/or by discipline-registered nurse (RN), therapist, or social worker. Examples include the following:
>
> • 6 reimbursable visits per RN each day.
>
> • 25 pediatric visits per therapist per week.
>
> • 120 reimbursable RN visits per week (Monday through Friday, 4 RNs at 30 visits each week, each RN averaging 6 visits per day) (p. 470).

This quantification of productivity data gives one better ways to "categorize, compare, trend, and analyze key budget indicators." Thus an administrator can better visualize how "actual labor, supply, and other costs compare to the expected cost for the volume and quality of procedures [or services] provided" (DiJerome, Dunham-Taylor, Ash, and Brown, p. 334).[4] Quantification is most effective when the data is computerized and readily available for the nurse administrator to use. For instance, when the volume of patients changes, the nurse administrator can evaluate the appropriate number of staff, and determine the appropriate staff mix needed to care for the change in patient volume based on available resources.

So if one was only *quantifying* the work output and one wanted to increase productivity, one could cut nursing staff FTEs for the same number of patients. The problem with this method, when used alone, is that it considers neither the acuity of the patient, nor the quality/value of the patient outcome. We do not advocate *just* quantifying the work output. After all, if cutting costs is not done carefully, this becomes an example of the slash-and-burn technique—the way *not* to do productivity measurement. This quantitative productivity measurement is very useful though, when used with other productivity data.

Case Mix Methods

As the industrial model was used, people began to realize that there were other important issues with productivity measurement that involved efficiency. For example, a patient day for a normal OB delivery versus a patient day for an intensive care unit patient requires different staffing. The same is true for home care or ambulatory visits; an initial visit usually takes longer because the staff have to get to know and assess a new patient, while a follow-up visit often takes less time. Somehow, this needed to be added to the productivity measurement equation.

---

[4] This article quantifies an endoscopy department's productivity.

This prompted the movement to use case mix methods. "Case mix is a method of clustering patients into groups that are homogeneous with respect to the use of resources. Factors used to cluster patients have included diagnosis, prognosis, resource utilization, organ system, hospital department, and patient demographic characteristics" (Sullivan and Decker, p. 120). Thus Medicare began to use case mix methods, such as diagnosis-related groups (DRGs) for hospital reimbursement, and resource utilization groups (RUGs) for long-term care reimbursement. Presently CMS has developed a case mix method for the ambulatory area using an Ambulatory Payment Classification system that has relative value units which reflect the complexity of each procedure. Same with home care. Various case mix numbers, such as x number of patients in the DRG category Heart Failure and Shock, can be substituted in the productivity equation for patient days.

The case mix cluster could also reflect patient acuity if the organization uses a patient classification system. These systems can be integrated with budgeting information, and used within the ratios. The predominant problem with this is that most often the finance department does not understand the importance of the patient classification system unless nurse administrators teach them about it. Patient classification systems are not covered in finance and accounting programs.

Case mix measurements are more likely to reflect a need for consistent staffing, for the population served, but the population can still can reflect fairly wide variation in patient needs. Here again, the productivity measurement does not include any measure of quality, acuity, or patient outcomes.

Cost Per Unit of Service

An important financial factor that nurses need to consider is how we can keep our practice costs within what the expected reimbursement will be. (Chapter 13, Comparing Reimbursements with Costs of Services Provided, outlines how to do this very nicely.) Costs are compounded because Medicare and Medicaid reimbursement is not made dollar for dollar. Often, reimbursement is actually about 50 percent of costs. This creates significant problems for us because our present practices are based upon giving extensive services to the patients. Part of our job, administratively, is to help all staff identify what is best to do with the resources that we have, based on what the patient needs most. (Then there is the issue of not feeling frustrated because we cannot do all that we used to do for patients! Actually, there are some things that we have done for patients that they have never wanted anyway!)

Thus the nurse manager needs to periodically evaluate the staffing plan. Having staff involvement in setting the plan is ideal because they are most familiar with what actually occurs, and because it is important to have staff buy-in when implementing the plan. The plan must consider issues related to specific types of patients; unit layout; support services available; daily, weekly, or seasonal census fluctuations; recent changes in patient mix; and so forth. The most efficient staffing plan occurs when the highest number of patients are present for the specified number of staff. For instance, if the staffing plan said that there needed to be three nursing staff present for 12 to 15 patients, and then four staff were needed when there were 16 to 18 patients, the best productivity is achieved when there are 15 patients or when there are 18 patients. Achieving maximum productivity on an inpatient unit is difficult because one cannot anticipate the number of patients one will have for a shift. Also, the total number of admissions and discharges, which take more nursing time, are not considered.

Based on this example, when there are 15 patients on the unit it may be best to admit a new patient to a different similar unit that is not up to the maximum number of patients to available staff.

If there are 14 patients on the unit and four staff are present, another productivity problem occurs because, according to the staffing plan, only three staff are necessary. The 14 patients may be of much higher acuity than anticipated, but just looking at the numbers, it looks like productivity levels are not desirable and that one staff member should not work on that shift.

Note here that the staffing plan is more accurate when it is based on patient acuity levels rather than number of patients with a specified staff mix.

This example also reflects the importance of people working together throughout the organization because efficiency will be effected if game playing occurs, (i.e., with units refusing patients just because they do not want to do more work). Instead, the system needs to be fairly administered. The unit is most effective if these numbers are used throughout a day, and if the nurse manager, and charge nurses, understand how this all works, and take care of staffing appropriately by shift.

Post the productivity level for each day where staff can see it. When staff understand the importance of this data, they will learn to automatically take care of staffing issues, helping the nurse manager and charge nurses to more effectively do their work. Everyone needs to discuss ahead what will happen, i.e., who is willing to float to another unit (be sure to provide orientation to the specified unit), who is willing to go home, and who is willing to work extra or be on call. All staff are adults and need to be involved in these decisions as equal partners.

Another productivity indicator for the nurse manager is the kind of staff labor used, i.e., regular staff, overtime paid, contract or agency nurses used, and whether other staff were floated to the unit. Chapter 12 on Budget Variances discusses how the nurse manager needs to work with this data.

Workload Index

Another productivity measurement, *workload index*, can show us the ratio between the budgeted staff hours and the actual worked staff hours. This gives an actual budget utilization figure. The workload index can be used to show budget adequacy. The workload index can be determined by dividing the budgeted staff hours by the actual staff hours worked. As long as the budgeted staff hours actually reflect a reasonable expectancy, this figure can be a useful quantitative reflection of productivity.

$$\frac{\textbf{\textit{Budgeted Staff Hours}}}{\textbf{\textit{Actual Staff Hours}}} = \textbf{\textit{Productivity Level or Workload Index}}$$

$$\frac{\textbf{\textit{1,326 Budgeted Staff Hours x 100*}}}{\textbf{\textit{1,296 Actual Staff Hours}}} = \textbf{\textit{102 percent Workload Index}}$$

*When we multiply by 100 we change the equation into a percentage.

In this example, the 102 percent represents the workload index or productivity level. Here staff productivity was better than expected, because the workload index is over 100 percent. (The 100 percent is what was actually budgeted, while the 2 percent was less than what was budgeted.) This means that the staff hours actually used were under what had been anticipated. (Another example is given in Chapter 12 on Budget Variances.)

It is dangerous just using these numbers without taking other contributing factors into consideration. For example, in this situation it is possible that the nursing unit was down three positions; everyone pitched in and contributed to get the work completed; part-time staff worked more hours; overtime was used; no agency or traveler staff were used; and staff had to work other shifts that were not their preference. Staff breathed a sigh of relief as they worked hard but managed to get the work done. It was good that the unit got through this but they would not want to continue having to work like this as it would burn out staff.

Still using this productivity measurement, let's say that someone in the finance department sees that the nursing unit has achieved 102 percent productivity, and thinks, "This is great. Less staff can do the work. Money can be saved. I'll set the new productivity level at the 102 percent level for the next budget year." Staff budgeted hours will now be 1,296, rather than 1,326. This frustrates the nurse manager and the staff as this means that staff will continue to have to work harder, work more hours, work more overtime, and work different shifts than they originally planned to do. Some staff may leave. Chances are, staff will continue to go about doing the work in the same way, and no time will be saved actually doing the work. Other factors—such as involving the nurse manager and the staff in the decision, and not making a decision without taking into account what actually happened—should have occurred before making the decision to cut staff FTEs. This is why we advocate continuous dialogue between nursing and finance.

With the current nursing shortage, overtime has increased. This becomes dangerous if it is over about 2 percent because staff are tired and will begin to make mistakes.

The opposite productivity measurement can occur. Let's say that the actual hours were above the budgeted hours as shown below. In this case the Workload Index becomes 92.6 percent, meaning that more staff were used than had been anticipated.

$$\frac{1,326\ Budgeted\ Staff\ Hours}{1,432\ Actual\ Staff\ Hours} \times 100 = 92.6\ percent\ Workload\ Index$$

Once again, it would be easy to jump to conclusions. But more facts are needed. For instance, let's say that there were more patients than had been anticipated so more staff were called in to work. Thus the actual worked hours were more than budgeted hours. On the other hand, if the census was down and the unit continued to staff the same way, it is a productivity problem.

What Is the Ideal Productivity Level?

It is generally recommended that the productivity level range between 95 percent and 100 percent. If the level gets too low, staff can become overwhelmed as there is too much work for them to do, and patient complications increase (Carter, 2000). We do not recommend continually staffing at productivity levels below 95 percent without beginning to add other things that will improve productivity, such as changing the work processes, or adding needed technology that will enable staff to complete the work in less time.

When one gets above 105 percent, staff are overwhelmed while if one gets below 95 percent staff do not have enough to do. When staff have extra time, they can start to create other problems in the work area. Staff will fill the extra time somehow. Some may be positive such as cleaning and organizing the unit; but some will start playing games that will cause more dissention on the unit.

This example looked at the unit as a whole. The nurse manager needs to look at individual staff productivity as well. For instance, if one observes that the RNs are always busy, rarely taking breaks, while the nurse aides are sitting around half the day, one would question if there was an appropriate staff mix. In this case, the RNs would seem to be very productive. However, it is possible that RNs will burn out and leave due to the heavy workload. The nurse aides in this example sound like they do not have enough to do. This group has time to get into game playing, which could affect morale. Thus, the skill mix needs to change. It might be a better use of the budget money to give up a couple aide positions for an RN position. One would also have to look into how effectively RNs were delegating to the aides, and whether both groups were working together effectively. Quick-fix solutions can be dangerous without taking into account all the factors involved.

FINANCIAL FACTORS

In health care, a number of financial productivity measurements evolved. These measurements typically relate to: *profitability*—total margin; return on investment, PLA; and operating margin; *liquidity and cash flow*—days cash on hand, all sources; current ratio of assets for one year; and days in accounts receivable; and *capital structure*—debt service coverage; average age of plant, and bad debt expense (Ohio Hospital Association, 2003). (For more detail see Chapter 18.)

Financially, a nurse manager must look at budget variances to see if there are variance issues that might be affecting productivity levels. (This is discussed in Chapter 12.) It really does not do much good to look at a variance report once the month is over because then it is too late to accomplish the daily staffing changes that are needed. Therefore, the nurse manager and charge nurses need to have this data readily available on an hourly basis. As explained in Chapter 12, the main use of a monthly variance report would be to see how accurately they accomplished the plan. It might indicate problems that the nurse executive would need to follow up on with the nurse manager.

What Else Is Missing in Productivity Measurement?

Do you see any problem with the methods—industrial, case mix, workload index, or financial measurements? The first issue is that we do not know much about the patients, what they want, if they are satisfied with the services given, whether there are patient safety issues, and what the patient outcomes were. There are also unknown factors with staff such as the skill mix and whether it was appropriate, if new staff were needing to attend orientation, and so forth.

Evaluate Factors Affecting Productivity

Thus when measuring productivity, it is important to always examine the factors that have affected current productivity levels. For instance, if one month our productivity level was not as good, what factors might have accounted for this change? Perhaps since the budgeted hours were established a significant event(s) has occurred that might increase or decrease the numbers of staff needed to accomplish the work. Factors might include such things as: a new procedure for patient safety was implemented, staff are caring for different, more acute patients; a new staff member is orienting; a new computerized documentation system has been implemented; a change has been made in a work process; a new physician is using different treatments; or more staff are needed temporarily while implementing a new change. Any of these factors could explain why the productivity level was not as high.

Nonproductive Time Another factor that can significantly change productivity measurement is nonproductive time. When determining productivity measurements, it is important to know whether nonproductive time is included. (Nonproductive time—non-worked time such as sick and vacation time, or annual leave time is further explained in the Budget Development and Evaluation Chapter.) If nonproductive time is figured into the productivity level, then anytime someone uses sick or vacation time the productivity level will drop. If this is the case, staff productivity may actually be the same from day to day, yet the productivity measurement may look like productivity has decreased whenever staff take nonproductive time. If one can actually have two separate staff budgets, one reflecting worked time and the other reflecting nonproductive time, productivity measurement is more accurate. If it is not possible to separate out the two, the nurse manager may have to manually refigure productivity just using productive time, and/or create a Microsoft™ Excel spreadsheet that will do this. (This is covered in more detail in Chapter 12, Budget Variances.)

Benchmark data, such as staff per patient ratios, nursing hours per patient day (NHPPD), and budget information used by facilities can also be affected, if one facility counts nonproductive time and another does not. If you are benchmarking with other organizations, be sure to clarify that all benchmark facilities are reporting nonproductive time in the same way, or you may be comparing apples and oranges. Benchmarking on productivity data can also be affected by other factors (i.e., staff get more vacation time at one facility, or staff getting education days at one location and not at another).

One other issue with productivity is that occasionally nonproductive time is *not* included *anywhere* in the budget. In this case, appropriate staffing will be impossible on most days as there will not be enough FTEs to cover staff who take annual leave time. Then the nurse manager must figure actual nonproductive time needed, immediately discuss this with the nurse executive and the finance department, and by the next budget year get the base budget recalculated to add a line for nonproductive time to the budget. In the meantime it could be dealt with as a variance.

LINKING QUANTITATIVE PRODUCTIVITY MEASURES WITH PERFORMANCE EVALUATION DATA

Productivity measurement in health care is most effective if it does not stand alone. It needs to be linked with patient outcomes. Otherwise, how do we know that the productivity levels have been effective? For instance, if productivity figures are wonderful but patients are having a lot of complications, something is wrong with the effectiveness component of productivity. This comparison is complicated by the fact that sometimes poor patient outcomes occur after a patient is discharged and we may never be aware that they occurred. Furthermore, we do not know, and have not measured, what the patient wants or values.

One way we have tried to add the effectiveness dimension is by using patient satisfaction instruments, discussed in Chapter 2. Patient satisfaction measurements provide additional data on how patients have viewed their health care experience. (This is discussed in more detail in Chapter 2 on Quality.) Unfortunately, most instruments are designed to find out historical data, so it is difficult to rectify problems as they occur. Ideally, more direct feedback is needed during the actual patient experience. Patients may be afraid to give negative information for fear that this will adversely affect their care. So we need more accurate data.

Although not ideal, today the most effective productivity evaluation measurements combine financial, organizational, and patient outcome data and are called *performance evaluation*. This includes patient-related outcome data such as length of stay, readmission rates, patient falls, adverse reactions, complications, infections, deaths, number of medications per patient, client condition on discharge, and consumer satisfaction/complaints. (Performance data are described in more detail in Chapters 2 and 15.) *Performance data does not yet measure whether the patient received what was wanted and valued.* It also may only measure complications that we are aware of while the patient is with us—*not what occurs after we have seen the client.* Then in performance evaluation, the outcome data (effectiveness) is compared with the processes influencing those outcomes (efficiencies). Process data measuring efficiency can include numbers and skill mix of staff; staff turnover; cost of the staffing; overhead costs; quality/safety measures implemented including adding technology; and/or equipment and supplies consumed.

Hall (2003) suggests a nursing productivity tool that measures *nursing knowledge indicators* (educational preparation, experience, career planning and development, autonomy, organizational trust, organizational commitment, and satisfaction), *nursing productivity system indicators* (nursing costs, turnover, absenteeism, orientation costs, and education costs), and *patient indicators* (nursing errors related to patient safety, and patient satisfaction). Unfortunately this still does not find out or measure whether the patient received what was wanted and valued.

When the payers realized that some patients at certain health care organizations seemed to be having more complications in certain facilities, payers started using this performance data as criteria for future contracts. If there was another provider available with better outcome data, payers would choose that provider's services, rather than contract with the provider whose patients were more at risk.

As more performance data, first called quality *report cards*, has become available on a national level through the Centers for Medicare and Medicaid Services (CMS). These published summaries of various performance measures have been developed to provide performance data to regulators, payers, and consumers via the internet. (Nursing report cards, linking nurse staffing and patient outcomes, are further discussed in Chapter 20, Staffing.) Payers use the performance data to compare the performance of providers—hospitals, physicians, ambulatory care, long-term care, home care—to determine who gives the best care (effectiveness) and who is less expensive (efficiency). This is called *performance-based reimbursement evaluation*. Consumers can choose their providers based on this data, if the consumer is aware the data exists.

When health care systems share this valuable historical performance data with employees for evaluation and improvement, everyone benefits. Enhanced productivity effectiveness results. So far, however, a lot of this is historical and is not capturing the information soon enough to rectify the situation immediately. Additionally, this data does not indicate *future* performance.

Although there are currently no absolute standards or guidelines as to actual criteria to use or how well a provider needs to perform, undoubtedly there will be considerable development in this arena. It will be exciting to see where this leads us as the research results have started to provide us with more effective assessment data, all essential for productivity measurement.

Performance data is just the first step, and, aside from the value question, brings up more questions, including: do the processes currently used and measured have an actual effect on the outcome? Let us give a couple examples: Does patient pre-operative teaching actually result in fewer complications, quicker recovery, and higher patient satisfaction following surgery? Are there fewer medication errors when patients give themselves their own medication(s) when possible? There are hundreds of these questions that we need to ask. We may think intuitively that we know the answer. However, our research does not prove it. Research results can surprise us! It would be nice to know what processes specifically make a difference in our patient outcomes. Effectiveness and efficiency need to be measured in tandem, and considered together, for the greatest effectiveness.

Productivity Evaluation Process

Productivity enhancement is most effective when *everyone* is involved in the process. This is preferable to the more haphazard process often used where supervisors and/or the finance department become very concerned with productivity, but where many workers do not think about it or even understand what it is.

By saying 'everyone,' board members, the executive team, every department, all within each department, physicians, suppliers, and even patients and their families are all included, because productivity is linked with patient care.

As we teach staff about productivity, encourage them to come up with ways that we can find out what each patient wants and values. Then we can determine what care is possible based on available resources.

Benefield (Harris, 1997) advocates going through an evaluation process, and developing or

---

Definition

Productivity Evaluation Process:

1) Analyze environmental factors that affect productivity.

2) Analyze staff factors that affect productivity.

3) Determine the current productivity of staff.

4) Develop a productivity standard(s).

changing productivity standards based on this evaluation. In this process, everyone is encouraged to *question everything* as they go through the following evaluation steps:
1. Analyze environmental factors that affect productivity.
2. Analyze staff factors that affect productivity.
3. Determine the current productivity of staff.
4. Develop a productivity standard(s) (p. 473).

ENVIRONMENTAL FACTORS

Environmental factors can include things that are occurring both within and external to the organization. *Internal factors* can include such things as:

- Staff scheduling;
- Career ladders are available to encourage staff to try new roles;
- How the building(s) is configured;
- Span of control of nurse managers;
- Leader's style;
- Group affiliations;
- What services are contracted;
- Paperwork;
- Meetings and other times for group work;
- Orientation program(s);
- Services that are offered;
- Times of operation;
- Policies and procedures (for instance, sick and vacation time may vary depending upon job classification or length of employment; or in home care staff may not be assigned to make visits in the neighborhoods where they live);
- Staff assignments (is there a difference in what a new staff member is expected to do as compared with an experienced worker, or is it difficult to find staff when needed throughout the shift);
- Staff turnover;
- Staff morale;
- Staff teamwork;
- Job responsibilities (maybe no one covers for the secretary when it is mealtime so other staff have to keep interrupting their work to answer the phone);
- Where are the supplies kept (are they easily accessible, can they be charged to the patient); and
- Is needed equipment readily available.

Organizational processes are other internal factors that should also be evaluated. Here we need to evaluate meeting time. Is it all necessary? Are the meetings accomplishing outcomes? We must also evaluate current work flow processes being used, i.e.,

- How many activities are necessary before a patient is admitted? Which activities are unnecessary, or duplicate work—what could we stop doing because it really does not accomplish anything?

- How could the work be done more efficiently? Is there a better way to do the work that would be more effective? Could the process be simplified?
- How long does the patient have to wait for us to do something?
- Have technology or payment structures changed how long patients are with us so that we do not have the time to do everything we used to do?
- What needs to be changed?
- Would additional supplies, equipment, or technology improve efficiency or effectiveness?
- Is the building configured in a way that is conducive to get the work accomplished?
- Are the appropriate staff doing certain activities or procedures?
- Are there less expensive ways to accomplish the work?
- Are there patient safety issues that need to be improved?
- Are current regulatory standards or laws being met?

External factors include:

- The geographic area served (a densely populated inner city, or rural area, perhaps part of the environment is unsafe or hazardous for some reason, and whether patients are local or may be coming from a great distance);
- Client demographics (elderly);
- Type of financial reimbursements made for services (what percentage is Medicare or Medicaid, private pay, or non-pay); and
- Is there a seasonal difference in numbers or types of patients, as well as other SWOT (Strengths-Weaknesses-Opportunities-Threats) analysis features. (A SWOT analysis is explained in Chapter 15.)

STAFF FACTORS

There are many issues with staff:

- How experienced they are,
- Whether staff have expertise with the various kinds of patient problems or with various technologies being used,
- Whether clinical nurse specialists or nurse practitioners are available to plan care for more complicated patients,
- Whether the orientation program properly prepares new staff to function effectively,
- Whether there is good morale and teamwork between staff, and
- Whether facility administrators/managers are competent.

Staff factors need to take into account situational temporary events as well, such as staffing shortages when a staff member needs sudden surgery or leave time—factors that could affect staffing, and productivity.

CURRENT STAFF PRODUCTIVITY

Current staff productivity measurements and standards need to be examined. Are staff aware that these standards exist and are being measured? Are staff productive? Are staff aware of ways that they contribute to the productivity standards? Are the present measurements accurate, reliable, and valid? If not, what needs to be changed? What do the measurements indicate? Do the measures examine both efficiency and effectiveness? Should other measurements be added? All this still needs to take into account what reimbursement amount can be expected so we stay within the budget. (Benefield [Harris, 1997] outlines how to do this for home care.)

Productivity measurement is easier to manage when a computerized system is available that can capture appropriate productivity data automatically as staffing occurs, patients are being given care, and documentation is completed (Carter, 2000; Harris, 1997; DiJerome, Dunham-Taylor, Ash, and Brown, 1999) Chapter 12 on Budget Variances, and Chapter 25, Acuity-Based Flexible Nursing Budgets also provide more information. The information systems programs are most helpful when integrated so they can talk to one another, and data does not need to be transferred or recopied to another program. (Another productivity issue!) Examples include:

- When what is documented is linked automatically to determine patient classification and budget data or for performance measurement, and
- When personnel data is linked with each department and with finance data.

Once the data is entered, staff do not need to enter it into a different document for another use—a great increase in efficiency.

WHAT DOES THE PATIENT WANT?

So far we have been discussing issues from the staff perspective. Before actually setting the standard(s), the patient perspective needs to be considered. What does the patient want, need, and value? What does the patient need to achieve safety and good patient outcomes? What can the patient afford? Was the patient satisfied with what s/he received? Does the patient value what staff currently do? Can staff reasonably give the patient what the patient wants?

PRODUCTIVITY STANDARDS

After this assessment, it is helpful to change, or set, the productivity standard(s). Performance data, discussed in Chapter 2 on Quality, should tie in with the productivity standard(s). For example, if one of the performance criteria is that the staffing is maintained at a certain level based on number of patients, this should also be the level used for the productivity standard. In addition, the standard must consider financial data, such as revenues over expenses. After all, productivity standards are useless unless we can meet both direct and indirect costs within the available budget. If the budget does not cover current costs, everyone must be involved in determining the appropriate action to take, and always remember the basic value, what is best for the patient? The standard, once set, becomes the benchmark that is measured against to see if the productivity level was achieved. The standard will need to be periodically evaluated and changed.

After the Initial Evaluation, What Comes Next?

While evaluating current practice and determining the productivity standard(s), the need for some changes or improvements may become obvious. In addition, once the productivity standard(s) is set, it is important to measure against that standard to make sure the standard is met, or exceeded. If not met, other productivity improvement measures may be needed. But productivity improvement does not stop there. It must permeate everything we do.

Then implementation begins. One strategy for implementation is discussed in the Budget Strategy Chapter. For example, new care paths may need to be developed for certain patients, educational programs may need to be implemented so staff are using the most efficient or effective approach with clients, paperwork may be eliminated or streamlined by purchasing new technology, new programs may be started with present programs being eliminated or revamped, or new incentives may be implemented to encourage staff to improve productivity.

Productivity Improvement

Productivity improvement is everyone's responsibility. In this book we stress the importance of involving staff at all levels in the decision making process. This continues to be true with productivity:

> Remember the basic assumptions when [improving] productivity. First, productivity improvement is not completed in a vacuum. Improving only one component of an agency will not increase overall productivity, so consider an agencywide program. Second, involve all staff, particularly direct caregivers, in planning and evaluating the productivity of an agency. Third, management holds the key to effective productivity through effective supervision and the ability to create environments that challenge and motivate staff (Benefield in Harris, p. 479).

As all staff are involved, it is important that they understand that productivity is linked with organizational viability.

Productivity improvement is more easily accomplished when we feel that we do meaningful work:

> What drives people to work at their best? How can health care leaders revitalize the lost passion of employees? What are the retention strategies that will support the rebuilding of a hopeful culture? Interestingly, the answer is simple. When employees believe their work is meaningful—productive in the sense of producing beneficial results—then they will be motivated to work harder and will experience a renewal of passion and hopefulness. Productivity is not only about quantity; it is also about quality.
>
> Optimizing employee performance takes on a whole new meaning in this context. All human beings have a need to express their uniqueness and their talents in the work they do and be recognized for their contributions (**Exhibit 21–4**). Therefore, employees are typically motivated by jobs that develop their skills and expand their minds, demand individual initiative, involve working on teams, benefit others, and spark a desire to make a difference in the world. Jobs that have these characteristics pos-

sess what Cedric Johnson (2000) called *fruitfulness*—work flows from one person to another in a way that is both respectful and valued. To ensure that health care workers possess fruitfulness, leaders need to do the following:

- Continually examine services, measures, and systems to assess their impact on patient outcomes. Retain those that improve patient outcomes, and eliminate those that have no effect or a negative effect.
- Believe that hope can be restored to care providers through restoring value to the work they do.
- Believe intensely that individuals will give their best when treated like adults.
- Be alive and be committed to doing what is best for patients.
- Consistently expect only value-adding services to be delivered to patients. Publicly recognize individuals who are able to focus on value, and guide those who require assistance in eliminating unnecessary and non-valued-adding work.
- Believe that all health care providers intuitively know that restoring value to work is the right path but have not been able to translate their perceptions into practice. Believe that most, but not all, will eventually make the transition. Believe that the health care system will not only support but will require increases in the value of health care services. Know that colleagues support caring, healing work that makes a difference (Porter-O'Grady and Malloch, pp. 317–318).

Exhibit 21–4 Optimizing Performance: Productivity or Fruitfulness?

Productivity

- Productivity is mechanistic.
- In a productivity-driven organization, employees are treated like machines and judged on the quantity of their output.
- The predominant concern is getting more "bang for the buck."
- Efforts to increase employee motivation are dependent on external sources, pay, benefits, etc.

Fruitfulness

- Fruitfulness is humanistic.
- Fruitfulness involves a respectful, holistic view of each person that recognizes values, beliefs, and expectations.
- Fruitfulness honors the inner need of each person to express his or her uniqueness and talents and to develop and expand.
- Fruitfulness engages the inner selves of employees and causes them to grow and be sustained naturally and enduringly.

From: Johnson, C. B. (2000). When working harder is not smarter, *Inner Edge*, 3(2), pp. 18–21.

So what is our goal for productivity enhancement? It is something like this: You are an excellent nurse manager. Your unit runs very efficiently. The staff stay because they like working there and can plan schedules that best meet the needs of both their patients and themselves. The physicians like their patients to be assigned to this unit. In fact, patients ask to be admitted to this unit. Patient length of stay is below the national average. Staff are proud that most patients do not experience complications because staff can quickly pick up on symptoms, alert physicians, and change the care for patients immediately when necessary. Actual productivity figures indicate that productivity has increased from last year even though the patient acuity has also increased. Staff turnover the past year was 2 percent. Staff costs are below other similar units yet the RN ratio is higher. In this year's performance evaluation, the nurse manager and the staff on that unit can be very proud of their accomplishments. Productivity is excellent. Money was saved. Everyone continues to work to find out what each patient wants, to improve quality and safety, to improve productivity, and to improve productivity measurement.

References

Brinkerhoff, R., & Dressler, D. (1990). Productivity measurement. *Applied Social Research Methods Series*, 19. Newbury Park, CA: Sage.

Carter, M. (September–October 2000). Use of a nursing labor computer productivity measurement tool. *Nursing Economic$, 18*(5), 237–242.

Chang, C., Price, S., & Pfoutz, S. (2001). *Economics and nursing: Critical professional issues*. Philadelphia: F.A. Davis.

Collins, J., & Porras, J. (1994). *Built to last*. New York: HarperBusiness.

DiJerome, L., Dunham-Taylor, J., Ash, D., & Brown, R. (November–December 1999). Evaluating cost center productivity. *Nursing Economic$, 17*(6), 334–340.

Druskat, V., & Wolff, S. (2001). Building the emotional intelligence of groups. *Harvard Business Review, 79*(3), 81–90.

Hall, L. (January–February 2003). Nursing intellectual capital: A theoretical approach for analyzing nursing productivity. *Nursing Economic$, 21*(1), 14–19.

Harris, M. (1997). *Handbook of home health care administration*. 2nd ed. Gaithersburg, MD: Aspen.

Health Care Education Associates. (1987). *Basic budgeting for nurse managers*. St. Louis: Mosby.

Hoffman, F. (1988). *Productivity assessment and costing out nursing services*. Philadelphia: Lippincott.

Hunt, V. (1993). *The Human Energy Field and Health*. Videotape available from: Malibu Publishing Company, P.O. Box 4234, Malibu, CA.

Johnson, C. (2000). When working harder is not smarter. *The Inner Edge, 3*(2), 18–21.

Linn, N., & (1982). Managing public health productivity–The art of taming conflict and chaos. *Public Productivity Review, 6*(3), 170–183.

Ohio Hospital Statewide Financial Performance. (2003). *Vital signs: Indicators of Ohio hospital financial viability*. Columbus, OH: Ohio Hospital Association.

Olson, V. (1983). *White collar waste: Gain the productivity edge.* Englewood Cliffs, NJ: Prentice-Hall.

Orsburn, J., Moran, J., Musselwhite, E., & Zenter, J. (1990). *Self-directed work teams.* Homewood, IL: Business One Irwin.

Porter-O'Grady, T., & Malloch, K. (2003). *Quantum leadership: A textbook of new leadership.* Sudbury, MA: Jones and Bartlett.

Roach, S. (September–October 1998). In search of productivity. *Harvard Business Review,* 153–160.

Sullivan, E., & Decker, P. (2001). *Effective leadership and management in nursing.* 5th ed. Upper Saddle River, NJ: Prentice Hall.

Swansburg, R. (1997). *Budgeting and financial management for nurse managers.* Sudbury, MA: Jones and Bartlett.

Van Slyck, A. (January 1999). Improving productivity: A payer/provider debate. *JONA, 29*(1), 51–56.

Walker, D. (October 1996). A "bottom-line" approach to nurse staffing. *Nursing Management, 27*(10), 31–32.

Index

G

M